Lung Inflammation in Health and Disease

Lung Inflammation in Health and Disease

Editor: Gage Phillips

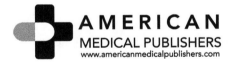

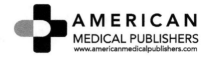

Cataloging-in-Publication Data

Lung inflammation in health and disease / edited by Gage Phillips.
   p. cm.
Includes bibliographical references and index.
ISBN 979-8-88740-576-6
1. Pneumonia. 2. Lungs--Diseases. 3. Lungs--Diseases--Treatment. I. Phillips, Gage.
RC771 .L86 2023
616.241--dc23

© American Medical Publishers, 2023

American Medical Publishers,
41 Flatbush Avenue,
1st Floor, New York,
NY 11217, USA

ISBN 979-8-88740-576-6 (Hardback)

This book contains information obtained from authentic and highly regarded sources. Copyright for all individual chapters remain with the respective authors as indicated. All chapters are published with permission under the Creative Commons Attribution License or equivalent. A wide variety of references are listed. Permission and sources are indicated; for detailed attributions, please refer to the permissions page and list of contributors. Reasonable efforts have been made to publish reliable data and information, but the authors, editors and publisher cannot assume any responsibility for the validity of all materials or the consequences of their use.

Trademark Notice: Registered trademark of products or corporate names are used only for explanation and identification without intent to infringe.

Contents

Preface...IX

Chapter 1   **The Role of Transient Receptor Potential Channel 6 Channels in the Pulmonary Vasculature**..1
Monika Malczyk, Alexandra Erb, Christine Veith, Hossein Ardeschir Ghofrani, Ralph T. Schermuly, Thomas Gudermann, Alexander Dietrich, Norbert Weissmann and Akylbek Sydykov

Chapter 2   **Cytokine–Ion Channel Interactions in Pulmonary Inflammation**......................12
Jürg Hamacher, Yalda Hadizamani, Michèle Borgmann, Markus Mohaupt, Daniela Narcissa Männel, Ueli Moehrlen, Rudolf Lucas and Uz Stammberger

Chapter 3   **Inflammatory Responses Regulating Alveolar Ion Transport during Pulmonary Infections**..57
Christin Peteranderl, Jacob I. Sznajder, Susanne Herold and Emilia Lecuona

Chapter 4   **TNF Lectin-Like Domain Restores Epithelial Sodium Channel Function in Frameshift Mutants Associated with Pseudohypoaldosteronism Type 1B**..........................65
Anita Willam, Mohammed Aufy, Susan Tzotzos, Dina El-Malazi, Franziska Poser, Alina Wagner, Birgit Unterköfler, Didja Gurmani, David Martan, Shahid Muhammad Iqbal, Bernhard Fischer, Hendrik Fischer, Helmut Pietschmann, Istvan Czikora, Rudolf Lucas, Rosa Lemmens-Gruber and Waheed Shabbir

Chapter 5   **Cytokine-Regulation of Na^+-K^+-Cl^- Cotransporter 1 and Cystic Fibrosis Transmembrane Conductance Regulator — Potential Role in Pulmonary Inflammation and Edema Formation**..80
Sarah Weidenfeld and Wolfgang M. Kuebler

Chapter 6   **Alveolar Fluid Clearance in Pathologically Relevant Conditions: *In Vitro* and *In Vivo* Models of Acute Respiratory Distress Syndrome**...88
Laura A. Huppert and Michael A. Matthay

Chapter 7   **Inhibition of the NOD-Like Receptor Protein 3 Inflammasome is Protective in Juvenile Influenza A Virus Infection**...94
Bria M. Coates, Kelly L. Staricha, Nandini Ravindran, Clarissa M. Koch, Yuan Cheng, Jennifer M. Davis, Dale K. Shumaker and Karen M. Ridge

Chapter 8   **Epithelial Sodium Channel-α Mediates the Protective Effect of the TNF-Derived TIP Peptide in Pneumolysin-Induced Endothelial Barrier Dysfunction**..........................106
Istvan Czikora, Abdel A. Alli, Supriya Sridhar, Michael A. Matthay, Helena Pillich, Martina Hudel, Besim Berisha, Boris Gorshkov, Maritza J. Romero, Joyce Gonzales, Guangyu Wu, Yuqing Huo, Yunchao Su, Alexander D. Verin, David Fulton, Trinad Chakraborty, Douglas C. Eaton and Rudolf Lucas

VI   Contents

Chapter 9   **FXYD5 is an Essential Mediator of the Inflammatory Response during Lung Injury** 115
Patricia L. Brazee, Pritin N. Soni, Elmira Tokhtaeva, Natalia Magnani, Alex Yemelyanov, Harris R. Perlman, Karen M. Ridge, Jacob I. Sznajder, Olga Vagin and Laura A. Dada

Chapter 10   **Hypercapnia Impairs ENaC Cell Surface Stability by Promoting Phosphorylation, Polyubiquitination and Endocytosis of β-ENaC in a Human Alveolar Epithelial Cell Line** 128
Paulina Gwoździńska, Benno A. Buchbinder, Konstantin Mayer, Susanne Herold, Rory E. Morty, Werner Seeger and István Vadász

Chapter 11   **Gas Exchange Disturbances Regulate Alveolar Fluid Clearance during Acute Lung Injury** 141
István Vadász and Jacob I. Sznajder

Chapter 12   **Involvement of Cytokines in the Pathogenesis of Salt and Water Imbalance in Congestive Heart Failure** 148
Zaher S. Azzam, Safa Kinaneh, Fadel Bahouth, Reem Ismael-Badarneh, Emad Khoury and Zaid Abassi

Chapter 13   **Inhibition of TNF Receptor p55 by a Domain Antibody Attenuates the Initial Phase of Acid-Induced Lung Injury in Mice** 161
Michael R. Wilson, Kenji Wakabayashi, Szabolcs Bertok, Charlotte M. Oakley, Brijesh V. Patel, Kieran P. O'Dea, Joanna C. Cordy, Peter J. Morley, Andrew I. Bayliffe and Masao Takata

Chapter 14   **Regulation of Lung Epithelial Sodium Channels by Cytokines and Chemokines** 173
Brandi M. Wynne, Li Zou, Valerie Linck, Robert S. Hoover, He-Ping Ma and Douglas C. Eaton

Chapter 15   **The Role of Transient Receptor Potential Vanilloid 4 in Pulmonary Inflammatory Diseases** 182
Rachel G. Scheraga, Brian D. Southern, Lisa M. Grove and Mitchell A. Olman

Chapter 16   **Role of Autophagy in Lung Inflammation** 189
Jacob D. Painter, Lauriane Galle-Treger and Omid Akbari

Chapter 17   **Extracellular Vesicle: An Emerging Mediator of Intercellular Crosstalk in Lung Inflammation and Injury** 207
Heedoo Lee, Eric Abston, Duo Zhang, Ashish Rai and Yang Jin

Chapter 18   **Mechanisms of Virus-Induced Airway Immunity Dysfunction in the Pathogenesis of COPD Disease, Progression and Exacerbation** 215
Hong Guo-Parke, Dermot Linden, Sinéad Weldon, Joseph C. Kidney and Clifford C. Taggart

Chapter 19   **Epigenetic Regulation of Airway Epithelium Immune Functions in Asthma** 225
Bilal Alashkar Alhamwe, Sarah Miethe, Elke Pogge von Strandmann, Daniel P. Potaczek and Holger Garn

Chapter 20 **Genetic Ablation of CXCR2 Protects against Cigarette Smoke-Induced Lung Inflammation and Injury**.. 233
Chad A. Lerner, Wei Lei, Isaac K. Sundar and Irfan Rahman

Permissions

List of Contributors

Index

Preface

Inflammation refers to the process through which the immune system fights with injury, infection and other harmful substances. Lung inflammation can develop from toxin exposure, cystic fibrosis, chronic obstructive pulmonary disease (COPD), acute respiratory distress syndrome (ARDS), and asthma. Some common symptoms of lung inflammation are breathing problems, wheezing, chest pain or tightness, fatigue, lung pain, unintended weight loss and decreased appetite. Various types of diagnostic tests, including blood culture, pulse oximetry, lung biopsy, saliva test, sweat chloride test, and pulmonary function test can be used for the diagnosis of lung inflammation. Its treatment may involve oxygen therapy, physical therapy, surgery and medications like leukotriene modifiers, antifungals, biologic medications, antibiotics, corticosteroids, anti-inflammatories and bronchodilators. This book provides significant information on lung inflammation to help develop a good understanding of its effects in health and disease. A number of latest researches have been included to keep the readers up-to-date with the global concepts on this medical condition. Students, researchers, experts and all associated with the study of lung inflammation will benefit alike from this book.

Significant researches are present in this book. Intensive efforts have been employed by authors to make this book an outstanding discourse. This book contains the enlightening chapters which have been written on the basis of significant researches done by the experts.

Finally, I would also like to thank all the members involved in this book for being a team and meeting all the deadlines for the submission of their respective works. I would also like to thank my friends and family for being supportive in my efforts.

Editor

The Role of Transient Receptor Potential Channel 6 Channels in the Pulmonary Vasculature

Monika Malczyk[1], Alexandra Erb[1], Christine Veith[1], Hossein Ardeschir Ghofrani[1], Ralph T. Schermuly[1], Thomas Gudermann[2], Alexander Dietrich[2], Norbert Weissmann[1]* and Akylbek Sydykov[1]*

[1] Excellence Cluster Cardio-Pulmonary System, Universities of Giessen and Marburg Lung Center (UGMLC), German Center for Lung Research (DZL), Justus Liebig University of Giessen, Giessen, Germany, [2] Walther Straub Institute for Pharmacology and Toxicology, Ludwig Maximilian University of Munich, German Center for Lung Research (DZL), Munich, Germany

*Correspondence:
Norbert Weissmann
norbert.weissmann@innere.med.
uni-giessen.de;
Akylbek Sydykov
akylbek.sydykov@innere.med.
uni-giessen.de

Canonical or classical transient receptor potential channel 6 (TRPC6) is a Ca^{2+}-permeable non-selective cation channel that is widely expressed in the heart, lung, and vascular tissues. The use of TRPC6-deficient ("knockout") mice has provided important insights into the role of TRPC6 in normal physiology and disease states of the pulmonary vasculature. Evidence indicates that TRPC6 is a key regulator of acute hypoxic pulmonary vasoconstriction. Moreover, several studies implicated TRPC6 in the pathogenesis of pulmonary hypertension. Furthermore, a unique genetic variation in the TRPC6 gene promoter has been identified, which might link the inflammatory response to the upregulation of TRPC6 expression and ultimate development of pulmonary vascular abnormalities in idiopathic pulmonary arterial hypertension. Additionally, TRPC6 is critically involved in the regulation of pulmonary vascular permeability and lung edema formation during endotoxin or ischemia/reperfusion-induced acute lung injury. In this review, we will summarize latest findings on the role of TRPC6 in the pulmonary vasculature.

Keywords: transient receptor potential channels, transient receptor potential channel 6, hypoxic pulmonary vasoconstriction, pulmonary hypertension, vascular permeability

INTRODUCTION

Regulation of the intracellular Ca^{2+} ($[Ca^{2+}]_i$) homeostasis is a crucial factor in many physiological processes (1). Altered Ca^{2+} homeostasis in both vascular endothelium and smooth muscle has been documented for a majority of pathophysiological conditions in the pulmonary vasculature. Changes in $[Ca^{2+}]_i$ play a pivotal role in the regulation of contraction, migration, and proliferation of vascular smooth muscle cells (2). Furthermore, Ca^{2+} signaling in endothelial cells (ECs) is essential for the maintenance of the endothelial barrier integrity (3).

Non-selective cation channels (NSCCs) play an important role in the regulation of vascular tone and vascular smooth muscle cell proliferation by mediating the entry of cations (4). Among the ion channels located in the pulmonary vasculature, members of the canonical or classical transient receptor potential (TRP) channels subfamily allow for the entry of Na^+ and Ca^{2+}. There is growing evidence that transient receptor potential channel 6 (TRPC6) mediates receptor-operated cation entry and is critically involved in numerous physiological processes. Recent studies have provided important insights into the role of TRPC6 in normal physiology and disease states of the pulmonary vasculature. We provide an overview on current knowledge regarding the role of TRPC6 channels in pulmonary vasculature and potential therapeutic strategies.

REGULATION OF CALCIUM HOMEOSTASIS

In general, Ca^{2+} enters cells from extracellular fluid through L-type voltage-dependent calcium channels or NSCCs, which can be divided into store-operated calcium channels (SOCCs) and receptor-operated calcium channels (ROCCs) (**Figure 1**). Stimulation of G-protein-coupled receptors initiates signaling mechanisms leading to activation of ROCC. These signaling pathways include phospholipase C (PLC) activation resulting in production of diacylglycerol (DAG) along with inositol 1,4,5-trisphosphate (IP_3) from phosphatidylinositol 4,5-bisphosphate (PIP_2). DAG regulates the activity of ROCC to induce receptor-operated Ca^{2+} entry, whereas IP_3 generation induces depletion of the intracellular Ca^{2+} stores in the endoplasmic reticulum, leading to induction of store-operated Ca^{2+} entry. Ca^{2+} entry through SOCCs plays a very important role in Ca^{2+} stores replenishment in the endoplasmic/sarcoplasmatic reticulum and maintaining Ca^{2+} homeostasis.

CLASSICAL TRANSIENT RECEPTOR POTENTIAL CHANNEL 6

Transient receptor potential (TRP) channels play a prominent role in the regulation of the cation homeostasis (5). TRP channels belong to a large and diverse family of mostly NSCCs. In this regard, they are non-selectively permeable to cations, including potassium (K^+), sodium (Na^+), calcium (Ca^{2+}), and magnesium (Mg^{2+}) (6). Based on amino acid sequence homology, the 28 mammalian TRP channels are grouped into six subfamilies, one of which is the TRPC (for classical or canonical) subfamily (6). The TRPC subfamily includes seven members, TRPC1 to TRPC7, and can be further divided into subfamilies on the basis of their structural and functional similarities. All TRPC proteins have a common structure. Mainly, they are composed of four N-terminal ankyrin repeats, six transmembrane domains with a putative pore between domains 5 and 6, and several protein-binding domains (4). TRPC proteins can form homomeric or heteromeric channels consisting of four monomers.

Transient receptor potential channel 6 is a NSCC, which is about six times more permeable for Ca^{2+} than for Na^+ (7). It belongs to the subfamily of ROCC and there is good evidence that TRPC6 is directly activated by DAG (8). TRPC6 is ubiquitously expressed in the whole vasculature (9). In the pulmonary circulation, TRPC6 is most prominent in pulmonary artery smooth muscle cells (PASMCs) and ECs (10). TRPC6 mRNA and protein were identified in PASMCs isolated from both proximal and distal pulmonary arteries (11–13). However, TRPC6 expression is higher in PASMCs isolated from distal pulmonary arteries than in those isolated from proximal vessels (14). Recently, expression of TRPC6 in pulmonary venous smooth muscle cells has also been demonstrated (15).

PULMONARY HYPERTENSION

Pulmonary hypertension (PH) is a pathophysiological disorder that may involve various clinical conditions and can complicate

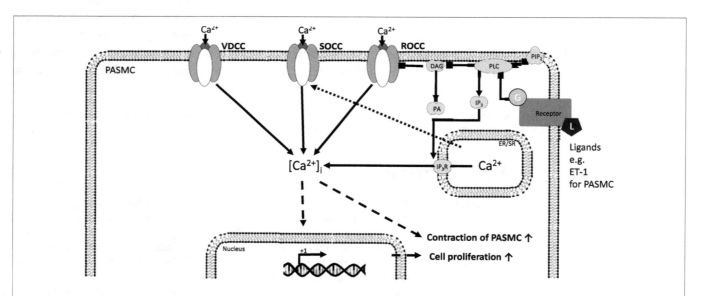

FIGURE 1 | $[Ca^{2+}]_i$ homeostasis regulation in precapillary pulmonary arterial smooth muscle cells (PASMCs) and ECs. Ca^{2+} enters cells from extracellular fluid through L-type voltage-dependent calcium channels or non-selective cation channels, which can be divided into SOCCs and ROCCs. The initiation of ROCC-mediated Ca^{2+}-influx from the extracellular space is thought to be induced by ligand-activated G-protein coupled receptors, starting a PLC-mediated hydrolyzation of PIP_2 to IP_3 and DAG. DAG regulates the activity of ROCC to induce receptor-operated Ca^{2+} entry, whereas IP_3 generation induces depletion of the intracellular Ca^{2+} stores in the endoplasmic reticulum, leading to induction of store-operated Ca^{2+} entry. The increased $[Ca^{2+}]_i$ drives different cellular responses. Ca^{2+}, calcium ion; $[Ca^{2+}]_i$, intracellular Ca^{2+} concentration; ROCC, receptor-operated calcium channel; SOCC, store-operated calcium channel; VDCC, L-type voltage-dependent calcium channel; DAG, diacylglycerol; DAGK, DAG kinase; EC, endothelial cell; ER/SR, endoplasmic/sarcoplasmic reticulum; IP_3, inositol trisphosphate; IP_3R, inositol trisphosphate receptor; L, ligand; PA, phosphatidic acid; PASMC, precapillary pulmonary arterial smooth muscle cells; PIP_2, phosphatidylinositol 4,5-bisphosphate; PLC, phospholipase C; VEGF, vascular endothelial growth factor; solid arrows indicate direct interactions; dotted arrows illustrate indirect interactions.

cardiovascular and respiratory diseases (16). PH is characterized by remodeling of the pulmonary vessels, leading to a progressive increase in pulmonary vascular resistance (PVR), right ventricular failure, and premature death. PH is defined as a resting mean pulmonary artery pressure ≥ 25 mmHg (17). The disorder has been classified into five clinical groups based on their similarities in clinical presentation, pathophysiological mechanisms, and therapeutic options: pulmonary arterial hypertension (PAH) (Group 1); PH due to left heart disease (Group 2); PH due to chronic lung disease and/or hypoxia (Group 3); chronic thromboembolic PH (Group 4); and PH due to unclear and/or multifactorial mechanisms (Group 5) (18).

Depending on the pulmonary artery wedge pressure values, PH is divided into precapillary and postcapillary forms. Pulmonary artery wedge pressure provides an indirect estimate of left atrial pressure and its elevation >15 mmHg in patients with PH indicates presence of postcapillary PH due to left heart disease (Group 2) (17). Precapillary PH is defined by the presence of PH and a pulmonary artery wedge pressure ≤ 15 mmHg and includes the clinical groups 1, 3, 4, and 5 (17).

Pulmonary arterial hypertension is a progressive disease characterized by the presence of precapillary PH and a PVR > 3 Wood units in the absence of other causes of precapillary PH (17). It includes idiopathic PAH (IPAH), hereditary PAH, and PAH associated with diseases, drugs, and toxins (APAH) (18). Sustained pulmonary vasoconstriction, *in situ* thrombosis, and pathological pulmonary vascular remodeling due to excessive vascular cell growth leading to intimal narrowing and vascular occlusion are the main causes for the increased PVR and pulmonary arterial pressure in IPAH patients. In addition, pulmonary vascular remodeling with increased muscularization contributes to elevated PVR as well as hyperreactivity of pulmonary vessels to various vasoconstrictor agents. Neointimal and medial hypertrophy in small and medium-sized pulmonary arteries is a key aspect of pulmonary vascular remodeling in IPAH patients.

Role of TRPC6 in Hypoxic Pulmonary Vasoconstriction (HPV)

Acute HPV is an adaptive response of the pulmonary circulation to a local alveolar hypoxia, by which local lung perfusion is matched to ventilation resulting in optimization of ventilation-perfusion ratio and thus gas exchange (19, 20). This dynamic mechanism is also known as von Euler–Liljestrand mechanism (21) and can be found in fish, reptiles, birds, and mammals. Acute HPV occurs throughout the pulmonary vascular bed, including arterioles, capillaries, and veins, but is most pronounced in small pulmonary arterioles (22, 23). In isolated pulmonary arteries and isolated perfused lungs, the HPV response is typically biphasic (24–26). The first phase is characterized by a fast but mostly transient vasoconstrictor response that starts within seconds and reaches a maximum within minutes. The following second phase is characterized by a sustained pulmonary vasoconstriction. Acute HPV in local alveolar hypoxia is limited to the affected lung segments and is not accompanied by an increase in pulmonary artery pressure.

A rise of $[Ca^{2+}]_i$ in PASMCs is a key element in HPV (27, 28). We have demonstrated that TRPC6 plays an essential role in acute HPV (29). We have shown that the first acute phase of HPV (<20 min of hypoxic exposure) was completely abolished in isolated, ventilated, and buffer-perfused lungs from TRPC6-deficient mice. However, the vasoconstrictor response during the second sustained phase (60–160 min of hypoxic exposure) in TRPC6$^{-/-}$ mice was not significantly different from that in wild-type mice (29). During hypoxia, DAG is accumulated in PASMCs and leads to activation of TRPC6 (29). Accumulation of DAG can result from PLC activation or from ROS-mediated DAG kinase (DAGK) inhibition (30, 31). Along these lines, inhibition of DAG synthesis by the PLC inhibitor U73122 inhibited acute HPV in wild-type mouse lungs (32). Blocking DAG degradation to phosphatidic acid through DAGKs or activation of TRPC6 with a membrane-permeable DAG analog 1-oleoyl-2-acetyl-sn-glycerol (OAG) resulted in normoxic vasoconstriction in wild-type but not in TRPC6$^{-/-}$ mice (32). Recently, the cystic fibrosis transmembrane conductance regulator and sphingolipids have been demonstrated to regulate TRPC6 activity in HPV, as both translocate TRPC6 channels to the caveolae and activate the PLC–DAG–TRPC6 pathway (33). Cytochrome P-450 epoxygenase-derived epoxyeicosatrienoic acids also induced translocation of TRPC6 to the caveolae during acute hypoxia (34). Consistent with these data, 11,12-epoxyeicosatrienoic acids increased pulmonary artery pressure in a concentration-dependent manner and potentiated HPV in heterozygous but not in TRPC6-deficient lungs (34). As the constriction of the pulmonary vessels in response to the thromboxane mimetic U46619 is not altered in TRPC6$^{-/-}$ mice, TRPC6 channels appear to be a key regulator of acute HPV. These studies are summarized in **Figure 2**.

In PASMCs isolated from small precapillary arteries of TRPC6-deficient mice, cation influx and currents induced by severe hypoxia (1% O_2) were completely absent (29). The rise of $[Ca^{2+}]_i$ in response to hypoxia was not dependent on Ca^{2+} release from internal stores, because, in the absence of extracellular Ca^{2+}, no hypoxia-induced increases in $[Ca^{2+}]_i$ were detected (29). Interestingly, blocking voltage-gated Ca^{2+} channels almost completely inhibited acute HPV in isolated wild-type mouse lungs and Ca^{2+} influx in wild-type PASMCs (29), suggesting that Na^+ influx through TRPC6 channels leads to membrane depolarization and activation of voltage-gated L-type Ca^{2+} channels mediating the bulk of the Ca^{2+} influx and contraction of smooth muscle cells (35). Importantly, the lack of acute HPV in TRPC6 KO mice has profound physiological relevance, because partial occlusion of alveolar ventilation provoked severe hypoxemia in TRPC6$^{-/-}$ but not in wild-type mice (29). These data provide compelling evidence that different molecular mechanisms regulate pulmonary vascular responses to acute and sustained hypoxia. TRPC6 channels may thus represent a potential therapeutic target for the control of pulmonary hemodynamics and gas exchange in hypoxic conditions.

Role of TRPC6 in Experimental PH

A variety of animal models are currently used to study PH. These models have provided a plethora of scientific information and

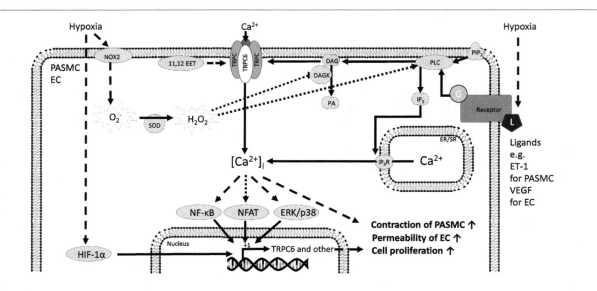

FIGURE 2 | Mechanisms of TRPC6 regulation and function in precapillary pulmonary arterial smooth muscle cells (PASMCs) and ECs in response to hypoxia. The TRPC6 protein forms homomeric and heteromeric channels composed of TRPC6 alone or TRPC6 and other TRPC proteins. TRPC6 is expressed in PASMCs from mice, rat, as well as humans and is suggested to play a significant role in human idiopathic PAH. The initiation of TRPC6-mediated Ca^{2+} influx from the extracellular space is thought to be induced by ligand-activated G-protein coupled receptors, starting a PLC-mediated hydrolyzation of PIP_2 to IP_3 and DAG. It has been already shown that DAG activates TRPC6-containing channels to induce Ca^{2+} influx from the extracellular space. Ca^{2+} entry through TRPC6 might be triggered by hypoxia-induced O_2^- production or hypoxia-induced DAG accumulation and that the increased $[Ca^{2+}]_i$ drives different cellular responses through ERK and p38, NFAT, and NF-κB downstream signaling. These pathways might be involved in the induction of TRPC6 expression and contribute to the modulated cellular response associated with hypoxia. Moreover, hypoxia leads to acute stabilization of HIF-1α, which might induce TRPC6 expression among other proteins. 11,12 EET, 11,12-epoxyeicosatrienoic acid; Ca^{2+}, calcium ion; $[Ca^{2+}]_i$, intracellular Ca^{2+} concentration; DAG, diacylglycerol; DAGK, DAG kinase; EC, endothelial cell; ER/SR, endoplasmic/sarcoplasmic reticulum; ERK, extracellular signal-regulated kinase; ET-1, endothelin-1; G, G-protein; H_2O_2, hydrogen peroxide; HIF-1α, hypoxia-inducible factor 1 alpha; IP_3, inositol trisphosphate; IP_3R, inositol trisphosphate receptor; L, ligand; NF-κB, nuclear factor kappa-light-chain enhancer of activated B-cells; NFAT, nuclear factor of activated T-cells; NOX2, NADPH (nicotinamide adenine dinucleotide phosphate) oxidase 2; O_2^-, superoxide; PA, phosphatidic acid; p38, p38 mitogen-activated protein kinase; PASMC, precapillary pulmonary arterial smooth muscle cells; PIP_2, phosphatidylinositol 4,5-bisphosphate; PLC, phospholipase C; SOD, superoxide dismutase; TRPC, classical transient receptor potential channel; TRPC6, classical transient receptor potential channel 6; VEGF, vascular endothelial growth factor; solid arrows indicate direct interactions; dotted arrows illustrate indirect interactions. Not all interaction partners have been identified.

made significant contribution to our understanding of molecular mechanisms in PH. In animals, PH can be induced by pharmacologic/toxic substances, genetic manipulations, exposure to environmental factors, or surgical interventions (36).

Exposure to chronic hypoxia is the most commonly used animal model of PH in biomedical research. In global alveolar hypoxia, which occurs at high altitude and chronic respiratory diseases, HPV involves the entire pulmonary vascular bed leading to elevation of pulmonary artery pressure. Chronic global alveolar hypoxia induces structural remodeling of pulmonary vessels due to smooth muscle cell proliferation and migration characterized by increased muscularization of smaller arteries with extension of smooth muscle cells into previously non-muscularized arterioles (37). This vascular remodeling has previously been thought to be a major determinant of the persistent elevation of PVR in chronic hypoxia-induced PH (38–40). However, recent studies have provided evidence that sustained vasoconstriction is an important contributor to chronic hypoxia-induced PH (41).

Although TRPC6 is important in the acute phase of HPV in mouse lungs, the data regarding its role in chronic hypoxic PH are controversial. We have previously shown that, despite disrupted acute HPV, TRPC6-deficient mice display sustained HPV and chronic hypoxia-induced PH with pulmonary vascular remodeling and RV hypertrophy after 3 weeks of hypoxia (10% O_2), which are indistinguishable from those in wild-type mice (29). Slightly but significantly lower right ventricular systolic pressure was observed in TRPC6$^{-/-}$ mice exposed to 1 week of hypoxia when compared to wild-type mice (42). Nevertheless, this difference was not significant after 3 weeks of exposure to hypoxia (42). In contrast, other authors have demonstrated attenuation of PH and pulmonary vascular remodeling in TRPC6 KO mice after 4 weeks of hypoxia (43). Although the exact reason is not clear, differences in age (44, 45), gender (46), strain, and substrain (47, 48) of mice can account for most of the discrepancies.

Excessive proliferation of PASMCs is the main cause of pulmonary arterial medial hypertrophy, which narrows the intraluminal diameter, increases the resistance to blood flow, and eventually leads to PH. Proliferation of PASMCs is regulated by $[Ca^{2+}]_i$. There is increasing evidence that elevated TRPC6 expression might be responsible for the elevated $[Ca^{2+}]_i$. Interestingly, it has been shown that enhanced expression of TRPC6, STIM2, and Orai2 as proteins of the store-operated Ca^{2+} influx underlies the change of the phenotype of PASMCs from the contractile to the proliferative (49). Furthermore, deletion of TRPC6 significantly attenuated Ca^{2+} currents in the proliferative phenotype of PASMCs (49).

Transient receptor potential channel 6 upregulation in PASMCs has been demonstrated to be dependent on hypoxia-inducible transcription factor 1 (HIF-1) (50). Overexpression of HIF-1 led to TRPC6 upregulation under normoxic conditions while partial deficiency in HIF-1 resulted in hypoxia-induced Ca^{2+} influx in PASMCs, suggesting an important role of HIF-1 for sustained expression of TRPC6 channels (50). Although short-term hypoxia (1% O_2 for 72 h) did not produce any changes in TRPC6 mRNA expression in isolated murine PASMCs (51), increased expression of TRPC6 on mRNA and protein level was detected in pulmonary arteries and PASMCs isolated from pulmonary arteries of mice and rats exposed to chronic hypoxia (42, 50, 52). Moreover, a Notch-dependent upregulation of TRPC6 channels in PASMCs in response to chronic hypoxia has recently been reported (43). It has been shown that TRPC6 is induced by BMP4 in rat PASMCs *via* the p38MAPK and ERK1/2 pathways (53, 54). Additionally, BMP4 may increase TRPC6 expression by elevating NOX4-mediated ROS levels in PASMCs (55). Interestingly, BMP4 expression has been shown to be dependent on HIF-1 as well (15).

Chronic lung diseases including chronic obstructive pulmonary disease (COPD) are often complicated by PH (56). Growing evidence implicates cigarette smoke (CS) products in the initiation of pulmonary vascular alterations in COPD (57). Recently, we have demonstrated the formation of PH in mice chronically exposed to tobacco smoke (58). Similarly, development of PH has been documented in rats chronically exposed to CS (59, 60). CS is an inflammatory stimulus, which upregulates Ca^{2+}-regulatory molecules. In this regard, TRPC6 was upregulated in rat lungs and isolated rat PASMCs after 4, 12, and 20 weeks of CS exposure (59). In another study, expression of TRPC1 and TRPC6 was increased in PASMCs isolated from distal pulmonary arteries of rats after 1, 3, and 6 months of CS exposure (60). Furthermore, PASMCs in rats exposed to CS for 3 and 6 months showed a higher basal $[Ca^{2+}]_i$ and an increased Ca^{2+} entry (60).

The role of TRPC6 in other models of PH has not been investigated in detail. Increased expression of TRPC6 protein in distal pulmonary arteries was observed in the monocrotaline-induced rat model of PH (61). Chronic thromboembolic PH in a rat model is associated with upregulation of TRPC1 and TRPC6 in PASMCs isolated from distal pulmonary arteries, elevated basal $[Ca^{2+}]_i$, and an increased Ca^{2+} entry (62).

There is growing evidence that in addition to TRPC6, other members of the TRPC family also contribute to the pulmonary vascular remodeling in PH. Culture of isolated PASMCs under hypoxic conditions led to upregulation of TRPC1 mRNA (50, 51, 63). Furthermore, enhanced expression of TRPC1 and TRPC4 mRNA and protein has been documented in pulmonary arteries and PASMCs isolated from mice and rats with PH induced by various stimuli (50, 59, 60, 62, 64, 65). Treatment of murine PASMCs with TRPC1-specific small interfering RNA resulted in significant attenuation of hypoxia-induced proliferation of cells (51). Consistent with this, PASMCs isolated from TRPC1$^{-/-}$ mice showed diminished proliferation under hypoxic conditions (51).

Additionally, TRPC1$^{-/-}$ mice exposed to chronic hypoxia were protected from development of PH, which was associated with attenuated pulmonary vascular remodeling (51). In line with our data, reduced chronic hypoxic vascular remodeling in TRPC1$^{-/-}$ mice has been demonstrated by an independent research group (42). Moreover, downregulation of TRPC1 expression by small interfering RNA attenuated PH and pulmonary vascular remodeling in a murine model of hypoxia-induced PH (66). Interestingly, in mice deficient for both TRPC1 and TRPC6, chronic hypoxia-induced changes in pulmonary arterial pressure, right ventricular hypertrophy, and pulmonary vascular remodeling are even more inhibited compared to those in mice with a deficiency for a single gene (42). In a recent study, deficiency for TRPC4 has been shown to confer a survival benefit, which was associated with diminished vasculopathy in a rat model of severe PAH (67).

Involvement of TRPC6 in IPAH

Pulmonary arterial hypertension is characterized by progressive adverse structural changes in the resistance pulmonary arteries driven mainly by excessive vascular cell growth (68). Vascular remodeling in PAH is mediated by multiple stimuli. It is widely recognized that PASMCs in IPAH patients have a hyperproliferative phenotype and contribute to the pro-proliferative microenvironment in the vascular wall of their pulmonary arteries (68, 69). The enhanced $[Ca^{2+}]_i$ plays an key role in PASMC growth (70). Furthermore, increased $[Ca^{2+}]_i$ levels have been observed in PASMCs from IPAH patients (71). Expression studies revealed that c-jun/STAT3-induced upregulation of TRPC6 expression underlies PDGF-mediated proliferation of PASMCs (72). The mRNA and protein expression of TRPC6 in lung tissues and PASMCs from IPAH patients has been shown to be much higher than in those from normotensive patients (73). Furthermore, inhibition of TRPC6 gene expression by small interfering RNA significantly diminished proliferation of PASMCs from IPAH patients suggesting that the abnormally increased PASMC proliferation in these patients may be due to enhanced expression of TRPC6 (73).

Mounting evidence implicates inflammatory mechanisms in the development of PAH (74, 75). A unique genetic variant of the TRPC6 gene promoter has been identified, which might link inflammatory responses to the upregulation of TRPC6 expression and ultimate development of pulmonary vascular abnormality in IPAH (76). Sequencing TRPC6 regulatory regions of 268 patients with IPAH revealed three biallelic single-nucleotide polymorphisms (SNPs): −361(A>T), −254(C>G), and −218(C>T) (76). Among these three SNPs, only the −254(C>G) SNP was associated with IPAH by increasing basal TRPC6 gene promoter activity. Furthermore, the −254(C>G) SNP introduces a new binding site for the inflammatory transcription factor nuclear factor κB (NF-κB) in the promoter region of the TRPC6 gene and thus enhances NF-κB-mediated promoter activity and stimulates TRPC6 expression in PASMCs (76). In addition, this SNP has functional relevance as it also affects TRPC6 channel activity. In PASMCs from IPAH patients with the −254(C>G) SNP, TNF-α-induced activation of NF-κB significantly increased TRPC6 expression, elevated the resting $[Ca^{2+}]_i$, and enhanced OAG-induced Ca^{2+}

influx (76). In contrast, inhibition of nuclear translocation of NF-κB by overexpression of an IκBα super-repressor significantly diminished TNF-α-mediated enhancement of TRPC6 expression, resting $[Ca^{2+}]_i$, and agonist-induced elevation of $[Ca^{2+}]_i$. The importance of NF-κB has been demonstrated in experimental models of PAH (77–79). More importantly, activation of NF-κB has recently been observed in the pulmonary vessels of patients with end-stage IPAH (80). Thus, in the presence of inflammatory triggers, individuals carrying the −254(C>G) SNP may have an increased risk of developing IPAH (81). Although the functional significance of the two other SNPs, −361(A>T) and −218(C>T), is not clear, it has been shown that patients with IPAH and APAH carrying all three SNPs develop a more severe disease (82).

TRPC6 As a Therapeutic Target in PH

Transient receptor potential channel 6 is predominantly expressed in tissues harboring smooth muscle cells including the lungs (83, 84). However, TRPC6$^{-/-}$ mice do not have any major pathological phenotypes probably because TRPC6 channels have little basal activity and modest importance under physiological conditions (85). Moreover, loss of TRPC6 is compensated by the activity of closely related TRPC3 channels in the systemic vasculature (86) and airway smooth muscle (87). Nevertheless, TRPC6 channels are specifically activated in various disease conditions suggesting their pathophysiological relevance and thus represent attractive therapeutic targets. Importantly, systemic application of TRPC inhibitors in mice was not associated with any serious side effects (88, 89).

A number of non-selective small molecule inhibitors of TRPC6 channel activities including 2-APB and SKF-96365 have become available during recent years (85, 90). Also, antagonists including synthetic gestagen norgestimate and compound 8009-5364 with IC50 values in a low micromolar range and with higher selectivity for TRPC6 have been identified (91, 92). As the members of the TRPC3/6/7 subfamily have very similar biochemical and biophysical properties, most of the TRPC6-selective blockers exhibit poor selectivity between the subfamily members (85, 90). A continuous search for selectively acting pharmacological TRPC6 has recently identified new highly potent TRPC6 inhibitors with subtype selectivity, SAR7334, and larixyl acetate (93, 94). Most importantly, these drugs effectively blocked acute HPV in isolated mouse lungs (92–94). However, the only inhibitor that has been tested in experimental PH is the non-specific TRPC blocker 2-APB, which prevented development of PH in mice exposed to chronic hypoxia (43).

Evidence supporting the role of TRPC6 in the pathogenesis of IPAH suggests that it might serve as a pharmacologic target. Although the selective TRPC6 inhibitors represent promising drug candidates for the treatment of PH, they have not yet been tested in experimental models of PH. It would be highly desirable to confirm the therapeutic efficacy and safety of the new potent and selective TRPC6 blockers in animal models of PH with the ultimate goal of development of new therapeutic strategies for patients with PH.

Recent studies suggest that specific drugs approved for PAH treatments can also target TRPC6 expression and activity. In a small number of PAH patients with a positive response to acute vasodilator testing, initial therapy includes high doses of calcium channel blockers. However, most of the PAH patients do not react to calcium channel blockers, and they are treated with drugs approved for PAH therapy. Currently, established clinical practice treatments of PAH target three signaling pathways that are involved in the pathogenesis of PH: endothelin, nitric oxide, and prostacyclin (95). These therapies include endothelin receptor antagonists, phosphodiesterase type 5 inhibitors, soluble guanylate cyclase stimulators, prostacyclin receptor agonists, and epoprostenol. Bosentan has been found to directly downregulate TRPC6 expression in addition to its well-known blockade of endothelin receptors (96).

In PASMCs from chronically hypoxic rats, the potent phosphodiesterase type 5 inhibitor sildenafil decreased acutely basal $[Ca^{2+}]_i$ (97). Chronic treatment of rats exposed to 10% O_2 for 21 days with sildenafil showed a decreased right ventricular pressure and right ventricular hypertrophy, which is related to decreased TRPC6 mRNA and protein expression in pulmonary arteries (63). Furthermore, knockdown of TRPC6 gene by small interference RNA diminished the hypoxic increases of basal $[Ca^{2+}]_i$ and Ca^{2+} influx in PASMCs exposed to hypoxia for 60 h (63). It has been shown that inhibition of the Ca^{2+}/NFAT pathway is involved in the antiproliferative effect of sildenafil on PASMCs (98). More recent studies have revealed that sildenafil inhibits hypoxia-induced TRPC6 protein expression in PASMCs *via* the cGMP–PKG–PPARγ axis (99).

TRPC6 IN ACUTE LUNG INJURY (ALI)

Acute lung injury is characterized by lung edema due to increased lung vascular permeability of the alveolar-capillary barrier and subsequent impairment of arterial oxygenation. Ca^{2+} homeostasis has been shown to be essential in the mechanism of barrier disruption and endothelial contraction (3). Elevated $[Ca^{2+}]_i$ leads to changes in EC morphology and increased endothelial permeability. Recent studies have shown that Ca^{2+} entry through TRPC6 is essential for increased endothelial permeability and compromised barrier function in pulmonary vasculature (100).

In ALI, lung vascular barrier disruption usually coincides with the invasion of immune cells and activation of inflammatory signaling pathways (101). Various mediators, including platelet-activating factor (PAF), vascular endothelial growth factor (VEGF), thrombin, tumor necrosis factor-α (TNF-α), and others, induce changes in EC shape and consequently an increase in endothelial permeability (3, 102). PAF, a critical mediator in numerous experimental models of ALI, has been shown to increase lung vascular permeability by activation of acid sphingomyelinase (ASM) (103). In an extension of that study, the authors provided evidence that ASM activation by PAF causes rapid recruitment of TRPC6 channels into caveolae of lung ECs, thus facilitating endothelial Ca^{2+} entry and subsequent increases in endothelial permeability (104). Translocation of the TRPC6 to caveolin-rich areas in the plasma membrane in response to bradykinin has also been shown to be facilitated by 11,12-epoxyeicosatrienoic acids (105). TRPC6 has also been implicated in the VEGF-mediated increase in $[Ca^{2+}]_i$ and subsequent downstream signaling in microvascular ECs (106–108). In human pulmonary ECs, interaction of a protein called phosphatase and tensin homolog with TRPC6 enables cell surface expression of the channel in ECs and OAG-induced Ca²⁺ entry through TRPC6 as well as a subsequent increase in monolayer permeability (109). Thrombin-mediated Ca²⁺ entry through TRPC6 in human pulmonary artery ECs activated RhoA in a protein kinase C-α-dependent manner and thereby induced EC shape change and an increase in endothelial permeability (100).

A novel function for TRPC6 in pulmonary ECs in ALI induced by the endotoxin lipopolysaccharide (LPS) has also been indentified (110). In that study, LPS induced generation of DAG by binding to toll-like receptor 4 (TLR4), and DAG in turn directly activated TRPC6 and increased Ca²⁺ entry in ECs resulting in enhanced lung vascular permeability. Most interestingly, TRPC6 signaling was also important for the LPS/TLR4-mediated NF-κB activation and lung inflammation (110).

Lung edema and endothelial injury are accompanied by an influx of neutrophils into the interstitium and alveolar space (111). Therefore, activation and recruitment of polymorphonuclear neutrophils are thought to play key roles in the progression of ALI. When neutrophils are recruited to inflamed tissue, they become migratory and traverse the walls of blood vessels. It is known that the stimulation of CXC-type Gq-protein-coupled chemokine receptors activates PLC and induces a sustained increase in [Ca²⁺]ᵢ (112). An important role of TRPC6 signaling was demonstrated in CXCR2-induced intermediary chemotaxis (113). A deficiency for TRPC6 in neutrophil granulocytes negatively affects macrophage inflammatory protein-2 and OAG-induced cell migration (114). It has also been shown that TRPC6 expressed in ECs promotes leukocyte transendothelial migration by mediating trafficking of the lateral border recycling compartment membrane (115).

Recently, we have investigated the role of TRPC6 in lung ischemia-reperfusion edema (LIRE) formation in mice (31). Remarkably, global TRPC6⁻/⁻ mice were fully protected from LIRE, whereas global TRPC1- and TRPC4-deficient mice showed no protection. Bone marrow transplantation experiments using TRPC6 KO and wild-type mice allowed us to exclude the involvement of TRPC6 in immune cells. In line with our *in vivo* findings, pulmonary ECs isolated from TRPC6 KO mice displayed reduced permeability in response to hypoxia. A detailed analysis of signaling pathways underlying TRPC6 activation showed that mice lacking NOX2, but not NOX1 and NOX4, were also protected from LIRE. Moreover, mice deficient for NOX2 specifically in pulmonary arterial ECs displayed protection from LIRE. Consistent with our *in vivo* findings, we observed enhanced O_2^- production by endothelial NOX2 during the ischemic (hypoxic) phase. We have shown that after extracellular conversion to hydrogen peroxide (H_2O_2), H_2O_2 penetrates into the cell, where it inhibits DAGK $\eta_{1/2}$ activity and activates PLCγ, resulting in DAG accumulation and activation of TRPC6. Furthermore, elevation in [Ca²⁺]ᵢ was diminished in ECs lacking either NOX2 or TRPC6, indicating that NOX2 influences TRPC6-dependent Ca²⁺ homeostasis. Our studies provided a unique mechanistic insight into the pathogenesis of LIRE involving production of superoxide by endothelial Nox2, activation of PLCγ, inhibition of DAGK, and DAG-mediated activation of TRPC6 (31). These studies are summarized in **Figure 3**.

CONCLUDING REMARKS

In summary, TRPC6 channels are involved in various physiological and pathophysiological processes in the pulmonary vasculature. There is a clear evidence for the importance of

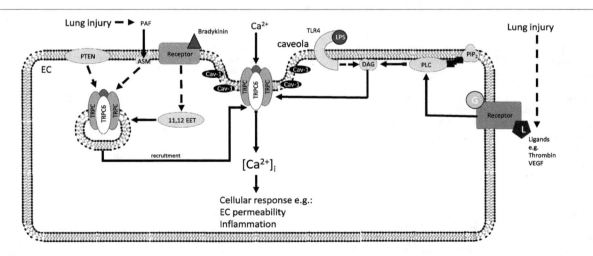

FIGURE 3 | Additional TRPC6 signaling pathways in ECs after lung injury. Recruitment of TRPC6 by the indicated factors increases the density of TRPC6 channels at the plasma membrane (left), which open after activation of endothelial receptors (right) and increase endothelial permeability and inflammatory processes inducing endothelial dysfunction. 11,12 EET, 11,12-epoxyeicosatrienoic acid; ASM, acid sphingomyelinase; Ca²⁺, calcium ion; [Ca²⁺]ᵢ, intracellular Ca²⁺ concentration; Cav-1, caveolin-1; DAG, diacylglycerol; EC, endothelial cell; G, G-protein; HIF-1α, hypoxia-inducible factor 1 alpha; L, ligand; LPS, lipopolysaccharide; PAF, platelet-activating factor; PTEN, phosphatase and tensin homolog; PIP₂, phosphatidylinositol 4,5-bisphosphate; PLC, phospholipase C; TLR4, toll-like receptor 4; TRPC, classical transient receptor potential channel; TRPC6, classical transient receptor potential channel 6; VEGF, vascular endothelial growth factor; solid arrows indicate direct interactions; dotted arrows illustrate indirect interactions. Not all interaction partners have been identified.

TRPC6 in the mechanism of acute HPV. Although the role of TRPC6 in chronic hypoxia-induced PH is controversial, there is evolving evidence for an important function of TRPC6 in pulmonary vascular remodeling in IPAH and endothelial barrier disruption in ALI. Therefore, TRPC6 is a promising target for pharmacological interventions. In physiological processes like acute HPV, TRPC6 activators may be useful to redirect blood flow from non-ventilated regions to oxygen-rich regions of the lungs to avoid life-threatening arterial hypoxemia. In pathophysiological processes like excessive vascular remodeling, PH, or enhanced endothelial permeability, inhibitors of TRPC6 channels might represent a valuable approach. Thus, specific drugs designed to

target TRPC6 channels have to be identified as a prerequisite to develop new therapeutic strategies in diseases coupled to physiological and pathological functions of TRPC6 channels.

AUTHOR CONTRIBUTIONS

MM, AE, CV, and AS drafted the manuscript. MM, AE, CV, HG, RS, TG, AD, NW, and AS revised the manuscript critically for important intellectual content and approved the final version of the manuscript submitted.

REFERENCES

1. Clapham DE. Calcium signaling. *Cell* (2007) 131:1047–58. doi:10.1016/j.cell.2007.11.028
2. Morrell NW, Adnot S, Archer SL, Dupuis J, Jones PL, MacLean MR, et al. Cellular and molecular basis of pulmonary arterial hypertension. *J Am Coll Cardiol* (2009) 54:S20–31. doi:10.1016/j.jacc.2009.04.018
3. Mehta D, Malik AB. Signaling mechanisms regulating endothelial permeability. *Physiol Rev* (2006) 86:279–367. doi:10.1152/physrev.00012.2005
4. Dietrich A, Kalwa H, Fuchs B, Grimminger F, Weissmann N, Gudermann T. In vivo TRPC functions in the cardiopulmonary vasculature. *Cell Calcium* (2007) 42:233–44. doi:10.1016/j.ceca.2007.02.009
5. Clapham DE. TRP channels as cellular sensors. *Nature* (2003) 426:517–24. doi:10.1038/nature02196
6. Earley S, Brayden JE. Transient receptor potential channels in the vasculature. *Physiol Rev* (2015) 95:645–90. doi:10.1152/physrev.00026.2014
7. Dietrich A, Mederos y Schnitzler M, Emmel J, Kalwa H, Hofmann T, Gudermann T. N-linked protein glycosylation is a major determinant for basal TRPC3 and TRPC6 channel activity. *J Biol Chem* (2003) 278:47842–52. doi:10.1074/jbc.M302983200
8. Hofmann T, Obukhov AG, Schaefer M, Harteneck C, Gudermann T, Schultz G. Direct activation of human TRPC6 and TRPC3 channels by diacylglycerol. *Nature* (1999) 397:259–63. doi:10.1038/16711
9. Inoue R, Jensen LJ, Shi J, Morita H, Nishida M, Honda A, et al. Transient receptor potential channels in cardiovascular function and disease. *Circ Res* (2006) 99:119–31. doi:10.1161/01.RES.0000233356.10630.8a
10. Dietrich A, Mederos y Schnitzler M, Kalwa H, Storch U, Gudermann T. Functional characterization and physiological relevance of the TRPC3/6/7 subfamily of cation channels. *Naunyn Schmiedebergs Arch Pharmacol* (2005) 371:257–65. doi:10.1007/s00210-005-1052-8
11. McDaniel SS, Platoshyn O, Wang J, Yu Y, Sweeney M, Krick S, et al. Capacitative Ca(2+) entry in agonist-induced pulmonary vasoconstriction. *Am J Physiol Lung Cell Mol Physiol* (2001) 280:L870–80.
12. Ng LC, Gurney AM. Store-operated channels mediate Ca(2+) influx and contraction in rat pulmonary artery. *Circ Res* (2001) 89:923–9. doi:10.1161/hh2201.100315
13. Wang J, Shimoda LA, Sylvester JT. Capacitative calcium entry and TRPC channel proteins are expressed in rat distal pulmonary arterial smooth muscle. *Am J Physiol Lung Cell Mol Physiol* (2004) 286:L848–58. doi:10.1152/ajplung.00319.2003
14. Lu W, Wang J, Shimoda LA, Sylvester JT. Differences in STIM1 and TRPC expression in proximal and distal pulmonary arterial smooth muscle are associated with differences in Ca2+ responses to hypoxia. *Am J Physiol Lung Cell Mol Physiol* (2008) 295:L104–13. doi:10.1152/ajplung.00058.2008
15. Wang Q, Wang D, Yan G, Sun L, Tang C. TRPC6 is required for hypoxia-induced basal intracellular calcium concentration elevation, and for the proliferation and migration of rat distal pulmonary venous smooth muscle cells. *Mol Med Rep* (2016) 13:1577–85. doi:10.3892/mmr.2015.4750

16. Galie N, Humbert M, Vachiery JL, Gibbs S, Lang I, Torbicki A, et al. 2015 ESC/ERS Guidelines for the diagnosis and treatment of pulmonary hypertension: the Joint Task Force for the Diagnosis and Treatment of Pulmonary Hypertension of the European Society of Cardiology (ESC) and the European Respiratory Society (ERS): Endorsed by: Association for European Paediatric and Congenital Cardiology (AEPC), International Society for Heart and Lung Transplantation (ISHLT). *Eur Heart J* (2016) 37:67–119. doi:10.1093/eurheartj/ehv317
17. Hoeper MM, Bogaard HJ, Condliffe R, Frantz R, Khanna D, Kurzyna M, et al. Definitions and diagnosis of pulmonary hypertension. *J Am Coll Cardiol* (2013) 62:D42–50. doi:10.1016/j.jacc.2013.10.032
18. Galie N, Humbert M, Vachiery JL, Gibbs S, Lang I, Torbicki A, et al. 2015 ESC/ERS Guidelines for the diagnosis and treatment of pulmonary hypertension: the Joint Task Force for the Diagnosis and Treatment of Pulmonary Hypertension of the European Society of Cardiology (ESC) and the European Respiratory Society (ERS): Endorsed by: Association for European Paediatric and Congenital Cardiology (AEPC), International Society for Heart and Lung Transplantation (ISHLT). *Eur Respir J* (2015) 46:903–75. doi:10.1183/13993003.01032-2015
19. Rhodes J. Comparative physiology of hypoxic pulmonary hypertension: historical clues from brisket disease. *J Appl Physiol* (2005) 98:1092–100. doi:10.1152/japplphysiol.01017.2004
20. Sylvester JT, Shimoda LA, Aaronson PI, Ward JP. Hypoxic pulmonary vasoconstriction. *Physiol Rev* (2012) 92:367–520. doi:10.1152/physrev.00041.2010
21. Euler USv, Liljestrand G. Observations on the pulmonary arterial blood pressure in the cat. *Acta Physiol Scand* (1946) 12:301–20. doi:10.1111/j.1748-1716.1946.tb00389.x
22. Nagasaka Y, Bhattacharya J, Nanjo S, Gropper MA, Staub NC. Micropuncture measurement of lung microvascular pressure profile during hypoxia in cats. *Circ Res* (1984) 54:90–5. doi:10.1161/01.RES.54.1.90
23. Sonobe T, Schwenke DO, Pearson JT, Yoshimoto M, Fujii Y, Umetani K, et al. Imaging of the closed-chest mouse pulmonary circulation using synchrotron radiation microangiography. *J Appl Physiol (1985)* (2011) 111:75–80. doi:10.1152/japplphysiol.00205.2011
24. Bennie RE, Packer CS, Powell DR, Jin N, Rhoades RA. Biphasic contractile response of pulmonary artery to hypoxia. *Am J Physiol* (1991) 261:L156–63.
25. Weissmann N, Winterhalder S, Nollen M, Voswinckel R, Quanz K, Ghofrani HA, et al. NO and reactive oxygen species are involved in biphasic hypoxic vasoconstriction of isolated rabbit lungs. *Am J Physiol Lung Cell Mol Physiol* (2001) 280:L638–45.
26. Weissmann N, Akkayagil E, Quanz K, Schermuly RT, Ghofrani HA, Fink L, et al. Basic features of hypoxic pulmonary vasoconstriction in mice. *Respir Physiol Neurobiol* (2004) 139:191–202. doi:10.1016/j.resp.2003.10.003
27. Weigand L, Foxson J, Wang J, Shimoda LA, Sylvester JT. Inhibition of hypoxic pulmonary vasoconstriction by antagonists of store-operated Ca2+ and nonselective cation channels. *Am J Physiol Lung Cell Mol Physiol* (2005) 289:L5–13. doi:10.1152/ajplung.00044.2005

28. Wang J, Shimoda LA, Weigand L, Wang W, Sun D, Sylvester JT. Acute hypoxia increases intracellular [Ca2+] in pulmonary arterial smooth muscle by enhancing capacitative Ca2+ entry. *Am J Physiol Lung Cell Mol Physiol* (2005) 288:L1059–69. doi:10.1152/ajplung.00448.2004

29. Weissmann N, Dietrich A, Fuchs B, Kalwa H, Ay M, Dumitrascu R, et al. Classical transient receptor potential channel 6 (TRPC6) is essential for hypoxic pulmonary vasoconstriction and alveolar gas exchange. *Proc Natl Acad Sci U S A* (2006) 103:19093–8. doi:10.1073/pnas.0606728103

30. Liu H, Zhang H, Forman HJ. Silica induces macrophage cytokines through phosphatidylcholine-specific phospholipase C with hydrogen peroxide. *Am J Respir Cell Mol Biol* (2007) 36:594–9. doi:10.1165/rcmb.2006-0297OC

31. Weissmann N, Sydykov A, Kalwa H, Storch U, Fuchs B, Mederos y Schnitzler M, et al. Activation of TRPC6 channels is essential for lung ischaemia-reperfusion induced oedema in mice. *Nat Commun* (2012) 3:649. doi:10.1038/ncomms1660

32. Fuchs B, Rupp M, Ghofrani HA, Schermuly RT, Seeger W, Grimminger F, et al. Diacylglycerol regulates acute hypoxic pulmonary vasoconstriction via TRPC6. *Respir Res* (2011) 12:20. doi:10.1186/1465-9921-12-20

33. Tabeling C, Yu H, Wang L, Ranke H, Goldenberg NM, Zabini D, et al. CFTR and sphingolipids mediate hypoxic pulmonary vasoconstriction. *Proc Natl Acad Sci U S A* (2015) 112:E1614–23. doi:10.1073/pnas.1421190112

34. Keseru B, Barbosa-Sicard E, Popp R, Fisslthaler B, Dietrich A, Gudermann T, et al. Epoxyeicosatrienoic acids and the soluble epoxide hydrolase are determinants of pulmonary artery pressure and the acute hypoxic pulmonary vasoconstrictor response. *FASEB J* (2008) 22:4306–15. doi:10.1096/fj.08-112821

35. Gudermann T, Mederos y Schnitzler M, Dietrich A. Receptor-operated cation entry – more than esoteric terminology? *Sci STKE* (2004) 2004:e35. doi:10.1126/stke.2432004pe35

36. Pak O, Janssen W, Ghofrani HA, Seeger W, Grimminger F, Schermuly RT, et al. Animal models of pulmonary hypertension: role in translational research. *Drug Discov Today Dis Models* (2010) 7:89–97. doi:10.1016/j.ddmod.2011.02.002

37. Arias-Stella J, Saldana M. The muscular pulmonary arteries in people native to high altitude. *Med Thorac* (1962) 19:484–93.

38. Groves BM, Reeves JT, Sutton JR, Wagner PD, Cymerman A, Malconian MK, et al. Operation Everest II: elevated high-altitude pulmonary resistance unresponsive to oxygen. *J Appl Physiol (1985)* (1987) 63:521–30.

39. Canepa A, Chavez R, Hurtado A, Rotta A, Velasquez T. Pulmonary circulation at sea level and at high altitudes. *J Appl Physiol* (1956) 9:328–36.

40. Hultgren HN, Kelly J, Miller H. Effect of oxygen upon pulmonary circulation in acclimatized man at high altitude. *J Appl Physiol* (1965) 20:239–43.

41. Rowan SC, McLoughlin P. Hypoxic pulmonary hypertension: the paradigm is changing. *Exp Physiol* (2014) 99:837–8. doi:10.1113/expphysiol.2014.078485

42. Xia Y, Yang XR, Fu Z, Paudel O, Abramowitz J, Birnbaumer L, et al. Classical transient receptor potential 1 and 6 contribute to hypoxic pulmonary hypertension through differential regulation of pulmonary vascular functions. *Hypertension* (2014) 63:173–80. doi:10.1161/hypertensionaha.113.01902

43. Smith KA, Voiriot G, Tang H, Fraidenburg DR, Song S, Yamamura H, et al. Notch activation of Ca(2+) signaling in the development of hypoxic pulmonary vasoconstriction and pulmonary hypertension. *Am J Respir Cell Mol Biol* (2015) 53:355–67. doi:10.1165/rcmb.2014-0235OC

44. Tucker A, Migally N, Wright ML, Greenlees KJ. Pulmonary vascular changes in young and aging rats exposed to 5,486 m altitude. *Respiration* (1984) 46:246–57. doi:10.1159/000194696

45. Saker M, Lipskaia L, Marcos E, Abid S, Parpaleix A, Houssaini A, et al. Osteopontin, a key mediator expressed by senescent pulmonary vascular cells in pulmonary hypertension. *Arterioscler Thromb Vasc Biol* (2016) 36:1879–90. doi:10.1161/atvbaha.116.307839

46. Miller AA, Hislop AA, Vallance PJ, Haworth SG. Deletion of the eNOS gene has a greater impact on the pulmonary circulation of male than female mice. *Am J Physiol Lung Cell Mol Physiol* (2005) 289:L299–306. doi:10.1152/ajplung.00022.2005

47. Tada Y, Laudi S, Harral J, Carr M, Ivester C, Tanabe N, et al. Murine pulmonary response to chronic hypoxia is strain specific. *Exp Lung Res* (2008) 34:313–23. doi:10.1080/01902140802093204

48. Moreth K, Fischer R, Fuchs H, Gailus-Durner V, Wurst W, Katus HA, et al. High-throughput phenotypic assessment of cardiac physiology in four commonly used inbred mouse strains. *J Comp Physiol B* (2014) 184:763–75. doi:10.1007/s00360-014-0830-3

49. Fernandez RA, Wan J, Song S, Smith KA, Gu Y, Tauseef M, et al. Upregulated expression of STIM2, TRPC6, and Orai2 contributes to the transition of pulmonary arterial smooth muscle cells from a contractile to proliferative phenotype. *Am J Physiol Cell Physiol* (2015) 308:C581–93. doi:10.1152/ajpcell.00202.2014

50. Wang J, Weigand L, Lu W, Sylvester JT, Semenza GL, Shimoda LA. Hypoxia inducible factor 1 mediates hypoxia-induced TRPC expression and elevated intracellular Ca2+ in pulmonary arterial smooth muscle cells. *Circ Res* (2006) 98:1528–37. doi:10.1161/01.res.0000227551.68124.98

51. Malczyk M, Veith C, Fuchs B, Hofmann K, Storch U, Schermuly RT, et al. Classical transient receptor potential channel 1 in hypoxia-induced pulmonary hypertension. *Am J Respir Crit Care Med* (2013) 188:1451–9. doi:10.1164/rccm.201307-1252OC

52. Lin MJ, Leung GP, Zhang WM, Yang XR, Yip KP, Tse CM, et al. Chronic hypoxia-induced upregulation of store-operated and receptor-operated Ca2+ channels in pulmonary arterial smooth muscle cells: a novel mechanism of hypoxic pulmonary hypertension. *Circ Res* (2004) 95:496–505. doi:10.1161/01.RES.0000138952.16382.ad

53. Lu W, Ran P, Zhang D, Lai N, Zhong N, Wang J. Bone morphogenetic protein 4 enhances canonical transient receptor potential expression, store-operated Ca2+ entry, and basal [Ca2+]i in rat distal pulmonary arterial smooth muscle cells. *Am J Physiol Cell Physiol* (2010) 299:C1370–8. doi:10.1152/ajpcell.00040.2010

54. Zhang Y, Wang Y, Yang K, Tian L, Fu X, Wang Y, et al. BMP4 increases the expression of TRPC and basal [Ca2+]i via the p38MAPK and ERK1/2 pathways independent of BMPRII in PASMCs. *PLoS One* (2014) 9:e112695. doi:10.1371/journal.pone.0112695

55. Jiang Q, Fu X, Tian L, Chen Y, Yang K, Chen X, et al. NOX4 mediates BMP4-induced upregulation of TRPC1 and 6 protein expressions in distal pulmonary arterial smooth muscle cells. *PLoS One* (2014) 9:e107135. doi:10.1371/journal.pone.0107135

56. Seeger W, Adir Y, Barbera JA, Champion H, Coghlan JG, Cottin V, et al. Pulmonary hypertension in chronic lung diseases. *J Am Coll Cardiol* (2013) 62:D109–16. doi:10.1016/j.jacc.2013.10.036

57. Blanco I, Piccari L, Barbera JA. Pulmonary vasculature in COPD: the silent component. *Respirology* (2016) 21:984–94. doi:10.1111/resp.12772

58. Seimetz M, Parajuli N, Pichl A, Veit F, Kwapiszewska G, Weisel FC, et al. Inducible NOS inhibition reverses tobacco-smoke-induced emphysema and pulmonary hypertension in mice. *Cell* (2011) 147:293–305. doi:10.1016/j.cell.2011.08.035

59. Zhao L, Wang J, Wang L, Liang YT, Chen YQ, Lu WJ, et al. Remodeling of rat pulmonary artery induced by chronic smoking exposure. *J Thorac Dis* (2014) 6:818–28. doi:10.3978/j.issn.2072-1439.2014.03.31

60. Wang J, Chen Y, Lin C, Jia J, Tian L, Yang K, et al. Effects of chronic exposure to cigarette smoke on canonical transient receptor potential expression in rat pulmonary arterial smooth muscle. *Am J Physiol Cell Physiol* (2014) 306:C364–73. doi:10.1152/ajpcell.00048.2013

61. Wang J, Jiang Q, Wan L, Yang K, Zhang Y, Chen Y, et al. Sodium tanshinone IIA sulfonate inhibits canonical transient receptor potential expression in pulmonary arterial smooth muscle from pulmonary hypertensive rats. *Am J Respir Cell Mol Biol* (2013) 48:125–34. doi:10.1165/rcmb.2012-0071OC

62. Yun X, Chen Y, Yang K, Wang S, Lu W, Wang J. Upregulation of canonical transient receptor potential channel in the pulmonary arterial smooth muscle of a chronic thromboembolic pulmonary hypertension rat model. *Hypertens Res* (2015) 38:821–8. doi:10.1038/hr.2015.80

63. Lu W, Ran P, Zhang D, Peng G, Li B, Zhong N, et al. Sildenafil inhibits chronically hypoxic upregulation of canonical transient receptor potential expression in rat pulmonary arterial smooth muscle. *Am J Physiol Cell Physiol* (2010) 298:C114–23. doi:10.1152/ajpcell.00629.2008

64. Liu XR, Zhang MF, Yang N, Liu Q, Wang RX, Cao YN, et al. Enhanced store-operated Ca(2)+ entry and TRPC channel expression in pulmonary arteries of monocrotaline-induced pulmonary hypertensive rats. *Am J Physiol Cell Physiol* (2012) 302:C77–87. doi:10.1152/ajpcell.00247.2011

65. Yang K, Lu W, Jia J, Zhang J, Zhao M, Wang S, et al. Noggin inhibits hypoxia-induced proliferation by targeting store-operated calcium entry and transient receptor potential cation channels. *Am J Physiol Cell Physiol* (2015) 308:C869–78. doi:10.1152/ajpcell.00349.2014

66. Sun CK, Zhen YY, Lu HI, Sung PH, Chang LT, Tsai TH, et al. Reducing TRPC1 expression through liposome-mediated siRNA delivery markedly attenuates hypoxia-induced pulmonary arterial hypertension in a murine model. *Stem Cells Int* (2014) 2014:316214. doi:10.1155/2014/316214

67. Alzoubi A, Almalouf P, Toba M, O'Neill K, Qian X, Francis M, et al. TRPC4 inactivation confers a survival benefit in severe pulmonary arterial hypertension. *Am J Pathol* (2013) 183:1779–88. doi:10.1016/j.ajpath.2013.08.016

68. Schermuly RT, Ghofrani HA, Wilkins MR, Grimminger F. Mechanisms of disease: pulmonary arterial hypertension. *Nat Rev Cardiol* (2011) 8:443–55. doi:10.1038/nrcardio.2011.87

69. Grimminger F, Schermuly RT, Ghofrani HA. Targeting non-malignant disorders with tyrosine kinase inhibitors. *Nat Rev Drug Discov* (2010) 9:956–70. doi:10.1038/nrd3297

70. Golovina VA, Platoshyn O, Bailey CL, Wang J, Limsuwan A, Sweeney M, et al. Upregulated TRP and enhanced capacitative Ca(2+) entry in human pulmonary artery myocytes during proliferation. *Am J Physiol Heart Circ Physiol* (2001) 280:H746–55.

71. Yuan JX, Aldinger AM, Juhaszova M, Wang J, Conte JV Jr, Gaine SP, et al. Dysfunctional voltage-gated K+ channels in pulmonary artery smooth muscle cells of patients with primary pulmonary hypertension. *Circulation* (1998) 98:1400–6. doi:10.1161/01.CIR.98.14.1400

72. Yu Y, Sweeney M, Zhang S, Platoshyn O, Landsberg J, Rothman A, et al. PDGF stimulates pulmonary vascular smooth muscle cell proliferation by upregulating TRPC6 expression. *Am J Physiol Cell Physiol* (2003) 284:C316–30. doi:10.1152/ajpcell.00125.2002

73. Yu Y, Fantozzi I, Remillard CV, Landsberg JW, Kunichika N, Platoshyn O, et al. Enhanced expression of transient receptor potential channels in idiopathic pulmonary arterial hypertension. *Proc Natl Acad Sci U S A* (2004) 101:13861–6. doi:10.1073/pnas.0405908101

74. Hassoun PM, Mouthon L, Barbera JA, Eddahibi S, Flores SC, Grimminger F, et al. Inflammation, growth factors, and pulmonary vascular remodeling. *J Am Coll Cardiol* (2009) 54:S10–9. doi:10.1016/j.jacc.2009.04.006

75. Savai R, Pullamsetti SS, Kolbe J, Bieniek E, Voswinckel R, Fink L, et al. Immune and inflammatory cell involvement in the pathology of idiopathic pulmonary arterial hypertension. *Am J Respir Crit Care Med* (2012) 186:897–908. doi:10.1164/rccm.201202-0335OC

76. Yu Y, Keller SH, Remillard CV, Safrina O, Nicholson A, Zhang SL, et al. A functional single-nucleotide polymorphism in the TRPC6 gene promoter associated with idiopathic pulmonary arterial hypertension. *Circulation* (2009) 119:2313–22. doi:10.1161/circulationaha.108.782458

77. Hosokawa S, Haraguchi G, Sasaki A, Arai H, Muto S, Itai A, et al. Pathophysiological roles of nuclear factor kappaB (NF-kB) in pulmonary arterial hypertension: effects of synthetic selective NF-kB inhibitor IMD-0354. *Cardiovasc Res* (2013) 99:35–43. doi:10.1093/cvr/cvt105

78. Wang Q, Zuo XR, Wang YY, Xie WP, Wang H, Zhang M. Monocrotaline-induced pulmonary arterial hypertension is attenuated by TNF-alpha antagonists via the suppression of TNF-alpha expression and NF-kappaB pathway in rats. *Vascul Pharmacol* (2013) 58:71–7. doi:10.1016/j.vph.2012.07.006

79. Sawada H, Mitani Y, Maruyama J, Jiang BH, Ikeyama Y, Dida FA, et al. A nuclear factor-kappaB inhibitor pyrrolidine dithiocarbamate ameliorates pulmonary hypertension in rats. *Chest* (2007) 132:1265–74. doi:10.1378/chest.06-2243

80. Price LC, Caramori G, Perros F, Meng C, Gambaryan N, Dorfmuller P, et al. Nuclear factor kappa-B is activated in the pulmonary vessels of patients with end-stage idiopathic pulmonary arterial hypertension. *PLoS One* (2013) 8:e75415. doi:10.1371/journal.pone.0075415

81. Hamid R, Newman JH. Evidence for inflammatory signaling in idiopathic pulmonary artery hypertension: TRPC6 and nuclear factor-kappaB. *Circulation* (2009) 119:2297–8. doi:10.1161/circulationaha.109.855197

82. Pousada G, Baloira A, Valverde D. Molecular and clinical analysis of TRPC6 and AGTR1 genes in patients with pulmonary arterial hypertension. *Orphanet J Rare Dis* (2015) 10:1. doi:10.1186/s13023-014-0216-3

83. Hofmann T, Schaefer M, Schultz G, Gudermann T. Transient receptor potential channels as molecular substrates of receptor-mediated cation entry. *J Mol Med (Berl)* (2000) 78:14–25. doi:10.1007/s001099900070

84. Beech DJ, Muraki K, Flemming R. Non-selective cationic channels of smooth muscle and the mammalian homologues of *Drosophila* TRP. *J Physiol* (2004) 559:685–706. doi:10.1113/jphysiol.2004.068734

85. Bon RS, Beech DJ. In pursuit of small molecule chemistry for calcium-permeable non-selective TRPC channels – mirage or pot of gold? *Br J Pharmacol* (2013) 170:459–74. doi:10.1111/bph.12274

86. Dietrich A, Mederos YSM, Gollasch M, Gross V, Storch U, Dubrovska G, et al. Increased vascular smooth muscle contractility in TRPC6-/- mice. *Mol Cell Biol* (2005) 25:6980–9. doi:10.1128/mcb.25.16.6980-6989.2005

87. Sel S, Rost BR, Yildirim AO, Sel B, Kalwa H, Fehrenbach H, et al. Loss of classical transient receptor potential 6 channel reduces allergic airway response. *Clin Exp Allergy* (2008) 38:1548–58. doi:10.1111/j.1365-2222.2008.03043.x

88. Kiyonaka S, Kato K, Nishida M, Mio K, Numaga T, Sawaguchi Y, et al. Selective and direct inhibition of TRPC3 channels underlies biological activities of a pyrazole compound. *Proc Natl Acad Sci U S A* (2009) 106:5400–5. doi:10.1073/pnas.0808793106

89. Kim MS, Lee KP, Yang D, Shin DM, Abramowitz J, Kiyonaka S, et al. Genetic and pharmacologic inhibition of the Ca2+ influx channel TRPC3 protects secretory epithelia from Ca2+-dependent toxicity. *Gastroenterology* (2011) 140:2107–15, 2115.e1–4. doi:10.1053/j.gastro.2011.02.052

90. Harteneck C, Gollasch M. Pharmacological modulation of diacylglycerol-sensitive TRPC3/6/7 channels. *Curr Pharm Biotechnol* (2011) 12:35–41. doi:10.2174/138920111793937943

91. Miehe S, Crause P, Schmidt T, Lohn M, Kleemann HW, Licher T, et al. Inhibition of diacylglycerol-sensitive TRPC channels by synthetic and natural steroids. *PLoS One* (2012) 7:e35393. doi:10.1371/journal.pone.0035393

92. Urban N, Hill K, Wang L, Kuebler WM, Schaefer M. Novel pharmacological TRPC inhibitors block hypoxia-induced vasoconstriction. *Cell Calcium* (2012) 51:194–206. doi:10.1016/j.ceca.2012.01.001

93. Maier T, Follmann M, Hessler G, Kleemann HW, Hachtel S, Fuchs B, et al. Discovery and pharmacological characterization of a novel potent inhibitor of diacylglycerol-sensitive TRPC cation channels. *Br J Pharmacol* (2015) 172:3650–60. doi:10.1111/bph.13151

94. Urban N, Wang L, Kwiek S, Rademann J, Kuebler WM, Schaefer M. Identification and validation of larixyl acetate as a potent TRPC6 inhibitor. *Mol Pharmacol* (2016) 89:197–213. doi:10.1124/mol.115.100792

95. Galie N, Ghofrani AH. New horizons in pulmonary arterial hypertension therapies. *Eur Respir Rev* (2013) 22:503–14. doi:10.1183/09059180.00006613

96. Kunichika N, Landsberg JW, Yu Y, Kunichika H, Thistlethwaite PA, Rubin LJ, et al. Bosentan inhibits transient receptor potential channel expression in pulmonary vascular myocytes. *Am J Respir Crit Care Med* (2004) 170:1101–7. doi:10.1164/rccm.200312-1668OC

97. Pauvert O, Bonnet S, Rousseau E, Marthan R, Savineau JP. Sildenafil alters calcium signaling and vascular tone in pulmonary arteries from chronically hypoxic rats. *Am J Physiol Lung Cell Mol Physiol* (2004) 287:L577–83. doi:10.1152/ajplung.00449.2003

98. Wang C, Li JF, Zhao L, Liu J, Wan J, Wang YX, et al. Inhibition of SOC/Ca2+/NFAT pathway is involved in the anti-proliferative effect of sildenafil on pulmonary artery smooth muscle cells. *Respir Res* (2009) 10:123. doi:10.1186/1465-9921-10-123

99. Wang J, Yang K, Xu L, Zhang Y, Lai N, Jiang H, et al. Sildenafil inhibits hypoxia-induced transient receptor potential canonical protein expression in pulmonary arterial smooth muscle via cGMP-PKG-PPARgamma axis. *Am J Respir Cell Mol Biol* (2013) 49:231–40. doi:10.1165/rcmb.2012-0185OC

100. Singh I, Knezevic N, Ahmmed GU, Kini V, Malik AB, Mehta D. Galphaq-TRPC6-mediated Ca2+ entry induces RhoA activation and resultant endothelial cell shape change in response to thrombin. *J Biol Chem* (2007) 282:7833–43. doi:10.1074/jbc.M608288200

101. Mehta D, Ravindran K, Kuebler WM. Novel regulators of endothelial barrier function. *Am J Physiol Lung Cell Mol Physiol* (2014) 307:L924–35. doi:10.1152/ajplung.00318.2014

102. Ahmmed GU, Malik AB. Functional role of TRPC channels in the regulation of endothelial permeability. *Pflugers Arch* (2005) 451:131–42. doi:10.1007/s00424-005-1461-z

103. Yang Y, Yin J, Baumgartner W, Samapati R, Solymosi EA, Reppien E, et al. Platelet-activating factor reduces endothelial nitric oxide production: role of acid sphingomyelinase. *Eur Respir J* (2010) 36:417–27. doi:10.1183/09031936.00095609

104. Samapati R, Yang Y, Yin J, Stoerger C, Arenz C, Dietrich A, et al. Lung endothelial Ca2+ and permeability response to platelet-activating factor is mediated by acid sphingomyelinase and transient receptor potential classical 6. *Am J Respir Crit Care Med* (2012) 185:160–70. doi:10.1164/rccm.201104-0717OC

105. Fleming I, Rueben A, Popp R, Fisslthaler B, Schrodt S, Sander A, et al. Epoxyeicosatrienoic acids regulate Trp channel dependent Ca2+ signaling and hyperpolarization in endothelial cells. *Arterioscler Thromb Vasc Biol* (2007) 27:2612–8. doi:10.1161/atvbaha.107.152074

106. Pocock TM, Foster RR, Bates DO. Evidence of a role for TRPC channels in VEGF-mediated increased vascular permeability in vivo. *Am J Physiol Heart Circ Physiol* (2004) 286:H1015–26. doi:10.1152/ajpheart.00826.2003

107. Hamdollah Zadeh MA, Glass CA, Magnussen A, Hancox JC, Bates DO. VEGF-mediated elevated intracellular calcium and angiogenesis in human microvascular endothelial cells in vitro are inhibited by dominant negative TRPC6. *Microcirculation* (2008) 15:605–14. doi:10.1080/10739680802220323

108. Cheng HW, James AF, Foster RR, Hancox JC, Bates DO. VEGF activates receptor-operated cation channels in human microvascular endothelial cells. *Arterioscler Thromb Vasc Biol* (2006) 26:1768–76. doi:10.1161/01.ATV.0000231518.86795.0f

109. Kini V, Chavez A, Mehta D. A new role for PTEN in regulating transient receptor potential canonical channel 6-mediated Ca2+ entry, endothelial permeability, and angiogenesis. *J Biol Chem* (2010) 285:33082–91. doi:10.1074/jbc.M110.142034

110. Tauseef M, Knezevic N, Chava KR, Smith M, Sukriti S, Gianaris N, et al. TLR4 activation of TRPC6-dependent calcium signaling mediates endotoxin-induced lung vascular permeability and inflammation. *J Exp Med* (2012) 209:1953–68. doi:10.1084/jem.20111355

111. Zhou X, Dai Q, Huang X. Neutrophils in acute lung injury. *Front Biosci (Landmark Ed)* (2012) 17:2278–83. doi:10.2741/4051

112. Wettschureck N, Offermanns S. Mammalian G proteins and their cell type specific functions. *Physiol Rev* (2005) 85:1159–204. doi:10.1152/physrev.00003.2005

113. Lindemann O, Umlauf D, Frank S, Schimmelpfennig S, Bertrand J, Pap T, et al. TRPC6 regulates CXCR2-mediated chemotaxis of murine neutrophils. *J Immunol* (2013) 190:5496–505. doi:10.4049/jimmunol.1201502

114. Damann N, Owsianik G, Li S, Poll C, Nilius B. The calcium-conducting ion channel transient receptor potential canonical 6 is involved in macrophage inflammatory protein-2-induced migration of mouse neutrophils. *Acta Physiol (Oxf)* (2009) 195:3–11. doi:10.1111/j.1748-1716.2008.01918.x

115. Weber EW, Han F, Tauseef M, Birnbaumer L, Mehta D, Muller WA. TRPC6 is the endothelial calcium channel that regulates leukocyte transendothelial migration during the inflammatory response. *J Exp Med* (2015) 212:1883–99. doi:10.1084/jem.20150353

Cytokine–Ion Channel Interactions in Pulmonary Inflammation

Jürg Hamacher[1,2,3], Yalda Hadizamani[1,3†], Michèle Borgmann[1,3†], Markus Mohaupt[4],
Daniela Narcissa Männel[5], Ueli Moehrlen[6], Rudolf Lucas[7†] and Uz Stammberger[3,8†]*

[1]*Internal Medicine and Pneumology, Lindenhofspital, Bern, Switzerland,* [2]*Internal Medicine V – Pneumology, Allergology, Respiratory and Environmental Medicine, Faculty of Medicine, Saarland University, Saarbrücken, Germany,* [3]*Lungen- und Atmungsstiftung Bern, Bern, Switzerland,* [4]*Internal Medicine, Sonnenhofspital Bern, Bern, Switzerland,* [5]*Faculty of Medicine, Institute of Immunology, University of Regensburg, Regensburg, Germany,* [6]*Paediatric Visceral Surgery, Universitäts-Kinderspital Zürich, Zürich, Switzerland,* [7]*Department of Pharmacology and Toxicology, Vascular Biology Center, Medical College of Georgia, Augusta, GA, United States,* [8]*Novartis Institutes for Biomedical Research, Translational Clinical Oncology, Novartis Pharma AG, Basel, Switzerland*

*Correspondence:
Jürg Hamacher
hamacher@greenmail.ch

[†]*These authors have contributed
equally to this work.*

The lungs conceptually represent a sponge that is interposed in series in the bodies' systemic circulation to take up oxygen and eliminate carbon dioxide. As such, it matches the huge surface areas of the alveolar epithelium to the pulmonary blood capillaries. The lung's constant exposure to the exterior necessitates a competent immune system, as evidenced by the association of clinical immunodeficiencies with pulmonary infections. From the *in utero* to the postnatal and adult situation, there is an inherent vital need to manage alveolar fluid reabsorption, be it postnatally, or in case of hydrostatic or permeability edema. Whereas a wealth of literature exists on the physiological basis of fluid and solute reabsorption by ion channels and water pores, only sparse knowledge is available so far on pathological situations, such as in microbial infection, acute lung injury or acute respiratory distress syndrome, and in the pulmonary reimplantation response in transplanted lungs. The aim of this review is to discuss alveolar liquid clearance in a selection of lung injury models, thereby especially focusing on cytokines and mediators that modulate ion channels. Inflammation is characterized by complex and probably time-dependent co-signaling, interactions between the involved cell types, as well as by cell demise and barrier dysfunction, which may not uniquely determine a clinical picture. This review, therefore, aims to give integrative thoughts and wants to foster the unraveling of unmet needs in future research.

Keywords: epithelial sodium channel, Na$^+$/K$^+$-ATPase, tumor necrosis factor, TNF tip peptide, pneumonia, acute respiratory distress syndrome, lung transplantation, ischemia–reperfusion injury

INTRODUCTION

Acute lung injury (ALI) and acute respiratory distress syndrome (ARDS) are both clinical syndromes with a high morbidity and mortality rate. Although of a different degree of severity, both ARDS and ALI are characterized by critical gas exchange disturbances, an inflammatory reaction, and an associated alveolar fluid overload (edema). The etiology of ALI and ARDS can be differentiated between direct and indirect lung injury.

The conceptual work presented here discusses the mechanisms regulating alveolar fluid clearance (AFC) during inflammation. As recently demonstrated by several groups, the interaction between cytokines and ion channels may play a critical role in this setting. The presented review does not cover all cytokines and ion channels, but rather focuses on a selection of mainly pre-clinical pathophysiological models and addresses clinical needs and difficulties to effectively translate pre-clinical data into the clinical field. **Tables 1–3** give an overview on ion channels and mediator interaction. The ultimate aim of this translational research should be to improve patient care and to reduce morbidity and mortality. This can be achieved by reducing long-term residual sequelae and time on the ventilator, which can improve long-term lung function and health status or health-related quality of life.

The main task of the lungs is to account for the efficient external gas exchange between air and the blood. Only a thin barrier of several micrometers separates the pulmonary capillaries from the immense alveolar surface, mainly made up by alveolar type I cells. An intimately fine, deformable, tensible, flexible, and continuous net of interstitial tissue integrates the interstitial net around vessels and bronchi. The whole system has to be "breathable," i.e., has to be efficiently moved by the thoracic cage to transport fresh air in the alveolar space that matches to the vascular bed for gas exchange. A number of structural and physiological features prevent alveolar flooding. These protective mechanisms include the very low vascular resistance in the pulmonary circulation, the high capillary colloid-osmotic pressure and, on the other hand, the diminished interstitial colloid-osmotic pressure in case of increased filtration. The minimal mechanic stress of alveolar septa due to surface tension reduction by surfactant as well as the optimal active fluid reabsorption out of the alveolar space are further measures that optimize fluid clearance. Structurally, a rather tight pulmonary microvascular endothelium allows for a minimal continuous filtration of water, micro-and macromolecules, with an even tighter alveolar epithelium (1). All three fluid compartments, the capillaries, the interstitium, and the alveoli are in a complex dynamic equilibrium. The continuous pulmonary interstitial space is a drainable continuum that is ultimately emptied by the lymphatic vessels. There is a basal transendothelial filtration of about 10 ml/h that increases up to tenfold during physical activity. When such filtered fluid enters the alveolar interstitial space, it moves proximally to the peri-bronchovascular space (2). Under normal conditions, most of this filtered fluid will be removed by the lymphatics from the interstitium and returns to the systemic circulation (2).

The interstitial compartment is a reversible store of excess fluid. In the adult lung, interstitial fluid—or interstitial edema—can mount up to a volume of 500 ml. However, at that volume there is usually already some alveolar edema (3). It was formerly wrongfully postulated that the Starling filtration forces, which essentially represent the balance between oncotic and hydrostatic pressures in the capillaries and the interstitial space, are the only driving forces for liquid flow from the bloodstream into the extravascular space. In the last four decades, four important refinements have been made. The first one is that fluid reabsorption from the alveolar space is mainly performed by active vectorial Na^+ transport (4). Moreover, also Cl^- transport was suggested to be important, leading to consecutive counter-ion transport, as well as to an osmotic water shift. In the last few years, a second refinement has been made which mainly occurs in heart failure, namely that pumps which usually free the alveolus of ions can also provide inverse transport (5). This biological "emergency plan" in case of hydrostatic pulmonary edema widens the scope of mechanisms in cardiogenic lung edema, as one can argue that in heart failure these mechanisms could be rescue fluid shifts including into the alveolar space, and that a concerted fluid management in vascular, renal, and intestinal and pulmonary vascular beds might occur in severe cardiac failure or fluid overload, taking into account some degree of alveolar pulmonary edema. A third rather novel field is the research on emptying of the alveolar space from its protein load; but so far only few insights in this clinical topic exist (6). The fourth refinement is the close relationship of ion channel activation with barrier tightness. Interactions between the lectin-like domain of tumor necrosis factor (TNF), mimicked by its amino acid-identic TNF tip peptide (a.k.a. AP301 and Solnatide) and the epithelial sodium channel (ENaC) were shown to have a clear effect on epithelial (7) and endothelial barrier tightness (8, 9). As such, ion channel activity and barrier tightness may be key survival factors for tissue function, be it the lung or the kidney, the brain or other organs, and for tissue stability (9–11).

Alveolar fluid reabsorption is a very physiological process that is even required directly after birth where the lung has to be cleared from liquid as it has been so far immersed in the amnionic fluid. In premature infant, insufficient clearance of lung liquid at birth may lead to respiratory distress syndrome (RDS). The key clinical relevance of the physiological role of αENaC in the lungs has been confirmed in the mouse in which the ENaC-α gene was deleted by a homologous recombination. These animals were not able to remove alveolar fluid from their lungs and died shortly after birth (12). Surprisingly, in humans this situation seems more complex, as a child with an inactive homozygous ENaC-α mutation did not suffer perinatal respiratory failure (13).

Likewise in adults with heart failure or RDS, while they show no active fluid clearance greater morbidity and mortality rate is probable (14). In clinical studies using quantification of protein in alveolar liquid, prognosis was dependent on the estimated AFC. In a recent study, 56% had impaired AFC, and only 13% a maximal AFC rate (**Figure 1**). Survival was higher and days on mechanical ventilation were less in those patients with maximal alveolar clearance rate compared to patients with impaired clearance rate. With hydrostatic edema, by contrast, 75% of patients had submaximal to maximal AFC (15). Of note is that in hydrostatic edema alveolar fluid shift may even actively be reversed (5, 16) as discussed above.

PULMONARY EDEMA

Pulmonary alveolar edema is a life-threatening state that results from an imbalance between passive and active forces driving fluid into the airspaces and those mechanisms involved in its removal (1, 4). Based on the underlying cause, in the next two chapters we will discuss two main fundamentally different types of pulmonary edema occur in humans (2).

TABLE 1 | Role of different mediators on fluid transport through impacting on ion channels in the apical and basolateral membrane of epithelial cells.

Channel name	Mediator	Impact on pulmonary barrier function	Mechanism of action
Apical membrane			
Epithelial sodium channel (ENaC)	Transforming growth factor beta (TGF-β)	−/+	Decrease in expression during bacterial infection (132) Decreases expression of the αENaC mRNA and protein (132) Internalization of αβγENaC complex from the lung epithelial cell surface and, hence, block the sodium-transporting capacity of alveolar epithelial cells (AECs) (133) Increases the function of ENaC (134)
	Tumor necrosis factor (TNF) receptor binding site	−	Decreases the expression of ENaC mRNA in AECs *in vitro* (135)
	TNF lectin-like domain	+	Activates ENaC (37, 136) Increases ENaC open probability (102)
	Interleukin-1β (IL-1β)	−/+	Decreases the expression of ENaC during bacterial infection (113) Decreases expression of αENaC *via* a p38 MAPK-dependent signaling pathway (113) Suppresses expression of βENaC (137) Decreases ENaC function (138) Augments *in vitro* alveolar epithelial repair (139) Increases ENaC subunits expression in a specific fetal context (140)
	Interleukin-4 (IL-4)	−	Decreases in ENaC expression during bacterial infection (141) Decreases ENaC activity by decreasing the mRNA levels of γENaC and, to a lesser extent, that of the β subunit (142)
	Keratinocyte growth factor (FGF-7)	−	Decreases the expression of αENaC (143)
	Protein kinase C (PKC)	−	Inhibits ENaC function (144–147)
	Cycloheximide (CHX)	−	Downregulate αENaC mRNA abundance similarly *via* the ERK and p38 MAPK pathway (148); Chx effect involves post-transcriptional mechanisms (148)
	Lipopolysaccharide (LPS)	−	Downregulates αENaC mRNA abundance similarly *via* the ERK and p38 MAPK pathways (148); inhibits αENaC promoter activity (148)
	Pneumolysin (PLY)	−	Inhibits ENaC expression upon activation of ERK (102) and inhibits ENaC open probability, by reducing its association with myristoylated alanine-rich C kinase substrate (10, 149)
	Glutathione disulfide (GSSG)	−	Inhibits ENaC activity in primary AECs (150, 151)
	Reactive oxygen species (ROS)	−/+	Inhibit ENaC (150, 152) Decrease channel activity (117) Increases ENaC activity through: (i) Enhancing ENaC gating (153) (ii) Increasing channel abundance (153)
	Ethanol	+	Increases ENaC open-state probability (153) Increases ENaC abundance (153)
	Superoxide (O_2^a)	+	Elevating endogenous (O_2^-) levels with a superoxide dismutase inhibitor, prevents NO inhibition of ENaC activity (111)
	Nitric oxide (NO)	−	Inhibits highly selective sodium channels (52, 53)
	Inter-α-inhibitor (Iαl)	−	Inhibits ENaC activity in CF patients (154)
	NEDD4-2	−	Decreases the expression of the epithelial ENaC (155)
	Hypoxia	−	Decreases apical expression of ENaC subunits (especially beta and gamma) (156)
	Purinergic receptors (P2YR)	−	Inhibits ENaC expression (157, 158)
	Muscarinic cholinergic	+	Increases ENaC activity. RhoA activity is essential for this process (159)
	Estriadol	+	Increases activity of the non-selective ENaC channels, and these effects are mediated through the G protein-coupled estrogen receptor (160)
	Glucocorticoids	+	Increased in expression of ENaC during bacterial infection (161–164)
	Thyroid hormone	+	Thyroid hormone in concert with glucocorticoids increased the expression of ENaC (165, 166)
	Corticosteroids	+	Increase expression of the γ-ENaC subunit which leads to increase ENaC activity (167)

(Continued)

TABLE 1 | Continued

Channel name	Mediator	Impact on pulmonary barrier function	Mechanism of action
	Prostasin [channel activating protease 1 (168)]	+	Activates ENaC (169)
	Urokinase-like plasminogen activator	+	Increases the ENaC activity (154, 170–173)
	Cyclic adenosine monophosphate (cAMP)	+	Increases channel activity either by increasing its open probability or by increasing the number of channels at the apical membrane (174)
	Cystic fibrosis transmembrane conductance regulator (CFTR)	+	Activated CFTR can inhibit ENaC (175)
	Dopamine	+	Increases ENaC activity by a cAMP-mediated alternative signaling pathway involving EPAC and Rap1, signaling molecules usually associated with growth-factor-activated receptors (176)
	β2-agonists	+	Activates ENaC (159) Enhancing the insertion of ENaC subunits into the membrane of AECs (156)
	Human AGEs (receptor for advanced glycation end product ligand)	+	Increases ENaC activity through oxidant-mediated signaling (177)
CFTR (Cl⁻ channel)	Interferon-gamma (IFN-γ)	−	Decreases the expression of CFTR mRNA (142, 178)
	TGF-β	−	Decrease CFTR expression and function (179)
	Interleukin-4 (IL-4)	+	Increases the expression and function of CFTR (142)
	Interleukin-13 (IL-13)	+	Increases the CFTR expression (180)
	Interleukin-1β (IL-1β)	+	Increases CFTR expression trough increasing mRNA levels (138, 181)
	β2-agonists	+	β2AR mediates enhancement of AFC via increasing Cl⁻ flux through CFTR (182, 183) It activates CFTR by raising cAMP intracellular levels and mediating protein kinase A (PKA) activation (184)
	Na⁺/K⁺ ATPase (Na⁺/K⁺-ATPase)	−	Inhibition of the Na⁺/K⁺-ATPase lead to a reduced transcription of CFTR (185) CFTR dysfunction occurs through Na⁺/K⁺-ATPase inhibition by ouabain (186)
Cyclic nucleotide-gated cation channels (CNG) (Na⁺ channel)	Glucocorticoids	+	Increases mRNA for alphaCNG1 (187)
	mineralocorticoids	+	Increases mRNA for alphaCNG1 (187)
TMEM 16a (CaCC) (Ca⁺ activated Cl⁻ channel)	CFTR	−	Can inhibit TMEM 16a through attenuation of ionophore-induced rise in Ca^{2+} (188)
	IL-4	+	Increases the expression of CaCC (189)
	IL-9	+	Increases the expression of CaCC (189)
	IL-13	+	Increases the expression of CaCC (189)
ClC-2 (Cl⁻ channel)	TNF	−	Inhibits Aquaporin 5 (AQ-5) Expression (190)
AQ-5 (H₂O channel)	Transient receptor potential vanilloid 4 (TRPV4)	−	Reduction of AQP5 abundance (191)
	IFN-γ	+	Increases ClC-2 transcripts via mRNA stabilization (192)
	cAMP	+	Increasing synthesis of AQP5 mRNA (193) Triggering translocation of AQP5 to the plasma membrane (193)
	Progesterone	+	Increases abundance of AQP5 (194)
	Estradiol	+	Increases in the AQP5 protein level (194)
Basolateral membrane			
Na⁺/K⁺ ATPase (Na⁺, K⁺ pump)	IFN-γ	−	Inhibits Na⁺/K⁺-ATPase activity (195)
	Interleukin-1β (IL-1β)	+	Increases Na⁺/K⁺-ATPase subunit expression (140)
	TNF lectin-like domain	+	Increased Na⁺/K⁺-ATPase activity (196) Activation of Na⁺/K⁺-ATPase by TIP probably occurs indirectly upon prior activation of ENaC

(Continued)

TABLE 1 | Continued

Channel name	Mediator	Impact on pulmonary barrier function	Mechanism of action
	TGF-β	−/+	Decrease in Na⁺/K⁺-ATPase β1 subunit expression, resulting in decreased Na⁺/K⁺-ATPase activity(197, 198) Increases the expression of Na⁺/K⁺-ATPase α 1- and β 1-subunits (134)
	TNF-related apoptosis-inducing ligand (TRAIL)	−	Influenza A virus (IAV)-induced reduction of Na⁺/K⁺-ATPase is mediated by a host signaling pathway that involves epithelial type I IFN and an IFN-dependent elevation of macrophage TRAIL (199)
	Leukotriene D4	+	Activates Na⁺/K⁺-ATPase (200)
	Acetylcholine	+	Activates Na⁺/K⁺-ATPase (201)
	NO	−	Inhibits Na⁺/K⁺-ATPase (53, 202)

aThere is growing evidence that ROS are important regulators of ENaC activity and, hence, of epithelial Na⁺ absorption (153). But there is an important question here. Why does ROS increase ENaC activity under some circumstances (e.g., ethanol) but inhibit ENaC under others (e.g., influenza) (153)?

Cardiogenic or Hydrostatic Edema

Cardiogenic pulmonary edema (also called hydrostatic or hemodynamic edema) (2) is caused by an increased capillary hydrostatic pressure, secondary to an elevated pulmonary venous pressure (18) (**Figure 2**, left panel). This type of edema can occur following left ventricular heart failure, renal failure, or fluid overload, or arteriovenous shunts or fistulas. Left heart failure is most commonly caused by myocardial ischemia with or without myocardial infarction, exacerbation of chronic systolic or diastolic heart failure, or dysfunction of the mitral or aortic valve. Acute cardiogenic pulmonary edema is a frequent medical emergency that accounts for up to 1 million hospital admissions per year in the United States and for about 6.5 million hospital days each year, and is typically present during acute cardiac failure in 75–80% of patients (19). Coronary heart disease may account for about half to two-thirds of heart failures. There has been an increase in cardiac failure patients as well as in hospitalization rate during the last decade (20). As a matter of fact, heart failure is the most rapidly growing cardiovascular condition globally. The reported Western world life time risk is typically about 33% for men and 29% for women for our population, and depends, besides sex, on comorbidities and cardiovascular risk factors, such as arterial hypertension, diabetes, obesity, sleep related disorders, smoking, sedentary lifestyle, and ethnic background (20). In patients aged 65 years and older, more than 10% suffer from congestive heart failure (21). Interstitial pulmonary edema and alveolar flooding impair lung mechanics and gas exchange, thus causing dyspnea and tachypnea, which ultimately results in an age-dependent in-hospital mortality rate of about 15% (22).

The development of pulmonary edema is characterized by increased transcapillary hydrostatic pressure gradients. Moreover, a reversed and active electrolyte flow and its resulting active fluid transport can be involved (5, 23). This is possible by the bidirectional permeation permitting anion channels cystic fibrosis transmembrane conductance regulator (CFTR) and NKCC1 (16), which seems to account for up to 70% of the total alveolar fluid influx at elevated hydrostatic pressure. It is supporting the concept that alveolar fluid secretion is a secondary consequence of impaired alveolar Na⁺ uptake (16). Both CFTR

and NKCC1 are inhibited by furosemide. This might explain why in the clinical heart failure setting furosemide immediately relieves patients, i.e., by inhibition ion and, thus, fluid transport into the alveolus during alveolar lung edema generation when furosemide is administered, and not only after a huger delay of about half an hour or more when the renal effect of relevant diuresis has occurred. However, also a venous vasodilation, direcly reducing preload, occurs immediately after systemic furosemide administration (24).

A rapid increase in hydrostatic pressure in the pulmonary capillaries, leading to increased transvascular fluid filtration, and even active fluid transport as mentioned above, is the sign of acute cardiogenic or volume-overload edema (**Figure 2**, left panel). Such an increase could be usually due to elevated pulmonary venous pressure from increased left ventricular end-diastolic pressure and left atrial pressure (2). Mild elevations of left atrial pressure (18–25 mmHg) cause edema in the peri-microvascular and peri-bronchovascular interstitial spaces (1). Excess interstitial fluid is transported by lung lymphatics into the vascular system. A negative interstitial pressure gradient, even under conditions of edema, is the major force for the removal of pulmonary interstitial edema fluid into the lymphatics (25). If left atrial pressure rises further (>25 mmHg), edema fluid passes through the lung epithelium, in part by active transport, flooding the alveolar space with protein-poor fluid (**Figure 2**, left panel) (1, 2, 5). By contrast, non-cardiogenic pulmonary edema is based on increased pulmonary vascular permeability, resulting in an increased flux of fluid and macromolecules into the pulmonary interstitium and airspaces (**Figure 2**, right panel) (2).

There is a considerable link between inflammation and heart failure. The Val-HeFT study demonstrated a direct correlation between elevated levels of C-reactive protein and heart failure severity, and C-reactive protein predicts the risk of death and early readmission in acutely decompensated heart failure (26). As reviewed by Azzam et al. in this topic issue, one hypothesis is that heart failure is accompanied by systemic and mesenteric venous congestion, which may in turn cause bowel edema and a consecutive increased permeability, leading to bacterial translocation, endotoxin release, and resultant systemic inflammation. A second hypothesis postulates that the failing, but not the healthy,

Cytokine–Ion Channel Interactions in Pulmonary Inflammation

TABLE 2 | Impact of different factors on the alveolar–capillary barrier.

Mediator	Impact on pulmonary barrier function	Mechanism of action
Alveolar epithelium		
TGFβ1	–	Decreases lung epithelial barrier function (203–205) Increases the permeability of pulmonary endothelial monolayers (206) Increases the permeability of alveolar epithelial monolayers (206)
Tumor necrosis factor (TNF)	–	Causes alveolar epithelial dysfunction (207)
Lectin-like domain of TNF	+	Increases occludin expression, and improved gas–blood barrier function (7)
TNF-related apoptosis-inducing ligand (TRAIL)	–	Disruption of alveolar epithelial barrier (199, 208, 209)
Interleukin-1β (IL-1β)	+	Augments in vitro alveolar epithelial repair (139)
Protein kinase D3	–	Dysfunction of airway epithelial barrier through downregulation of a key tight junctional protein claudin-1 (210)
Claudin-3	–	Decreases alveolar epithelial barrier function (211)
Claudin-4	+	Improves the barrier function of pulmonary epithelial barrier by promoting pulmonary fluid–clearance function (211, 212)
Transient receptor potential vanilloid 4 (TRPV4)	–	Disruption of alveolar type I epithelial cells leading to lung vascular leak and alveolar edema (213)
Ethanol	–	Disruption of alveolar epithelial barrier function by activation of macrophage-derived TGFβ1 (214)
Acetoin (butter), diacetyl, pentanedione, maltol (malt), ortho-vanillin (vanilla), coumarin, and cinnamaldehyde	–	Impairment of epithelial barrier function in human bronchial epithelial cells (215)
Asbestos	–	Increases lung epithelial permeability through increasing epithelial fibrinolytic activity (216)
Pneumolysin (PLY)	–	Impairs epithelial barrier (217)
Fas-ligand system	–	Causes alveolar epithelial injury in humans with ALI or ARDS (218) Impairs alveolar epithelial function in mouse lungs by mechanisms involving caspase-dependent apoptosis (219) Inducing apoptosis of cells of the distal pulmonary epithelium during ALI (57)
CO	–	Enhances pulmonary epithelial permeability (220, 221)
Tight junctions (TJ)		
Purinergic receptor	+	Preserving integrity of endothelial cell (EC)-cell junctions (222)
Na+/K+ ATPase	+ +	Formation of TJs through RhoA GTPase and stress fibers (223) Gene transfer of β1-Na+, K+-ATPase upregulates TJs formation by enhancing expression of TJ protein zona occludins-1 and occludin and reducing pre-existing increase of lung permeability (224)
Nitric oxide (NO)	–	Decreases expression and mistargeting of TJ proteins in lung (225)
Influenza A virus (IAV)	–	Disruption epithelial cell TJs (226)
Caveolin-1	+	Regulates the expression of TJ proteins during hyperoxia-induced pulmonary epithelial barrier breakdown (227)
IL-4	–	Causes TJ disassembly and epithelial barrier permeability alteration via an EGFR-dependent MAPK/ERK1/2-pathway (228) Reduce protein density at the TJ without causing major changes in cldn1, cldn2, cldn3, and occludin protein levels (229)
IL-13	–	Reduction of protein density at the TJ without causing major changes in cldn1, cldn2, cldn3, and occludin protein levels (229)
TNF	–	Causes TJ permeability (230)
Interferon-gamma (IFN-γ)	–/+	Disorganization of the TJ and an increase in paracellular permeability (231) Promotes epithelial restitution by enhancing barrier function and wound healing (232) It can also reverse IL-4- and IL-13-induced barrier disruption (232)
Trypsin	–	Destroys the TJs which lead to airway leakage
Cigaret smoke	–	Causes disassembly of TJs, modulated through the EGFR–ERK1/2 signaling pathway (233)
Cadmium	–	Causes disruption of TJ integrity in human ALI airway cultures both through occludin hyperphosphorylation via kinase activation and by direct disruption of the junction-interacting complex (234)

(Continued)

TABLE 2 | Continued

Mediator	Impact on pulmonary barrier function	Mechanism of action
Capillary endothelium		
TGFβ 1	−	Induces endothelial barrier dysfunction *via* Smad2-dependent p38 activation (235)
TNF	−	Disruption of the lung vascular barrier (236, 237) Augmenting endothelial permeability (67, 238) Apoptosis of lung microvascular ECs (39, 239, 240)
Lectin-like domain of TNF	+	Strengthens barrier function or increasing endothelial barrier tightness (9) Protective effect in PLY-Induced endothelial barrier dysfunction (9) Can reduce PLY-induced RhoA/Rac-1 balance impairment and MLC phosphorylation (10) Protects from listeriolysin-induced hyperpermeability in human pulmonary microvascular ECs (241) Reducing vascular permeability (196) Increases in membrane conductance in primary lung microvascular ECs (242)
IFN-γ	−	Increases vascular permeability (243)
Interleukin-1β (IL-1β)	−	Given intratracheally, IL-1β increased endothelial permeability and lung leak (244–247) Increases vascular permeability (243)
Interleukin-2 (IL-2)	−	Increases vascular permeability (248)
Interleukin-6 (IL-6)	−	Increases endothelial permeability (249)
Interleukin-8 (IL-8)	−	Increases endothelial permeability (250)
Interleukin -12 (IL-12)	−	Upregulate the release of the vascular permeability factor which is a lymphokine derived from LN peripheral blood mononuclear cells (251)
Neutrophils	−	Inducing endothelial barrier disruption through secretion of leukotrienes or heparin-binding protein, direct signaling into the EC *via* adhesion-dependent mechanisms and production of ROS (252)
ENaC	+	ENaC-α can strengthen capillary barrier function (9)
TRPV4	−	Increases in vascular permeability thus promoting protein and fluid leak (253) Applying TRPV4 inhibitors exhibits vasculoprotective effects, inhibiting vascular leakage, and improving blood oxygenation (254)
Thrombin	−	Increase in endothelial permeability (255)
Platelet-activating factor	−	Increase in endothelial permeability (256)
Hydrogen peroxide	−	Increase vascular permeability through enhancing vascular endothelial growth factor expression (257)
Integrin αvβ5	−	Increases pulmonary vascular permeability (258)
T-cadherin	−	Causes enhancement of endothelial permeability (259)
Myosin light chain kinase	−	Vascular hyperpermeability (260)
Lipopolysaccharide (LPS)	−	Induces lung endothelial barrier dysfunction (261)
PLY	−	Impairs endothelial barrier (10, 262)
P2Y receptors	+	Regulators of lung endothelial barrier integrity (263)
CO	−	Enhances pulmonary epithelial permeability (221)
Soluble receptor for advanced glycation end products	−	Increase in alveolar–capillary barrier permeability (264)
EC adhesion		
Podocalyxin	+	Decreases vascular permeability of ECs by altering EC adhesion (265)
NLRP3	+	Protects alveolar barrier integrity by an inflammasome-independent increase of epithelial cell adherence (266)

heart has the ability to produce pro-inflammatory TNF during dilated myopathy. Third, decreased cardiac output could cause systemic tissue hypoxia with subsequent systemic inflammation, which might be the primary stimulus for increased TNF production (21).

Soluble TNF receptor-1 and interleukin-8 (IL-8) are independently associated with cardiovascular mortality, as is endothelin-1. In transgenic mice overexpressing TNF the left ventricular ejection fraction was depressed depending on TNF gene dosage (21). TNF has been associated with worsened prognosis. However, two studies aiming to neutralize the cytokine in heart failure, using the soluble human TNF receptor 2 construct etanercept, were stopped because of lack of clinical benefit and patients receiving the highest dose even had increased adverse

TABLE 3 | Comparison of the properties of highly selective and non-selective channels.

	Highly Selective	Non-selective
Na/K selectivity (267, 268)	>40	1.1
Unit conductance, pS (267–269)	6	21
Amiloride K_i, nM (268, 270)	38	2,300
Increased cellular cyclic adenosine monophosphate or β-adrenergic stimulation (271, 272)	Channel surface density increases	P_o increases
Increased cGMP or NO (273)	P_o decreases	P_o decreases
Protein kinase C activation (274, 275)	P_o decreases, surface density decreases	Channel surface density increases
Increased intracellular Ca^{2+} (271)	No effect	P_o increases
Purinergic stimulation (276–279)	P_o decreases	P_o increases
Dopaminergic stimulation (176, 280)	P_o increases	No effect
Superoxide production (111)	P_o increases	Channel surface density increases
Hypoxia (268)	Channel surface density decreases	Channel surface density increases

P_o, channel open probability; K_i, inhibitory constant, i.e., the dose that reduces open probability by 50%.

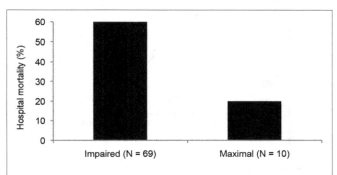

FIGURE 1 | Hospital mortality is increased in patients with acute lung injury or the acute respiratory distress syndrome with impaired fluid clearance (17).

outcomes (27). Similar results were observed with the neutralizing antibody infliximab (28). Whether the negative results are explained by inappropriate blocking of a "physiological" inflammation linked with tissue-reparative processes such as cardiac remodeling, or whether other mechanisms like too advanced heart failure, infections, toxicity of treatment, or genetic polymorphisms are involved, remains open, and should be further studied (21). Recently, it was suggested that beneficial or detrimental effects of TNF neutralizing agents depend on whether they spared or rather blunted discrete amounts of TNF that preconditioned cardiomyocytes to make them more resistant to high concentrations of the cytokine (29). The results, however, put forward that cytokines are effectors and not solely biomarkers in heart failure. Furthermore, reparative processes in the myocardium are accompanied by reactive or replacement fibrosis, mediated by TGF-β1, endothelin-1, and angiotensin-II (21). Angiotensin-II decreases AFC *via* cyclic adenosine monophosphate (cAMP) effect on the Na^+/K^+-ATPase pathway.

It is involved through p38 and possibly p42/44 MAP kinases with myocardial hypertrophy, inflammation, and neurotransmitter and catecholamine synthesis and release in the brain. Angiotensin-II regulates the NF-κB-dependent gene expression in response to IL-1β stimulation by controlling the duration of ERK and NF-κB activation (21). Many immune cell functions are moreover coupled to intracellular pH. As such, a higher pH represents an important signal for cytokine and chemokine release, and a low pH can induce an efficient antigen presentation. The pH regulating Na^+/H^+ exchanger isoforms may play a role in these events (30).

The kidney is a major target organ and a modulator in the pathogenesis of heart failure at least partially by means of the renin–angiotensin system. In initial heart failure, it aims at blood pressure maintenance by direct systemic vasoconstriction, *via* augmentation of the sympathetic nervous system activity and by promoting renal Na^+ retention. The latter mechanism is deleterious in the progress of cardiac failure and is characterized by enhanced Na^+ reabsorption in the proximal tubule and collecting duct induced by effects of angiotensin-II and aldosterone on NHE3 and ENaC, respectively (21). Two-thirds of filtered Na^+ is reabsorbed in the proximal tubule *via* transporters for amino acids, glucose, phosphate and *via* NHE3. At the distal tubule, Na^+ is reabsorbed by Na^+, K^+ co-transporter, which is sensitive to thiazide. In the collecting ducts, a minimal amount of sodium is reabsorbed by ENaC and this is increased by aldosterone. The counterbalance by the natriuretic and vasodilatory atrial natriuretic peptide is dominated at that point by angiotensin-II and aldosterone effects, attenuates endothelial-dependent renal vasodilation and leads to endothelial dysfunction characteristic of cardiac heart failure (21). Heart failure also causes a vasopressin-dependent water reabsorption which maintains blood pressure in the failing heart and further increases fluid retention. The renin–angiotensin system, especially angiotensin-II, activates the immune system and *vice versa*. TNF and IL-6 stimulate the generation of angiotensinogen, exaggerate sodium retention and enhance renal fibrosis. Angiotensin-II enhances TNF and IL-6 in cardiomyocytes and in renal cortical and tubular cells, impairs mitochondrial function, and is pro-oxidative (21). CRP also directly activates endothelin and by this may potentiate a pulmonary vasoconstriction. The review by Azzam et al. in this issue further discusses the causative role of cytokines in the development of cardiogenic edema.

Non-Cardiogenic or Permeability Pulmonary Edema

Non-cardiogenic pulmonary edema, also known as permeability pulmonary edema, accompanies ALI, pneumonia, pulmonary reimplantation response after lung transplantation, or ARDS (2, 31) (**Figure 2**, right panel). During the course of these diseases, the interstitium and the alevolus are sites of intense inflammation by an innate immune cell-mediated damage of the alveolar endothelial and alveolar epithelial barrier, with consecutive exudation of protein-rich pulmonary edema fluid (31–33), as recently reviewed by Thompson et al. (31).

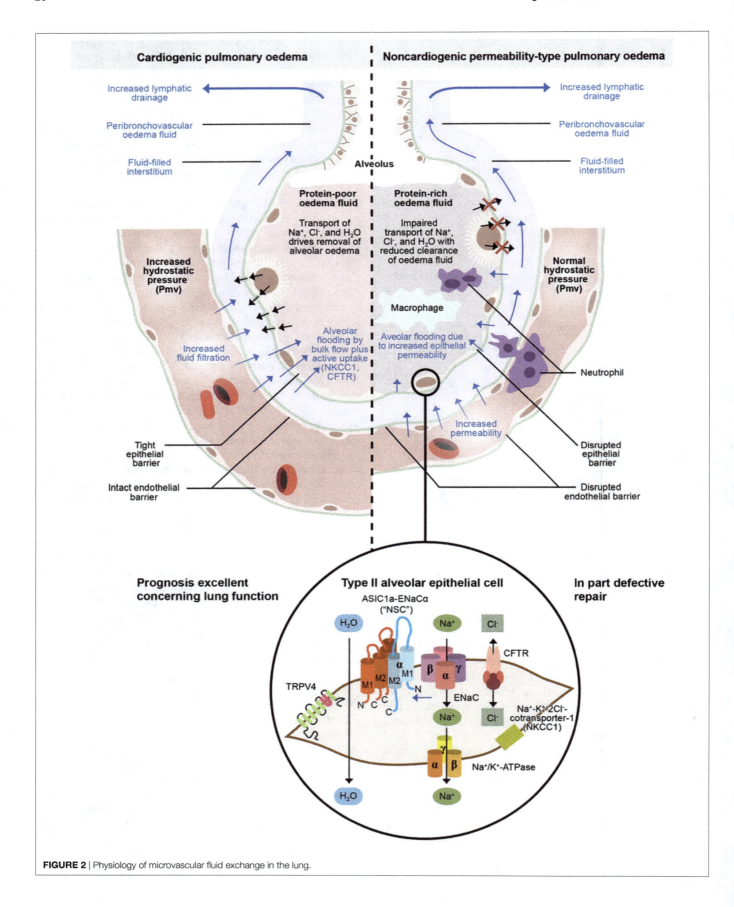

FIGURE 2 | Physiology of microvascular fluid exchange in the lung.

This type of pulmonary edema occurs due to modifications in barrier function of the pulmonary capillary or alveolar epithelial compartments as a consequence of either a direct or an indirect pathological process (31). There is some evidence that direct injury, such as pneumonia, aspiration, or pulmonary contusion, mainly affects epithelial barriers, whereas indirect blood-borne insults such as severe sepsis, non-thoracic trauma, pancreatitis, or burns may predominantly target the capillary endothelium (34). Permeability edema accompanies a spectrum of illnesses, ranging from the less severe form of ALI to ARDS (18). Variations in histology and in fluid management strategies suggest different ARDS subphenotypes (31). Apart from ARDS, ALI and severe pneumonia, also lung transplantation can be accompanied by acute pulmonary edema by the pulmonary reimplantation response (35). Ischemic vascular injury of the allograft results in increased permeability of the lung after reperfusion and in turn leads to interstitial and alveolar edema (33).

The extent of alveolar edema depends on the competing effects of increased permeability and the active edema fluid clearance from the alveolar space in regions where the epithelium is undamaged (31, 36). Inflammation plays a key role in the pathogenesis of permeability edema (37, 38) and can lead to the orchestration of a great variety of inflammatory and non-inflammatory cells, the former of which can locally release pro-inflammatory mediators such as TNF, LTD4 (32). There may also be endothelial and alveolar epithelial cell (AECs) death, which can further contribute to organ dysfunction and leak (39, 40). Moreover, a cascade of inflammation and a downregulation of repair mechanisms may occur (**Figures 3, 4**).

Cells of the innate immune system, such as activated alveolar macrophages and recruited polymorphonuclear granulocytes (PMN) and also cells from the adaptive immune system, such as T_H17 cells can interact in ALI and ARDS and release huge amounts of mediators (31). Thrombo-coagulative processes ensue, e.g., TNF-mediated by tissue factor, with a proaggregatory role for platelets. Preventive aspirin was recently shown to protect from ARDS (41). Regional tissue overdistension especially during ventilation and repetitive opening and closing of inflamed alveolar spaces amplify the regional inflammation, further denaturing surfactant, underlining the vital importance of protective ventilation strategies and positions.

Although pulmonary edema is one of the most frequent medical emergencies, clinically it is sometimes difficult to differentiate between its two main subtypes: cardiogenic and non-cardiogenic edema (2). Moreover, to date, no proven drug therapy is available for permeability edema associated with ALI and ARDS (2, 31, 38). Morbidity and mortality inversely correlate with AFC capacity in this setting (42, 43). The severity of shock in sepsis-induced ARDS is associated with lower AFC (44).

As mentioned above, 56% of patients with permeability pulmonary had an impaired AFC, and only 13% a maximal AFC rate (**Figure 1**). Survival of patients with maximal alveolar clearance rate was higher, as compared to patients with abnormal clearance rate, and the days on mechanical ventilation was less in this group. Clinically impressive is also a series of post-lung transplant patients showing a relation between total ischemic time and the degree of post-transplantation protein-rich and

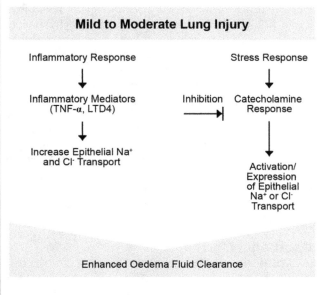

FIGURE 3 | Mild-to-moderate lung injury. Mild-to-moderate lung injury may lead to enhanced edema clearance. This response is due to an activation of epithelial Na⁺ transport probably based on the increased endogenous catecholamine production associated with the insult. However, in certain types of injury, other pathways may be involved. Other inflammatory mediators such as tumor necrosis factor (TNF) potentially participate (4).

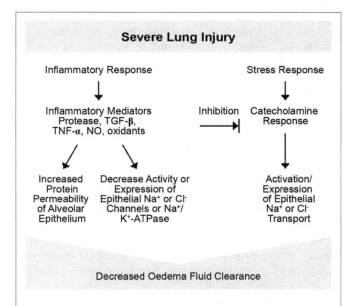

FIGURE 4 | Severe lung injury. Severe lung injury may usually lead to decreased edema clearance. Severe injury usually includes alveolar epithelial injury and, thus, increases epithelial permeability and electrolytes and is associated with reduced epithelial Na⁺ transport. Inflammatory mediators are involved in this response, such as proteases, tumor necrosis factor (TNF), TGF-β, nitric oxide (NO), and oxidants. Possibly the intensity of the inflammatory response may transform a mild to a severe lung injury form by inducing changes in function and integrity of the alveolar epithelium and endothelium (4).

highly neutrophil-rich (71–99% of cells) permeability edema. Those patients with the best AFC had the best clinical outcomes, including the least and the fastest resolving pulmonary reimplantation response (45). Thus, the ability to reabsorb fluid from the alveolar space was a marker of less severe reperfusion injury. These findings indicate that intact alveolar epithelial fluid transport is critically important for a timely recovery from post-transplantation reperfusion pulmonary edema.

PULMONARY FLUID BALANCE THROUGH BARRIERS

Airways normally have a critically regulated fluid layer essential for normal gas exchange and removal of foreign particulates from the airway. Maintaining this fluid layer in the alveoli also depends critically on sodium reabsorption. The pulmonary epithelium serves as a barrier to prevent access of the inspired luminal contents to the subepithelium (11) and modulates the initial responses of the airways and lung to both infectious and non-infectious stimuli (11). One mechanism by which the epithelium achieves this is by coordinating transport of diffusible molecules across the epithelial barrier, both through and between cells (11). Specific elements of pulmonary alveoli play different roles as a barrier maintaining the pulmonary fluid balance (38). These barriers will be discussed in more detail below.

Epithelial Barrier

Lung epithelium is a mucosal surface composed of ciliated cells, mucus-producing cells, and undifferentiated basal and progenitor cells. This dynamic barrier forms the interface between the lumen and the parenchyma from the upper airways to the alveoli. The lung epithelium constantly responds to luminal stimuli and coordinates its response to maintain homeostasis in the lung (11). A breakdown in this coordinated response can cause different lung diseases (11). The alveolar epithelium (0.1–0.2 μm) covers 99% of the airspace surface area in the lung (46) and contains a number of important cell types. Type I cells (AT1) cover at least 95% of the alveolar surface and are the apposition between the alveolar epithelium and the vascular endothelium. This provides a tight barrier that facilitates efficient gas exchange and which is involved in fluid and protein movement from the interstitial and vascular sites (38, 47) and its reabsorption *vice versa* (4, 5). The role of aquaporin 5 (AQ-5) in AFC is not clear, in view of the normal AFC capacity in physiological situations in AQ-5 knock out mice (48). The osmotic clearance of water secondary to the ion transport gradient across the alveolar epithelium probably occurs by paracellular pathways and not by the assumed transcellular using aquaporin 5 (25); however, their role in injury is not fully excluded (4). Type II cells (AT2) cover about 5% of the alveolar surface and are known especially for their key function in surfactant secretion and in vectorial transport of Na^+ (49), a major driving force for fluid removal from the alveolar space. Amiloride-sensitive sodium channels on the apical, "air-faced," surface, mainly the ENaC, are key channels in alveolar fluid transport (50, 51), with the driving force stemming from the Na^+/K^--ATPase on the basolateral, "blood-faced," surface (46). Dysfunction of these Na^+ transporters during inflammation can contribute to pulmonary edema (52–54). Tight junctions (TJ) that connect adjacent epithelial cells near their apical surfaces and maintain apical and basolateral cell polarity are fundamental to create a permeability barrier required to preserve distinct compartments in the lung (55).

Alveolar and distal airway epithelia are surprisingly resistant to injury, particularly if compared to the adjacent lung endothelium. When lung endothelium gets injured, the alveolar epithelial barrier may retain its normal impermeability and its normal fluid transport capacity, as seen in animal models with LPS given intravenously or intratracheally (4). This might explain why in mild-to-moderate lung injury AFC may not only be preserved, but even upregulated by stress hormones—an effect that may be inhibited by amiloride or propranolol.

However, in severe ALI, ARDS, and pneumonia, epithelial cell death may occur, as has been shown in a seminal morphological study published 4 decades ago by Bachofen and Weibel (56). A central role for soluble Fas ligand (FasL) has been proposed in AT1 and AT2 cell death, and an association between its levels in bronchoalveolar lavage level on day 1 of ARDS and patient death has been proposed (57, 58). However, there may be extensive crosstalk between injurious, inflammatory, and death cascades and repair in the lungs, as well as in other organs in patients with ARDS. Direct alveolar cell death may probably also occur due to bacterial exotoxins or stresses like overdistension. Such epithelial cell death may make the lungs prone to increased permeability and thus disturb AFC, as well as to the danger of disordered repair, such as in fibroproliferative ARDS.

Recent work on different predictors of ARDS suggests that the degree of AT1 cell injury is a central determinant of outcome in ALI and ARDS. Receptor for advanced glycation end products (RAGE) is an immunoglobulin superfamily member, involved in propagating inflammation. RAGE is abundant in the lungs and can be primarily found in AT1 cells. Higher baseline plasma levels of RAGE were found to be associated with worse outcome, including less ventilator-free days and increased mortality, and it excellently discriminated in sepsis patients for the diagnosis of ARDS. Higher levels in bronchoalveolar lavage also predicted post-lung-transplant primary graft failure and correlated with its grade of severity (59). Apart from RAGE, also surfactant protein D level, an AT2 cell product, was, together with the neutrophil chemokine IL-8 (CXCL8), the best performing biomarker for poorer outcome in terms of mortality (60).

Endothelial Barrier

The capillary endothelial barrier also functions as a key component to maintain the integrity of the vascular boundaries in the lung. The gas exchange surface area of the alveolar–capillary membrane is extremely huge and optimized to facilitate perfusion–ventilation matching (61). Pulmonary endothelium separates also the intravascular marginated pool of polymorphonuclear neutrophils from the airspaces. The endothelium, the most abundant cell relative to the total cell population in the lung, has additional key regulatory roles apart from gas exchange,

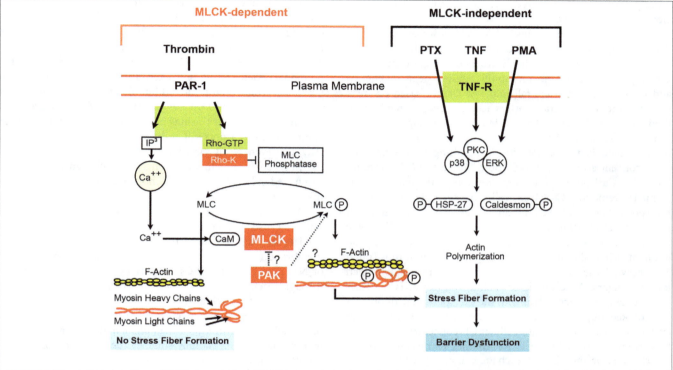

FIGURE 5 | Myosin light chain kinase (MLCK)-dependent and MLCK-independent pathways involved in endothelial cell (EC) barrier dysfunction (66). Adapted from Ware and Matthay (2).

namely vascular tone *via* nitric oxide (NO) and endothelin-1, and coagulation, as recently discussed in depth in a review on the endothelium and ARDS (34).

In the pulmonary microvasculature, the endothelial cells (ECs) form a semi-permeable barrier between the blood and the lung interstitium (38). Disruption of this barrier may occur during inflammatory disease such as pneumonia, ALI, ARDS, or ischemia–reperfusion injury. In sepsis, early microcirculatory perfusion indices are more markedly impaired in non-survivors, as compared to survivors and correlate with increasing severity of vascular dysfunction (62). Lung ECs are considered orchestrators of the inflammatory response. These cells can directly sense pathogens *via* toll-like receptors and may contain local bacterial spreading by coagulation, leading to capillary thrombosis and extravascular fibrin deposition (34). This contributes to an increased dead-space fraction that correlates with clinical outcome (63). In sepsis, overwhelming EC activation can lead to apoptosis within minutes to hours (64), which in turn increases barrier permeability and subsequent mortality (65). In ARDS, EC death can occur in by mechanical insults, like shear stress, and by pro-inflammatory mediators, including TNF, angiostatin, and TGF-β (39).

Intercellular junctions act as dynamic structures and do not statically resist entry to all substances. They that can open or close in response to physiological or pathological stimuli. **Figure 5** presents some potential pathways regulating EC barrier function (66). Endothelial barrier dysfunction can result in the movement of both fluid and macromolecules into the interstitium and pulmonary air spaces. This can contribute to important morbidity and mortality (66). TNF can reduce capillary endothelial barrier function (67, 68).

REGULATION OF AFC

In the normal lung, fluid and protein leakage is thought to occur primarily through small gaps between capillary ECs (2, 3). Since both capillary endothelial and AECs have TJ, fluid, and macromolecules that are filtered from the circulation into the alveolar interstitial space normally do not enter the alveoli (2).

The hydrophobic plasma membranes composed of phospholipids, act as a huge energy barrier for transporting ions (69–71). Yet, physiological processes assure for the continuous in- and outflow of ions, as such overcoming the plasma membrane barrier, which is impermeable to ions. Due to their biological complexity, interactions between cytokines and ion channels may be under-recognized (72). A group of plasma membrane proteins, including active transporters, generate and maintain ion concentration gradients for particular ions. These active transporters carry out this task by forming complexes with the ions they are translocating. The process of ion binding and unbinding for transport typically requires several milliseconds. As a result, ion translocation by active transporters is much slower than ion movement through ion channels, which can conduct thousands of ions across a membrane each millisecond. Active transporters effectively store energy in the form of ion concentration gradients, whereas the opening of ion channels rapidly dissipates this stored energy during relatively brief electrical signaling events.

Several types of active transporters have now been identified. Although the specific roles of these transporters differ, all must translocate ions against their electrochemical gradients (energetically "uphill"). Moving ions uphill requires the use of energy, and neuronal transporters fall into two classes based on their energy sources. Some transporters acquire energy directly from the hydrolysis of ATP and are called ATPase pumps. The most prominent example of an ATPase pump is the Na^+/K^+-ATPase pump, which is responsible for maintaining transmembrane (TM) concentration gradients for both Na^+ and K^+ (73). Another one is the Ca^{2+} pump, which provides one of the main mechanisms for removing Ca^{2+} from cells. The second class of active transporters does not use ATP directly as an energy source, but rather the electrochemical gradients of other ions. This type of transporter carries one or more ions up its electrochemical gradient, while simultaneously taking another ion, most often Na^+, down its gradient. These transporters are usually called ion exchangers. An example of such a transporter is the Na^+/Ca^{2+} exchanger, which shares with the Ca^{2+} pump the important task of keeping intracellular Ca^{2+} concentrations low. Other exchangers regulate both intracellular Cl^- concentration and pH by swapping intracellular Cl^- for another extracellular anion, bicarbonate, or the Na^+/H^+ exchanger that regulates intracellular pH, by regulating the concentration of H^+. Although the electrochemical gradient of Na^+ (or other counter ions) is the immediate source of energy for ion exchangers, these gradients ultimately depend on the hydrolysis of ATP by ATPase pumps, such as the Na^+/K^+ ATPase pump (74).

Alveolar fluid clearance is mainly regulated by Na^+ uptake through the apically expressed ENaC and the basolaterally localized Na^+/K^+-ATPase in type II AECs (**Figure 2**, lower panel) (54). Dysfunction of these Na^+ transporters during pulmonary inflammation can contribute to pulmonary edema (54). In this context, the movement of larger plasma proteins is restricted (2). The hydrostatic force for fluid filtration across the lung microcirculation is approximately equal to the hydrostatic pressure in the pulmonary capillaries, which is partly compensated by a protein osmotic pressure gradient (2). The net quantity of accumulated pulmonary edema is logically determined by the balance between the rate at which fluid is filtered into the lung (1) and the rate at which fluid is removed from the air spaces and lung interstitium (46). In mild-to-moderate lung injury, the capacity of the alveolar epithelium to transport salt and water is not only preserved but may also even be upregulated by stress hormones (**Figure 3**) (4). In severe lung injury, pulmonary fluid clearance can also be stimulated in lung injury by catecholamine-independent mechanisms (**Figure 4**) (4).

Moderate hypoxemia was shown to reduce AFC by 50%. This is caused by decreasing apical sodium uptake, at least partially through impaired trafficking of ENaC to the surface membrane (75–77). Hypoxia, moreover, inhibits the function of Na^+/K^+-ATPase in AECs, in part by triggering endocytosis through reactive oxygen species (ROS) and phosphorylation of the α1 subunit (78) (**Figure 6**). Restoration of normoxia rapidly reversed the depressant effects of hypoxemia in rats. Therefore, the simple administration of supplemental oxygen to patients with pulmonary edema may enhance the resolution of alveolar edema. As discussed more in detail in a contribution by Vadasz and Sznajder in this topic issue, hypercapnia can also impair AFC by the mechanisms of ubiquitination-mediated retrieval of ENaC from the plasma membrane, i.e., a post-translational modification of βENaC by regulating trafficking and stability, thereby modifying, and in this case reducing cell surface expression of the channel through βENaC ubiquitinylation in the alveolar epithelium (78–80). This mechanism seems of importance in ARDS as well in COPD. Hypercapnia and the associated acidosis have been shown to have anti-inflammatory effects, which might be advantages at sites of excessive inflammation, whereas

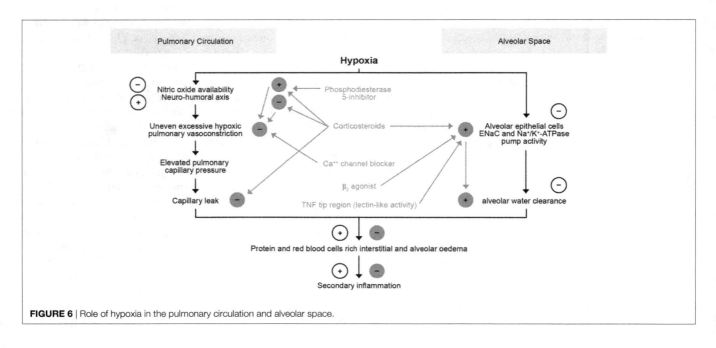

FIGURE 6 | Role of hypoxia in the pulmonary circulation and alveolar space.

on the other hand, ARDS and COPD studies showed that both patient groups had worse outcome when they were hypercapnic (78). In a randomized controlled trial Köhnlein, Windisch et al. showed that in severely sick, chronic hypercapnic COPD patients non-invasive ventilation, when targeted to reach noromocapnia (PaCO2 < 6.5 kPa/48.1 mmHg) or to improve hypercapnia by at least 20%, is associated with much better outcome (81). Survival was impressively improved, and also quality of life and lung function in terms of FEV1 improved. Possibly further effects exist such as sometimes improved cardiac output (82, 83), although interactions between ventilation and cardiac output are complex.

Ion Channels and Pumps/Transporters and AFC

Ion channels are integral membrane proteins that form a pore to allow the passage of specific ions by passive diffusion (84). Most ion channels undergo conformational changes from closed to open states. Once open, ion channels allow the passage of thousands of ions (84). This distinguishes them from transporters and pumps, which can also transport ions, but only a few at a time (84). The opening and closing of channels can be controlled by various means, including voltage, the binding of ligands such as intracellular Ca^{2+} or extracellular neurotransmitters, and post-translational modifications such as phosphorylation (84).

Ion channels and pumps also play multiple important roles in cell homeostasis (84). Their function promotes passive, agonist-induced, or voltage-dependent flux of specific ions in and out of the cell (84, 85). The mchanisms of removing the infiltrated fluid from the alveoli is called AFC (84).

The ENaC in Type I and II Alveolar Epithelial Cells

Epithelial sodium channel, a member of the ENaC/degenerin (ENaC/DEG) family of ion channels, constitutes the rate-limiting entry step in Na^+ reabsorption across epithelial in colon, kidney, and lungs (86). ENaC is inhibited by the drugs amiloride, benzamil, and triamterene, some of which are clinically used as potassium-sparing diuretics (87, 88). ENaC is a heteromultimeric protein (89) and is composed of at least four homologous subunits, α, β, γ, and δ (89–91) which are able to compose an ion channel (50, 92). A functional, pore-forming channel usually comprises one or two α subunits, together with a β - and a γ -subunit (89, 91, 93, 94). δ as a fourth unique subunit can form ion channels joining the β and γ subunits but exhibits biophysical and pharmacological features that are different compared to α ENaC channels (95). Investigations of the biological role of αENaC in the mouse lungs underlined the crucial role of this subunit in AFC (12). The β subunit is highly glycosylated and an important regulator of ENaC (4). In the lungs, ENaC is expressed not only in alveolar type II and type I cells (96), but also in capillary ECs (97).

Epithelial sodium channel was shown to exert a crucial role in pulmonary fluid reabsorption (46). Accordingly, ENaC is responsible for the maintenance of Na^+ balance, extracellular fluid volume and blood pressure (98). ENaC activity is determined by the number of channels in the surface membrane N, which can change according to membrane insertion, degradation, or retrieval, as well as by the open probability time Po of individual channels (86, 99, 100). The basolaterally expressed, ouabain-inhibitable Na^+/K^+-ATPase then further drives the vectorial transport into the interstitium and, finally, into the lymphatic and blood vessels (73).

In order to maintain the correct composition and volume of alveolar lining fluid, Na^+ transport through apically located ENaC in the alveolar epithelium is critical for gas exchange (92).

Epithelial sodium channel expression was shown to be decreased in transplanted lungs, both at the messenger RNA and protein level (8, 101).

Physiological ENaC Regulation

Epithelial sodium channel activity is important for fluid homeostasis and blood pressure control, but its regulation is complex and remains in many aspects incompletely understood (102) (**Table 1**). ENaC channels are also called highly selective cation (HSC) channels, and are presumed to be made up by the three ENaC subunits, α, β, and γ (103).

Epithelial sodium channel function can be affected by direct modulation of channel activity (92), subunit degradation, and membrane trafficking/recycling (104). cAMP indirectly increases ENaC activity, since it activates Cl^- uptake through CFTR (105). Intracellular as well as extracellular proteases, including prostasin and furin can affect the activity of the channel by modulating the Na^+ self-inhibition (106, 107). Another important system that modulates ENaC activity is trafficking of the channels to the membrane, which involves a complex system of ubiquitination and binding to Nedd-4-2 (108). Na^+ transport can also be regulated by gene expression (4). The two major hormonal modulators of pulmonary ENaC expression are catecholamines (50) and corticosteroids (109).

Many agents that increase Na^+/K^+-ATPase activity also increase ENaC activity (36). Negative ENaC regulators are activated purinergic P2Y receptors (110), NO (111, 112), Il-1β (113), hypoxia (46), and TGF-β (46).

ENaC Dysfunction

Dysfunction of the ENaC, which regulates salt and water homeostasis in epithelial, causes several human pathological conditions, including pulmonary edema (114). As ENaC regulates the airway surface liquid layer, its exaggerated activity might lead to airway dehydration, mucus stasis and bacterial overgrowth, as can be seen in cystic fibrosis and chronic bronchitis (115–117). ENaC hypo-activity, by contrast, can dramatically impair AFC, which is particularly important in conditions of pulmonary edema and correlates with mortality and morbidity in patients with ALI and ARDS (33).

The significant role of ENaC in inherited diseases associated with mutations in ENaC which increase or decrease channel activity regarding salt and water homeostasis has been well-documented (118). Mutations in the PPxY motif of β- and γ-subunits cause a severe form of hypertension, associated with ENaC in Liddle's syndrome (OMIM: 177200) (119–123). A decrease in ENaC function can also cause a rare, life-threatening salt-wasting syndrome in pseudohypoaldosteronism type 1B

(PHA1B) (OMIM: 264350) (124–127). This disease does not improve with age and patients are at risk from life-threatening, salt-losing crises, combined with severe hyperkalemia and dehydration throughout their entire lives (128, 129). Additionally, dysregulation of channel function and/or expression can lead to organ dysfunction and severe disease (84, 85, 130).

The Hybrid Acid-Sensing Ion Channel 1a (ASIC1a)/α-ENaC (NSC) Channels in Alveolar Type I and Type II Cells

Apart from ENaC, another apically expressed channel was recently shown to promote AFC. This hybrid channel is relatively non-selective for Na^+ over K^+, has a larger conductance, and shorter mean open and closed times (103, 131). In elegant assays, Trac et al. showed that the channel included ASIC1a as the mandatory counterpart to α-ENaC. These hybrid channels are, thus, composed of, at a minimum, one α-ENaC subunit and one or more ASIC1a subunits. The biological significance is great, as the regulation of these NSC channels is dramatically different from ENaC. Thus, treatments to reduce alveolar flooding based on the known properties of ENaC (HSC) could be suboptimal because ASIC1a/α-ENaC-channels are regulated differently (see **Table 3**). Indeed, NSC channels are less sensitive to inhibition by amiloride than ENaC HSC channels.

As the proton-gated ASIC1a plays a role in the formation of channels, its properties determine the pharmacological ASIC1a/α-ENaC-channels (NSC) modulation. The MitTx agonist, derived from Texas coral snake toxin, strongly activates ASIC1a/α-ENaC-channels (NSC) (**Table 3**).

Why Do Alveolar Epithelial Cells in the Lungs Have Several Types of Channels That Mediate Na^+ Uptake?

As shown, an important functional role of non-selective cation (NSC) channels, which consist of ASIC1a and of ENaC-α subunits (281), is Na^+ uptake by AT2 cells in the lung (103). By contrast, other sodium-transporting epithelial tissues such as the distal nephron of the kidney and the colon were not reported to have these functional NSC channels, and mainly transport Na^+ through ENaC. In the lungs, the alveolar fluid layer must be very tightly controlled. Therefore, it may be important to have alternative ion transport pathways that respond differently to physiological stimuli, such as to acidification, which accompanies ALI and which activates NSC channels (282). An alternative hypothesis is that NSC channels provide a stable driving force for cation and anion movement across the alveolar epithelium. Indeed, NSC channels contribute to the apical membrane potential, causing the membrane potential to be close to zero. This will ensure that there is a driving force for the unidirectional movement of anions, through CFTR and for movement of Na^+ through classical ENaC and NSC into cells. This is necessary because of the requirement to move salt, i.e., anions plus cations. Other epithelia tend to have counter-ion pathways for cations that obviate the need to maintain a strong potential driving force.

In an evolutionary context, the lung has been the most recent organ to adapt to a terrestrial environment. Typical for evolutionary processes is the modification of existing mechanisms to produce a different evolutionary outcome, in this case, the formation of a new channel type out of parts from two pre-existing channels of the same channel family. Of further evolutionary interest is that the activity of both HSC channels HSC (ENaC) and NSC channels is increased by a peptide mimicking the lectin-like region of TNF, which binds to ENaC-α, as shown below and in Czikora et al. (9), in this issue (9).

The Na^+/K^+-ATPase

Apart from apical ENaC and, potentially NSC, the basolaterally expressed Na^+/K^+-ATPase, a.k.a. the sodium-potassium pump is also a crucial driver of AFC (73, 78). Na^+/K^+-ATPase activity regulation also involves complex patterns, including modulation of the trafficking of the protein to the membrane (73). The Na^+/K^+-ATPase is a ubiquitous enzyme consisting of α and β subunits and a less well-characterized regulatory FXYD subunit. The Na^+/K^+-ATPase is responsible for the generation and preservation of the Na^+ and K^+ gradients across the cell membrane by transporting 3 Na^+ out and 2 K^+ into the cell (283).

Changes in intracellular Na^+ concentration and hormones, such as mineralocorticoids, glucocorticoids and thyroid hormones as well as adrenoceptor stimulants modulate Na^+/K^+-ATPase activity (284). Like ENaC, increase of Na^+/K^+-ATPase expression is considered central to enhance transepithelial Na^+ transport (4). In addition, thyroid, mineralocorticoid and glucocorticoid hormones modulate Na^+/K^+-ATPase expression (4). Likewise, β adrenoceptor activation upregulates Na^+/K^+-ATPase expression in AECs (50).

The Na^+/K^+-ATPase contains one principal catalytic subunit, designated α and one sugar-rich auxiliary subunit, designated β. There is also a regulatory subunit FXYD subunit, which was recently shown to play an important role in regulation of lung inflammation (285). The α-subunit carries the catalytic function of the enzyme, and this is reflected in its possession of several binding and functional domains (283). The α subunit (4) transports Na^+ out of the cell, providing the driving force for Na^+ reabsorption (286). It is clear that an essential role for β subunit lies in the delivery and the appropriate insertion of the α subunit in the membrane (287). In recent years, a variety of studies have suggested that the β subunit may be more intimately involved in the mechanism of active transport (287–290).

FXYD5 or Dysadherin or RIC is a pro-inflammatory type I membrane protein, which belongs to seven members of the FXYD family named by their shared TM amino acid motif. FXYD5 is an established tissue-specific modulatory subunit of Na^+/K^+-ATPase, expressed in a variety of epithelial cells. Recent work shows a role for FXYD5 as a key mediator of the inflammatory response during ALI (285). It impairs adherens junctions by downregulating the markers zona occludins-1 (ZO-1) and occludin and redistributing beta catenin (291). It is required for the secretion of NF-κB, e.g., upon lipopolysaccharide (LPS), and inflammatory mediators, including TNF and interferon-α (IFN-α) and C-C chemokine ligand-2 (CCL2) from AECs that activate alveolar macrophages, amplify lung injury by orchestrating an overly exuberant inflammatory response, and recruit monocytes into the alveolar compartment, or in bronchoalveolar lavage fluid (285). The presence of FXYD5 is an important component for NF-κB activation pathway as shown in AECs induced by LPS, TNF, or interferon-α, as its silencing prevented IκB-α phosphorylation and reduced cytokine secretion in response to these stimuli. Probably FXYD5 increases CCL2 transcription by inducing Akt-dependent activation of NF-κB signaling. Binding of IFN-α activated phosphoinositide 3-kinase (PI3K) *via* STAT5, which in turn activates NF-κB. Activation of PI3K seems downstream of TLR4 and TNFR1. Possibly, FXYD5 modulates NF-κB signaling by regulating the location of TNF receptor 1, by modulation associations with other proteins and their location and mobility in the membrane (285). It is of interest that FXYD5 regulates inflammation, activates NF-κB dependent cytokine secretion and infiltration of immune cells to the alveolar spaces as well as alveolar barrier tightness, and is closely linked to one key ion transport channel.

The Cystic Fibrosis Transmembrane Conductance Regulator

Cystic fibrosis transmembrane conductance regulator is a cAMP-regulated and post-translationally modified chloride channel of 1,480 amino acids, which is mainly expressed in epithelial cells. The non-glycosylated form of CFTR has a molecular weight of 127 kDa, with 160 kDa for the glycosylated form. CFTR can either take up or release Cl⁻ ions from the AT1 and AT2 cells. Apical to basolateral chloride transport may be important because the maximal rate of sodium and water transport from the airspaces appears to be limited by the concomitant chloride transport (115–117). An important part of transepithelial chloride transport occurs through the paracellular route in the alveolar epithelium. The selectivity and magnitude of paracellular ion conductance may influence net transport capacity. Upon increasing Cl⁻ influx, CFTR will activate ENaC-mediated Na⁺ uptake, as such activating AFC, but the channel will inhibit AFC upon increasing Cl⁻ efflux. Increased cAMP generation will open CFTR in the apical membrane of AT1 and AT2 cells for Cl⁻ uptake, as such increasing Na⁺ uptake and AFC. Therefore, factors that can activate cAMP-mediated Cl⁻ uptake by CFTR, such as β2 agonists, have been investigated as potential therapeutic candidates for pulmonary edema (105). Cystic fibrosis, a disease characterized by impaired airway dehydration, is caused by a loss of function of CFTR, accompanied by an excessive activity of ENaC. A peptide mimetic of SPLUNC, i.e., SPX-101, was shown to promote internalization of the three ENaC subunits and to restore mucus transport in a mouse and a sheep model of CF (292).

The Transient Receptor Potential Vanilloid 4 (TRPV4) Channel

Transient receptor potential vanilloid 4 is a TM cation channel and a vanilloid-type member of the transient receptor potential (TRP) protein superfamily (293). TRPV4 is ubiquitously expressed in many cell types in the respiratory system (294). It is part of an integrated system, consisting of ion channels and membrane pumps, which tightly regulates intracellular calcium levels in a spatiotemporal manner (295). TRPV4 counts 871 amino acids and contains six TM domains, an ion pore located between TM5 and 6, an NH2 terminal intracellular sequence with several ankyrin-type repeats, and a COOH-terminal intracellular tail (296, 297). Both the NH2 and COOH termini interact with signal kinases, other molecules (e.g., NO), and scaffolding proteins (298). The intracellular tails contain several activity-modifying phosphorylation sites (294). In the setting of pulmonary inflammation, TRPV4 has been found to be highly expressed and upregulated in airway smooth muscle, vascular ECs, AECs, as well as in immune cells, such as macrophages and neutrophils (298–303).

The Role of TRPV4 in Pulmonary Edema

Transient receptor potential vanilloid 4 mediates cellular responses to both physical (such as osmotic, mechanical, and heat) as well as chemical stimuli (304). It is also involved in lung diseases associated with parenchymal stretch and inflammation or infection (254, 294). Target diseases include cough, asthma, cancer, and pulmonary edema associated with ARDS (253, 294, 305–310).

These studies support a role for TRPV4 in a broad spectrum of lung and airway functions and disease processes. TRPV4 also has been implicated as a key regulator of lung endothelial barrier integrity, specifically, the integrity of the lung alveolar–capillary endothelium, which is most relevant to alveolar edema generation in ALI (311). TRPV4 activation increases vascular permeability, thus promoting protein and fluid leak (254).

Several studies have shown that TRPV4 can regulate generation of inflammatory cytokines that play key roles in orchestrating lung tissue homeostasis and inflammatory lung disease (301, 307, 309, 310, 312–314). Therefore, TRPV4 could be considered a potential target for lung disease pathogenesis, including to alveolar–capillary barrier function (300). TRPV4 has been proposed as a candidate target for the management of ALI that develops as a consequence of aspiration of gastric contents, or acute chlorine gas exposure (254). Protection from the ALI response to intratracheal HCl and a key role *in vivo* of polymorphonuclear neutrophil TRPV4 (294) was noted in mice that lack TRPV4 (TRPV4 KO), or in mice that were treated with three different small molecule inhibitors of TRPV4 (253, 301, 307, 309, 312, 313, 315).

However, in view of its ubiquitous expression, and the multitude of functions attributed to the channel, including its role in pulmonary vasomotor control, endothelial barrier tightness, inflammatory response and systemic blood pressure regulation, TRPV4 blockade may represent a double-edged sword. Therapeutic benefits of TRPV4 inhibition have, therefore, to be carefully weighed against potential adverse effects (254).

Transient receptor potential vanilloid 4 activation and its downstream signaling pathways differ in response to varying stimuli, cell types, and contexts (294). For instance in asthma, TRPV4 mediates hypotonicity-induced airway hyperresponsiveness, but not release of Th2 cytokines (312, 316). In CF, TRPV4 appears to play paradoxical roles in CBF/mucociliary clearance and epithelial cell pro-inflammatory chemokine (IL-8/KC) secretion (317, 318). Depending on the underlying etiology, TRPV4 may play different roles in ARDS (307, 310, 314, 319). Also, in pulmonary fibrosis, TRPV4 has been shown to mediate the

TRPV4 and Macrophage Function in Lung Injury

Alveolar macrophages are known to be effector cells in bacterial and particle clearance but also in any injury and repair process (320). Since intracellular Ca^{2+} is known to be required for the phagocytic process, and because TRPV4 plays a role in force-dependent cytoskeletal changes in other systems/cell types, the role of TRPV4 in macrophage phagocytosis was extensively studied by Scheraga and colleagues (213, 253, 307, 315, 321–323). The process of phagocytosis in macrophages requires integration of signals from macrophage surface receptors, pathogens, and the extracellular matrix (324–326). However, the effects of matrix stiffness on the macrophage phenotypic response or its signal transduction pathways have yet to be fully elucidated (294). TRPV4 mediates LPS-stimulated macrophage phagocytosis of both opsonized particles [immunoglobulin G (IgG)-coated latex beads] and non-opsonized particles (Escherichia coli) *in vitro* (294). Inhibition of TRPV4 by siRNA or pharmacologic inhibitors completely abrogated both the LPS effect and the matrix stiffness effect on phagocytosis (294). These data indicate that both the LPS and stiffness effect on macrophage phagocytosis are TRPV4 dependent (310). Concordant with their *in vitro* data, also LPS-induced alveolar macrophage phagocytosis was proposed to be TRPV4 dependent (294).

Collectively, obtained data demonstrate that TRPV4 responds to extracellular matrix stiffness, thereby altering the LPS signal to mediate macrophage phagocytosis and cytokine production (310). Furthermore, TRPV4 regulates a feed-forward mechanism of phagocytosis in activated lung tissue macrophages when they interact with stiffened infection/injury-associated lung matrix. This concept is further supported by the observation that surfactant protein B-deficient mice have altered alveolar macrophage shape and function in association with increased alveolar surface tension (327).

Other Ion Channels

Recent research has given much more detail to a number of further ion channels and their interactions, such as Cl⁻ regulators in the paracellular TJ area including claudin-4 and -18 implicated in epithelial ion and fluid transport and ARDS regulation in specific infectious, inflammatory, or other stimulatory situations. The reader is referred to further reviews as that of Brune et al (11). and Weidenfeld and Kübler (5). The transient receptor potential channel 6 (TRPC6), a Ca^{2+}-permeable non-selective cation channel, widely expressed in the lungs, was proposed to be a key regulator of acute hypoxic pulmonary vasoconstriction and was demonstrated to be implicated in pulmonary hypertension. TRPC6 is also involved in pulmonary vascular permeability and lung edema formation during LPS- or ischemia/reperfusion-induced ALI as discussed in this topic issue (328).

CYTOKINE-ION CHANNEL INTERACTION

Cytokines, which are organized in a cytokine network, play a major role in maintaining lymphocyte and leukocyte homeostasis under both steady-state and inflammatory conditions (329). Regulatory cytokines have to function in combination with other environmental signals to properly modulate the function and the extent of lymphocyte and leukocyte activation (329). Increased generation of pro-inflammatory cytokines represents a first-line defense mechanism against bacterial infections of the lung (102). Dysregulation of cytokine generation leads to alterations in cell–cell interactions (330). Cytokines, such as TNF, IL-1, IL-6 activate host defense by promoting the production of a wide spectrum of other cytokines and chemokines, including GM-CSF, G-CSF and IL-8 in inflammatory processes (331, 332). They moreover mediate the increase of surface adhesion molecule expression through activation of leukocytes and ECs (38). As such, cytokines can contribute to the pathogenesis and development of pulmonary edema (37, 99, 333–338). During the acute phases of ARDS, higher levels of TNF were detected in the BALF from patients with early-stage ARDS (39).

The Dichotomous Yin and Yang Effects of TNF in Pulmonary Edema

Tumor necrosis factor is a homotrimeric 51 kDa protein, binding to two types of membrane receptors: TNF receptor 1, which signals either apoptosis, necroptosis or inflammation; and TNF receptor 2, which is mainly implicated in inflammation and which is devoid of a death domain (239, 339, 340). TNF is one of the central cytokines in inflammation and moreover modulates ion channel activity (341–344). An intriguing feature of the ligands of the TNF and TNFR family is that when certain members are shed, they inhibit the function of the ligand-receptor complex and act as inhibitors (345). A central regulatory process may, therefore, be the proteolytic release of soluble bioactive oligomers from membrane-bound forms, e.g., for TNF by the protease TACE. The existence of TM forms of most of the TNF-superfamily ligands indicates that they are meant to act locally. Only under non-physiological conditions, when these ligands are released, they may prove to be harmful (345) or beneficial, as is the case of immune defense to bacterial infection (346). As a consequence, long-term treatment with TNF neutralizing substances can cause increased sensitivity to tuberculosis (346).

Tumor necrosis factor contributes to the pathogenesis and development of pulmonary edema (38), but, paradoxically, also plays an important role in edema reabsorption (347–350). It was assumed for a long time that cytokines exert their activities solely upon activating their respective receptors, but in the case of TNF, this is not true, which broadens this concept (38). TNF was shown to exert a lytic, i.e., killing effect on certain bloodstream stages of African trypanosomes, by means of a lectin-like interaction with trimannoses and *N,N'*-diacetylchitobiose oligosaccharide residues in the variant surface glycoprotein on the surface of the parasites (344). Later investigations could demonstrate that this lectin-like activity can be attributed to a special 17 amino acid long domain, named the lectin-like domain of TNF in the molecule's tip region (351, 352) (**Figure 7**). This special region is spatially distinct from its receptor binding sites (353) and is not present in lymphotoxin, which has a highly similar tertiary structure as TNF. Comparative sequence analysis of TNF and

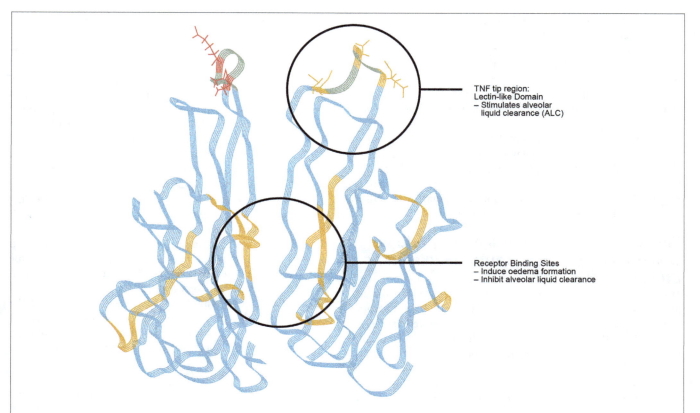

FIGURE 7 | Tumor necrosis factor. Tumor necrosis factor (TNF) as a "moonlighting" or dual role, or dichotomal yin-yang cytokine. The TNF receptor 1 binding sites within the TNF homotrimer mediate edema formation and blunt edema reabsorption. The lectin-like domain of the same cytokine activates epithelial sodium channel function and as such promotes alveolar fluid clearance and acts on endothelial cell barrier tightness (360).

LT allowed for the identification of the lectin-like domain of TNF (353).

For experimental purposes to mimic the TNF lectin-like domain, the amino acid sequence-identic synthetic 17 amino acid peptide which has shown to biologically mimic the lectin-like tip domain of TNF (353–355), as described above, has been used in a variety of experimental researches. It, moreover, gave rise to a therapeutic candidate that was recently evaluated in clinical trials (a.k.a AP301 and Solnatide) (356–358).

There are conflicting data about the critical involvement of TNF in the regulation of AFC (359). *In situ* and *in vivo* investigations conducted by Braun et al. in flooded rat lungs demonstrated a dual role for TNF in pulmonary edema (37, 38). This is possibly due to the opposite effects of, on the one hand, the classical TNF receptor 1 binding sites and, on the other hand, the lectin-like domain of TNF on pulmonary fluid reabsorption (37). In fact, the TNF tip region with its lectin-like activity is spatially distinct from the cytokine's receptor binding sites and causes an increase of alveolar fluid reabsorption, which is completely independent of the TNF receptors type 1 and 2, and further increases the cell–cell barrier tightness as shown in the alveolar EC barrier (**Figure 7**) (38, 99).

As discussed more in detail in this issue (361), in murine models of ventilator-induced ALI, TNF receptor 2 can have protective effects, whereas TNF receptor 1 is deleterious, thus adding another level of complexity to the role of TNF in edema (362). As such, the complex between soluble TNF receptor 1 and TNF can stimulate fluid reabsorption. TNF causes receptor-mediated edema formation in part by decreasing the expression of ENaC mRNA in AECs *in vitro* (135) leading to decreased amiloride-sensitive sodium uptake (135). Moreover, TNF receptor 1 signaling initiates the process of neutrophil migration (363) which can also contribute to the formation of pulmonary edema. It is also involved in orchestrating mechanisms, such as complement activation, cytokine regulation, chemokine production, and activation of adhesion molecules as well as their respective adhesion molecule receptors (364).

A TNF-dependent and amiloride-sensitive increase in AFC occurs in a rat model of *Pseudomonas aeruginosa* pneumonia (365). Other studies have shown in rats that intestinal ischemia–reperfusion leads to stimulation of AFC. This stimulation is at least in part mediated by a TNF-dependent mechanism which is independent of catecholamine release, because propranolol did not influence the AFC, and there was no observed cAMP stimulation (366). This indicates a protective effect of TNF-dependent stimulation of AFC in the early phase of injury (366).

Fukuda et al. could show that in ventilated rats TNF increased AFC by about 67% (136). This increase was inhibited by amiloride, but not by propranolol, indicating the mechanism is catecholamine-independent. A triple TNF mutant, in which three crucial residues for the lectin-like activity were mutated to alanines, did not show any increase in AFC. The effect of TNF occurred within 30 s from the onset of perfusion in A549 cells and within 1 h in the distal airspaces of the rat. This shows that the primary mechanism does not depend on a transcriptional effect of TNF. This indicates that TNF increased AFC most probably by an amiloride-sensitive mode of action, independent of any TNF receptor binding and mediated through the lectin-like region.

These antagonistic functions of the same molecule on pulmonary edema refer to the complex biology of the TNF molecule (361). Indeed the TNF receptor 1 binding sites of TNF inhibit, whereas its lectin-like domain activates edema reabsorption (**Figure 7**) (37), and, as described above, tightens intercellular epithelial and endothelial barrier function (8, 9).

The Impact of TNF on Pulmonary Edema Generation by TNF Receptor-Mediated Effects

Tumor necrosis factor is mainly known for its receptor-mediated pro-inflammatory functions in the systemic inflammatory response and the induction of apoptosis on a cellular level (339, 367). Both of these activities of TNF are implicated in the pathogenesis of pulmonary edema, which is often associated with ALI (37).

Tumor necrosis factor promotes pulmonary dysfunction through edema formation and inhibition of edema reabsorption by several procedures (37), for instance:

- TNFR-dependent upregulation of chemokine production (338, 363) and adhesion molecule expression (333, 334, 368), which leads to neutrophil attraction and sequestration.
- Decrease in barrier function in human pulmonary artery ECs and rearrangement of microtubules (67).
- Induction of reactive oxygen intermediates (336).
- Down-regulation of ENaC expression in alveolar type 2 cells (135)

TNF Inhibits Transcription of All Three ENaC Subunits

Seminal studies conducted by Dagenais et al. clearly demonstrated the involvement of TNF in modulation of Na^+ absorption in cultured AECs is investigated. The results show that TNF decreased the expression of the α-, β-, and γ-subunits of ENaC mRNA after 24-h treatment and reduced to 50% the amount of ENaC-α protein in these cells (135). There was no impact, however, on $\alpha 1$ and $\beta 1$ Na^+/K^+-ATPase mRNA expression (135). Amiloride-sensitive currents and ouabain-sensitive Rb^+ uptake were reduced. A strong correlation was found at different TNF concentrations between the decrease of amiloride-sensitive current and ENaC-α mRNA expression (135). All these data show that TNF has a profound effect on the capacity of AECs to transport Na^+ (135). In another study performed by Yamagata et al., mRNA expression of all three ENaC subunits in whole lung tissue was inhibited by TNF (359). TNF also inhibited ENaC function, as indicated by the reduction of amiloride-sensitive current (359). These data suggest that TNF may affect the pathophysiology of ALI and pulmonary edema through the inhibition of AFC and sodium transport (359).

TNF Increases Permeability of the Epithelial–Endothelial Barrier

The activation of TNF receptor 1 by TNF modulates the integrity of the alveolar barrier, in addition to its direct effects on ion channels and pumps of the alveolar epithelium. TNF increases the endothelial expression of chemo-attractants and adhesion molecules including IL-8 (formerly called neutrophil chemotactic factor), the IL-8- receptor 2, the intercellular adhesion molecule-1 (ICAM-1), platelet endothelial cell adhesion molecule-1 (PECAM-1), and vascular adhesion molecule-1, thus promoting excessive recruitment of mononuclear phagocytes and neutrophils during lung inflammation (71, 369–371).

Tumor necrosis factor is released in acute inflammatory lung syndromes linked to the extensive vascular dysfunction associated with increased permeability and EC apoptosis (372). The critical importance of the pulmonary vascular barrier function is shown by the balance between competing EC contractile forces, which generate centripetal tension, and adhesive cell–cell and cell matrix tethering forces, which regulate cell shape. Both competing forces in this model are intimately linked through the endothelial cytoskeleton, a complex network of actin microfilaments, microtubules, and intermediate filaments, which combine to regulate shape change and transduce signals within and between ECs (66).

Tumor necrosis factor can activate ECs, cause acute pulmonary vascular endothelial (VE) injury or even EC death and increase pulmonary vascular permeability *in vivo* as well as *in vitro* (39, 67, 373). Also, TNF increases the permeability of EC monolayers to macromolecules and lower molecular weight solutes by involving pertussis toxin-sensitive regulatory G protein (374). Furthermore, it is reported that TNF can increase the permeability of lung EC monolayers and that fibronectin can blunt this effect (375). In addition, TNF-induced increase in endothelial permeability involves the loss of fibronectin and remodeling of the extracellular matrix (376). Moreover, it has also been shown that TNF can increase capillary permeability causing transcapillary filtration *in vivo* (377).

TNF Increases ROS Generation

In addition to the above-mentioned mechanisms, TNF can induce pulmonary edema indirectly through increasing ROS (336). ROS have been shown to be able to disrupt the pulmonary endothelial barrier (336) and to decrease Na^+ channel activity (378).

Identification of the Alveolar Liquid Clearance-Promoting Effects of TNF
Lung Transplantation and Primary Graft Dysfunction (PGD)/Ischemia–Reperfusion Injury

The receptor-independent lectin-like domain of murine TNF has a potential physiological role in the resolution of alveolar edema in an *in situ* mouse lung model and an *ex vivo* rat lung model (99). The lectin-like domain of TNF can activate amiloride-sensitive sodium uptake in type II AECs (99, 100). Therefore this TNF domain is a potential therapeutic candidate (360).

As there is no specific treatment for ischemia–reperfusion-mediated lung injury, which is accompanied by a disrupted capillary barrier integrity and an impeded AFC, the capacity of the TNF tip peptide to improve lung function after unilateral orthotopic lung iso-transplantation was tested *in vivo* in adult rats (8).

The unilateral rat transplant study showed that a highly severe lung injury with blood gas parameters qualifying for severe ARDS could be virtually prevented by the activation of the TNF lectin-like region. Furthermore, a significant reduction in polymorphonuclear neutrophilic leukocytes (PMN) infiltration in the bronchoalveolar lavage fluid was observed. The TNF tip peptide reduced ROS generation in the transplanted rat lungs *in vivo* and diminished ROS generation in pulmonary artery ECs *in vitro* under hypoxia and reoxygenation (8). ROS, the generation of which is increased during ischemia–reperfusion ALI (379–381), have been shown to be able both to disrupt pulmonary endothelial barrier integrity (378) and to inhibit ENaC activity (382).

Moreover, the effect of the lectin-like domain of TNF likely has physiologic relevance during inflammation and infection (8). As the soluble TNF receptors are cleaved by the same enzyme that generates soluble TNF, i.e., TACE (383), complexes between soluble TNF receptors and TNF can form (8). Soluble TNF receptors do not inhibit the activity of the lectin-like domain of TNF and complexes between these receptors and TNF are even able to stimulate AFC in *in situ* flooded rat lungs (37, 99, 353). At the same time, unfavorable actions of TNF on edema reabsorption and formation that are mediated by TNF receptor 1 activation are being blocked by the soluble receptors (37). Therefore, the favorable actions of the lectin-like domain of TNF might occur in conditions where both TNF and its soluble receptors are being generated (8).

A recent pilot study of 20 patients on treatment of PGD by twice daily nebulized 125 mg inhalation of the TNF tip peptide (AP301, solnatide) randomized 1:1 showed an improved gas exchange (mean and SD, daily measured up to 72 h, PaO2/FiO2 365.6 ± 90.4 versus 335.2 ± 42.3 mm Hg; $p = 0.049$) and clearly less time intubated (2 ± 0.82 versus 3.7 ± 1.95 days, p = 0.02) in the verum group, which also seems clinically relevant (357).

In summary, the lectin-like activity of TNF, and thus, the TNF tip peptide significantly improves lung function after lung transplantation in the rat. Pilot studies confirm a relevant effect in clinical treatment (8, 357). The experimental model showed a reduced alveolar neutrophil content and less ROS generation. It exerts a favorable effect on organ function in terms of gas exchange (8). It was furthermore shown that the apically expressed ENaC was found to be decreased at the messenger ribonucleic acid and the protein level in transplanted lungs, suggesting that ENaC, rather than the basolaterally expressed Na^+/K^+-ATPase, is important in the abnormal AFC (101). These studies reinforce the idea that the TNF tip peptide acts as an agent with potential therapeutic traits against the ischemia–reperfusion injury associated with lung transplantation.

The Lectin-Like Region of TNF Ameliorates High-Altitude Pulmonary Edema (HAPE) in Rats
About 100 million people live at altitudes greater than 2,500 m, about 15 million above 3,000 m, and some above 5,000 m (384).

Most of these individuals have developed the ability to live and reproduce at elevation as high as 5,000 m, but in some cases, develop chronic medical problems due to their high-altitude residence. At 5,500 m barometric pressure is about only half of the one at sea level. Furthermore, many lowlanders venture to high altitude for work and recreation. The prevalence of HAPE depends on an individual's susceptibility, the rate of ascent, the final altitude, but also on heavy and prolonged exercise, and is higher in males (385). Although the mechanism underlying HAPE remains incompletely understood, it appears that the elevated pulmonary artery pressure plays a pivotal role in the process. Multiple studies demonstrated that susceptible individuals have abnormally high pulmonary artery pressure in response to hypoxic breathing, during normoxic and hypoxic exercise, and on high altitude before the onset of edema. Increased sympathetic tone, and alteration in vasoactive mediators such as endothelin-1, NO produced by pulmonary ECs, may also lead to stronger hypoxic pulmonary vasoconstriction (384). In autopsies, a red cell rich proteinaceous alveolar exudate with hyaline membrane is characteristic. In all autopsies, areas of pneumonitis with neutrophil accumulation but no evidence of bacterial accumulation have been observed. The estimated death rate of altitude illness is about 7.7/100,000 trekkers, with increasing mortality during the last decade (386). Treatment of HAPE consists, if ever possible, in descent from altitude, rest, oxygen supplementation, and administration of drugs like corticosteroids and furosemide.

Prophylactic inhalation of salmeterol, an inhalative β2-adrenergic receptor (β2AR) agonist, decreased the incidence of HAPE by more than 50% (387). The most pertinent explanation was that salmeterol would enhance the clearance of alveolar fluid since β2-adrenergic agonists upregulate AFC by stimulating transepithelial sodium transport. This hypothesis is supported by the fact that the level of sodium transport in the respiratory epithelium is lower in patients prone to HAPE. However, the study results cannot exclude the possibility that the β2 agonist could have modulated vascular permeability or the hemodynamic response associated with hypoxemia and HAPE (4).

In an experimental rat model simulating HAPE by hypobaric and hypoxic conditions equivalent to an altitude of 4,500 m with exhaustive treadmill exercise of 15 m per minute for 24 h, then for an equivalent of altitude of 6,000 m for further 48 h, the TNF tip peptide reduced pulmonary edema and increased expression of the epithelial TJ protein occludin, as compared to high-altitude controls. Compared to untreated high-altitude control animals, TNF tip peptide significantly lowered levels of the inflammatory cytokines TNF, IL-1β, IL-6 and the chemokine IL-8 in bronchoalveolar lavage. TNF tip peptide-treated animals experienced less pulmonary edema, as compared to dexamethasone-treated animals, and was more effective than its comparators in reduction of bronchoalveolar lavage protein content and inflammatory parameters (7).

Identification of the Mechanism of ENaC Activation by the Lectin-Like Region of TNF
It has been shown that the lectin-like domain of TNF can activate ENaC (353) and increases sodium uptake capacity in type II AEC (38). Intriguingly, the TNF tip peptide was shown to directly

bind to the α subunit of ENaC (54, 102) in a two-hit manner, first interacting with the glycosylated extracellular loop of the subunit and subsequently in the TM 2 domain, where the actual activation of the channel occurs (54, 102, 114). The former interaction was proposed to increase the expression of ENaC at the surface membrane in the presence of bacterial toxins, whereas the latter increases the channel's open probability time (102). Indeed, the binding of ENaC to the lectin-like domain of TNF or to the TNF tip peptide stabilizes the channel's complex formation with myristoylated alanine-rich C kinase substrate and with phosphatidylinositol 4,5-bisphosphate, both of which are important for the open conformation of the channel (388), in the presence of the pneumococcal pore-forming toxin pneumolysin (PLY), an important mediator of permeability edema in pneumococcal pneumonia (54). Knock-in mice expressing a TNF mutant lacking a functional lectin-like domain was shown to be more prone to develop capillary leak and permeability edema than their wild-type counterparts after instillation of a low dose of PLY, which did not induce significant barrier dysfunction in control mice (54). In short, these results demonstrate a novel TNF-mediated mechanism of direct ENaC activation and indicate a physiological role for the lectin-like domain of TNF in the resolution of alveolar edema during inflammation (54).

The Lectin-Like Region of TNF Increases Activity of Na$^+$/K$^+$-ATPase

Vadasz et al. investigated the impact of the TNF tip peptide on fluid balance in experimental lung injury. Alveolar–capillary permeability and fluid clearance were assessed in adult male rabbits. Aerosolized TNF tip peptide improved ALC by both reducing vascular permeability and by enhancing the absorption of excess alveolar fluid in experimental lung injury. TNF tip peptide increased Na$^+$/K$^+$-ATPase activity by promoting its exocytosis to the AEC surface and increased amiloride-sensitive sodium uptake, which increased the active Na$^+$ transport 2.2-fold and consecutively the AFC (196). Together with its previously discussed effects on ENaC, these data suggest a role for the TNF tip peptide as a potential therapeutic agent in pulmonary edema (196), since the two main mediators of Na$^+$ transport are both activated by the TNF tip peptide. It should be noted that the primary target is likely ENaC and that the activation of Na$^+$/K$^+$-ATPase could be through the indirect increase in intracellular Na$^+$ upon prior stimulation of ENaC (8). Moreover, the TNF tip peptide was recently also shown to increase the activity of NSC channels (9).

The Lectin-Like Region of TNF Restores ENaC Function in PHA1B Mutants

The lectin-like domain of human TNF activates the ENaC in various cell- and animal-based studies. The synthetically produced cyclic peptides Solnatide (a.k.a. tip peptide or AP301) and its congener AP318 possess molecular structures that mimic the TNF tip region. AP318-mediated ENaC activation was shown to rescue loss of function in a phenotype of ENaC carrying mutations and restored the amiloride-sensitive Na$^+$ current to physiological levels or even higher (118). This implies that the TNF tip domain can activate ENaC by a mechanism which remains intact even in the presence of various mutations occurring in different subunits, because binding to the putative binding site in the TM 2 domain of the glycosylated α subunit apparently remains basically unaffected in all tested point mutations or was compensated in frame shift mutations *via* a moderate activation of αβ- and βγ-ENaC, respectively (389). Apart from the mechanism responsible for loss of the ENaC performance in the studied ENaC mutations, the synthetic TIP and AP318 peptides could restore ENaC function up to or even higher than current levels of wild-type ENaC (118). As therapy of PHA1B is only symptomatic so far, these TNF tip peptides, which directly target ENaC, are promising candidates for the treatment of the channelopathy-caused disease PHA1B (118).

Clinical Trials on the Effect of the Lectin-Like Region of TNF

In a recent phase 2a clinical trial with ALI, patients received inhalable TNF tip peptide in the ventilator twice daily over a 7-day period. There was no significant improvement in lung liquid clearance over all patients, as assessed by the PiCCO method. However, there was a significant increase in extravascular lung water removal in those patients with a sequential organ failure assessment score higher than or equal to 11, representing more than 50% of the subjects in this trial (358). One hypothesis for this observation is that patients in this group, apart from suffering from impaired AFC capacity, might also suffer from more severe capillary barrier dysfunction. The TNF tip peptide was recently shown to not only improve AFC (54, 102), but also capillary barrier function (97) in the presence of bacterial toxins.

As mentioned before, in a randomized pilot study performed with 20 patients on the treatment of established PGD after lung transplantation by twice daily inhalation of the TNF tip peptide (AP301, solnatide) versus placebo, the TNF tip peptide improved gas exchange and clearly reduced the intubation—and thus mechanical ventilation—time in a probably clinically relevant manner (357).

TNF-Related Apoptosis-Inducing Ligand (TRAIL)

TNF-related apoptosis-inducing ligand, a member of the superfamily of TNF ligands, is a homotrimeric type II TM protein with a conserved C-terminal extracellular domain that mediates receptor binding and which can be cleaved by metalloproteinases to generate a soluble mediator (390). TRAIL is produced by several cell types, including immune cells such as macrophages and T cells and can be induced by both type I and type III Interferons (IFNs), a family of cytokines with fundamental importance in the innate immune response to viral infections (209, 391). Macrophages generate both soluble and membrane-bound TRAIL, which operate through distinct receptors on infected and non-infected, neighboring cells (209). TRAIL is a potent activator of cell death in transformed cells and activates cellular stress pathways in epithelial cells, as such finally leading to caspase-dependent or -independent cell death (209). In view of the prominent role of IFNs in antiviral response, IFN-dependent induction of TRAIL is a prominent regulator of disease outcome especially in respiratory viral infection, enters into the scene (209). As such, the IFN/TRAIL signaling axis is of potential interest in disease progression and attenuation of tissue injury during respiratory viral infection (209). Here we focused on the role of TRAIL in edema reabsorption and in alveolar epithelial function.

TRAIL Disrupts the Alveolar Epithelial Barrier

TRAIL plays adverse roles in viral infection (392–394). On the one hand, TRAIL drives infected cells into apoptosis in order to limit virus distribution (209). On the other hand TRAIL can induce functional and structural damage not only in infected cells, but also in bystander cells, such as uninfected cells of the alveolar epithelium (199, 208). As such TRAIL can at the same time prevent viral spreading, but also cause lung injury in acute respiratory viral infection (209). Accordingly, in influenza A virus (IAV) infection, TRAIL acts as a detrimental factor contributing to tissue injury and impaired inflammation resolution when released in excessive amounts by recruited immune cells (209). The activation of proapoptotic and pro-necroptotic pathways in respiratory infection can result in a structural disruption of the airway and the alveolar epithelial barrier, which is a major hallmark of respiratory disease and its progression to the ARDS (395, 396).

TRAIL Decreases Na$^+$/K$^+$-ATPase Expression and Impairs AFC

Peteranderl et al (199). have investigated whether IAV infection alters Na$^+$/K$^+$-ATPase expression and function in AECs and the ability of the lung to clear edema. IAV infection reduced α1 Na$^+$/K$^+$-ATPase expression in the plasma membrane of human and murine AECs and in distal lung epithelium of infected mice. Accordingly, the decreased Na$^+$/K$^+$-ATPase expression impaired AFC in IAV-infected mice. A paracrine cell communication network between infected and non-infected AECs and alveolar macrophages was identified, which led to decreased alveolar epithelial Na$^+$/K$^+$-ATPase function, thus to AFC inhibition (199). The IAV-induced reduction of Na$^+$/K$^+$-ATPase was mediated by a host signaling pathway that involved epithelial type I IFN and an IFN-dependent elevation of macrophage TRAIL (199). In non-infected cells within the IAV-infected lung, TRAIL severely compromised the function of the ion channel Na$^+$/K$^+$-ATPase, which was mediated by induction of the stress kinase AMPK (199) thereby potentially revealing a cross-link to TRAIL-induced autophagic cell stress pathways in bystander cells both *in vitro* and *in vivo* (199). The TRAIL-induced and AMPK-mediated downregulation of the Na$^+$/K$^+$-ATPase, a major driver of vectorial ion and fluid transport from the alveolar airspace toward the interstitium, resulted in a reduced capacity of IAV-infected mice to clear excessive fluid from the alveoli (395). Thus, TRAIL signaling contributes to intensive edema formation, a hallmark of disease in virus-induced ARDS (395). Notably, this effect of TRAIL on Na$^+$/K$^+$-ATPase expression was induced independently of cell death pathways elicited by caspases, as treatment of cells and mice with a specific caspase-3 inhibitor diminished apoptosis in AECs but still allowed for the reduction of the Na$^+$/K$^+$-ATPase (199).

Transforming Growth Factor-β (TGF-β)

Transforming growth factor-β is a pleiotropic cytokine with a broad regulatory role in the immune system. Three highly homologous isoforms - TGFβ1, TGFβ2, and TGFβ3—share a receptor complex and signal transduction pathway, but their tissue expression levels are different (397). All are produced as inactive complexes, which must be activated to bind to their receptors (398). Platelets, T lymphocytes, macrophages, ECs, keratinocytes, smooth muscle cells, fibroblasts, i.e., a wide range of cells, can produce TGF (399). Following wounding or inflammation, all these cells are potential sources of TGF-β (400). Receptors for TGF-β have been found almost on every cell type tested so far, which enables this cytokine to exert its effects on almost any body tissue (401). Classically, TGF-β receptor signaling occurs by activating the Smad-dependent intracellular signaling pathway (398). The TGFβ receptor complex consists of two receptor subunits, TGF-β receptor (TGF-βR) I and II (398). These receptors mediate multiple responses (401).

TGFβ Context-Dependent Mode of Action

Transforming growth factor-β action is highly context-dependent and can be influenced by cell type, culture condition, interaction with other signaling pathways, developmental or disease stage *in vivo* and innate genetic variation among individuals (402). As such, TGF-β can be both a pro- and anti-inflammatory cytokine, which affects the growth and proliferation of many cell types (399). During inflammation, TGF-β1 is also able to effectively inhibit inflammatory response (403). The action of TGF-β following inflammatory responses is characterized by increased production of extracellular matrix components, as well as mesenchymal cell proliferation, migration, and accumulation (404). Pleiotropic nature of TGF-β modulates expression of adhesion molecules, provides a chemotactic gradient for leukocytes and other cells participating in an inflammatory response in one hand and, in contrast, inhibits them once they have become activated (405). Also in autoimmunity, TGFβ represents a double-edged sword (406). It can cause both T-cell growth promotion, as well as immune suppression (406).

Role of TGF-β Role in Pulmonary Edema

Transforming growth factor-β has a dual role in pulmonary edema. It can up- or downregulate alveolar ion and fluid transport, through its impact on ion channels/pumps (ENaC, CFTR and Na$^+$/K$^+$-ATPase) or on the pulmonary barrier. As such, TGF-β can decrease the expression of ENaC through decreasing expression of its α subunit mRNA and protein during bacterial infection (132). During ALI/ARDS, increased TGF-β1 activity in the distal airspaces promotes alveolar edema by reducing distal airway epithelial sodium and fluid clearance (132). Moreover, TGF-β can induce the internalization of βENaC from the lung epithelial cell surface and, hence, block the sodium-transporting capacity of AECs (133). In fact, TGF-β causes the subsequent activation of phospholipase D1, phosphatidylinositol- 4-phosphate 5-kinase 1α, and NADPH oxidase 4 (Nox4) (133). Nox4 activation moreover results in the production of ROS, which in turn reduces cell surface stability of the αβγENaC complex and thus leads to edema fluid accumulation (371). Apart from its effects on ENaC expression, TGF-β can also decrease CFTR expression and function (179) and it, moreover, impairs expression of the Na$^+$/K$^+$-ATPase β1 subunit, resulting in decreased Na$^+$/K$^+$-ATPase activity in lung epithelial cells (197, 198).

Transforming growth factor-β decreases lung epithelial barrier function (203–205) *in vitro* by a mechanism that involves depletion of intracellular glutathione (206, 407). The cytokine moreover induces endothelial barrier dysfunction *via* Smad2-dependent p38 activation (235).

The integrin αvβ6 (408) can activate latent TGF-β in the lungs and skin (409). Using this clue, Pittet et al. have shown that mice lacking integrin αvβ6 are completely protected from pulmonary edema in bleomycin-induced ALI. Furthermore, pharmacologic inhibition of TGF-β also protected wild-type mice from pulmonary edema induced by bleomycin or *Escherichia coli* endotoxin (206). In short, integrin-mediated local activation of TGF-β is critical for the development of pulmonary edema in ALI, and blocking TGF-β or its activation attenuates pulmonary edema. This neutralization can be done e.g., by the administration of a soluble type II TGF-β receptor, which sequesters free TGF-β during lung injury (206).

All of the deleterious actions of TGF-β discussed above will ultimately lead to decreased ion transport and may, therefore, promote and worsen pulmonary edema. However, TGF-β can also positively impact pulmonary edema. Intriguingly, TGF-β was proposed to increase the function of ENaC, *via* enhancing the expression of Na$^+$/K$^+$-ATPase α1- and β1-subunits (134).

Interleukin-8

Interleukin-8 is a pro-inflammatory chemokine produced by a variety of tissue and blood cells (410), including bronchial epithelial cells (411), that correlates with neutrophil accumulation in distal airspaces of patients with ARDS. IL-8 is also a predictor of mortality in ALI (412–414). As such, significantly higher concentrations of IL-8 are found in the pulmonary edema fluid and plasma of patients with a septic versus a non-septic etiology of ARDS (415). Moreover, IL-8 promotes edema formation by blocking AFC (105).

The Role of IL-8 in Inhibiting β2AR Agonist

Roux et al (105). have shown that IL-8 or its rat analog cytokine-induced neutrophil chemokine-1 significantly decreased β2AR agonist-stimulated vectorial Cl$^-$ and net fluid transport across rat and human alveolar epithelial type II cells, through reducing CFTR activity and biosynthesis (105). This reduction process was mediated by heterologous β2AR desensitization and downregulation (50%) *via* the G-protein-coupled receptor kinase 2 (GRK2)/PI3K signaling pathway (105) (**Figure 8**). Consistent with the experimental results, high pulmonary edema fluid levels of IL-8 (>4,000 pg/ml) were associated with impaired AFC in patients with ALI. Taken together, these results suggest a role for IL-8 in inhibiting β2AR agonist-stimulated alveolar epithelial fluid transport *via* a GRK2/PI3K-dependent mechanism (105). On top of this, IL-8 can promote edema formation by increasing endothelial permeability (250).

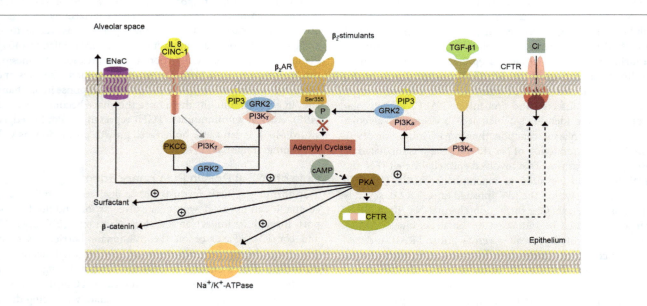

FIGURE 8 | Rationale for the problematic role of β2 adrenergic agonists in clinical trials. Schematic representation of the mechanisms by which interleukin-8 (IL-8)/cytokine-induced neutrophil chemokine (CINC)-1 and transforming growth factor (TGF)-β1 have a synergistic inhibitory effect on the β2-adrenergic receptor (β2AR) signaling pathway in type II alveolar (ATII) cells. IL-8/CINC-1 and TGF-β1 cause the activation of different phosphoinositide 3-kinase (PI3K) isoforms. However, IL-8/CINC-1 but not TGF-β1 phosphorylates G-protein-coupled receptor kinase 2 (GRK2) *via* a protein kinase C-zeta (PKC-ζ)-dependent mechanism explaining why the blockade of IL-8/CINC-1 prevents the TGF-β1-mediated inhibition of the β2AR signaling pathway in ATII cells. This results in the translocation of the protein complex GRK2 and PI3K to the cell membrane. This protein complex causes phosphorylation at the Ser355 heterologous desensitization and downregulation of the β2AR in ATII cells. IL-8/CINC-1 and TGF-β1 then prevent the activation of 3′-5′-cyclic adenosine monophosphate (cAMP)/protein kinase A (PKA) pathway that upregulates the vectorial fluid transport across the alveolar epithelium *via* phosphorylation and increased expression of cystic fibrosis transmembrane conductance regulator (CFTR) at the plasma membrane of ATII cells. The solid lines indicate the pathways stimulated by IL-8/CINC-1 and the dashed lines indicate the pathways inhibited by these mediators (416).

Interleukin-1β

Interleukin-1β is associated with decreased alveolar fluid reabsorption and thus with worse outcome in ALI and sepsis. IL-1β primarily decreases alveolar fluid reabsorption *via* a p38 MAPK, reducing the expression of the α-subunit of ENaC (113) as well as the β-subunit (137). In ARDS patients, the mean initial plasma levels of TNF IL-1β, IL-6, and IL-8 were significantly higher in non-survivors and in patients with sepsis. High plasma levels of IL-1β were associated with poor patient outcome (417). Likewise, high levels of IL-1β in the lungs of patients with ARDS were associated with an increased risk of mortality (417). The FAS/CD95 system acts together with TNF and IL-1β (57, 219, 418–420), leading to NF-κB production and neutrophil accumulating IL-8 secretion. Of note, an epithelial repair effect for type II pneumocytes *via* IL-1β was described in the injured alveolus (139), possibly in a specific context of cytokines, mediators and growth factors (139). Only in a specific fetal context IL-1β may increase alveolar fluid reabsorption by a hypothalamus-pituitary-adrenal gland axis (421) and an increase of both ENaC and Na^+/K^+-ATPase expression (140).

Fas/FasL System (CD95/CD95 Ligand System)

Fas is a 45-kDa type I cell surface receptor that belongs to the TNF receptor family. It can cause cytokine and chemokine release, especially the neutrophil attractant IL-8, *via* MAP kinase activation in lung epithelial cells, as such promoting inflammation (219). Binding of FasL to membrane Fas activates apoptosis through activation of caspases, which seems the key to AEC apoptosis, thus epithelial barrier breakdown and its consequences in ALI (57, 418).

Keratinocyte Growth Factor (KGF, FGF-7)

KGF is an epithelial cell-specific growth factor that has been shown to exert beneficial actions in many animal models of ALI and ARDS as well as in the *ex vivo* human lung (143, 422–430). Rats in which KGF was intratracheally administered increased AFC by about up to 50%, and this was further increased by the β2 agonist terbutaline (427). *In vitro* studies using mesenchymal stem cell-derived medium suggested that this growth factor plays a dominant role in tissue repair, even in the presence of the inflammatory cytokines IL-1β, TNF-α, and interferon-gamma, as well as in hypoxia. The observation that no downregulation of ENaC-α expression occurred despite of the presence of three key inflammatory cytokines suggested a dominant biological role of KGF in the acutely injured alveolar milieu (431). There is a currently a large interest in stem cell therapies as therapeutic approaches in clinical disorders like myocardial infarction, limb ischemia, diabetes, hepatic and renal failure, and ALI/ARDS. Stem and progenitor cell therapies as well as work with factors influencing those cells to reduce injury and increase repair have been performed. KGF has been proposed to be one of the main candidates to promote the repair capacity of stem cells in ALI. A recently performed double-blind, placebo-controlled phase 2 clinical trial—the KARE trial—tested the effects of KGF in 29 verum patients versus 31 placebo patients (432). There was no difference in the primary outcome variable, the oxygenation index, at day 7, and the treatment group had a trend to higher mortality, and more adverse events in terms of pyrexia. Nevertheless, these data do not exclude that the combined use of KGF and stem cells might provide protection in ALI.

Soluble Receptor for Advanced Glycation End Products (sRAGE)

Receptor for advanced glycation end products, first characterized in 1992 by Neeper et al. is a 35 kDa TM receptor which belongs to the immunoglobulin superfamily (433). RAGE is one of the AT1 cell-associated proteins in the lungs (434, 435). RAGE and its ligands have been recognized to be involved in the pathobiology of a wide range of diseases which are accompanied by symptoms, like enhanced oxidative stress, immune/inflammatory responses, and altered cell functions (436). RAGE is highly expressed in the lungs at readily measurable levels and its level increases quickly at sites of inflammation, mainly in inflammatory and epithelial cells (437). RAGE has three forms, consisting of N-truncated, dominant-negative, and soluble RAGE, which can be produced either by natural alternative splicing or by the action of membrane-associated proteases (438). The correlation between sRAGE levels and AFC rate was investigated in both a clinical study of patients with ARDS, as well as in an experimental model of acid-induced lung injury in mice (264). The results obtained showed a correlation between elevated levels of sRAGE with lung injury and an impairment of AFC (264). Accordingly, an increase in alveolar–capillary barrier permeability, arterial oxygenation impairment, lung injury scores, and the extent of human lung damage on CT scan are all associated with sRAGE levels (264). Conversely, it has been shown that RAGE regulates lung fluid balance *via* protein kinase C-gp91(phox) signaling to ENaC (177). In fact, hAGE, a RAGE ligand, increases ENaC activity through oxidant-mediated signaling, which can ultimately impact lung fluid clearance (177).

β2ARs AS IMPORTANT MODULATORS OF AFC

Structure and Subtypes

β2-adrenergic receptors are G protein-coupled receptors with seven-TM domains (439). Their three subtypes are β1, predominantly found in the heart, β2 in the respiratory system, and β3 in adipose tissue (440). β2 adrenergic agonists activate the β2-adrenoceptors (β2AR) on airway smooth muscle and are used to treat bronchoconstriction in asthma and chronic obstructive pulmonary disease (COPD) (441). In their canonical signaling pathway, agonist binding couples the β2AR to the Gs subtype of G protein. Gs activation leads to adenylyl cyclase, production of cAMP and activation of the cAMP-dependent protein kinase A (PKA), which mediates most of the functional consequences of Gs-coupled receptor activation (442). In airway smooth muscle, β2AR-stimulated PKA activity mediates relaxation through phosphorylation of multiple proteins involved in regulating intracellular calcium levels, calcium sensitivity, and cross-bridge cycling (442).

The Role of β2AR Agonists in AFC

The presence of pulmonary β2ARs includes the alveolar space and provides the possibility to modulate the active Na^+ transport. β2adrenoceptors and the β-adrenergic agonists accelerate AFC (439) due to Na^+ transport *via* an amiloride-sensitive pathway (443) as shown *in vitro* (444), *ex vivo* (445), and *in vivo* in rat (446), dog (447), sheep (448), guinea pig (449), mouse (443, 450), and human lung tissue (451). β2AR knockout mice results suggest that the β2AR is responsible for most of the β-adrenergic–mediated upregulation of AFC (452). Therefore, β2ARs appear to be responsible for the bulk of the β-receptor–sensitive alveolar active Na^+ transport likely due to direct and indirect up-regulation of the alveolar active Na^+ transport (445, 449, 452–454). β-agonists *via* activation of β2ARs regulate necessary key proteins for the process of alveolar epithelial active Na^+ transport such as ENaC, Na^+/K^+-ATPase and CFTR in animal models as well as in human lung tissue (445, 449, 453, 455). β2ARs mediate short-term regulation of Na^+ pumps which occurs within minutes of receptor engagement *via* highly regulated recruitment of assembled Na^+/K^+-ATPase from intracellular compartments through phosphorylation of intermediary proteins and RhoA-kinase (456, 457). Long-term regulation is carried out *via* transcription (458) and translation of α1-subunit of Na^+/K^+-ATPase and ENaC subunits through PKA induced phosphorylation of cAMP-responsive elements and post-transcriptional regulation *via* mitogen-activated protein kinase/extracellular signal–regulated kinase and rapamycin sensitive pathways (455, 459) by direct modulation of Na^+ channels at the apical surface of the cells (460) or an activation of PKA to modulate a cation channel (92, 453).

Impact of β2AR Agonists on ENaC

Protein kinase A-mediated β2-agonist action phosphorylates cytoskeleton proteins and promotes trafficking of Na^+ channels through the cell membrane and direct phosphorylation of epithelial Na^+ channel β and γ subunits stimulate the β2AR and increases the number of epithelial Na^+ channels and their open time in alveolar type II cells (453) and enhances the expression of the α-subunit of the epithelial Na^+ channel ENaC (458). β-agonists and cAMP analogs increase the open probability and open time of amiloride-sensitive Na^+ channels (161). β2AR agonists thus increase Na^+ flux across the apical cell membrane by increasing both membrane-bound channel abundance and Na^+ flux through ENaC (439).

Impact of β2AR Agonists on Na^+/K^+-ATPase

β-adrenergic agonist modulate Na^+/K^+-ATPase partially through adenosine 3′,5′-cyclic monophosphate (461). β2-adrenergic agonists increase the gene expression of Na^+/K^+-ATPase which leads to:

- Increased expression of α1-Na^+/K^+-ATPase mRNA and protein (458).
- Increase of the quantity of Na^+/K^+-ATPase (458)
- Increased activity of Na^+/K^+-ATPase (456, 458, 462–464).

Impact of β2AR Agonists on CFTR

Cystic fibrosis transmembrane conductance regulator is required for cAMP-mediated upregulation of fluid clearance, but is not necessary for basal fluid absorption (183), thus for alveolar fluid homeostasis in the uninjured lung (182, 183). β2-adrenergic stimulation activates CFTR by cAMP and PKA activation (184). In airway epithelial cells, the interaction of β2-AR with CFTR is mediated by scaffold proteins, such as NHERF1, allowing its interaction with PKA and stabilizing it on the plasma membrane (465). β2-adrenergic stimulation increases CFTR regulator expression in human airway epithelial cells through a cAMP/PKA-independent pathway (466).

β2-Adrenergic Agonists Are at Least in Part Not of Clinical Benefit in ALI/ARDS Studies and May Increase Mortality

In mild-to-moderate lung injury, alveolar edema fluid clearance is often preserved by catecholamine-dependent or -independent mechanisms (467). Stimulation of AFC is then related to activation or increased expression of sodium channels like ENaC or the Na^+/K^+-ATPase pump and may involve CFTR (467). In severe lung injury, AFC perturbation result through increased endothelial-interstitial-epithelial alveolar permeability and changes in activity or expression of sodium or chloride transport molecules (467). Improved barrier function and increased alveolar fluid reabsorption, theoretically by β-adrenergic agonists or the lectin-like TNF activity or alternatives, vasoactive drugs, regenerative or repair measures are therefore therapeutic alternatives (467). Whereas in the BALTI-2 study with salbutamol given as an intravenous infusion for up to 7 days, compared with a placebo, more than 160 patients [age 55 (SD 17) years] per group were studied, the study was stopped as salbutamol treatment was associated with increased 28-day mortality of 34% compared to 23% (risk ratio 1.47, 95% confidence interval 1.03 to 2.08) (468).

Salbutamol early in the course of ARDS was poorly tolerated. The authors concluded that such a β2-agonist therapy is unlikely to be beneficial and could worsen outcomes. Follow-up data further suggested worse outcome at 6 and 12 months in ARDS patients treated with salbutamol. They discussed that further trials of β-agonists in patients with ARDS were therefore unlikely to be conducted.

Some questions remained open, such as whether or not there may be benefit at a different dose or in specific populations (468). The survival curves for salbutamol and placebo appeared to continue to diverge after the end of the study drug infusion after 7 days, suggesting that the mechanisms may involve indirect effects as, e.g., more systemic disease under and after intravenous salbutamol. Concerning morbidity and mortality, Salbutamol can cause arrhythmia and tachycardia, and electrolyte and metabolic disturbances such as hypokalemia, hypomagnesemia, and lactic acidosis, which was observed in the study, and led to more salbutamol discontinuation. The used salbutamol dose of 15 µg/kg ideal body weight/hour i.v. was considered the maximum that critically ill patients could receive without an increase in ventricular or atrial tachycardia or ectopy. It was at the higher end of the recommended dosing regimen, and it is possible that lower doses might have been better tolerated and caused fewer adverse outcomes (468).

Rather similar results were observed in the USA in the ALTA trial (Albuterol for the Treatment of ALI). ALTA was a placebo-controlled multicentre study of nebulized salbutamol in patients with ALI. Patients were randomized to receive either salbutamol 5 mg every 4 h or saline placebo, for up to 10 days. The primary outcome was ventilator-free days. Recruitment started 2007 with a target sample size of 1,000 patients. It was terminated after 282 patients had been enrolled because of futility. There was no clear difference observed in both ventilator-free days between the salbutamol and placebo arms (14.4 versus 16.6 days; 95% CI −4.7 to 0.3 days) or in hospital mortality (salbutamol 23.0% versus placebo 17.7%; 95% CI −4.0% to 14.7%). Although the β2 stimulator intervention was delivered by a different route in ALTA, and the early termination of recruitment caused that confidence intervals are wide, the results seemed much consistent with the BALTI-2 trial.

One alternative way was to use combination of inhaled corticosteroid and inhaled β2 agonist. In a recently published pilot study, a typical asthma treatment combination of twice daily inhaled formoterol and budesonide for 5 days showed its feasibility and promising results. The rationale was to reduce by both budesonide and formoterol alveolar inflammation, and to further improve by formoterol AFC. The aim was to reduce ARDS. More patients in the placebo group developed ARDS (7 versus 0) and required mechanical ventilation (53% versus 21%) (469).

Further Potentially Critical Mechanisms of Action β-Adrenergic Agonists

Besides two futile ARDS trials, further factors might restrict the β2 receptor agonist usage as a therapy to increase the resolution of pulmonary edema (467). Prolonged stimulation of β-adrenergic receptors with endogenous catecholamines could desensitize the β-receptors and prevent their stimulation with exogenous catecholamines (467). For instance, in some patients the alveolar epithelium might be too injured to respond to β-adrenergic agonist therapy (467), likewise circulating factors could limit the action of β-adrenergic agonists (467). Also, in the presence of left atrial hypertension, atrial natriuretic peptide can inhibit the stimulatory effect (467). Similarly in prolonged hemorrhagic shock and resuscitation, cAMP agonists may not stimulate AFC because oxidant-mediated injury may reduce the response of the alveolar epithelium to β-2 agonists (467).

An important clinical aspect is the potential to increase cardiac index by β2 receptor agonists (470), by both cardiac stimulation and pulmonary arterial vasodilation. Cardiac stimulation can lead to a higher cardiac index. This is potentially dangerous, as due to the injured lung put in the circulation in series, there is an increase in filtration, which further increases alveolar fluid and gas exchange disturbance. An interrelated second, and in ALI most probably untoward "Robin Hood effect" of potential opening of vascular beds that are closed by vasoconstriction is, e.g., observed in COPD patients inhaling β2 receptor agonists and developing more hypoxemia (471). This is probably due to increased perfusion in badly ventilated ALI/ARDS alveolar areas. As shown by Briot et al., β2 receptor agonist therapy seems therefore to have the potential to heighten the protein leakage from plasma to alveoli in the acutely injured lung (470).

PROTEIN CLEARANCE OUT OF THE ALVEOLAR SPACE

Clearance of serum and inflammatory proteins from the alveolar space is an important and possibly vital process in recovery from pulmonary edema. Albumin and IgG are present in pulmonary edema fluid in concentrations that are 40–65% of plasma levels in hydrostatic pulmonary edema and 75–95% in non-cardiogenic pulmonary edema. Concentrations of albumin, for example, may be 5 g/100 ml or more. Protein concentrations rise during recovery from alveolar edema because the salt and water fraction of edema fluid is cleared much faster than albumin and IgG. Clearance of alveolar protein occurs by paracellular pathways in the setting of pulmonary edema. Transcytosis may be important in regulating the alveolar milieu under nonpathological circumstances. Alveolar protein degradation may become important in long-term protein clearance, clearance of insoluble proteins, or under pathological conditions such as immune reactions or ALI.

Early since the first descriptions of ARDS, we know that protein content is high, "haemorrhagic," and about the same as plasma proteins. Plasma and coagulative products such as fibrin strands are degraded or modified, e.g., also to hyaline membranes in a high number of patients (31). They are observed in ARDS, are especially covering denuded basement membranes where pneumocytes are missing, and may be related to adverse outcome (56).

Recent research hints to a better understanding of the resolution of those alveolar proteinaceous contents and debris out of the distal airways. Counterintuitively, neither macrophages, nor the mucociliary transport processes seem to play major roles in protein clearance also over several days time (472). Protein clearance from the distal air spaces is in part facilitated by active endocytotic processes including for albumin by the 600 kDa TM glycoprotein called megalin or LDL-receptor related protein-2, a member of the low-density lipoprotein-receptor superfamily (6). Again, its important functional inhibition seems TGF-beta1 related. Megalin seems negatively regulated by glycogen synthase kinase 3b (GSK3b). An important regulator for this protein kinase signaling molecule seems the RNA binding protein Embryonic Lethal, Abnormal Vision, Drosophila Like 1/Human antigen R (ELAVL-1/HuR) as an upstream regulator of GSK3b (6). ELAVL-1/HuR is an RNA binding protein that increases mRNA stability. Its importance has been shown in ventilator-induced and acid-induced mouse lung injury. In EC lines it induces ICAM-1 and IL-8 after TNF stimulation.

Endocytosis of macromolecules can be mediated by a nonselective fluid phase uptake, which is a very slow process in alveolar epithelium. A receptor-mediated endocytosis is much faster and occurs when specific high-affinity receptors are implicated. Two pathways are described, called caveolae-mediated and clathrin-mediated endocytosis.

Detailed research on alveolar protein and debris clearance have only recently begun. Judging their roles is more complex, as hyperosmotic stimuli might be of anti-inflammatory action, and possibly there is even more biological signaling as formerly assumed that may influence underlying lung disease.

POTENTIAL NOVEL APPROACHES TO UNDERSTANDING THE EFFECTS OF ION CHANNEL STIMULANTS IN LUNG DISEASE

Hyperosmolarity, High Na⁺ Content, or High Oncotic Pressure

One biological effect that has, to our knowledge, not yet been assessed is the question whether due to fluid reabsorption out of the alveolus the hyperosmolarity or hyper-oncotic situation is of biological effect. Several limitations have to be mentioned: Certainly the pulmonary surfaces including the mucus and the surfactant system and its layers are complex and disease-prone systems, as suggested in cystic fibrosis. Dose- and time response have to be taken into account. Actually, there are contradictory results on those effects: Some observations described anti-inflammatory effects of hyperosmolarity in the airways, as in the nose and sinuses with a few randomized controlled trials that compared isoosmotic versus hyperosmotic irrigating solutions (473, 474). Honey is hyperosmotic and antibacterial, and in wound healing it seems frequently beneficial (475). This is also the case for hyperosmotic salt pastilles in throat and neck infections. However, nebulized hypertonic saline is still disputed in infants with acute viral bronchiolitis (476). There are also *in vitro* cell model results showing a switch from adaptive to inflammatory gene expression by hyperosmotic stress by protein kinase R activation, NF-kappaB p65 activation with responsive genes including inducible NO synthase, interleukin-6, and interleukin-1β (477), others with some protection *via* p53 gene regulation (478). In a rat seawater drowning model, alveolar hypertonicity, but not iso-or hypotonicity-induced inflammation and vascular leak, thus edema probably by hypoxia-inducible factor-1 and including ataxia telangiectasia mutated kinase and PI3 kinase (479).

Local Na⁺ accumulation and enhanced availability have been linked to activation of tonicity-responsive enhancer binding protein (TonEBP) *via* the mononuclear phagocyte system in the skin (480), a system also widely represented in the lung. Enhanced local Na⁺ has been shown to boost pro-inflammatory TH17 cell production and, finally, IL-17 release (481). The pro-inflammatory phenotype is maintained in high-salt conditions with upregulation of TNF-α and IL-2. As it is currently unclear what is the mechanism of enhanced Na⁺ presentation to activate the TonEBP, an enhanced Na⁺ accumulation in the extracellular matrix (482), the activation of Na⁺ channels or even a permissive role of an altered Na⁺/K⁺-ATPase activity *via* endogenous ouabain have to be considered (483). As all of these mechanisms are also represented in the lung, both Na⁺ presentation and availability should, therefore, be considered in pulmonary fluid regulation.

Briefly, there may be important, but so far not yet well understood anti-, or even pro-inflammatory, stimuli, or signals by hyperosmotic stimulation, underlining the importance to investigate this subject further.

SPECIFIC CLINICAL SETTINGS WITH POTENTIAL SIGNIFICANCE OF ALVEOLAR FLUID REABSORPTION IN INFLAMED LUNGS

RDS in the Newborn

Respiratory distress syndrome is one of the most important causes of morbidity and mortality in newborns and has a prevalence of about 1%. It is clinically manifesting as respiratory distress accompanied by abnormal pulmonary function and hypoxemia directly in the first minutes or hours after birth. RDS prevalence increases with decreasing gestational age. As such the incidence of RDS is highest in extremely preterm infants, affecting more than 90% of infants at a gestational age of 28 weeks or less. In a birth cohort of more than 230,000 deliveries, the syndrome was observed at 34 weeks gestation in 10.5%, at 35 weeks in 6%, at 36 weeks in 2.8%, at 37 weeks in 1%, at 38, and more in 0.3%. Therapy is supportive, includes surfactant replacement, fluid restriction, and glucocorticoids. Whereas a viewpoint has been that qualitative and quantitative surfactant deficiency, inflammation including alveolar neutrophil influx, and fluid overload (in part by low urine output) account for this syndrome, some reports hint to a suboptimal Na⁺ transport. During gestation, the lung epithelium secretes Cl⁻ and fluid and develops the ability to actively reabsorb Na⁺ only during late gestation. At birth, the mature lung switches from active Cl⁻ and consecutive fluid secretion to active Na⁺ and consecutive fluid absorption in response to circulating catecholamines. Changes in oxygen tension augment the Na⁺-uptake capacity of the epithelium and increase ENaC gene expression. The inability of the immature fetal lung to switch from fluid secretion to fluid absorption results, at least in large part, from an immaturity in terms of low expression of ENaC, where all three ENaC subunits are low in preterm relative to full-term infants. ENaC-α is increased in the respiratory epithelium by therapeutic glucocorticosteroids (484, 485).

However, in the last years the incidence of near-term and term infants with RDS has increased, and their clinical characteristics differ from those of premature infants with RDS. Li et al. found that death was virtually inevitable for some babies, despite intensive care and surfactant replacement therapy, particularly in near-term and term infants. Lung tissue slices taken during autopsies of near-term and term infants who died of neonatal RDS showed that some alveoli were obviously dilated, with a large amount of lung fluid. This was in addition to an alveolar collapse from a lack of surfactant, and suggested that lung fluid absorption disorders might be an important additional cause of RDS by influencing gas exchange or surfactant function (486). In their study on 120 neonates with RDS and 129 controls, 7 newborns died despite of intensive care and surfactant replacement therapy. All of them received surfactant more than once and four of them were near-term or term infants. Preterm babies (less than 35 weeks of gestational age) had a better response to surfactant treatment than near-term and term babies. These results were consistent with the finding that the surfactant therapy was not effective for all newborns with RDS. The authors assessed the relationship between RDS and 7 candidate polymorphisms of the SCNN1A gene that encodes α-ENaC. One single nucleotide polymorphism (rs4149570) of the SCNN1A gene was associated with RDS. Moreover, in a group of term infants (gestational age was 37 weeks or greater), another single nucleotide polymorphism locus (rs7956915) was associated with RDS. These results are consistent with the hypothesis that the causes of RDS are multifactorial, and that in term infants it might differ from those in preterm infants (487). Alveolar fluid reabsorption and, thus, α-ENaC might play a key role in the pathogenesis by influencing the amount of lung liquid absorption, especially in term infants with RDS.

Acute Infection-Related Respiratory Failure

Pulmonary infections are the most prevalent infections worldwide, most of bacterial or viral origin. Community-acquired pneumonia is a frequent infectious respiratory disease with an annual incidence of about 5–12/1,000, and leads to hospitalization in 20–50% of patients. Mortality in hospitalized patients ranges from 5 to 15%. The most common reason for hospital admission in childhood is pneumonia and accounts for up to 50% of admissions. The high morbidity, mortality, and epidemiologic dangers with viral or bacterial pneumonias are of high concern. Pneumonia mortality is typically caused by flooding of the pulmonary alveoli preventing normal gas exchange and consequent hypoxemia. We refer to excellent recent reviews (117, 371). Of note is that pneumonia and sepsis are by far the leading causes of ALI and ARDS. Sepsis is a major healthcare burden, mirrored by up to 45% of intensive care unit costs (64) and bearing a high mortality of about 30%. Cytokines and ion channels are key elements in this common health problem.

Lung Transplantation

Lung transplantation is a substitutive treatment of various end-stage pulmonary disease. Cystic fibrosis, COPD, and idiopathic pulmonary fibrosis (IPF) are the most important transplanted patient groups (488). The high mortality rate relative to other solid-organ transplants is in part due to chronic rejection. The limited availability of donor lungs results in a highly limited treatment strategy for patients in whom a survival benefit—estimated 5-year survival is about 60%—is expected (488).

Primary graft dysfunction (PGD) is termed the development of allograft infiltrates within 72 h of transplantation together with impaired oxygenation, when other identifiable insults such as volume overload, pneumonia, acute rejection, atelectasis or vascular compromises are excluded. PGD is usually referred to ischemia–reperfusion injury, but additionally to any further mechanical, surgical or chemical trauma such as inflammatory, neural or hormonal events of the donor, high oxygen fraction during reperfusion, or lymphatic disruption. PGD is mild and transient in most cases, but 10–20% of patient situations are sufficiently severe to cause life-threatening hypoxemia similar to ARDS, based on the same mediators and cytokines and a diffuse alveolar damage resembling ARDS. Similar to ARDS, it is considered a systemic disease, not only affecting the lung, but the whole patient. Thereby, the increased occurrence of cerebral dysfunction, i.e., patient delirium, worsens prognosis. Severe PGD quadruples perioperative mortality, the leading cause of early death of lung transplant recipients. In one study it is associated with a 30 day mortality of 63 versus 9%, and associated duration of mechanical ventilation is 15 versus 1 day (489) (**Figures 9** and **10**). The risk of higher morbidity and death risk persists even after an often protracted recovery, suggesting that PGD triggers an increased risk for bronchiolitis obliterans syndrome as a manifestation of chronic allograft rejection (490).

Ischemia–reperfusion injury is the main mechanism for PGD (503, 504). With logarithmic function ischemia time is associated with reperfusion injury: Whereas 4 h ischemia is associated with about 13% more risk than 2 h, 6 h ischemia increases the risk by more than 50%, 8 h by a factor of 3, and 10 h by a factor of about 8 (494). The hypothermic preservation increases oxidative stress, leads to accumulation of intracellular sodium and loss of intracellular potassium and an intracellular calcium overload, cell death with apoptosis (240) and necrosis. The release of pro-and anti-inflammatory cytokines such as TNF, INF-γ, IL-8, IL-10, IL-12, and IL-18 and complement cause smooth muscle contraction and increase vascular permeability, amplify by C5a the inflammatory response and are chemoattractant. Soluble complement receptor-1 is an accepted, but underused treatment based on a placebo-controlled clinical trial with 59 patients (505).

A huge part of the ischemia–reperfusion injury of lung allografts is mediated by the change in vascular shear stress due to the blood flow cessation. The endothelial sensing mechanism called mechanosome chiefly consists of PECAM-1, VEGR receptor-2 (VEGFR2) and VE cadherin in the EC caveolae (499). It closes the K_{ATP} channel of the EC membrane, depolarizes it and leads to NADPH oxidase 2 activation as the main source to generate ROS. EC depolarization results in opening of T-type voltage-gated Ca^{2+} channels, increase intracellular calcium, and NO synthase activation and consecutive NO-mediated vasodilation, and an overproduction of ROS that causes oxidative injury which triggers inflammation or even cell death (499). PI3K-Akt leads to NADPH activation, producing ROS. With ischemia, there is also an NO production by endothelial NO synthase, probably as a physiological response to the loss of blood flow. The ROS generated in ECs interact with signaling-related proteins and thus with enzymatic activity. NF-ƙB, activator protein 1 (AP-1), and c-Jun and c-Fos and the redox-sensitive HIF-1α, Nrf2, ATR/CREB are increased (499). Even although PMN are then recruited into lungs, the production of ROS by the endothelium is the initial signal.

Reperfusion further activates NADPH oxidase-2 leading to lipid peroxidation, which can be several fold more extensive than ischemia alone. Opening of an inward K^+ channel was accompanied with hyperpolarization and ROS as well as NO production. Mainly a PMN influx and macrophage activation contribute to that injury. There is a strong correlation between excessive oxidative stress markers and the acute donor lung injury extent, and immunological rejection including later chronic rejection in terms of bronchitis obliterans syndrome as both the major causes for lung graft failure (499) (**Figure 9**).

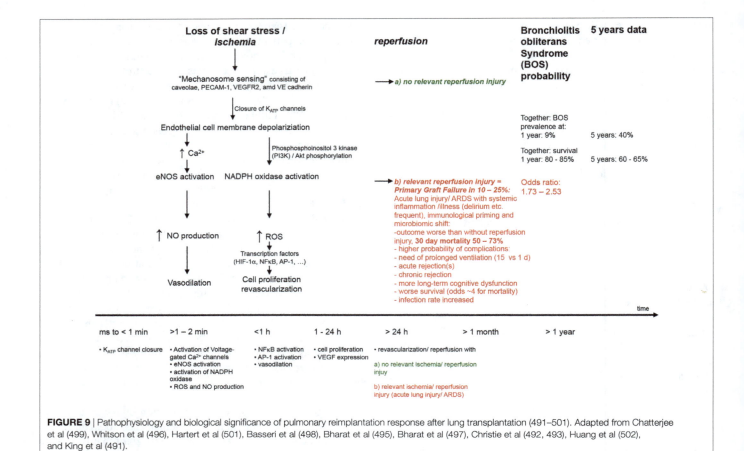

FIGURE 9 | Pathophysiology and biological significance of pulmonary reimplantation response after lung transplantation (491–501). Adapted from Chatterjee et al (499), Whitson et al (496), Hartert et al (501), Basseri et al (498), Bharat et al (495), Bharat et al (497), Christie et al (492, 493), Huang et al (502), and King et al (491).

The success of lung transplantation is much tempered by the limited organ supply. Many potential recipients are dying on the waiting list or being removed from the list because of clinical decline (506). Groups have therefore tried to expand the donor polls using extended criteria donors, with efforts to suggest rates of PGD, bronchiolitis obliterans syndrome, early morbidity and mortality to have equivalent to those with standard criteria donors (506). Most lung grafts come from brain-dead donors, but only about 15–20% of donors provide lungs that are satisfactory for lung transplantation (506). Strategies to expand the donor pool include the use of donation after cardiocirculatory death by doing a normothermic *ex vivo* lung perfusion (507), resulting in a study an about 28% increase in lungs suitable for transplantation. Problems are the increased risk of perioperative hypotension, warm ischemia time, a higher rate of aspiration, and more uncertainty to predict the lung's usability for transplantation. *Ex vivo* assessment and reconditioning might overcome some issues in the longer term (506) (**Figure 9**).

As shown before, using TNF tip peptide as preventative strategy in the left-sided unilateral orthotopic rat lung transplant model of prolonged cold ischemia we could show important biological effects, as highly severe lung injury with blood gas parameters qualifying for severe ARDS could be virtually prevented by the activation of the TNF lectin-like region (8) (**Figure 11**). The clinical pilot study of Aigner et al. suggests relevant improvement during established PGD by the TNF tip peptide (357). Both studies underline the biological potential of the TNF lectin-like region, i.e., the cytokine's ion channel activation, thus its potent modulation of ALI, and thus its potential effect to prevent untoward long-term effects.

Interstitial Lung Disease, Especially Acute Exacerbation of Idiopathic Pulmonary Fibrosis (aeIPF)

Idiopathic pulmonary fibrosis is a chronic and progressive lung disease of unknown etiology that occurs primarily in adults in their 50s and 60s and higher. Annual incidence is about 7–16 cases per 100,000 in the USA and 0.2 – 7 per 100,000 in Europe. Prognosis is severe with a median survival of about 2–3 years after diagnosis (508).

Acute exacerbation of idiopathic pulmonary fibrosis is a highly important disease progression of high morbidity and an extremely high mortality of 50–90% (509). It is typically reported to have an annual incidence of 5–15 or more %, with a higher incidence in advanced disease, and is defined as an acute worsening of dyspnea and lung function without an identifiable cause. Intriguingly, aeIPF has quite similar clinical features and similar prognosis compared with non-idiopathic causes of acute respiratory worsening in IPF such as infection or aspiration. It is, therefore, debated whether etiologies are to be separated (509).

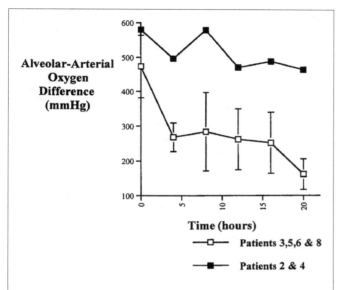

FIGURE 10 | Time course of mean AaPO2 after the onset of reperfusion pulmonary edema. Comparison of mean AaPO2 in four patients with intact alveolar epithelial fluid clearance (open squares) to the patients with no net alveolar epithelial fluid clearance (solid squares). The data for Patients 3, 5, 6, and 8 are expressed as mean 6 SD. The data for Patients 2 and 4 are expressed as the average of the AaPO2 at each time point (45).

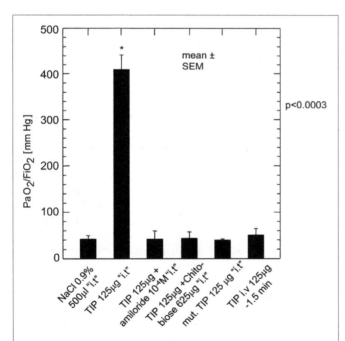

FIGURE 11 | Oxygenation at 24 h after transplantation. At sacrifice, 24 h after reperfusion of the left-sided lung transplant, the PaO2/FIO2 ratio was measured after excluding the native right-sided lung by clipping the right-sided stem bronchus and right-sided pulmonary artery. The animals were tracheotomized and ventilated with an FIO2 of 1.0. The tumor necrosis factor tip peptide significantly increased gas exchange compared with all other study groups. *$p < 0.003$ versus NaCl. Data are mean ± SEM. i.t., intratracheally (8).

There is some similarity between aeIPF and ARDS. However, the biological backgrounds are even much less understood. Gene expression profiles mainly show primarily infections or overwhelming inflammatory etiology, but more epithelial injury and proliferation as main profile, including gene expression of CCNA2, alpha-defensin, and apoptosis. Histopathologically, diffuse alveolar damage seems frequently observed in aeIPF. This finding is similar to ARDS and also has systemic multiorgan disease consequences, as evidenced by autopsy findings (510).

A number of current pharmacotherapies are under investigation for the therapeutic challenge of aeIPF as reviewed by Juarez et al., but no substance, combination of substances, or treatment modality (such as non-invasive ventilation which seems beneficial) has demonstrated such a clear benefit to become a new standard of therapy. This leaves clinicians with polypragmatic, mainly supportive care. Novel approaches are actually developed concerning immune suppression including calcineurin inhibitors, rituximab, removal of immune cells and mediators by either therapeutic plasma exchange or haemoperfusions with polymycin-B immobilized fibers aimed to remove not primarily endotoxin, but also contributing cytokines, and maybe hemostasis modulating agents such as intravenous recombinant thrombomodulin (508). The option of modulating the inflammation and to protect barrier function with, e.g., the biological action of TNF tip region is actually conceptualized in this group of severely sick patients.

Pre-eclampsia

Pre-eclampsia refers to the new onset of the combination of hypertension and proteinuria or of hypertension and end-organ dysfunction without or with proteinuria in previously normotensive pregnant women after at least 20 weeks of gestation. About 4–5% of pregnancies worldwide are complicated with pre-eclampsia, and first pregnancies are more frequently associated with this disease. Together with hemorrhage, thromboembolism, and cardiovascular disease, pre-eclampsia is one of the four leading causes of maternal death, accounting for 15% of them in the Western world. Prevalence is about 1 maternal death per 100,000 live births. When pre-eclampsia occurs, the fatality rate is about 6 per 10,000. Severe acute diastolic dysfunction in severe pre-eclampsia can lead to pulmonary edema in this patient group. Maternal and fetal/placental factors seem responsible, such as abnormal trophoblast invasion of the spiral arteria of the decidua and myometrium early in pregnancy, a suboptimal uteroplacental blood flow possibly leading to high oxidative placental stress, altering placental angiogenesis, poor feto-placental vasculature and abnormal vascular reactivity. Endothelial dysfunction can be caused by systemic anti-angiogenic signals by anti-angiogenic factors. Elevated levels of soluble fms-like tyrosine kinase 1 (sFlt-1; an inhibitor of vascular endothelial growth factor), reduced levels of placental growth factor (PlGF), and an increased sFlt-1:PlGF ratio have been reported both in women with established pre-eclampsia and in women before the development of pre-eclampsia (511). This is moreover accompanied by increased pro-inflammatory cytokine production, which in turn promotes renal and pulmonary barrier dysfunction and impaired ion channel activity. As a consequence, pulmonary edema is a severe feature of the disease. In this case, the edema can be multifactorial, due to left heart failure, and thus excessive pulmonary vascular hydrostatic pressure, to decreased plasma oncotic pressure, to capillary leak, or to iatrogenic volume overload (511, 512).

High-Altitude Pulmonary Edema

About 100 million people live at altitudes greater than 2,500 m, about 15 million above 3,000 m, and some above 5,000 m (384). Most have developed the ability to live and reproduce at elevation as high as 5,000 m, but in some cases, develop chronic medical problems due to their high-altitude residence. At 5,500 m the pressure is about only half the normal. Furthermore, many lowlanders venture to high altitude for work and recreation. These more acute exposures also pose the hazards of acute altitude illness, e.g., in Colorado skiers in 15–40% of them with an incidence of HAPE then of 0.1–1%. The prevalence of HAPE depends on an individual's susceptibility, the rate of ascent, the final altitude, but also heavy and prolonged exercise, and is higher in male. At altitudes of 4,500 m the prevalence is between 0.2 and 6%, and at 5,500 m between 2 and 15% (385). Many adaptive processes can vastly reduce the risk of such sickness. Susceptibility to altitude illness varies considerably between individuals, but for a single individual, the symptoms are often reproducible given the same rate of ascent. High-altitude pulmonary odemea is the most important complication of high-altitude illness and its most common cause of death. It typically manifests with 2–4 days of ascent to altitudes above 2,400 m, most commonly beginning on the second night. In the early stage of disease, decreased exercise performance occurs and individuals require increased amount of time to recover from exertions. Individuals also complained of fatigue, weakness, and persistent dry cough, possibly combined with symptoms of acute sickness. As the disease progresses, individuals become short of breath with minimal exertion. Dyspnea at rest, audible chest congestion, generalized pallor, nail bed cyanosis and production of pink frothy sputum are late findings in severe disease. Even in the absence of concurrent high-altitude cerebral edema, severe hypoxemia may produce mental changes, ataxia, and altered levels of consciousness. In general blood gas analysis reveals severe hypoxemia. Pulmonary arterial pressure is high, but pulmonary wedge pressure is normal, and heart size is not increased. Although the mechanism underlying HAPE remains incompletely understood, it appears that the elevated pulmonary artery pressure plays a pivotal role in the process. Multiple studies demonstrated that susceptible individuals have abnormally high pulmonary artery pressure in response to hypoxic breathing, during normoxic and hypoxic exercise, and on high altitude before the onset of edema. Increased sympathetic tone, and alteration in vasoactive mediators-like endothelin-1, NO produced by pulmonary ECs may also lead to stronger hypoxic pulmonary vasoconstriction (384). In autopsies, a red cell rich proteinaceous alveolar exudate with hyaline membrane is characteristic. In all autopsies, areas of pneumonitis with neutrophil accumulation but no evidence of bacterial accumulation has been observed. Most reports mentioned capillary and arterial thrombi, fibrin deposits, hemorrhage, and infarcts. Uneven hypoxic vasoconstriction is discussed. Uneven perfusion is suggested clinically by the typical patchy radiographic appearance and by MRI studies in patients together with hypoxic blood gas parameters which demonstrates greater heterogeneous regional perfusion in HAPE-susceptible subjects (384). The estimated death rate of altitude illness is about 7.7/100,000 trekkers, with increasing mortality during the last decade (386).

Treatment of HAPE consists, if ever possible, in descent from altitude, rest, oxygen supplementation, and administration of drugs such as corticosteroids and furosemide.

Prophylactic inhalation the β2AR agonist salmeterol decreased the HAPE incidence by more than 50% (387). The most pertinent explanation was that salmeterol would enhance the clearance of alveolar fluid since β-adrenergic agonists upregulate the clearance of alveolar fluid by stimulating transepithelial sodium transport. This hypothesis is supported by the fact that the level of sodium transport in the respiratory epithelium is lower in patients susceptible to HAPE. However, the study results cannot exclude the possibility that the beta2 agonist could have modulated vascular permeability or the hemodynamic response associated with hypoxemia and HAPE (4).

In an experimental rat model simulating HAPE by hypobaric and hypoxic conditions equivalent to an altitude of 4,500 m with exhaustive treadmill exercise of 15 m per minute for 24 h, then for an equivalent of altitude of 6,000 m for further 48 h, it has been shown that the TNF tip peptide reduced pulmonary edema and increased the TJ occluding expression compared to high-altitude controls, dexamethasone, and aminophylline treated control animals (7). Compared to untreated high-altitude control animals, TNF tip peptide significantly lowered levels of the inflammatory cytokines TNF, IL-1β, IL-6 and IL-8 in bronchoalveolar lavage. TNF tip peptide-treated animals experienced less pulmonary edema also compared to dexamethasone-treated animals, and was more effective than its comparators in reduction of bronchoalveolar lavage protein content and inflammatory parameters (7). The higher expression of occludin may have translated in an increased stability of the alveolar–capillary barrier, probably related to the reduction in the extent of protein leakage in TNF tip peptide-treated animals. The results suggest that the biologic potential of the TNF tip region is more active in this model than dexamethasone as standard therapy on one hand, and as the glucocorticosteroids (7). The model suggests that HAPE can be treated with TNF tip peptide at least in a part of patients affected, and clinical studies are underway.

However, inhaled budesonide seems not consistently able to prevent acute mountain sickness and HAPE (513).

SUMMARY AND CONCLUSION

Alveolar fluid reabsorption is of high clinical importance in both cardiac and non-cardiac edema. Clinically, a conservative fluid strategy in ARDS patients resulted in more ventilator-free days (514). There is evidence that lower vascular pressures reduce pro-inflammatory pathways (515), and in chronic hydrostatic pulmonary edema tissue remodeling ensues (516).

Recent studies of cytokine-ion channel interactions have clearly shown that the concept of ion channel modulation to improve AFC has to be broadened, also taking into account previously ignored functions of these mediators. The concept of active interactions between barrier function and ion transporters to maintain lung fluid balance plays a pivotal biological role. TNF's lectin-like domain, mimicked by the TNF tip peptide, was demonstrated to strengthen capillary barrier function in the presence of bacterial toxins in vitro and in vivo. Indeed, influx, efflux, and tightness of the EC layer are all biologically interrelated. Such a relationship is also present in the alveolar epithelium with interactions with ion transporters and TJs (11). These observations suggest that the biologic potential of ion channel modulation with drugs or peptides is more relevant than initially presumed.

A conceptual problem in ALI and other inflammatory conditions is how fluid reabsorption can function in such an "un-tight system" as in partially destroyed endothelial-interstitial or interstitial-alveolar barriers, and what is the expression level of ion channels in those conditions (25). The same may hold true in the context of hypoxia and the decreased expression of ENaC. Regeneration and repair of injured, apoptotic or necrotic endothelial or AECs can be fostered endogenously by local or bone-marrow derived precursors or by exogenously administered factors, as formerly studied in animal models using progenitor cell populations and stimulants. Clinical refinements are underway and update outcome parameters, such as AFC (517).

In clinical situations with cardiogenic as well as with non-cardiogenic pulmonary edema, i.e., ALI and ARDS, we have to be extremely cautious with prescribing drugs that might interfere with alveolar fluid transports or inflammation. Furosemide might further be the mainstay of diuretic drug and the alveolar flooding stopper especially in cardiogenic edema due to its effect on NKCC1 and CFTR. Amiloride should not be taken. Many clinical questions will be open around beta blocking agents as well as beta stimulating agents in the context of pulmonary edema and will probably depend on their indication. cAMP may play some role, but from which point those two drug classes are counterproductive, remains actually open.

There has been much work focused on one ion channel without considering the interconnection between major biological ion channels or its modulators, which may limit the validity of conclusions or findings of much published work. In future research it would be important to try to better integrate these channels, as well as their interactions with cytokines present in the lung milieu during the various pathologies. Many parallels exist between different organ systems and ion channels, underlining that interdisciplinary network is promising.

As shown in lung transplant primary graft failure, and thus probably also true in ARDS, ALI causes important and systemic long-term injury, especially brain injury. The critical step of high ethical impact for the scientific community is to expand integrative translational research in terms of clinical investigation with the known targets to improve clinical outcome. This is especially important in lung transplantation, as donor shortage still leaves many patients worldwide dying without this therapeutic option, and possibly in ALI and ARDS.

AUTHOR CONTRIBUTIONS

All authors significantly contributed to the conceptual work, the writing and editing of the work.

ACKNOWLEDGMENTS

The authors acknowledge Sarah Lea Hipp, Graphics and Typography, www.sarahleahipp.ch, for designing and providing the **Figures 2, 4–8**. The authors also acknowledge the financial support of the Lungen-und Atmungsstiftung, Bern. The work is dedicated to Ellen Hamacher who died during the finalization of the manuscript.

REFERENCES

1. Staub NC. Pulmonary edema. *Physiol Rev* (1974) 54(3):678–811.
2. Ware LB, Matthay MA. Clinical practice. Acute pulmonary edema. *N Engl J Med* (2005) 353(26):2788–96. doi:10.1056/NEJMcp052699
3. Weibel ER, Taylor CR. Design and structure of the human lung. In: Fishman A, editor. *Pulmonary Diseases and Disorders*. New York: McGraw-Hill (1988). p. 11–60.
4. Berthiaume Y, Matthay MA. Alveolar edema fluid clearance and acute lung injury. *Respir Physiol Neurobiol* (2007) 159(3):350–9. doi:10.1016/j.resp.2007.05.010
5. Weidenfeld S, Kuebler WM. Cytokine-regulation of Na+-K+-Cl- cotransporter 1 and cystic fibrosis transmembrane conductance regulator-potential role in pulmonary inflammation and edema formation. *Front Immunol* (2017) 8:393. doi:10.3389/fimmu.2017.00393
6. Hoffman O, Burns N, Vadasz I, Eltzschig HK, Edwards MG, Vohwinkel CU. Detrimental ELAVL-1/HuR-dependent GSK3beta mRNA stabilization impairs resolution in acute respiratory distress syndrome. *PLoS One* (2017) 12(2):e0172116. doi:10.1371/journal.pone.0172116
7. Zhou Q, Wang D, Liu Y, Yang X, Lucas R, Fischer B. Solnatide demonstrates profound therapeutic activity in a rat model of pulmonary edema induced by acute hypobaric hypoxia and exercise. *Chest* (2017) 151(3):658–67. doi:10.1016/j.chest.2016.10.030
8. Hamacher J, Stammberger U, Roux J, Kumar S, Yang G, Xiong C, et al. The lectin-like domain of tumor necrosis factor improves lung function after rat lung transplantation – potential role for a reduction in reactive oxygen species generation. *Crit Care Med* (2010) 38(3):871–8. doi:10.1097/CCM.0b013e3181cdf725
9. Czikora I, Alli AA, Sridhar S, Matthay MA, Pillich H, Hudel M, et al. Epithelial sodium channel-α mediates the protective effect of the TNF-derived TIP peptide in pneumolysin-induced endothelial barrier dysfunction. *Front Immunol* (2017) 8:842. doi:10.3389/fimmu.2017.00842
10. Lucas R, Yang G, Gorshkov BA, Zemskov EA, Sridhar S, Umapathy NS, et al. Protein kinase C-alpha and arginase I mediate pneumolysin-induced pulmonary endothelial hyperpermeability. *Am J Respir Cell Mol Biol* (2012) 47(4):445–53. doi:10.1165/rcmb.2011-0332OC
11. Brune K, Frank J, Schwingshackl A, Finigan J, Sidhaye VK. Pulmonary epithelial barrier function: some new players and mechanisms. *Am J Physiol Lung Cell Mol Physiol* (2015) 308(8):L731–45. doi:10.1152/ajplung.00309.2014
12. Hummler E, Barker P, Gatzy J, Beermann F, Verdumo C, Schmidt A, et al. Early death due to defective neonatal lung liquid clearance in alpha-ENaC-deficient mice. *Nat Genet* (1996) 12(3):325–8. doi:10.1038/ng0396-325

13. Huppmann S, Lankes E, Schnabel D, Buhrer C. Unimpaired postnatal respiratory adaptation in a preterm human infant with a homozygous ENaC-alpha unit loss-of-function mutation. *J Perinatol* (2011) 31(12):802–3. doi:10.1038/jp.2011.46

14. O'Brodovich H. Pulmonary edema in infants and children. *Curr Opin Pediatr* (2005) 17(3):381–4. doi:10.1097/01.mop.0000159780.42572.6c

15. Verghese GM, Ware LB, Matthay BA, Matthay MA. Alveolar epithelial fluid transport and the resolution of clinically severe hydrostatic pulmonary edema. *J Appl Physiol (1985)* (1999) 87(4):1301–12.

16. Solymosi EA, Kaestle-Gembardt SM, Vadasz I, Wang L, Neye N, Chupin CJ, et al. Chloride transport-driven alveolar fluid secretion is a major contributor to cardiogenic lung edema. *Proc Natl Acad Sci U S A* (2013) 110(25): E2308–16. doi:10.1073/pnas.1216382110

17. Matthay MA, Clerici C. Alveolar epithelial and fluid transport. In: Broaddus VC, Mason RJ, Ernst JD, King TE Jr., Lazarus SC, Murray JF, Nadel JA, Slutsky SA, Gotway MB, editors. *Murray & Nadel's Textbook of Respiratory Medicine*. Philadelphia: Elsevier Saunders (2016). p. 150–6.

18. Ribeiro CM, Marchiori E, Rodrigues R, Gasparetto E, Souza AS Jr., Escuissato D, et al. Hydrostatic pulmonary edema: high-resolution computed tomography aspects. *J Bras Pneumol* (2006) 32(6):515–22. doi:10.1590/S1806-37132006000600008

19. Platz E, Jhund PS, Campbell RT, McMurray JJ. Assessment and prevalence of pulmonary oedema in contemporary acute heart failure trials: a systematic review. *Eur J Heart Fail* (2015) 17(9):906–16. doi:10.1002/ejhf.321

20. Roger VL. Epidemiology of heart failure. *Circ Res* (2013) 113(6):646–59. doi:10.1161/circresaha.113.300268

21. Azzam ZS, Kinaneh S, Bahouth F, Ismael-Badarneh R, Khoury E, Abassi Z. Involvement of cytokines in the pathogenesis of salt and water imbalance in congestive heart failure. *Front Immunol* (2017) 8:716. doi:10.3389/fimmu.2017.00716

22. Gray A, Goodacre S, Newby DE, Masson M, Sampson F, Nicholl J, et al. Noninvasive ventilation in acute cardiogenic pulmonary edema. *N Engl J Med* (2008) 359(2):142–51. doi:10.1056/NEJMoa0707992

23. Bove PF, Grubb BR, Okada SF, Ribeiro CM, Rogers TD, Randell SH, et al. Human alveolar type II cells secrete and absorb liquid in response to local nucleotide signaling. *J Biol Chem* (2010) 285(45):34939–49. doi:10.1074/jbc.M110.162933

24. Schmieder RE, Messerli FH, deCarvalho JG, Husserl FE. Immediate hemodynamic response to furosemide in patients undergoing chronic hemodialysis. *Am J Kidney Dis* (1987) 9(1):55–9. doi:10.1016/S0272-6386(87)80162-2

25. Matthay MA. Resolution of pulmonary edema. Thirty years of progress. *Am J Respir Crit Care Med* (2014) 189(11):1301–8. doi:10.1164/rccm.201403-0535OE

26. Lourenco P, Paulo Araujo J, Paulo C, Mascarenhas J, Frioes F, Azevedo A, et al. Higher C-reactive protein predicts worse prognosis in acute heart failure only in noninfected patients. *Clin Cardiol* (2010) 33(11):708–14. doi:10.1002/clc.20812

27. Mann DL, McMurray JJ, Packer M, Swedberg K, Borer JS, Colucci WS, et al. Targeted anticytokine therapy in patients with chronic heart failure: results of the Randomized Etanercept Worldwide Evaluation (RENEWAL). *Circulation* (2004) 109(13):1594–602. doi:10.1161/01.CIR.0000124490.27666.B2

28. Chung ES, Packer M, Lo KH, Fasanmade AA, Willerson JT, Anti-TNF Therapy Against Congestive Heart Failure Investigators. Randomized, double-blind, placebo-controlled, pilot trial of infliximab, a chimeric monoclonal antibody to tumor necrosis factor-alpha, in patients with moderate-to-severe heart failure: results of the anti-TNF Therapy Against Congestive Heart Failure (ATTACH) trial. *Circulation* (2003) 107(25):3133–40. doi:10.1161/01.CIR.0000077913.60364.D2

29. Cacciapaglia F, Salvatorelli E, Minotti G, Afeltra A, Menna P. Low level tumor necrosis factor-alpha protects cardiomyocytes against high level tumor necrosis factor-alpha: brief insight into a beneficial paradox. *Cardiovasc Toxicol* (2014) 14(4):387–92. doi:10.1007/s12012-014-9257-z

30. De Vito P. The sodium/hydrogen exchanger: a possible mediator of immunity. *Cell Immunol* (2006) 240(2):69–85. doi:10.1016/j.cellimm.2006.07.001

31. Thompson BT, Chambers RC, Liu KD. Acute respiratory distress syndrome. *N Engl J Med* (2017) 377(6):562–72. doi:10.1056/NEJMra1608077

32. Pittet JF, Mackersie RC, Martin TR, Matthay MA. Biological markers of acute lung injury: prognostic and pathogenetic significance. *Am J Respir Crit Care Med* (1997) 155(4):1187–205. doi:10.1164/ajrccm.155.4.9105054

33. Ware LB, Matthay MA. Alveolar fluid clearance is impaired in the majority of patients with acute lung injury and the acute respiratory distress syndrome. *Am J Respir Crit Care Med* (2001) 163(6):1376–83. doi:10.1164/ajrccm.163.6.2004035

34. Millar FR, Summers C, Griffiths MJ, Toshner MR, Proudfoot AG. The pulmonary endothelium in acute respiratory distress syndrome: insights and therapeutic opportunities. *Thorax* (2016) 71(5):462–73. doi:10.1136/thoraxjnl-2015-207461

35. Khan SU, Salloum J, O'Donovan PB, Mascha EJ, Mehta AC, Matthay MA, et al. Acute pulmonary edema after lung transplantation: the pulmonary reimplantation response. *Chest* (1999) 116(1):187–94. doi:10.1378/chest.116.1.187

36. Frank JA, Matthay MA. TGF-beta and lung fluid balance in ARDS. *Proc Natl Acad Sci U S A* (2014) 111(3):885–6. doi:10.1073/pnas.1322478111

37. Braun C, Hamacher J, Morel DR, Wendel A, Lucas R. Dichotomal role of TNF in experimental pulmonary edema reabsorption. *J Immunol* (2005) 175(5):3402–8. doi:10.4049/jimmunol.175.5.3402

38. Yang G, Hamacher J, Gorshkov B, White R, Sridhar S, Verin A, et al. The dual role of TNF in pulmonary edema. *J Cardiovasc Dis Res* (2010) 1(1):29–36. doi:10.4103/0975-3583.59983

39. Hamacher J, Lucas R, Lijnen HR, Buschke S, Dunant Y, Wendel A, et al. Tumor necrosis factor-alpha and angiostatin are mediators of endothelial cytotoxicity in bronchoalveolar lavages of patients with acute respiratory distress syndrome. *Am J Respir Crit Care Med* (2002) 166(5):651–6. doi:10.1164/rccm.2109004

40. Matute-Bello G, Liles WC, Frevert CW, Dhanireddy S, Ballman K, Wong V, et al. Blockade of the Fas/FasL system improves pneumococcal clearance from the lungs without preventing dissemination of bacteria to the spleen. *J Infect Dis* (2005) 191(4):596–606. doi:10.1086/427261

41. Chen W, Janz DR, Bastarache JA, May AK, O'Neal HR Jr., Bernard GR, et al. Prehospital aspirin use is associated with reduced risk of acute respiratory distress syndrome in critically ill patients: a propensity-adjusted analysis. *Crit Care Med* (2015) 43(4):801–7. doi:10.1097/CCM.0000000000000789

42. Sznajder JI. Alveolar edema must be cleared for the acute respiratory distress syndrome patient to survive. *Am J Respir Crit Care Med* (2001) 163(6): 1293–4. doi:10.1164/ajrccm.163.6.ed1801d

43. Matthay MA, Zemans RL. The acute respiratory distress syndrome: pathogenesis and treatment. *Annu Rev Pathol* (2011) 6:147–63. doi:10.1146/annurev-pathol-011110-130158

44. Zeyed YF, Bastarache JA, Matthay MA, Ware LB. The severity of shock is associated with impaired rates of net alveolar fluid clearance in clinical acute lung injury. *Am J Physiol Lung Cell Mol Physiol* (2012) 303(6):L550–5. doi:10.1152/ajplung.00190.2012

45. Ware LB, Golden JA, Finkbeiner WE, Matthay MA. Alveolar epithelial fluid transport capacity in reperfusion lung injury after lung transplantation. *Am J Respir Crit Care Med* (1999) 159(3):980–8. doi:10.1164/ajrccm.159.3.9802105

46. Matthay MA, Folkesson HG, Clerici C. Lung epithelial fluid transport and the resolution of pulmonary edema. *Physiol Rev* (2002) 82(3):569–600. doi:10.1152/physrev.00003.2002

47. Johnson MD, Widdicombe JH, Allen L, Barbry P, Dobbs LG. Alveolar epithelial type I cells contain transport proteins and transport sodium, supporting an active role for type I cells in regulation of lung liquid homeostasis. *Proc Natl Acad Sci U S A* (2002) 99(4):1966–71. doi:10.1073/pnas.042689399

48. Ma T, Fukuda N, Song Y, Matthay MA, Verkman AS. Lung fluid transport in aquaporin-5 knockout mice. *J Clin Invest* (2000) 105(1):93–100. doi:10.1172/JCI8258

49. Clements JA. Lung surfactant: a personal perspective. *Annu Rev Physiol* (1997) 59:1–21. doi:10.1146/annurev.physiol.59.1.1

50. Berthiaume Y, Lesur O, Dagenais A. Treatment of adult respiratory distress syndrome: plea for rescue therapy of the alveolar epithelium. *Thorax* (1999) 54(2):150–60. doi:10.1136/thx.54.2.150

51. Matalon ST, Shoenfeld Y, Blank M, Yacobi S, Blumenfeld Z, Ornoy A. The effects of IgG purified from women with SLE and associated pregnancy loss on rat embryos in culture. *Am J Reprod Immunol* (2002) 48(5):296–304. doi:10.1034/j.1600-0897.2002.01084.x

52. Althaus M, Clauss WG, Fronius M. Amiloride-sensitive sodium channels and pulmonary edema. *Pulm Med* (2011) 2011:830320. doi:10.1155/2011/830320

53. Althaus M, Pichl A, Clauss WG, Seeger W, Fronius M, Morty RE. Nitric oxide inhibits highly selective sodium channels and the Na+/K+-ATPase in H441 cells. *Am J Respir Cell Mol Biol* (2011) 44(1):53–65. doi:10.1165/2009-0335oc

54. Czikora I, Alli A, Bao HF, Kaftan D, Sridhar S, Apell HJ, et al. A novel tumor necrosis factor-mediated mechanism of direct epithelial sodium channel activation. *Am J Respir Crit Care Med* (2014) 190(5):522–32. doi:10.1164/rccm.201405-0833OC

55. Gon Y, Wood MR, Kiosses WB, Jo E, Sanna MG, Chun J, et al. S1P3 receptor-induced reorganization of epithelial tight junctions compromises lung barrier integrity and is potentiated by TNF. *Proc Natl Acad Sci U S A* (2005) 102(26):9270–5. doi:10.1073/pnas.0501997102

56. Bachofen M, Weibel ER. Alterations of the gas exchange apparatus in adult respiratory insufficiency associated with septicemia 1, 2. *Am J Respir Crit Care Med* (1977) 116(4):589–615. doi:10.1164/arrd.1977.116.4.589

57. Matute-Bello G, Liles WC, Steinberg KP, Kiener PA, Mongovin S, Chi EY, et al. Soluble Fas ligand induces epithelial cell apoptosis in humans with acute lung injury (ARDS). *J Immunol* (1999) 163(4):2217–25.

58. Martin TR, Hagimoto N, Nakamura M, Matute-Bello G. Apoptosis and epithelial injury in the lungs. *Proc Am Thorac Soc* (2005) 2(3):214–20. doi:10.1513/pats.200504-031AC

59. Hamilton BC, Kukreja J, Ware LB, Matthay MA. Protein biomarkers associated with primary graft dysfunction following lung transplantation. *Am J Physiol Lung Cell Mol Physiol* (2017) 312(4):L531–41. doi:10.1152/ajplung.00454.2016

60. Sharp C, Millar AB, Medford AR. Advances in understanding of the pathogenesis of acute respiratory distress syndrome. *Respiration* (2015) 89(5):420–34. doi:10.1159/000381102

61. Patterson CE, Lum H. Update on pulmonary edema: the role and regulation of endothelial barrier function. *Endothelium* (2001) 8(2):75–105. doi:10.3109/10623320109165319

62. Trzeciak S, Dellinger RP, Parrillo JE, Guglielmi M, Bajaj J, Abate NL, et al. Early microcirculatory perfusion derangements in patients with severe sepsis and septic shock: relationship to hemodynamics, oxygen transport, and survival. *Ann Emerg Med* (2007) 49(1):e1–2. doi:10.1016/j.annemergmed.2006.08.021

63. Nuckton TJ, Alonso JA, Kallet RH, Daniel BM, Pittet JF, Eisner MD, et al. Pulmonary dead-space fraction as a risk factor for death in the acute respiratory distress syndrome. *N Engl J Med* (2002) 346(17):1281–6. doi:10.1056/NEJMoa012835

64. Gill SE, Rohan M, Mehta S. Role of pulmonary microvascular endothelial cell apoptosis in murine sepsis-induced lung injury in vivo. *Respir Res* (2015) 16:109. doi:10.1186/s12931-015-0266-7

65. Mutunga M, Fulton B, Bullock R, Batchelor A, Gascoigne A, Gillespie JI, et al. Circulating endothelial cells in patients with septic shock. *Am J Respir Crit Care Med* (2001) 163(1):195–200. doi:10.1164/ajrccm.163.1.9912036

66. Dudek SM, Garcia JG. Cytoskeletal regulation of pulmonary vascular permeability. *J Appl Physiol (1985)* (2001) 91(4):1487–500.

67. Petrache I, Birukova A, Ramirez SI, Garcia JG, Verin AD. The role of the microtubules in tumor necrosis factor-alpha-induced endothelial cell permeability. *Am J Respir Cell Mol Biol* (2003) 28(5):574–81. doi:10.1165/rcmb.2002-0075OC

68. Lucas R, Verin AD, Black SM, Catravas JD. Regulators of endothelial and epithelial barrier integrity and function in acute lung injury. *Biochem Pharmacol* (2009) 77(12):1763–72. doi:10.1016/j.bcp.2009.01.014

69. Delany NS, Hurle M, Facer P, Alnadaf T, Plumpton C, Kinghorn I, et al. Identification and characterization of a novel human vanilloid receptor-like protein, VRL-2. *Physiol Genomics* (2001) 4(3):165–74.

70. Stevens T. Functional and molecular heterogeneity of pulmonary endothelial cells. *Proc Am Thorac Soc* (2011) 8(6):453–7. doi:10.1513/pats.201101-004MW

71. Herold S, Gabrielli NM, Vadasz I. Novel concepts of acute lung injury and alveolar-capillary barrier dysfunction. *Am J Physiol Lung Cell Mol Physiol* (2013) 305(10):L665–81. doi:10.1152/ajplung.00232.2013

72. Alberts B, Johnson A, Lewis J, Morgan D, Raff M, Roberts K, et al. *Molecular Biology of the Cell*. New York: Garland Science. Taylor & Francis Group (2014).

73. Sznajder JI, Factor P, Ingbar DH. Invited review: lung edema clearance: role of Na(+)-K(+)-ATPase. *J Appl Physiol (1985)* (2002) 93(5):1860–6. doi:10.1152/japplphysiol.00022.2002

74. Purves D, Augustine G, Fitzpatrick D. Neuroscience. In: Purves D, Augustine G, Fitzpatrick D, Katz L, LaMatina A, McNamara J, Williams S, editors. *Active*

Transporters Create and Maintain Ion Gradients. 2nd ed. Sunderland: Sinauer Associates (2001). p. 86–7.

75. Vivona ML, Matthay M, Chabaud MB, Friedlander G, Clerici C. Hypoxia reduces alveolar epithelial sodium and fluid transport in rats: reversal by beta-adrenergic agonist treatment. *Am J Respir Cell Mol Biol* (2001) 25(5):554–61. doi:10.1165/ajrcmb.25.5.4420

76. Urner M, Herrmann IK, Booy C, Roth-Z' Graggen B, Maggiorini M, Beck-Schimmer B. Effect of hypoxia and dexamethasone on inflammation and ion transporter function in pulmonary cells. *Clin Exp Immunol* (2012) 169(2):119–28. doi:10.1111/j.1365-2249.2012.04595.x

77. Gille T, Randrianarison-Pellan N, Goolaerts A, Dard N, Uzunhan Y, Ferrary E, et al. Hypoxia-induced inhibition of epithelial Na(+) channels in the lung. Role of Nedd4-2 and the ubiquitin-proteasome pathway. *Am J Respir Cell Mol Biol* (2014) 50(3):526–37. doi:10.1165/rcmb.2012-0518OC

78. Vadasz I, Raviv S, Sznajder JI. Alveolar epithelium and Na,K-ATPase in acute lung injury. *Intensive Care Med* (2007) 33(7):1243–51. doi:10.1007/s00134-007-0661-8

79. Gwozdzinska P, Buchbinder BA, Mayer K, Herold S, Morty RE, Seeger W, et al. Hypercapnia impairs ENaC Cell surface stability by promoting phosphorylation, polyubiquitination and endocytosis of beta-ENaC in a human alveolar epithelial cell line. *Front Immunol* (2017) 8:591. doi:10.3389/fimmu.2017.00591

80. Vadasz I, Sznajder JI. Gas exchange disturbances regulate alveolar fluid clearance during acute lung injury. *Front Immunol* (2017) 8:757. doi:10.3389/fimmu.2017.00757

81. Kohnlein T, Windisch W, Kohler D, Drabik A, Geiseler J, Hartl S, et al. Non-invasive positive pressure ventilation for the treatment of severe stable chronic obstructive pulmonary disease: a prospective, multicentre, randomised, controlled clinical trial. *Lancet Respir Med* (2014) 2(9):698–705. doi:10.1016/S2213-2600(14)70153-5

82. Windisch W, Storre JH, Kohnlein T. Nocturnal non-invasive positive pressure ventilation for COPD. *Expert Rev Respir Med* (2015) 9(3):295–308. doi:10.1586/17476348.2015.1035260

83. Schwarz SB, Magnet FS, Windisch W. Why high-intensity nppv is favourable to low-intensity NPPV: clinical and physiological reasons. *COPD* (2017) 14(4):389–95. doi:10.1080/15412555.2017.1318843

84. Jentsch TJ, Hubner CA, Fuhrmann JC. Ion channels: function unravelled by dysfunction. *Nat Cell Biol* (2004) 6(11):1039–47. doi:10.1038/ncb1104-1039

85. Hübner CA, Jentsch TJ. Ion channel diseases. *Hum Mol Genet* (2002) 11(20):2435–45. doi:10.1093/hmg/11.20.2435

86. Eaton DC, Helms MN, Koval M, Bao HF, Jain L. The contribution of epithelial sodium channels to alveolar function in health and disease. *Annu Rev Physiol* (2009) 71:403–23. doi:10.1146/annurev.physiol.010908.163250

87. Canessa CM, Horisberger JD, Rossier BC. Epithelial sodium channel related to proteins involved in neurodegeneration. *Nature* (1993) 361(6411):467–70. doi:10.1038/361467a0

88. Kellenberger S, Schild L. International union of basic and clinical pharmacology. XCI. structure, function, and pharmacology of acid-sensing ion channels and the epithelial Na+ channel. *Pharmacol Rev* (2015) 67(1):1–35. doi:10.1124/pr.114.009225

89. Canessa CM, Schild L, Buell G, Thorens B, Gautschi I, Horisberger JD, et al. Amiloride-sensitive epithelial Na+ channel is made of three homologous subunits. *Nature* (1994) 367(6462):463–7. doi:10.1038/367463a0

90. Waldmann R, Champigny G, Bassilana F, Voilley N, Lazdunski M. Molecular cloning and functional expression of a novel amiloride-sensitive Na+ channel. *J Biol Chem* (1995) 270(46):27411–4. doi:10.1074/jbc.270.46.27411

91. Ji HL, Su XF, Kedar S, Li J, Barbry P, Smith PR, et al. Delta-subunit confers novel biophysical features to alpha beta gamma-human epithelial sodium channel (ENaC) via a physical interaction. *J Biol Chem* (2006) 281(12):8233–41. doi:10.1074/jbc.M512293200

92. Matalon S, Lazrak A, Jain L, Eaton DC. Invited review: biophysical properties of sodium channels in lung alveolar epithelial cells. *J Appl Physiol (1985)* (2002) 93(5):1852–9. doi:10.1152/japplphysiol.01241.2001

93. McNicholas CM, Canessa CM. Diversity of channels generated by different combinations of epithelial sodium channel subunits. *J Gen Physiol* (1997) 109(6):681–92. doi:10.1085/jgp.109.6.681

94. Chalfant M, Denton J, Langloh A, Karlson K, Loffing J, Benos D, et al. The NH2 terminus of the epithelial sodium channel contains an endocytic motif. *J Biol Chem* (1999) 274:32889–96. doi:10.1074/jbc.274.46.32889

95. Ji H-L, Zhao R-Z, Chen Z-X, Shetty S, Idell S, Matalon S. δ ENaC: a novel divergent amiloride-inhibitable sodium channel. *Am J Physiol Lung Cell Mol Physiol* (2012) 303(12):L1013–26. doi:10.1152/ajplung.00206.2012

96. Guidot DM, Folkesson HG, Jain L, Sznajder JI, Pittet J-F, Matthay MA. Integrating acute lung injury and regulation of alveolar fluid clearance. *Am J Physiol Lung Cell Mol Physiol* (2006) 291(3):L301. doi:10.1152/ajplung.00153.2006

97. Czikora I, Sridhar S, Alli A, Verin A, Chakraborty T, Fulton D, et al. ENaC-a mediates the protective effect of the TNF-derived TIP peptide in pneumolysin-induced capillary barrier dysfunction. *FASEB J* (2017) 31(1 Suppl):978.6.

98. Garty H, Palmer LG. Epithelial sodium channels: function, structure, and regulation. *Physiol Rev* (1997) 77(2):359–96.

99. Elia N, Tapponnier M, Matthay MA, Hamacher J, Pache JC, Brundler MA, et al. Functional identification of the alveolar edema reabsorption activity of murine tumor necrosis factor-alpha. *Am J Respir Crit Care Med* (2003) 168(9):1043–50. doi:10.1164/rccm.200206-618OC

100. Hazemi P, Tzotzos SJ, Fischer B, Andavan GSB, Fischer H, Pietschmann H, et al. Essential structural features of TNF-α lectin-like domain derived peptides for activation of amiloride-sensitive sodium current in A549 cells. *J Med Chem* (2010) 53(22):8021–9. doi:10.1021/jm100767p

101. Sugita M, Ferraro P, Dagenais A, Clermont ME, Barbry P, Michel RP, et al. Alveolar liquid clearance and sodium channel expression are decreased in transplanted canine lungs. *Am J Respir Crit Care Med* (2003) 167(10): 1440–50. doi:10.1164/rccm.200204-312OC

102. Lucas R, Yue Q, Alli A, Duke BJ, Al-Khalili O, Thai TL, et al. The lectin-like domain of TNF increases ENaC open probability through a novel site at the interface between the second transmembrane and C-terminal domains of the alpha-subunit. *J Biol Chem* (2016) 291(45):23440–51. doi:10.1074/jbc.M116.718163

103. Trac PT, Thai TL, Linck V, Zou L, Greenlee M, Yue Q, et al. Alveolar nonselective channels are ASIC1a/alpha-ENaC channels and contribute to AFC. *Am J Physiol Lung Cell Mol Physiol* (2017) 312(6):L797–811. doi:10.1152/ajplung.00379.2016

104. Kamynina E, Staub O. Concerted action of ENaC, Nedd4-2, and Sgk1 in transepithelial Na(+) transport. *Am J Physiol Renal Physiol* (2002) 283(3):F377–87. doi:10.1152/ajprenal.00143.2002

105. Roux J, McNicholas CM, Carles M, Goolaerts A, Houseman BT, Dickinson DA, et al. IL-8 inhibits cAMP-stimulated alveolar epithelial fluid transport via a GRK2/PI3K-dependent mechanism. *FASEB J* (2013) 27(3):1095–106. doi:10.1096/fj.12-219295

106. Planes C, Leyvraz C, Uchida T, Angelova MA, Vuagniaux G, Hummler E, et al. In vitro and in vivo regulation of transepithelial lung alveolar sodium transport by serine proteases. *Am J Physiol Lung Cell Mol Physiol* (2005) 288(6):L1099–109. doi:10.1152/ajplung.00332.2004

107. Kleyman TR, Myerburg MM, Hughey RP. Regulation of ENaCs by proteases: an increasingly complex story. *Kidney Int* (2006) 70(8):1391–2. doi:10.1038/sj.ki.5001860

108. Snyder PM. Minireview: regulation of epithelial Na+ channel trafficking. *Endocrinology* (2005) 146(12):5079–85. doi:10.1210/en.2005-0894

109. Dagenais A, Denis C, Vives MF, Girouard S, Masse C, Nguyen T, et al. Modulation of alpha-ENaC and alpha1-Na+-K+-ATPase by cAMP and dexamethasone in alveolar epithelial cells. *Am J Physiol Lung Cell Mol Physiol* (2001) 281(1):L217–30.

110. Kunzelmann K, Bachhuber T, Regeer R, Markovich D, Sun J, Schreiber R. Purinergic inhibition of the epithelial Na+ transport via hydrolysis of PIP2. *FASEB J* (2005) 19(1):142–3. doi:10.1096/fj.04-2314fje

111. Helms MN, Jain L, Self JL, Eaton DC. Redox regulation of epithelial sodium channels examined in alveolar type 1 and 2 cells patch-clamped in lung slice tissue. *J Biol Chem* (2008) 283(33):22875–83. doi:10.1074/jbc.M801363200

112. Song W, Liu G, Bosworth CA, Walker JR, Megaw GA, Lazrak A, et al. Respiratory syncytial virus inhibits lung epithelial Na+ channels by up-regulating inducible nitric-oxide synthase. *J Biol Chem* (2009) 284(11): 7294–306. doi:10.1074/jbc.M806816200

113. Roux J, Kawakatsu H, Gartland B, Pespeni M, Sheppard D, Matthay MA, et al. Interleukin-1 beta decreases expression of the epithelial sodium channel alpha-subunit in alveolar epithelial cells via a p38 MAPK-dependent

114. signaling pathway. *J Biol Chem* (2005) 280(19):18579–89. doi:10.1074/jbc.M410561200

114. Shabbir W, Tzotzos S, Bedak M, Aufy M, Willam A, Kraihammer M, et al. Glycosylation-dependent activation of epithelial sodium channel by solnatide. *Biochem Pharmacol* (2015) 98(4):740–53. doi:10.1016/j.bcp.2015.08.003

115. Astrand AB, Hemmerling M, Root J, Wingren C, Pesic J, Johansson E, et al. Linking increased airway hydration, ciliary beating, and mucociliary clearance through ENaC inhibition. *Am J Physiol Lung Cell Mol Physiol* (2015) 308(1):L22–32. doi:10.1152/ajplung.00163.2014

116. Mall MA, Galietta LJ. Targeting ion channels in cystic fibrosis. *J Cyst Fibros* (2015) 14(5):561–70. doi:10.1016/j.jcf.2015.06.002

117. Matalon S, Bartoszewski R, Collawn JF. Role of epithelial sodium channels in the regulation of lung fluid homeostasis. *Am J Physiol Lung Cell Mol Physiol* (2015) 309(11):L1229–38. doi:10.1152/ajplung.00319.2015

118. Willam A, Aufy M, Tzotzos S, Evanzin H, Chytracek S, Geppert S, et al. Restoration of epithelial sodium channel function by synthetic peptides in pseudohypoaldosteronism type 1B mutants. *Front Pharmacol* (2017) 8:85. doi:10.3389/fphar.2017.00085

119. Shimkets RA, Warnock DG, Bositis CM, Nelson-Williams C, Hansson JH, Schambelan M, et al. Liddle's syndrome: heritable human hypertension caused by mutations in the beta subunit of the epithelial sodium channel. *Cell* (1994) 79(3):407–14. doi:10.1016/0092-8674(94)90250-X

120. Hansson JH, Schild L, Lu Y, Wilson TA, Gautschi I, Shimkets R, et al. A de novo missense mutation of the beta subunit of the epithelial sodium channel causes hypertension and Liddle syndrome, identifying a proline-rich segment critical for regulation of channel activity. *Proc Natl Acad Sci U S A* (1995) 92(25):11495–9. doi:10.1073/pnas.92.25.11495

121. Schild L, Canessa CM, Shimkets RA, Gautschi I, Lifton RP, Rossier BC. A mutation in the epithelial sodium channel causing Liddle disease increases channel activity in the *Xenopus laevis* oocyte expression system. *Proc Natl Acad Sci U S A* (1995) 92(12):5699–703. doi:10.1073/pnas.92.12.5699

122. Snyder PM, Price MP, McDonald FJ, Adams CM, Volk KA, Zeiher BG, et al. Mechanism by which Liddle's syndrome mutations increase activity of a human epithelial Na+ channel. *Cell* (1995) 83(6):969–78. doi:10.1016/0092-8674(95)90212-0

123. Inoue J, Iwaoka T, Tokunaga H, Takamune K, Naomi S, Araki M, et al. A family with Liddle's syndrome caused by a new missense mutation in the beta subunit of the epithelial sodium channel. *J Clin Endocrinol Metab* (1998) 83(6):2210–3. doi:10.1210/jcem.83.6.5030

124. Chang SS, Grunder S, Hanukoglu A, Rosler A, Mathew PM, Hanukoglu I, et al. Mutations in subunits of the epithelial sodium channel cause salt wasting with hyperkalaemic acidosis, pseudohypoaldosteronism type 1. *Nat Genet* (1996) 12(3):248–53. doi:10.1038/ng0396-248

125. Strautnieks SS, Thompson RJ, Gardiner RM, Chung E. A novel splice-site mutation in the gamma subunit of the epithelial sodium channel gene in three pseudohypoaldosteronism type 1 families. *Nat Genet* (1996) 13(2):248–50. doi:10.1038/ng0696-248

126. Gründer S, Firsov D, Chang SS, Jaeger NF, Gautschi I, Schild L, et al. A mutation causing pseudohypoaldosteronism type 1 identifies a conserved glycine that is involved in the gating of the epithelial sodium channel. *EMBO J* (1997) 16(5):899–907. doi:10.1093/emboj/16.5.899

127. Boiko N, Kucher V, Stockand JD. Pseudohypoaldosteronism type 1 and Liddle's syndrome mutations that affect the single-channel properties of the epithelial Na+ channel. *Physiol Rep* (2015) 3(11):e12600. doi:10.14814/phy2.12600

128. Zennaro M-C, Lombès M. Mineralocorticoid resistance. *Trends Endocrinol Metab* (2004) 15(6):264–70. doi:10.1016/j.tem.2004.06.003

129. Riepe FG, van Bemmelen MX, Cachat F, Plendl H, Gautschi I, Krone N, et al. Revealing a subclinical salt-losing phenotype in heterozygous carriers of the novel S562P mutation in the alpha subunit of the epithelial sodium channel. *Clin Endocrinol (Oxf)* (2009) 70(2):252–8. doi:10.1111/j.1365-2265.2008.03314.x

130. Eisenhut M, Wallace H. Ion channels in inflammation. *Pflugers Arch* (2011) 461(4):401–21. doi:10.1007/s00424-010-0917-y

131. Meltzer RH, Kapoor N, Qadri YJ, Anderson SJ, Fuller CM, Benos DJ. Heteromeric assembly of acid-sensitive ion channel and epithelial sodium channel subunits. *J Biol Chem* (2007) 282(35):25548–59. doi:10.1074/jbc.M703825200

132. Frank J, Roux J, Kawakatsu H, Su G, Dagenais A, Berthiaume Y, et al. Transforming growth factor-beta1 decreases expression of the epithelial sodium channel alphaENaC and alveolar epithelial vectorial sodium and fluid transport via an ERK1/2-dependent mechanism. *J Biol Chem* (2003) 278(45):43939–50. doi:10.1074/jbc.M304882200

133. Peters DM, Vadász I, Wujak Ł, Wygrecka M, Olschewski A, Becker C, et al. TGF-β directs trafficking of the epithelial sodium channel ENaC which has implications for ion and fluid transport in acute lung injury. *Proc Natl Acad Sci U S A* (2014) 111(3):E374–83. doi:10.1073/pnas.1306798111

134. Willis BC, Kim KJ, Li X, Liebler J, Crandall ED, Borok Z. Modulation of ion conductance and active transport by TGF-beta 1 in alveolar epithelial cell monolayers. *Am J Physiol Lung Cell Mol Physiol* (2003) 285(6):L1192–200. doi:10.1152/ajplung.00379.2002

135. Dagenais A, Fréchette R, Yamagata Y, Yamagata T, Carmel J-F, Clermont M-E, et al. Downregulation of ENaC activity and expression by TNF-α in alveolar epithelial cells. *Am J Physiol Lung Cell Mol Physiol* (2004) 286(2):L301–11. doi:10.1152/ajplung.00326.2002

136. Fukuda N, Jayr C, Lazrak A, Wang Y, Lucas R, Matalon S, et al. Mechanisms of TNF-alpha stimulation of amiloride-sensitive sodium transport across alveolar epithelium. *Am J Physiol Lung Cell Mol Physiol* (2001) 280(6):1258–65.

137. Choi JY, Choi YS, Kim SJ, Son EJ, Choi HS, Yoon JH. Interleukin-1beta suppresses epithelial sodium channel beta-subunit expression and ENaC-dependent fluid absorption in human middle ear epithelial cells. *Eur J Pharmacol* (2007) 567(1–2):19–25. doi:10.1016/j.ejphar.2007.04.026

138. Gray T, Coakley R, Hirsh A, Thornton D, Kirkham S, Koo JS, et al. Regulation of MUC5AC mucin secretion and airway surface liquid metabolism by IL-1β in human bronchial epithelia. *Am J Physiol Lung Cell Mol Physiol* (2004) 286:L320–30. doi:10.1152/ajplung.00440.2002

139. Geiser T, Jarreau PH, Atabai K, Matthay MA. Interleukin-1beta augments in vitro alveolar epithelial repair. *Am J Physiol Lung Cell Mol Physiol* (2000) 279(6):L1184–90.

140. Nair PD, Li T, Bhattacharjee R, Ye X, Folkesson HG. Oxytocin-induced labor augments IL-1 beta-stimulated lung fluid absorption in fetal guinea pig lungs. *Am J Physiol Lung Cell Mol Physiol* (2005) 289(6):L1029–38. doi:10.1152/ajplung.00256.2004

141. Galietta LJV, Pagesy P, Folli C, Caci E, Romio L, Costes B, et al. IL-4 is a potent modulator of ion transport in the human bronchial epithelium in vitro. *J Immunol* (2002) 168(2):839. doi:10.4049/jimmunol.168.2.839

142. Galietta LJ, Folli C, Caci E, Pedemonte N, Taddei A, Ravazzolo R, et al. Effect of inflammatory stimuli on airway ion transport. *Proc Am Thorac Soc* (2004) 1(1):62–5. doi:10.1513/pats.2306017

143. Zhou L, Graeff RW, McCray PB Jr., Simonet WS, Whitsett JA. Keratinocyte growth factor stimulates CFTR-independent fluid secretion in the fetal lung in vitro. *Am J Physiol* (1996) 271(6 Pt 1):L987–94.

144. Ling B, DC E. Effects of luminal Na+ on single Na+ channels in A6 cells, a regulatory role for protein kinase C. *Am J Physiol Renal Fluid Electrolyte Physiol* (1989) 256:F1094–103.

145. Frindt G, Palmer LG, Windhager EE. Feedback regulation of Na channels in rat CCT. IV. Mediation by activation of protein kinase C. *Am J Physiol* (1996) 270(2 Pt 2):F371–6.

146. Stockand JD, Bao HF, Schenck J, Malik B, Middleton P, Schlanger LE, et al. Differential effects of protein kinase C on the levels of epithelial Na+ channel subunit proteins. *J Biol Chem* (2000) 275(33):25760–5. doi:10.1074/jbc.M003615200

147. Soukup B, Benjamin A, Orogo-Wenn M, Walters D. Physiological effect of protein kinase C on ENaC-mediated lung liquid regulation in the adult rat lung. *Am J Physiol Lung Cell Mol Physiol* (2012) 302(1):L133–9. doi:10.1152/ajplung.00031.2011

148. Migneault F, Boncoeur E, Morneau F, Pascariu M, Dagenais A, Berthiaume Y. Cycloheximide and lipopolysaccharide downregulate alphaENaC mRNA via different mechanisms in alveolar epithelial cells. *Am J Physiol Lung Cell Mol Physiol* (2013) 305(10):L747–55. doi:10.1152/ajplung.00023.2013

149. Lucas R, Sridhar S, Rick FG, Gorshkov B, Umapathy NS, Yang G, et al. Agonist of growth hormone-releasing hormone reduces pneumolysin-induced pulmonary permeability edema. *Proc Natl Acad Sci U S A* (2012) 109(6):2084–9. doi:10.1073/pnas.1121075109

150. Downs CA, Helms MN. Regulation of ion transport by oxidants. *Am J Physiol Lung Cell Mol Physiol* (2013) 305(9):L595. doi:10.1152/ajplung.00212.2013

151. Downs CA, Kreiner L, Zhao XM, Trac P, Johnson NM, Hansen JM, et al. Oxidized glutathione (GSSG) inhibits epithelial sodium channel activity in primary alveolar epithelial cells. *Am J Physiol Lung Cell Mol Physiol* (2015) 308(9):L943–52. doi:10.1152/ajplung.00213.2014

152. Zhu S, Ware LB, Geiser T, Matthay MA, Matalon S. Increased levels of nitrate and surfactant protein a nitration in the pulmonary edema fluid of patients with acute lung injury. *Am J Respir Crit Care Med* (2001) 163(1):166–72. doi:10.1164/ajrccm.163.1.2005068

153. Snyder PM. Intoxicated Na(+) channels. Focus on "Ethanol stimulates epithelial sodium channels by elevating reactive oxygen species". *Am J Physiol Cell Physiol* (2012) 303(11):C1125–6. doi:10.1152/ajpcell.00301.2012

154. Lazrak A, Jurkuvenaite A, Ness EC, Zhang S, Woodworth BA, Muhlebach MS, et al. Inter-α-inhibitor blocks epithelial sodium channel activation and decreases nasal potential differences in ΔF508 mice. *Am J Respir Cell Mol Biol* (2014) 50(5):953–62. doi:10.1165/rcmb.2013-0215OC

155. Zhou R, Patel SV, Snyder PM. Nedd4-2 catalyzes ubiquitination and degradation of cell surface ENaC. *J Biol Chem* (2007) 282(28):20207–12. doi:10.1074/jbc.M611329200

156. Planes C, Blot-Chabaud M, Matthay MA, Couette S, Uchida T, Clerici C. Hypoxia and beta 2-agonists regulate cell surface expression of the epithelial sodium channel in native alveolar epithelial cells. *J Biol Chem* (2002) 277(49):47318–24. doi:10.1074/jbc.M209158200

157. Poulsen AN, Klausen TL, Pedersen PS, Willumsen NJ, Frederiksen O. Regulation of ion transport via apical purinergic receptors in intact rabbit airway epithelium. *Pflugers Arch* (2005) 450(4):227–35. doi:10.1007/s00424-005-1388-4

158. Burnstock G, Brouns I, Adriaensen D, Timmermans J-P. Purinergic signaling in the airways. *Pharmacol Rev* (2012) 64(4):834. doi:10.1124/pr.111.005389

159. Takemura Y, Helms MN, Eaton AF, Self J, Ramosevac S, Jain L, et al. Cholinergic regulation of epithelial sodium channels in rat alveolar type 2 epithelial cells. *Am J Physiol Lung Cell Mol Physiol* (2013) 304(6):L428–37. doi:10.1152/ajplung.00129.2012

160. Greenlee MM, Mitzelfelt JD, Yu L, Yue Q, Duke BJ, Harrell CS, et al. Estradiol activates epithelial sodium channels in rat alveolar cells through the G protein-coupled estrogen receptor. *Am J Physiol Lung Cell Mol Physiol* (2013) 305(11):L878–89. doi:10.1152/ajplung.00008.2013

161. Lazrak A, Nielsen VG, Matalon S. Mechanisms of increased Na(+) transport in ATII cells by cAMP: we agree to disagree and do more experiments. *Am J Physiol Lung Cell Mol Physiol* (2000) 278(2):L233–8.

162. Itani OA, Liu KZ, Cornish KL, Campbell JR, Thomas CP. Glucocorticoids stimulate human sgk1 gene expression by activation of a GRE in its 5′-flanking region. *Am J Physiol Endocrinol Metab* (2002) 283(5):E971–9. doi:10.1152/ajpendo.00021.2002

163. Dagenais A, Gosselin D, Guilbault C, Radzioch D, Berthiaume Y. Modulation of epithelial sodium channel (ENaC) expression in mouse lung infected with Pseudomonas aeruginosa. *Respir Res* (2005) 6:2. doi:10.1186/1465-9921-6-2

164. Dagenais A, Frechette R, Clermont ME, Masse C, Prive A, Brochiero E, et al. Dexamethasone inhibits the action of TNF on ENaC expression and activity. *Am J Physiol Lung Cell Mol Physiol* (2006) 291(6):L1220–31. doi:10.1152/ajplung.00511.2005

165. Brodovich H, Canessa C, Ueda J, Rafii B, Rossier BC, Edelson J. Expression of the epithelial Na+ channel in the developing rat lung. *Am J Physiol* (1993) 265(2):C491.

166. Tchepichev S, Ueda J, Canessa C, Rossier BC, Brodovich H. Lung epithelial Na channel subunits are differentially regulated during development and by steroids. *Am J Physiol Cell Physiol* (1995) 269(3):C805.

167. Husted RF, Volk KA, Sigmund RD, Stokes JB. Discordant effects of corticosteroids and expression of subunits on ENaC activity. *Am J Physiol Renal Physiol* (2007) 293(3):F813–20. doi:10.1152/ajprenal.00225.2007

168. Aggarwal S, Dabla PK, Arora S. Prostasin: an epithelial sodium channel regulator. *J Biomark* (2013) 2013:9. doi:10.1155/2013/179864

169. Bruns JB, Carattino MD, Sheng S, Maarouf AB, Weisz OA, Pilewski JM, et al. Epithelial Na+ channels are fully activated by furin- and prostasin-dependent release of an inhibitory peptide from the gamma-subunit. *J Biol Chem* (2007) 282(9):6153–60. doi:10.1074/jbc.M610636200

170. Booth RE, Stockand JD. Targeted degradation of ENaC in response to PKC activation of the ERK1/2 cascade. *Am J Physiol Renal Physiol* (2003) 284(5):F938–47. doi:10.1152/ajprenal.00373.2002

171. Hughey RP, Mueller GM, Bruns JB, Kinlough CL, Poland PA, Harkleroad KL, et al. Maturation of the epithelial Na+ channel involves proteolytic processing of the alpha- and gamma-subunits. *J Biol Chem* (2003) 278(39): 37073–82. doi:10.1074/jbc.M307003200

172. Sheng S, Carattino MD, Bruns JB, Hughey RP, Kleyman TR. Furin cleavage activates the epithelial Na+ channel by relieving Na+ self-inhibition. *Am J Physiol Renal Physiol* (2006) 290(6):F1488–96. doi:10.1152/ajprenal.00439.2005

173. Passero CJ, Mueller GM, Rondon-Berrios H, Tofovic SP, Hughey RP, Kleyman TR. Plasmin activates epithelial Na(+) channels by cleaving the γ subunit. *J Biol Chem* (2008) 283(52):36586–91. doi:10.1074/jbc.M805676200

174. Eaton DC, Chen J, Ramosevac S, Matalon S, Jain L. Regulation of Na+ channels in lung alveolar type II epithelial cells. *Proc Am Thorac Soc* (2004) 1(1):10–6. doi:10.1513/pats.2306008

175. Kunzelmann K. ENaC is inhibited by an increase in the intracellular Cl(-) concentration mediated through activation of Cl(-) channels. *Pflugers Arch* (2003) 445(4):504–12. doi:10.1007/s00424-002-0958-y

176. Helms MN, Chen XJ, Ramosevac S, Eaton DC, Jain L. Dopamine regulation of amiloride-sensitive sodium channels in lung cells. *Am J Physiol Lung Cell Mol Physiol* (2006) 290(4):L710–22. doi:10.1152/ajplung.00486.2004

177. Downs CA, Kreiner LH, Johnson NM, Brown LA, Helms MN. Receptor for advanced glycation end-products regulates lung fluid balance via protein kinase C-gp91(phox) signaling to epithelial sodium channels. *Am J Respir Cell Mol Biol* (2015) 52(1):75–87. doi:10.1165/rcmb.2014-0002OC

178. Besancon F, Przewlocki G, Baro I, Hongre AS, Escande D, Edelman A. Interferon-gamma downregulates CFTR gene expression in epithelial cells. *Am J Physiol* (1994) 267(5 Pt 1):C1398–404.

179. Pruliere-Escabasse V, Fanen P, Dazy AC, Lechapt-Zalcman E, Rideau D, Edelman A, et al. TGF-beta 1 downregulates CFTR expression and function in nasal polyps of non-CF patients. *Am J Physiol Lung Cell Mol Physiol* (2005) 288(1):L77–83. doi:10.1152/ajplung.00048.2004

180. Danahay H, Atherton H, Jones G, Bridges RJ, Poll CT. Interleukin-13 induces a hypersecretory ion transport phenotype in human bronchial epithelial cells. *Am J Physiol Lung Cell Mol Physiol* (2002) 282(2):L226–36. doi:10.1152/ajplung.00311.2001

181. Cafferata EG, Gonzalez-Guerrico AM, Giordano L, Pivetta OH, Santa-Coloma TA. Interleukin-1beta regulates CFTR expression in human intestinal T84 cells. *Biochim Biophys Acta* (2000) 1500(2):241–8. doi:10.1016/S0925-4439(99)00105-2

182. Jiang X, Ingbar DH, O'Grady SM. Adrenergic stimulation of Na+ transport across alveolar epithelial cells involves activation of apical Cl- channels. *Am J Physiol* (1998) 275(6 Pt 1):C1610–20.

183. Fang X, Fukuda N, Barbry P, Sartori C, Verkman AS, Matthay MA. Novel role for CFTR in fluid absorption from the distal airspaces of the lung. *J Gen Physiol* (2002) 119(2):199–207. doi:10.1085/jgp.119.2.199

184. Trotta T, Guerra L, Piro D, d'Apolito M, Piccoli C, Porro C, et al. Stimulation of β2-adrenergic receptor increases CFTR function and decreases ATP levels in murine hematopoietic stem/progenitor cells. *J Cyst Fibros* (2015) 14(1):26–33. doi:10.1016/j.jcf.2014.08.005

185. Baudouin-Legros M, Brouillard F, Tondelier D, Hinzpeter A, Edelman A. Effect of ouabain on CFTR gene expression in human Calu-3 cells. *Am J Physiol Cell Physiol* (2003) 284(3):C620–6. doi:10.1152/ajpcell.00457.2002

186. Welsh MJ, Smith JJ. cAMP stimulation of HCO3– secretion across airway epithelia. *JOP* (2001) 2(4 Suppl):291–3.

187. Qiu W, Laheri A, Leung S, Guggino SE. Hormones increase mRNA of cyclic-nucleotide-gated cation channels in airway epithelia. *Pflugers Arch* (2000) 441(1):69–77. doi:10.1007/s004240000359

188. Ousingsawat J, Kongsuphol P, Schreiber R, Kunzelmann K. CFTR and TMEM16A are separate but functionally related Cl- channels. *Cell Physiol Biochem* (2011) 28(4):715–24. doi:10.1159/000335765

189. Zhou Y, Dong Q, Louahed J, Dragwa C, Savio D, Huang M, et al. Characterization of a calcium-activated chloride channel as a shared target of Th2 cytokine pathways and its potential involvement in asthma. *Am J Respir Cell Mol Biol* (2001) 25(4):486–91. doi:10.1165/ajrcmb.25.4.4578

190. Towne JE, Krane CM, Bachurski CJ, Menon AG. Tumor necrosis factor-alpha inhibits aquaporin 5 expression in mouse lung epithelial cells. *J Biol Chem* (2001) 276(22):18657–64. doi:10.1074/jbc.M100322200

191. Sidhaye VK, Guler AD, Schweitzer KS, D'Alessio F, Caterina MJ, King LS. Transient receptor potential vanilloid 4 regulates aquaporin-5 abundance under hypotonic conditions. *Proc Natl Acad Sci U S A* (2006) 103(2):4747–52. doi:10.1073/pnas.0511211103

192. Chu S, Blaisdell CJ, Bamford P, Ferro TJ. Interferon-gamma regulates ClC-2 chloride channel in lung epithelial cells. *Biochem Biophys Res Commun* (2004) 324(1):31–9. doi:10.1016/j.bbrc.2004.09.026

193. Yang F, Kawedia JD, Menon AG. Cyclic AMP regulates aquaporin 5 expression at both transcriptional and post-transcriptional levels through a protein kinase A pathway. *J Biol Chem* (2003) 278(34):32173–80. doi:10.1074/jbc.M305149200

194. Csanyi A, Bota J, Falkay G, Gaspar R, Ducza E. The effects of female sexual hormones on the expression of aquaporin 5 in the late-pregnant rat uterus. *Int J Mol Sci* (2016) 17(8):E1300. doi:10.3390/ijms17081300

195. Sugi K, Musch MW, Field M, Chang EB. Inhibition of Na+,K+-ATPase by interferon gamma down-regulates intestinal epithelial transport and barrier function. *Gastroenterology* (2001) 120(6):1393–403. doi:10.1053/gast.2001.24045

196. Vadasz I, Schermuly RT, Ghofrani HA, Rummel S, Wehner S, Muhldorfer I, et al. The lectin-like domain of tumor necrosis factor-alpha improves alveolar fluid balance in injured isolated rabbit lungs. *Crit Care Med* (2008) 36(5):1543–50. doi:10.1097/CCM.0b013e31816f485e

197. Wujak LA, Becker S, Seeger W, Morty RE. TGF-β regulates Na,K-ATPase activity by changing the regulatory subunit stoichiometry of the Na,K-ATPase complex. *FASEB J* (2011) 25(1 Suppl):1039.

198. Wujak LA, Blume A, Baloglu E, Wygrecka M, Wygowski J, Herold S, et al. FXYD1 negatively regulates Na(+)/K(+)-ATPase activity in lung alveolar epithelial cells. *Respir Physiol Neurobiol* (2016) 220:54–61. doi:10.1016/j.resp.2015.09.008

199. Peteranderl C, Morales-Nebreda L, Selvakumar B, Lecuona E, Vadasz I, Morty RE, et al. Macrophage-epithelial paracrine crosstalk inhibits lung edema clearance during influenza infection. *J Clin Invest* (2016) 126(4):1566–80. doi:10.1172/JCI83931

200. Sloniewsky DE, Ridge KM, Adir Y, Fries FP, Briva A, Sznajder JI, et al. Leukotriene D4 activates alveolar epithelial Na,K-ATPase and increases alveolar fluid clearance. *Am J Respir Crit Care Med* (2004) 169(3):407–12. doi:10.1164/rccm.200304-472OC

201. Li X, Yan XX, Li HL, Li RQ. Endogenous acetylcholine increases alveolar epithelial fluid transport via activation of alveolar epithelial Na,K-ATPase in mice. *Respir Physiol Neurobiol* (2015) 217:25–31. doi:10.1016/j.resp.2015.05.005

202. Pittet JF, Lu M, Morris DG, Modelska K, Welch WJ, Carey HV, et al. Reactive nitrogen species inhibit alveolar epithelial fluid transport after hemorrhagic shock in rats. *J Immunol* (2001) 166. doi:10.4049/jimmunol.166.10.6301

203. Bechara RI, Brown LA, Roman J, Joshi PC, Guidot DM. Transforming growth factor beta1 expression and activation is increased in the alcoholic rat lung. *Am J Respir Crit Care Med* (2004) 170(2):188–94. doi:10.1164/rccm.200304-478OC

204. Bechara RI, Pelaez A, Palacio A, Joshi PC, Hart CM, Brown LA, et al. Angiotensin II mediates glutathione depletion, transforming growth factor-beta1 expression, and epithelial barrier dysfunction in the alcoholic rat lung. *Am J Physiol Lung Cell Mol Physiol* (2005) 289(3):L363–70. doi:10.1152/ajplung.00141.2005

205. Sheppard D. Transforming growth factor beta: a central modulator of pulmonary and airway inflammation and fibrosis. *Proc Am Thorac Soc* (2006) 3(5):413–7. doi:10.1513/pats.200601-008AW

206. Pittet JF, Griffiths MJ, Geiser T, Kaminski N, Dalton SL, Huang X, et al. TGF-beta is a critical mediator of acute lung injury. *J Clin Invest* (2001) 107(12):1537–44. doi:10.1172/jci11963

207. Patel BV, Wilson MR, O'Dea KP, Takata M. TNF-induced death signaling triggers alveolar epithelial dysfunction in acute lung injury. *J Immunol* (2013) 190(8):4274–82. doi:10.4049/jimmunol.1202437

208. Hogner K, Wolff T, Pleschka S, Plog S, Gruber AD, Kalinke U, et al. Macrophage-expressed IFN-beta contributes to apoptotic alveolar epithelial cell injury in severe influenza virus pneumonia. *PLoS Pathog* (2013) 9(2):e1003188. doi:10.1371/journal.ppat.1003188

209. Peteranderl C, Herold S. The impact of the interferon/TNF-related apoptosis-inducing ligand signaling axis on disease progression in

209. respiratory viral infection and beyond. *Front Immunol* (2017) 8:313. doi:10.3389/fimmu.2017.00313

210. Gan H, Wang G, Hao Q, Wang QJ, Tang H. Protein kinase D promotes airway epithelial barrier dysfunction and permeability through down-regulation of claudin-1. *J Biol Chem* (2014) 289(30):20489. doi:10.1074/jbc.A113.511527

211. Mitchell LA, Overgaard CE, Ward C, Margulies SS, Koval M. Differential effects of claudin-3 and claudin-4 on alveolar epithelial barrier function. *Am J Physiol Lung Cell Mol Physiol* (2011) 301(1):L40-9. doi:10.1152/ajplung.00299.2010

212. Wray C, Mao Y, Pan J, Chandrasena A, Piasta F, Frank JA. Claudin-4 augments alveolar epithelial barrier function and is induced in acute lung injury. *Am J Physiol Lung Cell Mol Physiol* (2009) 297(2):L219-27. doi:10.1152/ajplung.00043.2009

213. Alvarez DF, King JA, Weber D, Addison E, Liedtke W, Townsley MI. Transient receptor potential vanilloid 4-mediated disruption of the alveolar septal barrier: a novel mechanism of acute lung injury. *Circ Res* (2006) 99(9):988-95. doi:10.1161/01.res.0000247065.11756.19

214. Curry-McCoy TV, Venado A, Guidot DM, Joshi PC. Alcohol ingestion disrupts alveolar epithelial barrier function by activation of macrophage-derived transforming growth factor beta1. *Respir Res* (2013) 14:39. doi:10.1186/1465-9921-14-39

215. Gerloff J, Sundar IK, Freter R, Sekera ER, Friedman AE, Robinson R, et al. Inflammatory response and barrier dysfunction by different e-cigarette flavoring chemicals identified by gas chromatography–mass spectrometry in e-liquids and e-vapors on human lung epithelial cells and fibroblasts. *Appl In Vitro Toxicol* (2017) 3(1):28-40. doi:10.1089/aivt.2016.0030

216. Peterson MW, Walter ME, Gross TJ. Asbestos directly increases lung epithelial permeability. *Am J Physiol Lung Cell Mol Physiol* (1993) 265(3):L308.

217. Statt S, Ruan JW, Hung LY, Chang CY, Huang CT, Lim JH, et al. Statin-conferred enhanced cellular resistance against bacterial pore-forming toxins in airway epithelial cells. *Am J Respir Cell Mol Biol* (2015) 53(5):689-702. doi:10.1165/rcmb.2014-0391OC

218. Albertine KH, Soulier MF, Wang Z, Ishizaka A, Hashimoto S, Zimmerman GA, et al. Fas and Fas ligand are up-regulated in pulmonary edema fluid and lung tissue of patients with acute lung injury and the acute respiratory distress syndrome. *Am J Pathol* (2002) 161(5):1783-96. doi:10.1016/S0002-9440(10)64455-0

219. Herrero R, Tanino M, Smith LS, Kajikawa O, Wong VA, Mongovin S, et al. The Fas/FasL pathway impairs the alveolar fluid clearance in mouse lungs. *Am J Physiol Lung Cell Mol Physiol* (2013) 305(5):L377-88. doi:10.1152/ajplung.00271.2012

220. Fein A, Grossman RF, Jones JG, Hoeffel J, McKay D. Carbon monoxide effect on alveolar epithelial permeability. *Chest* (1980) 78(5):726-31. doi:10.1378/chest.78.5.726

221. Wilson MR, O'Dea KP, Dorr AD, Yamamoto H, Goddard ME, Takata M. Efficacy and safety of inhaled carbon monoxide during pulmonary inflammation in mice. *PLoS One* (2010) 5(7):e11565. doi:10.1371/journal.pone.0011565

222. Kolosova IA, Mirzapoiazova T, Moreno-Vinasco L, Sammani S, Garcia JG, Verin AD. Protective effect of purinergic agonist ATPgammaS against acute lung injury. *Am J Physiol Lung Cell Mol Physiol* (2008) 294(2):L319-24. doi:10.1152/ajplung.00283.2007

223. Rajasekaran AK, Rajasekaran SA. Role of Na-K-ATPase in the assembly of tight junctions. *Am J Physiol Ren Physiol* (2003) 285(3):F388. doi:10.1152/ajprenal.00439.2002

224. Lin X, Barravecchia M, Kothari P, Young JL, Dean DA. [beta]1-Na+,K+-ATPase gene therapy upregulates tight junctions to rescue lipopolysaccharide-induced acute lung injury. *Gene Ther* (2016) 23(6):489-99. doi:10.1038/gt.2016.19

225. Han X, Fink MP, Uchiyama T, Delude RL. Increased iNOS activity is essential for pulmonary epithelial tight junction dysfunction in endotoxemic mice. *Am J Physiol Lung Cell Mol Physiol* (2003) 286(2):L259-67. doi:10.1152/ajplung.00187.2003

226. Short KR, Kasper J, van der Aa S, Andeweg AC, Zaaraoui-Boutahar F, Goeijenbier M, et al. Influenza virus damages the alveolar barrier by disrupting epithelial cell tight junctions. *Eur Respir J* (2016) 47(3):954. doi:10.1183/13993003.01282-2015

227. Xu S, Xue X, You K, Fu J. Caveolin-1 regulates the expression of tight junction proteins during hyperoxia-induced pulmonary epithelial barrier breakdown. *Respir Res* (2016) 17(1):50. doi:10.1186/s12931-016-0364-1

228. Petecchia L, Sabatini F, Usai C, Caci E, Varesio L, Rossi GA. Cytokines induce tight junction disassembly in airway cells via an EGFR-dependent MAPK/ERK1/2-pathway. *Lab Invest* (2012) 92(8):1140-8. doi:10.1038/labinvest.2012.67

229. Saatian B, Rezaee F, Desando S, Emo J, Chapman T, Knowlden S, et al. Interleukin-4 and interleukin-13 cause barrier dysfunction in human airway epithelial cells. *Tissue Barriers* (2013) 1(2):e24333. doi:10.4161/tisb.24333

230. Mazzon E, Cuzzocrea S. Role of TNF-alpha in lung tight junction alteration in mouse model of acute lung inflammation. *Respir Res* (2007) 8:75. doi:10.1186/1465-9921-8-75

231. Youakim A, Ahdieh M. Interferon-gamma decreases barrier function in T84 cells by reducing ZO-1 levels and disrupting apical actin. *Am J Physiol* (1999) 276(5 Pt 1):G1279-88.

232. Ahdieh M, Vandenbos T, Youakim A. Lung epithelial barrier function and wound healing are decreased by IL-4 and IL-13 and enhanced by IFN-gamma. *Am J Physiol Cell Physiol* (2001) 281(6):C2029-38.

233. Petecchia L, Sabatini F, Varesio L, Camoirano A, Usai C, Pezzolo A, et al. Bronchial airway epithelial cell damage following exposure to cigarette smoke includes disassembly of tight junction components mediated by the extra-cellular signal-regulated kinase 1/2 pathway. *Chest* (2009) 135(6):1502-12. doi:10.1378/chest.08-1780

234. Cao X, Lin H, Muskhelishvili L, Latendresse J, Richter P, Heflich RH. Tight junction disruption by cadmium in an in vitro human airway tissue model. *Respir Res* (2015) 16:30. doi:10.1186/s12931-015-0191-9

235. Lu Q, Harrington EO, Jackson H, Morin N, Shannon C, Rounds S. Transforming growth factor-beta1-induced endothelial barrier dysfunction involves Smad2-dependent p38 activation and subsequent RhoA activation. *J Appl Physiol (1985)* (2006) 101(2):375-84. doi:10.1152/japplphysiol.01515.2005

236. van der Poll T, Lowry SF. Tumor necrosis factor in sepsis: mediator of multiple organ failure or essential part of host defense? *Shock* (1995) 3(1):1-12. doi:10.1097/00024382-199503010-00001

237. Tracey KJ, Fong Y, Hesse DG, Manogue KR, Lee AT, Kuo GC, et al. Anti-cachectin/TNF monoclonal antibodies prevent septic shock during lethal bacteraemia. *Nature* (1987) 330(6149):662-4. doi:10.1038/330662a0

238. Koss M, Pfeiffer GR II, Wang Y, Thomas ST, Yerukhimovich M, Gaarde WA, et al. Ezrin/radixin/moesin proteins are phosphorylated by TNF-alpha and modulate permeability increases in human pulmonary microvascular endothelial cells. *J Immunol* (2006) 176(2):1218-27. doi:10.4049/jimmunol.176.2.1218

239. Lucas R, Garcia I, Donati YR, Hribar M, Mandriota SJ, Giroud C, et al. Both TNF receptors are required for direct TNF-mediated cytotoxicity in microvascular endothelial cells. *Eur J Immunol* (1998) 28(11):3577-86. doi:10.1002/(SICI)1521-4141(199811)28:11<3577::AID-IMMU3577>3.0.CO;2-#

240. Stammberger U, Gaspert A, Hillinger S, Vogt P, Odermatt B, Weder W, et al. Apoptosis induced by ischemia and reperfusion in experimental lung transplantation. *Ann Thorac Surg* (2000) 69(5):1532-6. doi:10.1016/S0003-4975(00)01228-5

241. Xiong C, Yang G, Kumar S, Aggarwal S, Leustik M, Snead C, et al. The lectin-like domain of TNF protects from listeriolysin-induced hyperpermeability in human pulmonary microvascular endothelial cells - a crucial role for protein kinase C-alpha inhibition. *Vascul Pharmacol* (2010) 52(5-6):207-13. doi:10.1016/j.vph.2009.12.010

242. Hribar M, Bloc A, van der Goot FG, Fransen L, De Baetselier P, Grau GE, et al. The lectin-like domain of tumor necrosis factor-alpha increases membrane conductance in microvascular endothelial cells and peritoneal macrophages. *Eur J Immunol* (1999) 29(10):3105-11. doi:10.1002/(SICI)1521-4141(199910)29:10<3105::AID-IMMU3105>3.0.CO;2-A

243. Martin S, Maruta K, Burkart V, Gillis S, Kolb H. IL-1 and IFN-gamma increase vascular permeability. *Immunology* (1988) 64(2):301-5.

244. Leff JA, Bodman ME, Cho OJ, Rohrbach S, Reiss OK, Vannice JL, et al. Post-insult treatment with interleukin-1 receptor antagonist decreases oxidative lung injury in rats given intratracheal interleukin-1. *Am J Respir Crit Care Med* (1994) 150(1):109-12. doi:10.1164/ajrccm.150.1.8025734

245. Repine JE. Interleukin-1-mediated acute lung injury and tolerance to oxidative injury. *Environ Health Perspect* (1994) 102(Suppl 10):75–8. doi:10.1289/ehp.94102s1075

246. Hybertson BM, Lee YM, Cho HG, Cho OJ, Repine JE. Alveolar type II cell abnormalities and peroxide formation in lungs of rats given IL-1 intratracheally. *Inflammation* (2000) 24(4):289–303. doi:10.1023/A:1007092529261

247. Lee YM, Hybertson BM, Cho HG, Terada LS, Cho O, Repine AJ, et al. Platelet-activating factor contributes to acute lung leak in rats given interleukin-1 intratracheally. *Am J Physiol Lung Cell Mol Physiol* (2000) 279(1):L75–80.

248. Ballmer-Weber BK, Dummer R, Küng E, Burg G, Ballmer PE. Interleukin 2-induced increase of vascular permeability without decrease of the intravascular albumin pool. *Br J Cancer* (1995) 71(1):78–82. doi:10.1038/bjc.1995.16

249. Maruo N, Morita I, Shirao M, Murota S. IL-6 increases endothelial permeability in vitro. *Endocrinology* (1992) 131(2):710–4. doi:10.1210/endo.131.2.1639018

250. Biffl WL, Moore EE, Moore FA, Carl VS, Franciose RJ, Banerjee A. Interleukin-8 increases endothelial permeability independent of neutrophils. *J Trauma* (1995) 39(1):98–102. doi:10.1097/00005373-199507000-00013; discussion 102-103,

251. Matsumoto K, Ohi H, Kanmatsuse K. Interleukin 12 upregulates the release of vascular permeability factor by peripheral blood mononuclear cells from patients with lipoid nephrosis. *Nephron* (1998) 78(4):403–9. doi:10.1159/000044968

252. DiStasi MR, Ley K. Opening the flood-gates: how neutrophil-endothelial interactions regulate permeability. *Trends Immunol* (2009) 30(11):547–56. doi:10.1016/j.it.2009.07.012

253. Thorneloe KS, Cheung M, Bao W, Alsaid H, Lenhard S, Jian MY, et al. An orally active TRPV4 channel blocker prevents and resolves pulmonary edema induced by heart failure. *Sci Transl Med* (2012) 4(159):159ra148. doi:10.1126/scitranslmed.3004276

254. Morty RE, Kuebler WM. TRPV4: an exciting new target to promote alveolocapillary barrier function. *Am J Physiol Lung Cell Mol Physiol* (2014) 307(11):L817–21. doi:10.1152/ajplung.00254.2014

255. Mehta D, Ahmmed GU, Paria BC, Holinstat M, Voyno-Yasenetskaya T, Tiruppathi C, et al. RhoA interaction with inositol 1,4,5-trisphosphate receptor and transient receptor potential channel-1 regulates Ca2+ entry. Role in signaling increased endothelial permeability. *J Biol Chem* (2003) 278(35):33492–500. doi:10.1074/jbc.M302401200

256. Lien DC, Worthen GS, Henson PM, Bethel RA. Platelet-activating factor causes neutrophil accumulation and neutrophil-mediated increased vascular permeability in canine trachea. *Am Rev Respir Dis* (1992) 145(3):693–700. doi:10.1164/ajrccm/145.3.693

257. Lee KS, Kim SR, Park SJ, Park HS, Min KH, Lee MH, et al. Hydrogen peroxide induces vascular permeability via regulation of vascular endothelial growth factor. *Am J Respir Cell Mol Biol* (2006) 35(2):190–7. doi:10.1165/rcmb.2005-0482OC

258. Su G, Hodnett M, Wu N, Atakilit A, Kosinski C, Godzich M, et al. Integrin αvβ5 regulates lung vascular permeability and pulmonary endothelial barrier function. *Am J Respir Cell Mol Biol* (2007) 36(3):377–86. doi:10.1165/rcmb.2006-0238OC

259. Semina EV, Rubina KA, Sysoeva VY, Rutkevich PN, Kashirina NM, Tkachuk VA. Novel mechanism regulating endothelial permeability via T-cadherin-dependent VE-cadherin phosphorylation and clathrin-mediated endocytosis. *Mol Cell Biochem* (2014) 387(1):39–53. doi:10.1007/s11010-013-1867-4

260. Shen Q, Rigor RR, Pivetti CD, Wu MH, Yuan SY. Myosin light chain kinase in microvascular endothelial barrier function. *Cardiovasc Res* (2010) 87(2):272–80. doi:10.1093/cvr/cvq144

261. Liu H, Yu X, Yu S, Kou J. Molecular mechanisms in lipopolysaccharide-induced pulmonary endothelial barrier dysfunction. *Int Immunopharmacol* (2015) 29(2):937–46. doi:10.1016/j.intimp.2015.10.010

262. Chen F, Kumar S, Yu Y, Aggarwal S, Gross C, Wang Y, et al. PKC-dependent phosphorylation of eNOS at T495 regulates eNOS coupling and endothelial barrier function in response to G+ -toxins. *PLoS One* (2014) 9(7):e99823. doi:10.1371/journal.pone.0099823

263. Zemskov E, Lucas R, Verin AD, Umapathy NS. P2Y receptors as regulators of lung endothelial barrier integrity. *J Cardiovasc Dis Res* (2011) 2(1):14–22. doi:10.4103/0975-3583.78582

264. Jabaudon M, Blondonnet R, Roszyk L, Bouvier D, Audard J, Clairefond G, et al. Soluble receptor for advanced glycation end-products predicts impaired alveolar fluid clearance in acute respiratory distress syndrome. *Am J Respir Crit Care Med* (2015) 192(2):191–9. doi:10.1164/rccm.201501-0020OC

265. Debruin EJ, Hughes MR, Sina C, Lu A, Cait J, Jian Z, et al. Podocalyxin regulates murine lung vascular permeability by altering endothelial cell adhesion. *PLoS One* (2014) 9(10):e108881. doi:10.1371/journal.pone.0108881

266. Kostadinova E, Chaput C, Gutbier B, Lippmann J, Sander LE, Mitchell TJ, et al. NLRP3 protects alveolar barrier integrity by an inflammasome-independent increase of epithelial cell adherence. *Sci Rep* (2016) 6:30943. doi:10.1038/srep30943

267. Marunaka Y, Tohda H, Hagiwara N, O'Brodovich H. Cytosolic Ca(2+)-induced modulation of ion selectivity and amiloride sensitivity of a cation channel and beta agonist action in fetal lung epithelium. *Biochem Biophys Res Commun* (1992) 187(2):648–56. doi:10.1016/0006-291X(92)91244-K

268. Jain L, Chen XJ, Ramosevac S, Brown LA, Eaton DC. Expression of highly selective sodium channels in alveolar type II cells is determined by culture conditions. *Am J Physiol Lung Cell Mol Physiol* (2001) 280(4):L646–58.

269. Johnson MD, Bao HF, Helms MN, Chen XJ, Tigue Z, Jain L, et al. Functional ion channels in pulmonary alveolar type I cells support a role for type I cells in lung ion transport. *Proc Natl Acad Sci U S A* (2006) 103(13):4964–9. doi:10.1073/pnas.0600855103

270. Wang X, Kleyman TR, Tohda H, Marunaka Y, O'Brodovich H. 5-(N-Ethyl-N-isopropyl)amiloride sensitive Na+ currents in intact fetal distal lung epithelial cells. *Can J Physiol Pharmacol* (1993) 71(1):58–62. doi:10.1139/y93-009

271. Chen XJ, Eaton DC, Jain L. Beta-adrenergic regulation of amiloride-sensitive lung sodium channels. *Am J Physiol Lung Cell Mol Physiol* (2002) 282(4):L609–20. doi:10.1152/ajplung.00356.2001

272. Downs CA, Kriener LH, Yu L, Eaton DC, Jain L, Helms MN. beta-adrenergic agonists differentially regulate highly selective and nonselective epithelial sodium channels to promote alveolar fluid clearance in vivo. *Am J Physiol Lung Cell Mol Physiol* (2012) 302(11):L1167–78. doi:10.1152/ajplung.00038.2012

273. Jain L, Chen XJ, Brown LA, Eaton DC. Nitric oxide inhibits lung sodium transport through a cGMP-mediated inhibition of epithelial cation channels. *Am J Physiol* (1998) 274(4 Pt 1):L475–84.

274. Chen XJ, Seth S, Yue G, Kamat P, Compans RW, Guidot D, et al. Influenza virus inhibits ENaC and lung fluid clearance. *Am J Physiol Lung Cell Mol Physiol* (2004) 287(2):L366–73. doi:10.1152/ajplung.00011.2004

275. Eaton AF, Yue Q, Eaton DC, Bao HF. ENaC activity and expression is decreased in the lungs of protein kinase C-alpha knockout mice. *Am J Physiol Lung Cell Mol Physiol* (2014) 307(5):L374–85. doi:10.1152/ajplung.00040.2014

276. Ma HP, Li L, Zhou ZH, Eaton DC, Warnock DG. ATP masks stretch activation of epithelial sodium channels in A6 distal nephron cells. *Am J Physiol Renal Physiol* (2002) 282(3):F501–5. doi:10.1152/ajprenal.00147.2001

277. Davis IC, Matalon S. Epithelial sodium channels in the adult lung – important modulators of pulmonary health and disease. *Adv Exp Med Biol* (2007) 618:127–40. doi:10.1007/978-0-387-75434-5_10

278. Pochynyuk O, Bugaj V, Vandewalle A, Stockand JD. Purinergic control of apical plasma membrane PI(4,5)P2 levels sets ENaC activity in principal cells. *Am J Physiol Renal Physiol* (2008) 294(1):F38–46. doi:10.1152/ajprenal.00403.2007

279. Stockand JD, Mironova E, Bugaj V, Rieg T, Insel PA, Vallon V, et al. Purinergic inhibition of ENaC produces aldosterone escape. *J Am Soc Nephrol* (2010) 21(11):1903–11. doi:10.1681/ASN.2010040377

280. Helms MN, Self J, Bao HF, Job LC, Jain L, Eaton DC. Dopamine activates amiloride-sensitive sodium channels in alveolar type I cells in lung slice preparations. *Am J Physiol Lung Cell Mol Physiol* (2006) 291(4):L610–8. doi:10.1152/ajplung.00426.2005

281. Kapoor N, Lee W, Clark E, Bartoszewski R, McNicholas CM, Latham CB, et al. Interaction of ASIC1 and ENaC subunits in human glioma cells and rat astrocytes. *Am J Physiol Cell Physiol* (2011) 300(6):C1246–59. doi:10.1152/ajpcell.00199.2010

282. Gessner C, Hammerschmidt S, Kuhn H, Seyfarth HJ, Sack U, Engelmann L, et al. Exhaled breath condensate acidification in acute lung injury. *Respir Med* (2003) 97(11):1188–94. doi:10.1016/S0954-6111(03)00225-7

283. Suhail M. Na(+), K(+)-ATPase: ubiquitous multifunctional transmembrane protein and its relevance to various pathophysiological conditions. *J Clin Med Res* (2010) 2(1):1–17. doi:10.4021/jocmr2010.02.263w

284. Ingbar D, Wendt C, Crandall E. ATPase and the clearance of pulmonary edema fluid. In: Matthay MA, Ingbar DH, editors. *Pulmonary Edema*. New York: Marcel Dekker (1998). p. 477–99.

285. Brazee PL, Soni PN, Tokhtaeva E, Magnani N, Yemelyanov A, Perlman HR, et al. FXYD5 is an essential mediator of the inflammatory response during lung injury. *Front Immunol* (2017) 8:623. doi:10.3389/fimmu.2017.00623

286. Kellenberger S, Schild L. Epithelial sodium channel/degenerin family of ion channels: a variety of functions for a shared structure. *Physiol Rev* (2002) 82(3):735–67. doi:10.1152/physrev.00007.2002

287. McDonough AA, Geering K, Farley RA. The sodium pump needs its beta subunit. *FASEB J* (1990) 4(6):1598–605.

288. Kaplan JH. Ion movements through the sodium pump. *Annu Rev Physiol* (1985) 47:535–44. doi:10.1146/annurev.ph.47.030185.002535

289. Kotyk A, Amler E. Na,K-adenosinetriphosphatase: the paradigm of a membrane transport protein. *Physiol Res* (1995) 44(5):261–74.

290. Geering K. The functional role of beta subunits in oligomeric P-type ATPases. *J Bioenerg Biomembr* (2001) 33(5):425–38. doi:10.1023/A:1010623724749

291. Lubarski Gotliv I. FXYD5: Na(+)/K(+)-ATPase regulator in health and disease. *Front Cell Dev Biol* (2016) 4:26. doi:10.3389/fcell.2016.00026

292. Scott DW, Walker MP, Sesma J, Wu B, Stuhlmiller TJ, Sabater JR, et al. SPX-101 is a novel epithelial sodium channel-targeted therapeutic for cystic fibrosis that restores mucus transport. *Am J Respir Crit Care Med* (2017) 196(6):734–44. doi:10.1164/rccm.201612-2445OC

293. Liedtke W. Molecular mechanisms of TRPV4-mediated neural signaling. *Ann N Y Acad Sci* (2008) 1144:42–52. doi:10.1196/annals.1418.012

294. Scheraga RG, Southern BD, Grove LM, Olman MA. The role of transient receptor potential vanilloid 4 in pulmonary inflammatory diseases. *Front Immunol* (2017) 8:503. doi:10.3389/fimmu.2017.00503

295. Berridge MJ, Bootman MD, Roderick HL. Calcium signalling: dynamics, homeostasis and remodelling. *Nat Rev Mol Cell Biol* (2003) 4(7):517–29. doi:10.1038/nrm1155

296. Strotmann R, Schultz G, Plant TD. Ca2+-dependent potentiation of the nonselective cation channel TRPV4 is mediated by a C-terminal calmodulin binding site. *J Biol Chem* (2003) 278(29):26541–9. doi:10.1074/jbc.M302590200

297. Zhu MX. Multiple roles of calmodulin and other Ca(2+)-binding proteins in the functional regulation of TRP channels. *Pflugers Arch* (2005) 451(1):105–15. doi:10.1007/s00424-005-1427-1

298. White DB. 104 - end-of-life care in respiratory failure A2 - Broaddus, V. Courtney. 6th ed. In: Mason RJ, Ernst JD, King TE, Lazarus SC, Murray JF, Nadel JA, Slutsky AS, Gotway MB, editors. *Murray and Nadel's Textbook of Respiratory Medicine*. Philadelphia: W.B. Saunders (2016). p. 1807–20.

299. Yang XR, Lin MJ, McIntosh LS, Sham JS. Functional expression of transient receptor potential melastatin- and vanilloid-related channels in pulmonary arterial and aortic smooth muscle. *Am J Physiol Lung Cell Mol Physiol* (2006) 290(6):L1267–76. doi:10.1152/ajplung.00515.2005

300. Moran MM, McAlexander MA, Biro T, Szallasi A. Transient receptor potential channels as therapeutic targets. *Nat Rev Drug Discov* (2011) 10(8):601–20. doi:10.1038/nrd3456

301. Yang XR, Lin AH, Hughes JM, Flavahan NA, Cao YN, Liedtke W, et al. Upregulation of osmo-mechanosensitive TRPV4 channel facilitates chronic hypoxia-induced myogenic tone and pulmonary hypertension. *Am J Physiol Lung Cell Mol Physiol* (2012) 302(6):L555–68. doi:10.1152/ajplung.00005.2011

302. Suresh K, Servinsky L, Reyes J, Baksh S, Undem C, Caterina M, et al. Hydrogen peroxide-induced calcium influx in lung microvascular endothelial cells involves TRPV4. *Am J Physiol Lung Cell Mol Physiol* (2015) 309(12):L1467. doi:10.1152/ajplung.00275.2015

303. Parpaite T, Cardouat G, Mauroux M, Gillibert-Duplantier J, Robillard P, Quignard JF, et al. Effect of hypoxia on TRPV1 and TRPV4 channels in rat pulmonary arterial smooth muscle cells. *Pflugers Arch* (2016) 468(1):111–30. doi:10.1007/s00424-015-1704-6

304. Borish LC, Nelson HS, Corren J, Bensch G, Whitmore JB, Busse WW. Efficacy of soluble IL-4 receptor for the treatment of adults with asthma. *J Allergy Clin Immunol* (2001) 107(6):963–70. doi:10.1067/mai.2001.115624

305. Hamanaka K, Jian MY, Weber DS, Alvarez DF, Townsley MI, Al-Mehdi AB, et al. TRPV4 initiates the acute calcium-dependent permeability increase during ventilator-induced lung injury in isolated mouse lungs. *Am J Physiol Lung Cell Mol Physiol* (2007) 293(4):L923–32. doi:10.1152/ajplung.00221.2007

306. Zhou G, Dada LA, Wu M, Kelly A, Trejo H, Zhou Q, et al. Hypoxia-induced alveolar epithelial-mesenchymal transition requires mitochondrial ROS and hypoxia-inducible factor 1. *Am J Physiol Lung Cell Mol Physiol* (2009) 297(6):L1120–30. doi:10.1152/ajplung.00007.2009

307. Balakrishna S, Song W, Achanta S, Doran SF, Liu B, Kaelberer MM, et al. TRPV4 inhibition counteracts edema and inflammation and improves pulmonary function and oxygen saturation in chemically induced acute lung injury. *Am J Physiol Lung Cell Mol Physiol* (2014) 307(2):L158–72. doi:10.1152/ajplung.00065.2014

308. Rahaman SO, Grove LM, Paruchuri S, Southern BD, Abraham S, Niese KA, et al. TRPV4 mediates myofibroblast differentiation and pulmonary fibrosis in mice. *J Clin Invest* (2014) 124(12):5225–38. doi:10.1172/jci75331

309. Henry CO, Dalloneau E, Perez-Berezo MT, Plata C, Wu Y, Guillon A, et al. In vitro and in vivo evidence for an inflammatory role of the calcium channel TRPV4 in lung epithelium: potential involvement in cystic fibrosis. *Am J Physiol Lung Cell Mol Physiol* (2016) 311(3):L664–75. doi:10.1152/ajplung.00442.2015

310. Scheraga RG, Abraham S, Niese KA, Southern BD, Grove LM, Hite RD, et al. TRPV4 mechanosensitive ion channel regulates lipopolysaccharide-stimulated macrophage phagocytosis. *J Immunol* (2016) 196(1):428–36. doi:10.4049/jimmunol.1501688

311. Cioffi DL, Lowe K, Alvarez DF, Barry C, Stevens T. TRPing on the lung endothelium: calcium channels that regulate barrier function. *Antioxid Redox Signal* (2009) 11(4):765–76. doi:10.1089/ars.2008.2221

312. Jia Y, Wang X, Varty L, Rizzo CA, Yang R, Correll CC, et al. Functional TRPV4 channels are expressed in human airway smooth muscle cells. *Am J Physiol Lung Cell Mol Physiol* (2004) 287(2):L272–8. doi:10.1152/ajplung.00393.2003

313. Dalsgaard T, Sonkusare SK, Teuscher C, Poynter ME, Nelson MT. Pharmacological inhibitors of TRPV4 channels reduce cytokine production, restore endothelial function and increase survival in septic mice. *Sci Rep* (2016) 6:33841. doi:10.1038/srep33841

314. Yin J, Michalick L, Tang C, Tabuchi A, Goldenberg N, Dan Q, et al. Role of transient receptor potential vanilloid 4 in neutrophil activation and acute lung injury. *Am J Respir Cell Mol Biol* (2016) 54(3):370–83. doi:10.1165/rcmb.2014-0225OC

315. Zhu G, Gulsvik A, Bakke P, Ghatta S, Anderson W, Lomas DA, et al. Association of TRPV4 gene polymorphisms with chronic obstructive pulmonary disease. *Hum Mol Genet* (2009) 18(11):2053–62. doi:10.1093/hmg/ddp111

316. McAlexander MA, Luttmann MA, Hunsberger GE, Undem BJ. Transient receptor potential vanilloid 4 activation constricts the human bronchus via the release of cysteinyl leukotrienes. *J Pharmacol Exp Ther* (2014) 349(1):118–25. doi:10.1124/jpet.113.210203

317. Satir P, Sleigh MA. The physiology of cilia and mucociliary interactions. *Annu Rev Physiol* (1990) 52:137–55. doi:10.1146/annurev.ph.52.030190.001033

318. Salathe M. Regulation of mammalian ciliary beating. *Annu Rev Physiol* (2007) 69:401–22. doi:10.1146/annurev.physiol.69.040705.141253

319. Jurek SC, Hirano-Kobayashi M, Chiang H, Kohane DS, Matthews BD. Prevention of ventilator-induced lung edema by inhalation of nanoparticles releasing ruthenium red. *Am J Respir Cell Mol Biol* (2014) 50(6):1107–17. doi:10.1165/rcmb.2013-0163OC

320. Wynn TA, Chawla A, Pollard JW. Macrophage biology in development, homeostasis and disease. *Nature* (2013) 496(7446):445–55. doi:10.1038/nature12034

321. Jian MY, King JA, Al-Mehdi AB, Liedtke W, Townsley MI. High vascular pressure-induced lung injury requires P450 epoxygenase-dependent activation of TRPV4. *Am J Respir Cell Mol Biol* (2008) 38(4):386–92. doi:10.1165/rcmb.2007-0192OC

322. Wu S, Jian MY, Xu YC, Zhou C, Al-Mehdi AB, Liedtke W, et al. Ca2+ entry via alpha1G and TRPV4 channels differentially regulates surface expression of P-selectin and barrier integrity in pulmonary capillary endothelium. *Am J Physiol Lung Cell Mol Physiol* (2009) 297(4):L650–7. doi:10.1152/ajplung.00015.2009

323. Hamanaka K, Jian MY, Townsley MI, King JA, Liedtke W, Weber DS, et al. TRPV4 channels augment macrophage activation and ventilator-induced

lung injury. *Am J Physiol Lung Cell Mol Physiol* (2010) 299(3):L353–62. doi:10.1152/ajplung.00315.2009

324. Van Goethem E, Poincloux R, Gauffre F, Maridonneau-Parini I, Le Cabec V. Matrix architecture dictates three-dimensional migration modes of human macrophages: differential involvement of proteases and podosome-like structures. *J Immunol* (2010) 184(2):1049–61. doi:10.4049/jimmunol. 0902223

325. Blakney AK, Swartzlander MD, Bryant SJ. The effects of substrate stiffness on the in vitro activation of macrophages and in vivo host response to poly(ethylene glycol)-based hydrogels. *J Biomed Mater Res A* (2012) 100(6): 1375–86. doi:10.1002/jbm.a.34104

326. Murray JF, Nadel JA. Preface to the sixth edition. In: Murray JF, Nadel JA, Broaddus VC, Mason RJ, Ernst JD, King TE Jr., editors. *Murray and Nadel's Textbook of Respiratory Medicine*. 6th ed. Philadelphia: Elsevier Saunders (2016). p. 1–3.

327. Akei H, Whitsett JA, Buroker M, Ninomiya T, Tatsumi H, Weaver TE, et al. Surface tension influences cell shape and phagocytosis in alveolar macrophages. *Am J Physiol Lung Cell Mol Physiol* (2006) 291(4):L572–9. doi:10.1152/ajplung.00060.2006

328. Malczyk M, Erb A, Veith C, Ghofrani HA, Schermuly RT, Gudermann T, et al. The role of transient receptor potential channel 6 channels in the pulmonary vasculature. *Front Immunol* (2017) 8:707. doi:10.3389/fimmu. 2017.00707

329. Sanjabi S, Zenewicz LA, Kamanaka M, Flavell RA. Anti-inflammatory and pro-inflammatory roles of TGF-beta, IL-10, and IL-22 in immunity and autoimmunity. *Curr Opin Pharmacol* (2009) 9(4):447–53. doi:10.1016/j. coph.2009.04.008

330. Kelley J. Cytokines of the lung. *Am Rev Respir Dis* (1990) 141(3):765–88. doi:10.1164/ajrccm/141.3.765

331. Fiers W. Tumor necrosis factor characterization at the molecular, cellular and in vivo level. *FEBS Lett* (1991) 285(2):199–212. doi:10.1016/0014-5793(91)80803-B

332. Szatmary Z. Tumor necrosis factor-alpha: molecular-biological aspects minireview. *Neoplasma* (1999) 46(5):257–66.

333. Hocking DC, Ferro TJ, Johnson A. Dextran sulfate inhibits PMN-dependent hydrostatic pulmonary edema induced by tumor necrosis factor. *J Appl Physiol (1985)* (1991) 70(3):1121–8.

334. Lo SK, Everitt J, Gu J, Malik AB. Tumor necrosis factor mediates experimental pulmonary edema by ICAM-1 and CD18-dependent mechanisms. *J Clin Invest* (1992) 89(3):981–8. doi:10.1172/jci115681

335. Horgan MJ, Palace GP, Everitt JE, Malik AB. TNF-alpha release in endotoxemia contributes to neutrophil-dependent pulmonary edema. *Am J Physiol* (1993) 264(4 Pt 2):H1161–5.

336. Faggioni R, Gatti S, Demitri MT, Delgado R, Echtenacher B, Gnocchi P, et al. Role of xanthine oxidase and reactive oxygen intermediates in LPS- and TNF-induced pulmonary edema. *J Lab Clin Med* (1994) 123(3):394–9.

337. Lo SK, Bevilacqua B, Malik AB. E-selectin ligands mediate tumor necrosis factor-induced neutrophil sequestration and pulmonary edema in guinea pig lungs. *Circ Res* (1994) 75(6):955–60. doi:10.1161/01.RES.75.6.955

338. Koh Y, Hybertson BM, Jepson EK, Repine JE. Tumor necrosis factor induced acute lung leak in rats: less than with interleukin-1. *Inflammation* (1996) 20:461. doi:10.1007/BF01487039

339. Wallach D, Varfolomeev EE, Malinin NL, Goltsev YV, Kovalenko AV, Boldin MP. Tumor necrosis factor receptor and Fas signaling mechanisms. *Annu Rev Immunol* (1999) 17:331–67. doi:10.1146/annurev.immunol.17.1.331

340. Wallach D. The cybernetics of TNF: old views and newer ones. *Semin Cell Dev Biol* (2016) 50:105–14. doi:10.1016/j.semcdb.2015.10.014

341. Mannel DN, Echtenacher B. TNF in the inflammatory response. *Chem Immunol* (2000) 74:141–61. doi:10.1159/000058757

342. Locksley RM, Killeen N, Lenardo MJ. The TNF and TNF receptor super-families: integrating mammalian biology. *Cell* (2001) 104(4):487–501. doi:10.1016/S0092-8674(01)00237-9

343. Keane J. TNF-blocking agents and tuberculosis: new drugs illuminate an old topic. *Rheumatology (Oxford)* (2005) 44(6):714–20. doi:10.1093/rheumatology/keh567

344. Hundsberger H, Verin A, Wiesner C, Pfluger M, Dulebo A, Schutt W, et al. TNF: a moonlighting protein at the interface between cancer and infection. *Front Biosci* (2008) 13:5374–86. doi:10.2741/3087

345. Aggarwal BB. Signalling pathways of the TNF superfamily: a double-edged sword. *Nat Rev Immunol* (2003) 3(9):745–56. doi:10.1038/nri1184

346. Harris J, Keane J. How tumour necrosis factor blockers interfere with tuberculosis immunity. *Clin Exp Immunol* (2010) 161(1):1–9. doi:10.1111/j.1365-2249.2010.04146.x

347. Berry MA, Hargadon B, Shelley M, Parker D, Shaw DE, Green RH, et al. Evidence of a role of tumor necrosis factor alpha in refractory asthma. *N Engl J Med* (2006) 354(7):697–708. doi:10.1056/NEJMoa050580

348. Mukhopadhyay S, Hoidal JR, Mukherjee TK. Role of TNFα in pulmonary pathophysiology. *Respir Res* (2006) 7(1):125. doi:10.1186/1465-9921-7-125

349. Balkwill F. Tumour necrosis factor and cancer. *Nat Rev Cancer* (2009) 9(5):361–71. doi:10.1038/nrc2628

350. Zhang H, Park Y, Wu J, Chen X, Lee S, Yang J, et al. Role of TNF-alpha in vascular dysfunction. *Clin Sci (Lond)* (2009) 116(3):219–30. doi:10.1042/cs20080196

351. Hession C, Decker JM, Sherblom AP, Kumar S, Yue CC, Mattaliano RJ, et al. Uromodulin (Tamm-Horsfall glycoprotein): a renal ligand for lymphokines. *Science* (1987) 237(4821):1479–84. doi:10.1126/science.3498215

352. Sherblom AP, Decker JM, Muchmore AV. The lectin-like interaction between recombinant tumor necrosis factor and uromodulin. *J Biol Chem* (1988) 263(11):5418–24.

353. Lucas R, Magez S, De Leys R, Fransen L, Scheerlinck J-P, Rambelberg M, et al. Mapping the lectin-like activity of tumor necrosis factor. *Science* (1994) 263(5148):814–8. doi:10.1126/science.8303299

354. Fronius M. Treatment of pulmonary edema by ENaC activators/stimulators. *Curr Mol Pharmacol* (2013) 6(1):13–27. doi:10.2174/1874467211306010003

355. Hartmann EK, Boehme S, Duenges B, Bentley A, Klein KU, Kwiecien R, et al. An inhaled tumor necrosis factor-alpha-derived TIP peptide improves the pulmonary function in experimental lung injury. *Acta Anaesthesiol Scand* (2013) 57(3):334–41. doi:10.1111/aas.12034

356. Schwameis R, Eder S, Pietschmann H, Fischer B, Mascher H, Tzotzos S, et al. A FIM study to assess safety and exposure of inhaled single doses of AP301-A specific ENaC channel activator for the treatment of acute lung injury. *J Clin Pharmacol* (2014) 54(3):341–50. doi:10.1002/jcph.203

357. Aigner C, Slama A, Barta M, Mitterbauer A, Lang G, Taghavi S, et al. Treatment of primary graft dysfunction after lung transplantation with orally inhaled AP301: a prospective, randomized pilot study. *J Heart Lung Transplant* (2017) pii: S1053-2498(17):32036–32033. doi:10.1016/j.healun.2017.09.021

358. Krenn K, Lucas R, Croize A, Boehme S, Klein KU, Hermann R, et al. Inhaled AP301 for treatment of pulmonary edema in mechanically ventilated patients with acute respiratory distress syndrome: a phase IIa randomized placebo-controlled trial. *Crit Care* (2017) 21(1):194. doi:10.1186/s13054-017-1795-x

359. Yamagata T, Yamagata Y, Nishimoto T, Hirano T, Nakanishi M, Minakata Y, et al. The regulation of amiloride-sensitive epithelial sodium channels by tumor necrosis factor-alpha in injured lungs and alveolar type II cells. *Respir Physiol Neurobiol* (2009) 166(1):16–23. doi:10.1016/j.resp.2008.12.008

360. Lucas R, Czikora I, Sridhar S, Zemskov E, Gorshkov B, Siddaramappa U, et al. Mini-review: novel therapeutic strategies to blunt actions of pneumolysin in the lungs. *Toxins* (2013) 5(7):1244–60. doi:10.3390/toxins5071244

361. Wilson MR, Wakabayashi K, Bertok S, Oakley CM, Patel BV, O'Dea KP, et al. Inhibition of TNF receptor p55 by a domain antibody attenuates the initial phase of acid-induced lung injury in mice. *Front Immunol* (2017) 8:128. doi:10.3389/fimmu.2017.00128

362. Wilson MR, Goddard ME, O'Dea KP, Choudhury S, Takata M. Differential roles of p55 and p75 tumor necrosis factor receptors on stretch-induced pulmonary edema in mice. *Am J Physiol Lung Cell Mol Physiol* (2007) 293(1):L60–8. doi:10.1152/ajplung.00284.2006

363. Wright TW, Pryhuber GS, Chess PR, Wang Z, Notter RH, Gigliotti F. TNF receptor signaling contributes to chemokine secretion, inflammation, and respiratory deficits during pneumocystis pneumonia. *J Immunol* (2004) 172(4):2511–21. doi:10.4049/jimmunol.172.4.2511

364. Guo RF, Ward PA. Mediators and regulation of neutrophil accumulation in inflammatory responses in lung: insights from the IgG immune complex model. *Free Radic Biol Med* (2002) 33(3):303–10. doi:10.1016/S0891-5849(02)00823-7

365. Rezaiguia S, Garat C, Delclaux C, Meignan M, Fleury J, Legrand P, et al. Acute bacterial pneumonia in rats increases alveolar epithelial fluid

clearance by a tumor necrosis factor-alpha-dependent mechanism. *J Clin Invest* (1997) 99(2):325–35. doi:10.1172/JCI119161

366. Borjesson A, Norlin A, Wang X, Andersson R, Folkesson HG. TNF-a stimulates alveolar liquid clearance during intestinal ischemia-reperfusion in rats. *Am J Physiol Lung Cell Mol Physiol* (2000) 278:L3–12.

367. Vilcek J, Feldmann M. Historical review: cytokines as therapeutics and targets of therapeutics. *Trends Pharmacol Sci* (2004) 25(4):201–9. doi:10.1016/j.tips.2004.02.011

368. Yi ES, Ulich TR. Endotoxin, interleukin-1, and tumor necrosis factor cause neutrophil-dependent microvascular leakage in postcapillary venules. *Am J Pathol* (1992) 140(3):659–63.

369. Hammond ME, Lapointe GR, Feucht PH, Hilt S, Gallegos CA, Gordon CA, et al. IL-8 induces neutrophil chemotaxis predominantly via type I IL-8 receptors. *J Immunol* (1995) 155(3):1428–33.

370. Narasaraju T, Yang E, Samy RP, Ng HH, Poh WP, Liew AA, et al. Excessive neutrophils and neutrophil extracellular traps contribute to acute lung injury of influenza pneumonitis. *Am J Pathol* (2011) 179(1):199–210. doi:10.1016/j.ajpath.2011.03.013

371. Peteranderl C, Sznajder JI, Herold S, Lecuona E. Inflammatory responses regulating alveolar ion transport during pulmonary infections. *Front Immunol* (2017) 8:446. doi:10.3389/fimmu.2017.00446

372. Petrache I, Verin AD, Crow MT, Birukova A, Liu F, Garcia JG. Differential effect of MLC kinase in TNF-alpha-induced endothelial cell apoptosis and barrier dysfunction. *Am J Physiol Lung Cell Mol Physiol* (2001) 280(6):L1168–78.

373. Goldblum SE, Hennig B, Jay M, Yoneda K, McClain CJ. Tumor necrosis factor alpha-induced pulmonary vascular endothelial injury. *Infect Immun* (1989) 57(4):1218–26.

374. Brett J, Gerlach H, Nawroth P, Steinberg S, Godman G, Stern D. Tumor necrosis factor/cachectin increases permeability of endothelial cell monolayers by a mechanism involving regulatory G proteins. *J Exp Med* (1989) 169(6):1977–91. doi:10.1084/jem.169.6.1977

375. Wheatley EM, Vincent PA, McKeown-Longo PJ, Saba TM. Effect of fibronectin on permeability of normal and TNF-treated lung endothelial cell monolayers. *Am J Physiol* (1993) 264(1 Pt 2):R90–6.

376. Partridge CA, Horvath CJ, Del Vecchio PJ, Phillips PG, Malik AB. Influence of extracellular matrix in tumor necrosis factor-induced increase in endothelial permeability. *Am J Physiol* (1992) 263(6 Pt 1):L627–33.

377. Jahr J, Grande PO. In vivo effects of tumor necrosis factor-alpha on capillary permeability and vascular tone in a skeletal muscle. *Acta Anaesthesiol Scand* (1996) 40(2):256–61. doi:10.1111/j.1399-6576.1996.tb04429.x

378. Lum H, Roebuck KA. Oxidant stress and endothelial cell dysfunction. *Am J Physiol Cell Physiol* (2001) 280(4):C719–41.

379. Hamvas A, Palazzo R, Kaiser L, Cooper J, Shuman T, Velazquez M, et al. Inflammation and oxygen free radical formation during pulmonary ischemia-reperfusion injury. *J Appl Physiol (1985)* (1992) 72(2):621–8.

380. Ischiropoulos H, al-Mehdi AB, Fisher AB. Reactive species in ischemic rat lung injury: contribution of peroxynitrite. *Am J Physiol* (1995) 269(2 Pt 1):L158–64.

381. Peralta C, Bulbena O, Xaus C, Prats N, Cutrin JC, Poli G, et al. Ischemic preconditioning: a defense mechanism against the reactive oxygen species generated after hepatic ischemia reperfusion. *Transplantation* (2002) 73(8):1203–11. doi:10.1097/00007890-200204270-00004

382. Guo Y, DuVall MD, Crow JP, Matalon S. Nitric oxide inhibits Na+ absorption across cultured alveolar type II monolayers. *Am J Physiol* (1998) 274(3 Pt 1):L369–77.

383. Peschon JJ, Slack JL, Reddy P, Stocking KL, Sunnarborg SW, Lee DC, et al. An essential role for ectodomain shedding in mammalian development. *Science* (1998) 282(5392):1281–4. doi:10.1126/science.282.5392.1281

384. Luks AM, Schoene RB, Swenson ER. High altitude. In: Broaddus VC, Mason RJ, Ernst JD, King TE, Lazarus SC, Murray JF, Slutsky AS, Gotway MB, editors. *Murray & Nadel's Texpbook of Respiratory Medicine.* Philadelphia, USA: Elsevier (2016). p. 1367–84.

385. Bartsch P, Mairbaurl H, Maggiorini M, Swenson ER. Physiological aspects of high-altitude pulmonary edema. *J Appl Physiol (1985)* (2005) 98(3):1101–10. doi:10.1152/japplphysiol.01167.2004

386. Leshem E, Pandey P, Shlim DR, Hiramatsu K, Sidi Y, Schwartz E. Clinical features of patients with severe altitude illness in Nepal. *J Travel Med* (2008) 15(5):315–22. doi:10.1111/j.1708-8305.2008.00229.x

387. Sartori C, Matthay MA. Alveolar epithelial fluid transport in acute lung injury: new insights. *Eur Respir J* (2002) 20(5):1299–313. doi:10.1183/09031936.02.00401602

388. Alli AA, Bao HF, Alli AA, Aldrugh Y, Song JZ, Ma HP, et al. Phosphatidylinositol phosphate-dependent regulation of Xenopus ENaC by MARCKS protein. *Am J Physiol Renal Physiol* (2012) 303(6):F800–11. doi:10.1152/ajprenal.00703.2011

389. Collier DM, Tomkovicz VR, Peterson ZJ, Benson CJ, Snyder PM. Intersubunit conformational changes mediate epithelial sodium channel gating. *J Gen Physiol* (2014) 144(4):337–48. doi:10.1085/jgp.201411208

390. Wiley SR, Schooley K, Smolak PJ, Din WS, Huang C-P, Nicholl JK, et al. Identification and characterization of a new member of the TNF family that induces apoptosis. *Immunity* (1995) 3(6):673–82. doi:10.1016/1074-7613(95)90057-8

391. Fensterl V, Sen GC. Interferons and viral infections. *Biofactors* (2009) 35(1):14–20. doi:10.1002/biof.6

392. Brincks EL, Katewa A, Kucaba TA, Griffith TS, Legge KL. CD8 T cells utilize TRAIL to control influenza virus infection. *J Immunol* (2008) 181(10):7428. doi:10.4049/jimmunol.181.10.7428-a

393. Herold S, Steinmueller M, von Wulffen W, Cakarova L, Pinto R, Pleschka S, et al. Lung epithelial apoptosis in influenza virus pneumonia: the role of macrophage-expressed TNF-related apoptosis-inducing ligand. *J Exp Med* (2008) 205(13):3065–77. doi:10.1084/jem.20080201

394. Ellis GT, Davidson S, Crotta S, Branzk N, Papayannopoulos V, Wack A. TRAIL+ monocytes and monocyte-related cells cause lung damage and thereby increase susceptibility to influenza-*Streptococcus pneumoniae* coinfection. *EMBO Rep* (2015) 16(9):1203–18. doi:10.15252/embr.201540473

395. Matthay MA, Ware LB, Zimmerman GA. The acute respiratory distress syndrome. *J Clin Invest* (2012) 122(8):2731–40. doi:10.1172/jci60331

396. Gonzales JN, Lucas R, Verin AD. The acute respiratory distress syndrome: mechanisms and perspective therapeutic approaches. *Austin J Vasc Med* (2015) 2(1):ii:1009.

397. Millan FA, Denhez F, Kondaiah P, Akhurst RJ. Embryonic gene expression patterns of TGF beta 1, beta 2 and beta 3 suggest different developmental functions in vivo. *Development* (1991) 111(1):131–43.

398. Worthington JJ, Fenton TM, Czajkowska BI, Klementowicz JE, Travis MA. Regulation of TGFβ in the immune system: an emerging role for integrins and dendritic cells. *Immunobiology* (2012) 217(12):1259–65. doi:10.1016/j.imbio.2012.06.009

399. Kumar V, Abbas A, Aster J. *Robbins Basic Pathology.* Tenth ed. Pennsylvania: Elsevier (2017).

400. Branton MH, Kopp JB. TGF-beta and fibrosis. *Microbes Infect* (1999) 1(15):1349–65. doi:10.1016/S1286-4579(99)00250-6

401. Massague J, Andres J, Attisano L, Cheifetz S, Lopez-Casillas F, Ohtsuki M, et al. TGF-beta receptors. *Mol Reprod Dev* (1992) 32(2):99–104. doi:10.1002/mrd.1080320204

402. Akhurst RJ, Hata A. Targeting the TGFβ signalling pathway in disease. *Nat Rev Drug Discov* (2012) 11(10):790–811. doi:10.1038/nrd3810

403. Yang H, Cao C, Wu C, Yuan C, Gu Q, Shi Q, et al. TGF-βl suppresses inflammation in cell therapy for intervertebral disc degeneration. *Sci Rep* (2015) 5:13254. doi:10.1038/srep13254

404. Pohlers D, Brenmoehl J, Löffler I, Müller CK, Leipner C, Schultze-Mosgau S, et al. TGF-β and fibrosis in different organs — molecular pathway imprints. *Biochim Biophys Acta* (2009) 1792(8):746–56. doi:10.1016/j.bbadis.2009.06.004

405. Letterio JJ, Roberts AB. Regulation of immune responses by TGF-beta. *Annu Rev Immunol* (1998) 16:137–61. doi:10.1146/annurev.immunol.16.1.137

406. Filippi CM, Juedes AE, Oldham JE, Ling E, Togher L, Peng Y, et al. Transforming growth factor-beta suppresses the activation of CD8+ T-cells when naive but promotes their survival and function once antigen experienced: a two-faced impact on autoimmunity. *Diabetes* (2008) 57(10):2684–92. doi:10.2337/db08-0609

407. Guidot DM, Modelska K, Lois M, Jain L, Moss IM, Pittet J-F, et al. Ethanol ingestion via glutathione depletion impairs alveolar epithelial barrier function in rats. *Am J Physiol Lung Cell Mol Physiol* (2000) 279(1):L127.

408. Annes JP, Munger JS, Rifkin DB. Making sense of latent TGFβ activation. *J Cell Sci* (2003) 116(2):217–24. doi:10.1242/jcs.00229

409. Munger JS, Huang X, Kawakatsu H, Griffiths MJD, Dalton SL, Wu J, et al. A mechanism for regulating pulmonary inflammation and fibrosis: the

integrin αvβ6 binds and activates latent TGF β1. *Cell* (1999) 96(3):319–28. doi:10.1016/S0092-8674(00)80545-0

410. Bickel M. The role of interleukin-8 in inflammation and mechanisms of regulation. *J Periodontol* (1993) 64(5 Suppl):456–60.

411. Chen Z, Shao X, Dou X, Zhang X, Wang Y, Zhu C, et al. Role of the *Mycoplasma pneumoniae*/interleukin-8/neutrophil axis in the pathogenesis of pneumonia. *PLoS One* (2016) 11(1):e0146377. doi:10.1371/journal.pone.0146377

412. Goodman RB, Strieter RM, Martin DP, Steinberg KP, Milberg JA, Maunder RJ, et al. Inflammatory cytokines in patients with persistence of the acute respiratory distress syndrome. *Am J Respir Crit Care Med* (1996) 154(3 Pt 1):602–11. doi:10.1164/ajrccm.154.3.8810593

413. Kurdowska A, Miller EJ, Noble JM, Baughman RP, Matthay MA, Brelsford WG, et al. Anti-IL-8 autoantibodies in alveolar fluid from patients with the adult respiratory distress syndrome. *J Immunol* (1996) 157(6):2699–706.

414. Pease JE, Sabroe I. The role of interleukin-8 and its receptors in inflammatory lung disease. *Am J Respir Med* (2002) 1(1):19–25. doi:10.1007/BF03257159

415. Miller EJ, Cohen AB, Matthay MA. Increased interleukin-8 concentrations in the pulmonary edema fluid of patients with acute respiratory distress syndrome from sepsis. *Crit Care Med* (1996) 24(9):1448–54. doi:10.1097/00003246-199609000-00004

416. Wagener BM, Roux J, Carles M, Pittet JF. Synergistic inhibition of beta2-adrenergic receptor-mediated alveolar epithelial fluid transport by interleukin-8 and transforming growth factor-beta. *Anesthesiology* (2015) 122(5):1084–92. doi:10.1097/ALN.0000000000000595

417. Meduri GU, Headley S, Kohler G, Stentz F, Tolley E, Umberger R, et al. Persistent elevation of inflammatory cytokines predicts a poor outcome in ARDS: plasma IL-1β and IL-6 levels are consistent and efficient predictors of outcome over time. *Chest* (1995) 107(4):1062–73. doi:10.1378/chest.107.4.1062

418. Matute-Bello G, Frevert CW, Liles WC, Nakamura M, Ruzinski JT, Ballman K, et al. Fas/Fas ligand system mediates epithelial injury, but not pulmonary host defenses, in response to inhaled bacteria. *Infect Immun* (2001) 69(9):5768–76. doi:10.1128/IAI.69.9.5768-5776.2001

419. Bem RA, Farnand AW, Wong V, Koski A, Rosenfeld ME, van Rooijen N, et al. Depletion of resident alveolar macrophages does not prevent Fas-mediated lung injury in mice. *Am J Physiol Lung Cell Mol Physiol* (2008) 295(2):L314–25. doi:10.1152/ajplung.00210.2007

420. Farnand AW, Eastman AJ, Herrero R, Hanson JF, Mongovin S, Altemeier WA, et al. Fas activation in alveolar epithelial cells induces KC (CXCL1) release by a MyD88-dependent mechanism. *Am J Respir Cell Mol Biol* (2011) 45(3):650–8. doi:10.1165/rcmb.2010-0153OC

421. Ye X, Acharya R, Herbert JB, Hamilton SE, Folkesson HG. IL-1beta stimulates alveolar fluid absorption in fetal guinea pig lungs via the hypothalamus-pituitary-adrenal gland axis. *Am J Physiol Lung Cell Mol Physiol* (2004) 286(4):L756–66. doi:10.1152/ajplung.00214.2003

422. Mason CM, Guery BP, Summer WR, Nelson S. Keratinocyte growth factor attenuates lung leak induced by alpha-naphthylthiourea in rats. *Crit Care Med* (1996) 24(6):925–31. doi:10.1097/00003246-199606000-00009

423. Guery BP, Mason CM, Dobard EP, Beaucaire G, Summer WR, Nelson S. Keratinocyte growth factor increases transalveolar sodium reabsorption in normal and injured rat lungs. *Am J Respir Crit Care Med* (1997) 155(5):1777–84. doi:10.1164/ajrccm.155.5.9154891

424. Borok Z, Danto SI, Dimen LL, Zhang XL, Lubman RL. Na(+)-K(+)-ATPase expression in alveolar epithelial cells: upregulation of active ion transport by KGF. *Am J Physiol* (1998) 274(1 Pt 1):L149–58.

425. Verghese GM, McCormick-Shannon K, Mason RJ, Matthay MA. Hepatocyte growth factor and keratinocyte growth factor in the pulmonary edema fluid of patients with acute lung injury. Biologic and clinical significance. *Am J Respir Crit Care Med* (1998) 158(2):386–94. doi:10.1164/ajrccm.158.2.9711111

426. Yi ES, Salgado M, Williams S, Kim SJ, Masliah E, Yin S, et al. Keratinocyte growth factor decreases pulmonary edema, transforming growth factor-beta and platelet-derived growth factor-BB expression, and alveolar type II cell loss in bleomycin-induced lung injury. *Inflammation* (1998) 22(3):315–25. doi:10.1023/A:1022304317111

427. Wang Y, Folkesson HG, Jayr C, Ware LB, Matthay MA. Alveolar epithelial fluid transport can be simultaneously upregulated by both KGF and beta-agonist therapy. *J Appl Physiol (1985)* (1999) 87(5):1852–60.

428. Viget NB, Guery BP, Ader F, Neviere R, Alfandari S, Creuzy C, et al. Keratinocyte growth factor protects against *Pseudomonas aeruginosa*-induced lung injury. *Am J Physiol Lung Cell Mol Physiol* (2000) 279(6):L1199–209.

429. Welsh DA, Summer WR, Dobard EP, Nelson S, Mason CM. Keratinocyte growth factor prevents ventilator-induced lung injury in an ex vivo rat model. *Am J Respir Crit Care Med* (2000) 162(3 Pt 1):1081–6. doi:10.1164/ajrccm.162.3.9908099

430. Welsh DA, Guery BP, Deboisblanc BP, Dobard EP, Creusy C, Mercante D, et al. Keratinocyte growth factor attenuates hydrostatic pulmonary edema in an isolated, perfused rat lung model. *Am J Physiol Heart Circ Physiol* (2001) 280(3):H1311–7.

431. Goolaerts A, Pellan-Randrianarison N, Larghero J, Vanneaux V, Uzunhan Y, Gille T, et al. Conditioned media from mesenchymal stromal cells restore sodium transport and preserve epithelial permeability in an in vitro model of acute alveolar injury. *Am J Physiol Lung Cell Mol Physiol* (2014) 306(11):975–85. doi:10.1152/ajplung.00242.2013

432. McAuley DF, Cross LM, Hamid U, Gardner E, Elborn JS, Cullen KM, et al. Keratinocyte growth factor for the treatment of the acute respiratory distress syndrome (KARE): a randomised, double-blind, placebo-controlled phase 2 trial. *Lancet Respir Med* (2017) 5(6):484–91. doi:10.1016/S2213-2600(17)30171-6

433. Neeper M, Schmidt AM, Brett J, Yan SD, Wang F, Pan YC, et al. Cloning and expression of a cell surface receptor for advanced glycosylation end products of proteins. *J Biol Chem* (1992) 267(21):14998–5004.

434. Fehrenbach H, Kasper M, Tschernig T, Shearman MS, Schuh D, Muller M. Receptor for advanced glycation endproducts (RAGE) exhibits highly differential cellular and subcellular localisation in rat and human lung. *Cell Mol Biol (Noisy-le-grand)* (1998) 44(7):1147–57.

435. Shirasawa M, Fujiwara N, Hirabayashi S, Ohno H, Iida J, Makita K, et al. Receptor for advanced glycation end-products is a marker of type I lung alveolar cells. *Genes Cells* (2004) 9(2):165–74. doi:10.1111/j.1356-9597.2004.00712.x

436. Vazzana N, Santilli F, Cuccurullo C, Davi G. Soluble forms of RAGE in internal medicine. *Intern Emerg Med* (2009) 4(5):389–401. doi:10.1007/s11739-009-0300-1

437. Sparvero LJ, Asafu-Adjei D, Kang R, Tang D, Amin N, Im J, et al. RAGE (receptor for advanced glycation endproducts), RAGE ligands, and their role in cancer and inflammation. *J Transl Med* (2009) 7:17–17. doi:10.1186/1479-5876-7-17

438. Lee EJ, Park JH. Receptor for advanced glycation endproducts (RAGE), its ligands, and soluble RAGE: potential biomarkers for diagnosis and therapeutic targets for human renal diseases. *Genomics Inform* (2013) 11(4):224–9. doi:10.5808/GI.2013.11.4.224

439. Mutlu GM, Factor P. Alveolar epithelial β(2)-adrenergic receptors. *Am J Respir Cell Mol Biol* (2008) 38(2):127–34. doi:10.1165/rcmb.2007-0198TR

440. Skeberdis VA. Structure and function of beta3-adrenergic receptors. *Medicina (Kaunas)* (2004) 40(5):407–13.

441. Billington CK, Ojo OO, Penn RB, Ito S. cAMP regulation of airway smooth muscle function. *Pulm Pharmacol Ther* (2013) 26(1):112–20. doi:10.1016/j.pupt.2012.05.007

442. Walker JK, Penn RB, Hanania NA, Dickey BF, Bond RA. New perspectives regarding beta(2) -adrenoceptor ligands in the treatment of asthma. *Br J Pharmacol* (2011) 163(1):18–28. doi:10.1111/j.1476-5381.2010.01178.x

443. Icard P, Saumon G. Alveolar sodium and liquid transport in mice. *Am J Physiol* (1999) 277(6 Pt 1):L1232–8.

444. Goodman BE, Brown SE, Crandall ED. Regulation of transport across pulmonary alveolar epithelial cell monolayers. *J Appl Physiol Respir Environ Exerc Physiol* (1984) 57(3):703–10.

445. Goodman BE, Kim KJ, Crandall ED. Evidence for active sodium transport across alveolar epithelium of isolated rat lung. *J Appl Physiol (1985)* (1987) 62(6):2460–6.

446. Jayr C, Garat C, Meignan M, Pittet JF, Zelter M, Matthay MA. Alveolar liquid and protein clearance in anesthetized ventilated rats. *J Appl Physiol (1985)* (1994) 76(6):2636–42.

447. Berthiaume Y, Broaddus VC, Gropper MA, Tanita T, Matthay MA. Alveolar liquid and protein clearance from normal dog lungs. *J Appl Physiol* (1988) 65(2):585.

448. Berthiaume Y. Effect of exogenous cAMP and aminophylline on alveolar and lung liquid clearance in anesthetized sheep. *J Appl Physiol (1985)* (1991) 70(6):2490–7.

449. Norlin A, Finley N, Abedinpour P, Folkesson HG. Alveolar liquid clearance in the anesthetized ventilated guinea pig. *Am J Physiol* (1998) 274(2 Pt 1): L235–43.

450. Fukuda N, Folkesson HG, Matthay MA. Relationship of interstitial fluid volume to alveolar fluid clearance in mice: ventilated vs. in situ studies. *J Appl Physiol (1985)* (2000) 89(2):672–9.

451. Sakuma T, Folkesson HG, Suzuki S, Okaniwa G, Fujimura S, Matthay MA. Beta-adrenergic agonist stimulated alveolar fluid clearance in ex vivo human and rat lungs. *Am J Respir Crit Care Med* (1997) 155(2):506–12. doi:10.1164/ajrccm.155.2.9032186

452. Mutlu GM, Dumasius V, Burhop J, McShane PJ, Meng FJ, Welch L, et al. Upregulation of alveolar epithelial active Na+ transport is dependent on beta2-adrenergic receptor signaling. *Circ Res* (2004) 94(8):1091–100. doi:10.1161/01.RES.0000125623.56442.20

453. Yue G, Shoemaker RL, Matalon S. Regulation of low-amiloride-affinity sodium channels in alveolar type II cells. *Am J Physiol* (1994) 267(1 Pt 1): L94–100.

454. Matalon S, O'Brodovich H. Sodium channels in alveolar epithelial cells: molecular characterization, biophysical properties, and physiological significance. *Annu Rev Physiol* (1999) 61:627–61. doi:10.1146/annurev.physiol. 61.1.627

455. Mutlu GMM, Sznajder JIM. β2-agonists for treatment of pulmonary edema: ready for clinical studies? *Crit Care Med* (2004) 32(7):1607–8. doi:10.1097/01.CCM.0000130825.84691.E2

456. Bertorello AM, Ridge KM, Chibalin AV, Katz AI, Sznajder JI. Isoproterenol increases Na+-K+-ATPase activity by membrane insertion of alpha-subunits in lung alveolar cells. *Am J Physiol* (1999) 276(1 Pt 1):L20–7.

457. Lecuona E, Ridge K, Pesce L, Batlle D, Sznajder JI. The GTP-binding protein RhoA mediates Na,K-ATPase exocytosis in alveolar epithelial cells. *Mol Biol Cell* (2003) 14(9):3888–97. doi:10.1091/mbc.E02-12-0781

458. Minakata Y, Suzuki S, Grygorczyk C, Dagenais A, Berthiaume Y. Impact of beta-adrenergic agonist on Na+ channel and Na+-K+-ATPase expression in alveolar type II cells. *Am J Physiol* (1998) 275(2 Pt 1):L414–22.

459. Pesce L, Comellas A, Sznajder JI. Beta-adrenergic agonists regulate Na-K-ATPase via p70S6k. *Am J Physiol Lung Cell Mol Physiol* (2003) 285(4): L802–7. doi:10.1152/ajplung.00266.2002

460. Berthiaume Y. Long-term stimulation of alveolar epithelial cells by beta-adrenergic agonists: increased Na+ transport and modulation of cell growth? *Am J Physiol Lung Cell Mol Physiol* (2003) 285(4):L798–801. doi:10.1152/ajplung.00166.2003

461. Suzuki S, Zuege D, Berthiaume Y. Sodium-independent modulation of Na(+)-K(+)-ATPase activity by beta-adrenergic agonist in alveolar type II cells. *Am J Physiol* (1995) 268(6 Pt 1):L983–90.

462. Berthiaume Y, Staub NC, Matthay MA. Beta-adrenergic agonists increase lung liquid clearance in anesthetized sheep. *J Clin Invest* (1987) 79(2): 335–43. doi:10.1172/JCI112817

463. Saldias FJ, Lecuona E, Comellas AP, Ridge KM, Rutschman DH, Sznajder JI. beta-adrenergic stimulation restores rat lung ability to clear edema in ventilator-associated lung injury. *Am J Respir Crit Care Med* (2000) 162(1): 282–7. doi:10.1164/ajrccm.162.1.9809058

464. Dumasius V, Sznajder JI, Azzam ZS, Boja J, Mutlu GM, Maron MB, et al. beta(2)-adrenergic receptor overexpression increases alveolar fluid clearance and responsiveness to endogenous catecholamines in rats. *Circ Res* (2001) 89(10):907–14. doi:10.1161/hh2201.100204

465. Naren AP, Cobb B, Li C, Roy K, Nelson D, Heda GD, et al. A macromolecular complex of β2 adrenergic receptor, CFTR, and ezrin/radixin/moesin-binding phosphoprotein 50 is regulated by PKA. *Proc Natl Acad Sci U S A* (2003) 100(1):342–6. doi:10.1073/pnas.0135434100

466. Taouil K, Hinnrasky J, Hologne C, Corlieu P, Klossek JM, Puchelle E. Stimulation of beta 2-adrenergic receptor increases cystic fibrosis transmembrane conductance regulator expression in human airway epithelial cells through a cAMP/protein kinase A-independent pathway. *J Biol Chem* (2003) 278(19):17320–7. doi:10.1074/jbc.M212227200

467. Berthiaume Y, Folkesson HG, Matthay MA. Lung edema clearance: 20 years of progress: invited review: alveolar edema fluid clearance in the injured lung. *J Appl Physiol (1985)* (2002) 93(6):2207–13. doi:10.1152/japplphysiol.01201.2001

468. Gates S, Perkins GD, Lamb SE, Kelly C, Thickett DR, Young JD, et al. Beta-Agonist Lung injury TrIal-2 (BALTI-2): a multicentre, randomised, double-blind, placebo-controlled trial and economic evaluation of intravenous infusion of salbutamol versus placebo in patients with acute respiratory distress syndrome. *Health Technol Assess* (2013) 17(38):v–vi,1–87. doi:10.3310/hta17380

469. Festic E, Carr GE, Cartin-Ceba R, Hinds RF, Banner-Goodspeed V, Bansal V, et al. Randomized clinical trial of a combination of an inhaled corticosteroid and beta agonist in patients at risk of developing the acute respiratory distress syndrome. *Crit Care Med* (2017) 45(5):798–805. doi:10.1097/CCM.0000000000002284

470. Briot R, Bayat S, Anglade D, Martiel JL, Grimbert F. Increased cardiac index due to terbutaline treatment aggravates capillary-alveolar macromolecular leakage in oleic acid lung injury in dogs. *Crit Care* (2009) 13(5):R166. doi:10.1186/cc8137

471. Sylvester JT, Shimoda LA, Aaronson PI, Ward JP. Hypoxic pulmonary vasoconstriction. *Physiol Rev* (2012) 92(1):367–520. doi:10.1152/physrev. 00041.2010

472. Berthiaume Y, Albertine KH, Grady M, Fick G, Matthay MA. Protein clearance from the air spaces and lungs of unanesthetized sheep over 144 h. *J Appl Physiol (1985)* (1989) 67(5):1887–97.

473. Friedman M, Vidyasagar R, Joseph N. A randomized, prospective, double-blind study on the efficacy of dead sea salt nasal irrigations. *Laryngoscope* (2006) 116(6):878–82. doi:10.1097/01.mlg.0000216798.10007.76

474. Khianey R, Oppenheimer J. Is nasal saline irrigation all it is cracked up to be? *Ann Allergy Asthma Immunol* (2012) 109(1):20–8. doi:10.1016/j.anai.2012.04.019

475. Mandal MD, Mandal S. Honey: its medicinal property and antibacterial activity. *Asian Pac J Trop Biomed* (2011) 1(2):154–60. doi:10.1016/S2221-1691(11)60016-6

476. Angoulvant F, Bellettre X, Milcent K, Teglas JP, Claudet I, Le Guen CG, et al. Effect of nebulized hypertonic saline treatment in emergency departments on the hospitalization rate for acute bronchiolitis: a randomized clinical trial. *JAMA Pediatr* (2017) 171(8):e171333. doi:10.1001/jamapediatrics.2017.1333

477. Farabaugh KT, Majumder M, Guan BJ, Jobava R, Wu J, Krokowski D, et al. Protein kinase R mediates the inflammatory response induced by hyperosmotic stress. *Mol Cell Biol* (2017) 37(4):e521–516. doi:10.1128/MCB.00521-16

478. Gamboni F, Anderson C, Mitra S, Reisz JA, Nemkov T, Dzieciatkowska M, et al. Hypertonic saline primes activation of the p53-p21 signaling axis in human small airway epithelial cells that prevents inflammation induced by pro-inflammatory cytokines. *J Proteome Res* (2016) 15(10):3813–26. doi:10.1021/acs.jproteome.6b00602

479. Liu Z, Zhang B, Wang XB, Li Y, Xi RG, Han F, et al. Hypertonicity contributes to seawater aspiration-induced lung injury: role of hypoxia-inducible factor 1alpha. *Exp Lung Res* (2015) 41(6):301–15. doi:10.3109/01902148.2015.1030803

480. Machnik A, Neuhofer W, Jantsch J, Dahlmann A, Tammela T, Machura K, et al. Macrophages regulate salt-dependent volume and blood pressure by a vascular endothelial growth factor-C-dependent buffering mechanism. *Nat Med* (2009) 15(5):545–52. doi:10.1038/nm.1960

481. Kleinewietfeld M, Manzel A, Titze J, Kvakan H, Yosef N, Linker RA, et al. Sodium chloride drives autoimmune disease by the induction of pathogenic TH17 cells. *Nature* (2013) 496(7446):518–22. doi:10.1038/nature11868

482. Titze J, Shakibaei M, Schafflhuber M, Schulze-Tanzil G, Porst M, Schwind KH, et al. Glycosaminoglycan polymerization may enable osmotically inactive Na+ storage in the skin. *Am J Physiol Heart Circ Physiol* (2004) 287(1):H203–8. doi:10.1152/ajpheart.01237.2003

483. Scaife PJ, Mohaupt MG. Salt, aldosterone and extrarenal Na+-sensitive responses in pregnancy. *Placenta* (2017) 56:53–8. doi:10.1016/j.placenta.2017.01.100

484. O'Brodovich HM. Immature epithelial Na+ channel expression is one of the pathogenetic mechanisms leading to human neonatal respiratory distress syndrome. *Proc Assoc Am Physicians* (1996) 108(5):345–55.

485. Helve O, Pitkanen OM, Andersson S, O'Brodovich H, Kirjavainen T, Otulakowski G. Low expression of human epithelial sodium channel in

airway epithelium of preterm infants with respiratory distress. *Pediatrics* (2004) 113(5):1267–72. doi:10.1542/peds.113.5.1267

486. Li W, Long C, Renjun L, Zhangxue H, Yin H, Wanwei L, et al. Association of SCNN1A single nucleotide polymorphisms with neonatal respiratory distress syndrome. *Sci Rep* (2015) 5:17317. doi:10.1038/srep17317

487. De Luca D, van Kaam AH, Tingay DG, Courtney SE, Danhaive O, Carnielli VP, et al. The Montreux definition of neonatal ARDS: biological and clinical background behind the description of a new entity. *Lancet Respir Med* (2017) 5(8):657–66. doi:10.1016/S2213-2600(17)30214-X

488. Mason JS, Becker JB, Garrity JR. Indications for lung transplantation and patient selection. *Lung Transplantation: Principles and Practice.* Boca Raton, FL: CRC Press, Taylor & Francis Group (2016). p. 29–54.

489. Christie JD, Kotloff RM, Pochettino A, Arcasoy SM, Rosengard BR, Landis JR, et al. Clinical risk factors for primary graft failure following lung transplantation. *Chest* (2003) 124(4):1232–41. doi:10.1378/chest.124.4.1232

490. Kotloff RM, Keshavjee RM. Lung transplantation. In: Broaddus CV, Mason RJ, Ernst JD, King TE, Lazarus SC, Murray JF, Nadel JA, Slutsky AS, Gotway MB, editors. *Murray & Nadel's Textbook fof Respiratory Medicine.* Philadelphia: Elsevier (2016). p. 1832–49.

491. King RC, Binns OA, Rodriguez F, Kanithanon RC, Daniel TM, Spotnitz WD, et al. Reperfusion injury significantly impacts clinical outcome after pulmonary transplantation. *Ann Thorac Surg* (2000) 69(6):1681–5. doi:10.1016/S0003-4975(00)01425-9

492. Christie JD, Carby M, Bag R, Corris P, Hertz M, Weill D, et al. Report of the ISHLT working group on primary lung graft dysfunction part II: definition. A consensus statement of the International Society for Heart and Lung Transplantation. *J Heart Lung Transplant* (2005) 24(10):1454–9. doi:10.1016/j.healun.2004.11.049

493. Christie JD, Kotloff RM, Ahya VN, Tino G, Pochettino A, Gaughan C, et al. The effect of primary graft dysfunction on survival after lung transplantation. *Am J Respir Crit Care Med* (2005) 171(11):1312–6. doi:10.1164/rccm.200409-1243OC

494. Thabut G, Mal H, Cerrina J, Dartevelle P, Dromer C, Velly JF, et al. Graft ischemic time and outcome of lung transplantation: a multicenter analysis. *Am J Respir Crit Care Med* (2005) 171(7):786–91. doi:10.1164/rccm.200409-1248OC

495. Bharat A, Narayanan K, Street T, Fields RC, Steward N, Aloush A, et al. Early posttransplant inflammation promotes the development of alloimmunity and chronic human lung allograft rejection. *Transplantation* (2007) 83(2):150–8. doi:10.1097/01.tp.0000250579.08042.b6

496. Whitson BA, Prekker ME, Herrington CS, Whelan TP, Radosevich DM, Hertz MI, et al. Primary graft dysfunction and long-term pulmonary function after lung transplantation. *J Heart Lung Transplant* (2007) 26(10):1004–11. doi:10.1016/j.healun.2007.07.018

497. Bharat A, Kuo E, Steward N, Aloush A, Hachem R, Trulock EP, et al. Immunological link between primary graft dysfunction and chronic lung allograft rejection. *Ann Thorac Surg* (2008) 86(1):189–95. doi:10.1016/j.athoracsur.2008.03.073; discussion 196-187,

498. Basseri B, Conklin JL, Pimentel M, Tabrizi R, Phillips EH, Simsir SA, et al. Esophageal motor dysfunction and gastroesophageal reflux are prevalent in lung transplant candidates. *Ann Thorac Surg* (2010) 90(5):1630–6. doi:10.1016/j.athoracsur.2010.06.104

499. Chatterjee S, Nieman GF, Christie JD, Fisher AB. Shear stress-related mechanosignaling with lung ischemia: lessons from basic research can inform lung transplantation. *Am J Physiol Lung Cell Mol Physiol* (2014) 307(9):L668–80. doi:10.1152/ajplung.00198.2014

500. Cohen DG, Christie JD, Anderson BJ, Diamond JM, Judy RP, Shah RJ, et al. Cognitive function, mental health, and health-related quality of life after lung transplantation. *Ann Am Thorac Soc* (2014) 11(4):522–30. doi:10.1513/AnnalsATS.201311-388OC

501. Hartert M, Senbaklavacin O, Gohrbandt B, Fischer BM, Buhl R, Vahld CF. Lung transplantation: a treatment option in end-stage lung disease. *Dtsch Arztebl Int* (2014) 111(7):107–16. doi:10.3238/arztebl.2014.0107

502. Huang HJ, Yusen RD, Meyers BF, Walter MJ, Mohanakumar T, Patterson GA, et al. Late primary graft dysfunction after lung transplantation and bronchiolitis obliterans syndrome. *Am J Transplant* (2008) 8(11):2454–62. doi:10.1111/j.1600-6143.2008.02389.x

503. De Perrot M, Liu M, Waddell TK, Keshavjee S. Ischemia–reperfusion-induced lung injury. *Am J Respir Crit Care Med* (2003) 167(4):490–511. doi:10.1164/rccm.200207-670SO

504. Tatham KC, O'Dea KP, Romano R, Donaldson HE, Wakabayashi K, Patel BV, et al. Intravascular donor monocytes play a central role in lung transplant ischaemia-reperfusion injury. *Thorax* (2017) 1–11. doi:10.1136/thoraxjnl-2016-208977

505. Keshavjee S, Davis RD, Zamora MR, de Perrot M, Patterson GA. A randomized, placebo-controlled trial of complement inhibition in ischemia-reperfusion injury after lung transplantation in human beings. *J Thorac Cardiovasc Surg* (2005) 129(2):423–8. doi:10.1016/j.jtcvs.2004.06.048

506. Borders C, Ellis J, Cantu EM III, Christie JD. Primary graft dysfunction. In: Vineswaran WT, Garrity JER, Odell JA, editors. *Lung transplantation. Principles and Practice.* Boca Raton, London, New York: Taylor & Francis Group (2016). p. 251–63.

507. Cypel M, Keshavjee S. Strategies for safe donor expansion: donor management, donations after cardiac death, ex-vivo lung perfusion. *Curr Opin Organ Transplant* (2013) 18(5):513–7. doi:10.1097/MOT.0b013e328365191b

508. Juarez MM, Chan AL, Norris AG, Morrissey BM, Albertson TE. Acute exacerbation of idiopathic pulmonary fibrosis-a review of current and novel pharmacotherapies. *J Thorac Dis* (2015) 7(3):499–519. doi:10.3978/j.issn.2072-1439.2015.01.17

509. Ryerson CJ, Cottin V, Brown KK, Collard HR. Acute exacerbation of idiopathic pulmonary fibrosis: shifting the paradigm. *Eur Respir J* (2015) 46(2):512–20. doi:10.1183/13993003.00419-2015

510. Emura I, Usuda H. Acute exacerbation of IPF has systemic consequences with multiple organ injury, with SRA+ and TNF-alpha+ cells in the systemic circulation playing central roles in multiple organ injury. *BMC Pulm Med* (2016) 16(1):138. doi:10.1186/s12890-016-0298-x

511. Seely EW, Solomon CG. Improving the prediction of preeclampsia. *N Engl J Med* (2016) 374(1):83–4. doi:10.1056/NEJMe1515223

512. Roberts JM, Lain KY. Recent insights into the pathogenesis of pre-eclampsia. *Placenta* (2002) 23(5):359–72. doi:10.1053/plac.2002.0819

513. Naeije R, Swenson ER. Inhaled budesonide for acute mountain sickness. *Eur Respir J* (2017) 50(3). doi:10.1183/13993003.01355-2017

514. Wiedemann HP, Wheeler AP, Bernard GR, Thompson BT, Hayden D, deBoisblanc B, et al. Comparison of two fluid-management strategies in acute lung injury. *N Engl J Med* (2006) 354(24):2564–75. doi:10.1056/NEJMoa062200

515. Kuebler WM, Ying X, Singh B, Issekutz AC, Bhattacharya J. Pressure is proinflammatory in lung venular capillaries. *J Clin Invest* (1999) 104(4):495–502. doi:10.1172/JCI6872

516. Bachofen H, Bachofen M, Weibel ER. Ultrastructural aspects of pulmonary edema. *J Thorac Imaging* (1988) 3(3):1–7. doi:10.1097/00005382-198807000-00005

517. Constantin J-M, Cayot-Constantin S, Roszyk L, Futier E, Sapin V, Dastugue B, et al. Response to recruitment maneuver influences net alveolar fluid clearance in acute respiratory distress syndrome. *Anesthesiology* (2007) 106(5):944–51. doi:10.1097/01.anes.0000265153.17062.64

3

Inflammatory Responses Regulating Alveolar Ion Transport during Pulmonary Infections

Christin Peteranderl[1]*, Jacob I. Sznajder[2], Susanne Herold[1] and Emilia Lecuona[2]

[1] *Department of Internal Medicine II, University of Giessen and Marburg Lung Center (UGMLC), Member of the German Center for Lung Research (DZL), Giessen, Germany, [2] Division of Pulmonary and Critical Care Medicine, Feinberg School of Medicine, Northwestern University, Chicago, IL, USA*

*Correspondence:
Christin Peteranderl
christin.peteranderl@innere.med.
uni-giessen.de

The respiratory epithelium is lined by a tightly balanced fluid layer that allows normal O_2 and CO_2 exchange and maintains surface tension and host defense. To maintain alveolar fluid homeostasis, both the integrity of the alveolar–capillary barrier and the expression of epithelial ion channels and pumps are necessary to establish a vectorial ion gradient. However, during pulmonary infection, auto- and/or paracrine-acting mediators induce pathophysiological changes of the alveolar–capillary barrier, altered expression of epithelial Na,K-ATPase and of epithelial ion channels including epithelial sodium channel and cystic fibrosis membrane conductance regulator, leading to the accumulation of edema and impaired alveolar fluid clearance. These mediators include classical pro-inflammatory cytokines such as TGF-β, TNF-α, interferons, or IL-1β that are released upon bacterial challenge with *Streptococcus pneumoniae*, *Klebsiella pneumoniae*, or *Mycoplasma pneumoniae* as well as in viral infection with influenza A virus, pathogenic coronaviruses, or respiratory syncytial virus. Moreover, the pro-apoptotic mediator TNF-related apoptosis-inducing ligand, extracellular nucleotides, or reactive oxygen species impair epithelial ion channel expression and function. Interestingly, during bacterial infection, alterations of ion transport function may serve as an additional feedback loop on the respiratory inflammatory profile, further aggravating disease progression. These changes lead to edema formation and impair edema clearance which results in suboptimal gas exchange causing hypoxemia and hypercapnia. Recent preclinical studies suggest that modulation of the alveolar–capillary fluid homeostasis could represent novel therapeutic approaches to improve outcomes in infection-induced lung injury.

Keywords: ion channel, ion pumps, edema, cytokines, Na-K-ATPase, cystic fibrosis membrane conductance regulator, epithelial sodium channel, lung injury

---

Abbreviations: AFC, alveolar fluid clearance; ALF, alveolar lining fluid; ALI, acute lung injury; AMPK, AMP-kinase; AQP, aquaporin; ARDS, acute respiratory distress syndrome; ASL, airway surface liquid; CaCC, Ca^{2+}-activated ion channels; cAMP, cyclic AMP; CFTR, cystic fibrosis membrane conductance regulator; CNG, cyclic nucleotide-gated cation channel; ENaC, epithelial sodium channel; IAV, influenza A virus; ICAM, intercellular adhesion molecule-1; IFN, interferons; IL, interleukin; L-NMMA, N(omega)-monomethyl-L-arginine; LPS, lipopolysaccharide; MERS-CoV, middle east respiratory syndrome coronavirus; mRNA, messenger RNA; NETs, neutrophil extracellular traps; NKCC, $Na^+/K^+/2Cl^-$ cotransporters; NO, nitric oxide; PECAM, platelet endothelial cell adhesion molecule-1; RONS, reactive oxygen and nitrogen species; ROS, reactive oxygen species; RSV, respiratory syncytial virus; SARS-CoV, severe acute respiratory syndrome coronavirus; TGF-β, transforming growth factor beta; TNFR1, TNF receptor 1; TNF-α, tumor necrosis factor alpha; TRAIL, TNF-related apoptosis-inducing ligand; VCAM, vascular adhesion molecule-1; β2AR, beta-2 adrenergic receptor.

INTRODUCTION

The major task of the respiratory tract is the exchange between inhaled atmospheric oxygen and carbon dioxide carried by the bloodstream, which is ensured by a thin but large surface area formed by type I and type II alveolar epithelial cells. Both the upper and the lower respiratory epithelia are lined by a thin (0.2 μM) aqueous layer (1), referred to as airway surface liquid (ASL) and alveolar lining fluid (AFL), respectively. This fluidic component serves—in concerted action with surfactant, mucus, and ciliary beat—to reduce alveolar surface tension and prevent atelectasis as well as to defend against invading pathogens. To maintain the composition of the ASL and AFL and to prevent alveolar flooding, lung fluid homeostasis is tightly controlled by the expression and activity of ion channels and pumps. These channels and pumps establish an osmotic gradient between airspace and interstitium, driving paracellular or aquaporin- (AQP3, 4, and 5) (2) mediated fluid movement across the respiratory epithelium. Among these, the apical amiloride-sensitive epithelial sodium channel (ENaC) and the amiloride-insensitive cyclic nucleotide-gated cation channel (CNG) acting together with the basolaterally located Na,K-ATPase (NKA) promote transcellular sodium transport (3), which is accompanied in the alveolar epithelium by chloride uptake from the apical cystic fibrosis membrane conductance regulator (CFTR) (4). However, in the airway, CFTR promotes chloride secretion to regulate mucus density (5). In addition, Ca^{2+}-activated ion channels (CaCC) promote apical chloride secretion, further supported by basolateral chloride uptake via $Na^+/K^+/2Cl^-$ cotransporters (NKCC) (6) as well as potassium ion channels such as Kv7.1, contributing to cellular membrane potential and buildup of an electrochemical gradient necessary for apical chloride secretion (7). Additional factors influencing fluid homeostasis are epithelial (im)permeability established by tight junction proteins as well as endothelial integrity limiting the extravasation of fluid from the blood vessels driven by changes in the capillary hydrostatic pressure (8, 9).

Pulmonary infections commonly disturb ion and thus fluid homeostasis, resulting in abnormal changes of ASL, AFL, and alveolar edema formation. Both viral and bacterial pathogens are common causative agents for acute lung injury (ALI) and the acute respiratory distress syndrome (ARDS), which are characterized by a widespread inflammation within the lungs, extensive flooding of the alveolar airspace with protein-rich exudate fluid and impaired gas exchange leading to respiratory failure and resulting in mortality rates of 40–58% (10, 11). Additionally, sepsis resulting from primary infections at other sites is often complicated by the development of severe lung injury during the onset of bacteremia, resulting in lung failure and accounting for as many as half of all cases of ARDS (12). Although some of the pathogen-derived effects on ion transport during lung injury have been reported to be caused directly by the pathogen–host cell interaction (13), accumulating evidence suggests that auto- and paracrine mediators of local and/or systemic inflammatory responses mounted upon pathogen recognition and replication induce—among other pathophysiological changes—impaired ion transport and alveolar fluid clearance (AFC), resulting in edema formation and persistence. Importantly, mortality in ARDS patients has repeatedly been found to correlate with persistence of alveolar edema (11, 14).

In this review, we will highlight advances in the understanding of how inflammatory responses in pulmonary infection affect ion transport, including common patterns and unique pathways activated by different respiratory pathogens, and how these mechanisms might be modulated to improve the outcomes of ARDS patients.

MEDIATORS MODULATING ION AND FLUID HOMEOSTASIS

There are numerous reports showing that pulmonary infection leads to loss of barrier integrity and edema accumulation as well as the role of distinct mediators on impairing ion channel or transporter function on the alveolar, bronchial, and gut epithelia. However, there have been few studies showing how infectious agents modulate soluble signaling molecules that affect ion and fluid homeostasis. Several reports from the last decade have reestablished an important role for soluble, inflammatory mediators in the progression of ARDS. For example, Lee et al. demonstrated that exposure of human ATII cells to pulmonary edema fluid derived from ARDS patients alone was sufficient to downregulate the ion channels and pumps involved in AFC, including ENaC, the NKA, and CFTR (15). Concomitantly, it was established that viral or bacterial lung infections lead to edema accumulation and impair clearance via the induction of paracrine factors. For example, influenza A virus (IAV) has been shown to increase apical potassium secretion by upregulation of the apical potassium channel KCNN4 by a paracrine signaling event, thus disturbing the osmotic gradient necessary for edema clearance (16). Similarly, *Pseudomonas aeruginosa* evokes a strong inflammatory response and lung edema accumulation related with the modulation of ENaC subunit expression (17, 18). In the next paragraphs, we will provide an overview on interconnections of mediators released in pulmonary infection and their effects on ion and fluid homeostasis (**Figure 1**).

Interferon

Once cells detect pathogens by their specific and specialized pattern recognition receptors, they produce interferons (IFN), which can be detected—if not actively suppressed by a given pathogen—in most pulmonary infection scenarios. Effects of IFN on fluid homeostasis seem to be mostly limited to gamma IFN (IFN-γ), which have been attributed a modulatory role in both innate and adaptive immunity (19, 20). IFN-γ has been reported to decrease sodium transport at levels as low as 10 U/ml (21). Moreover, IFN-γ can also directly decrease chloride currents along the bronchial epithelium by downregulating CFTR due to a posttranscriptional modulation of CFTR messenger RNA (mRNA) stability and thus half-life (21–23). In contrast, both class I IFN, IFN-α, and IFN-β that are usually implicated in mounting a direct cellular pathogen-restrictive response do not modulate CFTR mRNA or protein abundance (22). IFN-α appears to negatively impact NKA cell membrane protein abundance during IAV infection via activating the metabolic sensor AMP-kinase (AMPK) (24). However, to date,

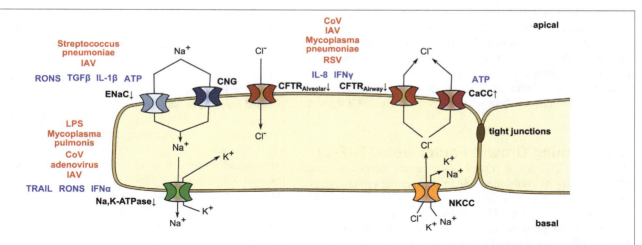

FIGURE 1 | **Mediators released in pulmonary infection and their effects on ion homeostasis.** Ion transport of the lung epithelial cell is mediated by various ion channels and pumps. Sodium enters the epithelial cell via the apical cyclic nucleotide-gated cation channel (CNG) or the epithelial sodium channel (ENaC), that can be downregulated by reactive oxygen and nitrogen species (RONS) and ATP, transforming growth factor beta (TGF-β) or interleukin-1 beta (IL-1β) upon *Streptococcus pneumoniae* and influenza A virus (IAV) infection. Sodium is secreted at the basolateral side by the Na,K-ATPase (NKA), which is modulated in lipopolysaccharide (LPS)-induced lung injury as well as upon *Mycoplasma pulmonis*, IAV, coronavirus (CoV), or adenovirus challenge. RONS, interferon-alpha (IFN-α), and TNF-related apoptosis-inducing ligand (TRAIL) lead to a decrease in NKA abundance or activity. In parallel, chloride is taken up (alveolar epithelium) or secreted (airway) by the cystic fibrosis membrane conductance regulator (CFTR) and secreted by apical Ca^{2+}-activated ion channels (CaCC), supported by basolateral potassium channels (not shown) and $Na^+/K^+/2Cl^-$ cotransporters (NKCC). While extracellular ATP enhances chloride secretion by CaCC, CFTR action is reduced by IFN-γ and interleukin-8 (IL-8) in CoV, IAV, respiratory syncytial virus (RSV), or *Mycoplasma pneumoniae* infection.

there is no data supporting whether this effect of IFN-α on ion transport is a generalized response during pulmonary infections.

Tumor Necrosis Factor Alpha (TNF-α)

Tumor necrosis factor alpha is a classical cytokine produced upon local or systemic inflammation, regulating differential processes such as proliferation and differentiation of immune cells as well as cell death (25–27). After initial conflicting studies, it has by now become clear that it plays a dichotomic role in lung fluid reabsorption (28). On one hand, TNF-α ligation to its receptor TNF receptor 1 (TNFR1, also named CD120a or p55) inhibits ENaC activity both *in vitro* and *in vivo via* a PKC-dependent mechanism (29). On the other hand, a distinct lectin-like domain of TNF different from the receptor-binding domain, which can be mimicked by the 17-amino acid circular TIP peptide (30), has been reported to increase edema reabsorption in rat bacterial pneumonia (31). Application of the TIP peptide has been demonstrated to elevate ENaC expression and open probability (32) resulting in enhanced AFC in *P. aeruginosa*-treated rats *in vivo* (31) and has furthermore been reported to increase NKA activity (33). In addition to its direct effects on ion channels and pumps of the alveolar epithelium, the TNF-α/TNFR1 interaction also modulates the integrity of the alveolar barrier, as it increases endothelial expression of chemoattractants and adhesion molecules including the interleukin-8 (IL-8; formerly called neutrophil chemotactic factor)/IL-8-receptor 2 axis, the intercellular adhesion molecule-1, platelet endothelial cell adhesion molecule-1, and vascular adhesion molecule-1, and thus promotes excessive recruitment of mononuclear phagocytes and neutrophils during lung inflammation (30, 34, 35). Importantly, besides cellular transmigration itself, neutrophil-derived proteases and neutrophil extracellular traps are central drivers of both endothelial and epithelial injury (36).

Interleukin-1 Beta (IL-1β)

Interleukin-1 beta is one of the most commonly found cytokines in pulmonary edema and bronchoalveolar lavage fluids in experimental and human ARDS (37, 38) and is, for example, induced during *Klebsiella pneumoniae* bacterial pneumonia (39–41). It is mainly produced by macrophages and, similarly to TNF-α, has a major impact on cell proliferation, differentiation, and cell death. In pulmonary inflammation, IL-1β increases lung barrier permeability in *in vitro* and *in vivo* models of ARDS (41, 42) and may contribute to alveolar edema in lung injury models by impairing fluid reabsorption from the lungs. This can in part be attributed to decreased sodium absorption due to a decrease in αENaC expression and trafficking to the apical membrane of ATII cells (43). In addition, IL-1β in *Streptococcus pneumonia* infection (44)—and also TNF-α and IFN-γ (45)—can influence ion transport processes *via* activation of the pro-coagulant factors (46). Thrombin in particular has been demonstrated to impair AFC by increasing the PKC-ζ-dependent endocytosis of the alveolar NKA (47).

Interleukin-8

Interleukin-8 is a chemotactic factor that correlates with neutrophil accumulation in distal airspaces of patients with ARDS and is a predictor of mortality (48–50). IL-8 is secreted by bronchial epithelial cells and can be induced by *Mycoplasma pneumoniae* antigen or live *M. pneumoniae* (51) as well as by severe acute respiratory syndrome coronavirus spike protein or respiratory syncytial virus infection (52, 53). The rate of AFC is impaired by high levels of IL-8 and is significantly lower in patients who have a pulmonary edema fluid concentration of IL-8 above 4,000 pg/ml (54). Mechanistically, IL-8 inhibits beta-2 adrenergic receptor (β2AR) agonist-stimulated fluid transport across rat and human alveolar epithelia. This inhibition is mediated by a PI3K-dependent desensitization and downregulation of the β2AR from the cell membrane associated with an inhibition of cyclic AMP generation normally observed in response to β2AR agonist stimulation (54).

Transforming Growth Factor Beta (TGF-β)

The cytokine TGF-β is a critical factor for the development of ARDS. Besides its established role in dampening inflammatory responses (55), e.g., by driving macrophages toward an anti-inflammatory phenotype (56), it increases alveolar epithelial permeability to promote edema formation upon lipopolysaccharide (LPS) stimulation (57). Furthermore, TGF-β has been shown to inhibit amiloride-sensitive sodium transport by an ERK1/2-dependent inhibition of the αENaC subunit promoter activity, decreasing αENaC mRNA and protein expression (58). In addition, Peters et al. (59) demonstrated that TGF-β leads to the subsequent activation of phospholipase D1, phosphatidyl-inositol-4-phosphate 5-kinase 1α, and NADPH oxidase 4 (Nox4). Nox4 activation results in the production of reactive oxygen species (ROS) that in turn reduce cell surface stability of the $\alpha\beta\gamma$ENaC complex and thus promote edema fluid accumulation. Moreover, TGF-β decreases NKA β1 subunit expression, resulting in decreased NKA activity in lung epithelial cells (60, 61). In further support of a role for TGF-β in lung injury, TGF-β levels are increased in lung fluids from patients with ALI/ARDS (62) and in murine models of *Streptococcus pneumoniae* and IAV infection (63, 64). Of note, TGF-β has been proposed to further aggravate edema formation in IAV infection by increasing epithelial cell death, causing a disruption of epithelial barrier integrity (64). Moreover, it has been implicated in the upregulation of cellular adhesins which increase host susceptibility to bacterial co-infections (65) posing a major risk for increased viral pneumonia-associated morbidity and mortality during influenza epidemics (66).

TNF-Related Apoptosis-Inducing Ligand (TRAIL)

The principal role of TRAIL, highly released by lung macrophages upon viral infection, is to drive infected cells into apoptosis to limit pathogen spread. TRAIL has been reported to be produced especially during viral respiratory infections, including IAV-, adenovirus-, and paramyxovirus infection, and cell sensitivity to TRAIL-induced apoptosis is enhanced in infected cells by increased TRAIL-receptor expression (67, 68). However, this process also affects alveolar epithelial barrier integrity leading to edema accumulation (67, 69). Moreover, TRAIL signaling leads to NKA downregulation in IAV infection in non-infected neighboring alveolar epithelial cells mediated by AMPK (24). Accordingly, TRAIL signaling reduces AFC and promotes edema formation. In addition, TRAIL release upon IAV infection further favors bacterial superinfection with *S. pneumoniae*, aggravating lung injury (70).

Nucleotides

During acute infection, extracellular nucleotides often serve as danger signals involved in recognition and control of pathogens by promoting the recruitment of inflammatory cells, stimulating pro-inflammatory cytokines, and increasing the production of ROS or nitric oxide (NO) (71, 72). Extracellular ATP, which can be released from the airway epithelia and is produced by endothelial cells upon acute inflammation, binds to P2 purinergic receptors to promote a calcium signaling-dependent stimulation of CaCC and a decreased open probability of ENaC (73, 74). Moreover, extracellular adenosine, produced from ATP by hydrolysis *via* the ecto-5'-nucleotidase CD73, is increased in bronchoalveolar lavage fluid of IAV-infected mice, and genetic deletion of the A1-adenosine-receptor is protective (75). However, CD73 is only to a limited extent involved in the progression of lung injury and has no effect on pulmonary edema formation (76).

Reactive Oxygen and Nitrogen Species (RONS)

Reactive oxygen and nitrogen species have been shown to be involved in the development of epithelial injury in pathologic situations, including LPS-/sepsis-induced lung injury as well as viral pneumonia, in which RONS are produced in large quantities by alveolar phagocytes (77). Studies in rabbit and piglet lungs further elucidated that RONS affect AFC and edema persistence by inhibiting both the activity of ENaC and alveolar epithelial NKA (78, 79).

EFFECTS OF ION CHANGES ON CYTOKINE PRODUCTION

To add to the complexity of airway and alveolar fluid regulation, it has been suggested that not only ion channels, pumps, and transporters are modulated by signaling factors released upon pulmonary infection but also changes in ion transport influence the respiratory inflammatory response. For example, the transporter NKCC1—which plays a critical role in basolateral ion transport—can affect the severity of pneumonia and sepsis and consequently severity of lung injury, by regulating the ability of the alveolar–capillary barrier to modulate neutrophil infiltration into the air spaces of the lung (80). Lack of NKCC1 in a mouse model of pneumonia infection with *K. pneumonia* or LPS resulted in increased numbers of neutrophils in the lavage fluid, decreased bacteremia, and importantly mortality. It has, therefore, been suggested that the activity of NKCC1 contributes to edema formation and decreased neutrophil migration into the lung air spaces, probably contributing to reduce bacterial killing and the subsequent development of severe sepsis (81–83). Similarly, mutations of CFTR can amplify lung inflammation by upregulating pro-inflammatory responses caused by an increase in cytokine production upon NFκB activation in lung epithelial cells (84). Lack of functional neutrophilic CFTR in a model of LPS-induced lung inflammation contributes to inflammatory imbalance with NFκB translocation and a reduction of anti-inflammatory cytokines such as IL-10, favoring the increase in lung vascular permeability (85). Also ion imbalances in

Inflammatory Responses Regulating Alveolar Ion Transport during Pulmonary Infections

response to expression of viral ion channels or viroporins, has been recognized as potential pathogen recognition pathway that favors inflammasome activation and the release of IL-1β, TNF, and IL-6, which might contribute to the limitation of virus spreading (86, 87).

THERAPEUTIC MODULATION OF THE ALVEOLAR–CAPILLARY FLUID BALANCE DURING PULMONARY INFECTION

As stated above, pulmonary infections—especially in severe cases—can lead to lung edema accumulation and impaired edema clearance. Lung edema results in impaired oxygenation and organ dysfunction which if not resolved leads to high mortality of patients with ARDS (11, 14). Current treatment options for infection-induced ARDS include antivirals and antibiotics. However, there is increased antibiotic resistance—reported for pathogens such as *K. pneumoniae*, *Escherichia coli*, *Staphylococcus aureus* and *P. aeruginosa* (82, 83, 88)—or lack of readily available treatment options for some acute emerging agents such as zoonotic influenza viruses or middle east respiratory syndrome coronavirus (89–91). Current approaches to treat ARDS patients include low tidal volume mechanical ventilation, positive end expiratory pressure, fluid management, and extracorporeal membrane oxygenation as measures to primarily improve oxygenation (92). Interestingly, lung-protective ventilation strategies have not only been reported to reduce mortality by 22% in patients with ARDS but also to diminish the number of neutrophils and the concentration of pro-inflammatory cytokines released in patient lavage fluids.

Novel approaches targeting host mediators known to promote lung edema formation and impair clearance such as studies on TIP peptide [see Tumor Necrosis Factor Alpha (TNF-α) above] administration in ARDS are being studied. Initial reports showed that AP301, a synthetic peptide mimicking TIP, induces ENaC activity in type II alveolar epithelial cells from dogs, pigs, and rats (93) and improves lung function in a porcine lung injury model (94). A subsequent phase II clinical trial with AP301 in ventilated ARDS patients resulted in improved AFC and oxygenation of

these patients (95). Also, mesenchymal stem cells, which have been reported to improve epithelial barrier integrity in human AEC II treated with a cytokine mix composed of a combination of IL-1β, TNFα, and IFNγ (96), are currently tested for safety and efficacy in phase II trials (clinical trial identifiers NCT02097641, NCT01775774, NCT02112500). Studies on β2-agonists, which had been previously shown to improve vectorial sodium transport and edema clearance (97, 98), did not improve ARDS outcomes (99, 100), possibly due to an enhanced inflammatory response driven by lung macrophages (101). Further treatment options targeting para- or autocrine signaling events affecting AFC in preclinical models include glucocorticoids that suppress inflammation and upregulate both NKA (102) and ENaC (103, 104), neutralizing antibodies directed against virus-specific release of macrophage TRAIL that improve NKA expression as well as AFC in IAV-infected mice (24) and nitric oxide synthase inhibitors aminoguanidine or N(omega)-monomethyl-L-arginine (L-NMMA) that protect against pulmonary edema in LPS-induced lung injury as well as in IAV infection (77, 105).

CONCLUSION

Pathogen-induced lung injury but also sepsis can lead to widespread respiratory inflammation that favors accumulation of lung edema leading to multiorgan dysfunction and poor outcomes. Recent advances in the development of novel treatment strategies targeting respiratory ion homeostasis show encouraging results, identifying them as promising candidates to improve AFC in ALI which could potentially improve the survival of patients with ARDS.

AUTHOR CONTRIBUTIONS

CP, SH, JS, and EL have performed bibliographic research and drafted the manuscript.

REFERENCES

1. Bastacky J, Lee CY, Goerke J, Koushafar H, Yager D, Kenaga L, et al. Alveolar lining layer is thin and continuous: low-temperature scanning electron microscopy of rat lung. *J Appl Physiol* (1995) 79:1615–28.
2. Verkman AS, Matthay MA, Song Y. Aquaporin water channels and lung physiology. *Am J Physiol Lung Cell Mol Physiol* (2000) 278:L867–79.
3. Bertorello AM, Komarova Y, Smith K, Leibiger IB, Efendiev R, Pedemonte CH, et al. Analysis of Na+,K+-ATPase motion and incorporation into the plasma membrane in response to G protein-coupled receptor signals in living cells. *Mol Biol Cell* (2003) 14:1149–57. doi:10.1091/mbc.E02-06-0367
4. Mutlu GM, Adir Y, Jameel M, Akhmedov AT, Welch L, Dumasius V, et al. Interdependency of beta-adrenergic receptors and CFTR in regulation of alveolar active Na+ transport. *Circ Res* (2005) 96:999–1005. doi:10.1161/01.RES.0000164554.21993.AC
5. Schwiebert EM, Kizer N, Gruenert DC, Stanton BA. GTP-binding proteins inhibit cAMP activation of chloride channels in cystic fibrosis airway

epithelial cells. *Proc Natl Acad Sci U S A* (1992) 89:10623–7. doi:10.1073/pnas.89.22.10623
6. Fischer H, Illek B, Finkbeiner WE, Widdicombe JH. Basolateral Cl channels in primary airway epithelial cultures. *Am J Physiol Lung Cell Mol Physiol* (2007) 292:L1432–43. doi:10.1152/ajplung.00032.2007
7. Mall M, Gonska T, Thomas J, Schreiber R, Seydewitz HH, Kuehr J, et al. Modulation of Ca²⁺-activated Cl- secretion by basolateral K+ channels in human normal and cystic fibrosis airway epithelia. *Pediatr Res* (2003) 53:608–18. doi:10.1203/01.PDR.0000057204.51420.DC
8. Koval M. Claudin heterogeneity and control of lung tight junctions. *Annu Rev Physiol* (2013) 75:551–67. doi:10.1146/annurev-physiol-030212-183809
9. Guidot DM, Folkesson HG, Jain L, Sznajder JI, Pittet JF, Matthay MA. Integrating acute lung injury and regulation of alveolar fluid clearance. *Am J Physiol Lung Cell Mol Physiol* (2006) 291:L301–6. doi:10.1152/ajplung.00153.2006
10. Brun-Buisson C, Minelli C, Bertolini G, Brazzi L, Pimentel J, Lewandowski K, et al. Epidemiology and outcome of acute lung injury in European intensive

10. care units. Results from the ALIVE study. *Intensive Care Med* (2004) 30:51–61. doi:10.1007/s00134-003-2136-x

11. Matthay MA, Zemans RL. The acute respiratory distress syndrome: pathogenesis and treatment. *Annu Rev Pathol* (2011) 6:147–63. doi:10.1146/annurev-pathol-011110-130158

12. Matthay MA, Ware LB, Zimmerman GA. The acute respiratory distress syndrome. *J Clin Invest* (2012) 122:2731–40. doi:10.1172/JCI60331

13. Londino JD, Lazrak A, Noah JW, Aggarwal S, Bali V, Woodworth BA, et al. Influenza virus M2 targets cystic fibrosis transmembrane conductance regulator for lysosomal degradation during viral infection. *FASEB J* (2015) 29:2712–25. doi:10.1096/fj.14-268755

14. Sznajder JI. Alveolar edema must be cleared for the acute respiratory distress syndrome patient to survive. *Am J Respir Crit Care Med* (2001) 163:1293–4. doi:10.1164/ajrccm.163.6.ed1801d

15. Lee JW, Fang X, Dolganov G, Fremont RD, Bastarache JA, Ware LB, et al. Acute lung injury edema fluid decreases net fluid transport across human alveolar epithelial type II cells. *J Biol Chem* (2007) 282:24109–19. doi:10.1074/jbc.M700821200

16. Waugh T, Ching JC, Zhou Y, Loewen ME. Influenza A virus (H1N1) increases airway epithelial cell secretion by up-regulation of potassium channel KCNN4. *Biochem Biophys Res Commun* (2013) 438:581–7. doi:10.1016/j.bbrc.2013.08.012

17. Morissette C, Skamene E, Gervais F. Endobronchial inflammation following *Pseudomonas aeruginosa* infection in resistant and susceptible strains of mice. *Infect Immun* (1995) 63:1718–24.

18. Dagenais A, Gosselin D, Guilbault C, Radzioch D, Berthiaume Y. Modulation of epithelial sodium channel (ENaC) expression in mouse lung infected with *Pseudomonas aeruginosa*. *Respir Res* (2005) 6:2. doi:10.1186/1465-9921-6-2

19. Schoenborn JR, Wilson CB. Regulation of interferon-gamma during innate and adaptive immune responses. *Adv Immunol* (2007) 96:41–101. doi:10.1016/S0065-2776(07)96002-2

20. Young HA, Hardy KJ. Role of interferon-gamma in immune cell regulation. *J Leukoc Biol* (1995) 58:373–81.

21. Galietta LJ, Folli C, Marchetti C, Romano L, Carpani D, Conese M, et al. Modification of transepithelial ion transport in human cultured bronchial epithelial cells by interferon-gamma. *Am J Physiol Lung Cell Mol Physiol* (2000) 278:L1186–94.

22. Besancon F, Przewlocki G, Baro I, Hongre AS, Escande D, Edelman A. Interferon-gamma downregulates CFTR gene expression in epithelial cells. *Am J Physiol* (1994) 267:C1398–404.

23. Resta-Lenert S, Barrett KE. Probiotics and commensals reverse TNF-alpha- and IFN-gamma-induced dysfunction in human intestinal epithelial cells. *Gastroenterology* (2006) 130:731–46. doi:10.1053/j.gastro.2005.12.015

24. Peteranderl C, Morales-Nebreda L, Selvakumar B, Lecuona E, Vadász I, Morty RE, et al. Macrophage-epithelial paracrine crosstalk inhibits lung edema clearance during influenza infection. *J Clin Invest* (2016) 126:1566–80. doi:10.1172/JCI83931

25. Gallipoli P, Pellicano F, Morrison H, Laidlaw K, Allan EK, Bhatia R, et al. Autocrine TNF-alpha production supports CML stem and progenitor cell survival and enhances their proliferation. *Blood* (2013) 122:3335–9. doi:10.1182/blood-2013-02-485607

26. Gaur U, Aggarwal BB. Regulation of proliferation, survival and apoptosis by members of the TNF superfamily. *Biochem Pharmacol* (2003) 66:1403–8. doi:10.1016/S0006-2952(03)00490-8

27. Micheau O, Tschopp J. Induction of TNF receptor I-mediated apoptosis via two sequential signaling complexes. *Cell* (2003) 114:181–90. doi:10.1016/S0092-8674(03)00521-X

28. Braun C, Hamacher J, Morel DR, Wendel A, Lucas R. Dichotomal role of TNF in experimental pulmonary edema reabsorption. *J Immunol* (2005) 175:3402–8. doi:10.4049/jimmunol.175.5.3402

29. Yamagata T, Yamagata Y, Nishimoto T, Hirano T, Nakanishi M, Minakata Y, et al. The regulation of amiloride-sensitive epithelial sodium channels by tumor necrosis factor-alpha in injured lungs and alveolar type II cells. *Respir Physiol Neurobiol* (2009) 166:16–23. doi:10.1016/j.resp.2008.12.008

30. Narasaraju T, Yang E, Samy RP, Ng HH, Poh WP, Liew AA, et al. Excessive neutrophils and neutrophil extracellular traps contribute to acute lung injury of influenza pneumonitis. *Am J Pathol* (2011) 179:199–210. doi:10.1016/j.ajpath.2011.03.013

31. Rezaiguia S, Garat C, Delclaux C, Meignan M, Fleury J, Legrand P, et al. Acute bacterial pneumonia in rats increases alveolar epithelial fluid clearance by a tumor necrosis factor-alpha-dependent mechanism. *J Clin Invest* (1997) 99:325–35. doi:10.1172/JCI119161

32. Czikora I, Alli A, Bao HF, Kaftan D, Sridhar S, Apell HJ, et al. A novel tumor necrosis factor-mediated mechanism of direct epithelial sodium channel activation. *Am J Respir Crit Care Med* (2014) 190:522–32. doi:10.1164/rccm.201405-0833OC

33. Vadász I, Schermuly RT, Ghofrani HA, Rummel S, Wehner S, Mühldorfer I, et al. The lectin-like domain of tumor necrosis factor-[alpha] improves alveolar fluid balance in injured isolated rabbit lungs. *Crit Care Med* (2008) 36:1543–50. doi:10.1097/CCM.0b013e31816f485e

34. Herold S, von Wulffen W, Steinmueller M, Pleschka S, Kuziel WA, Mack M, et al. Alveolar epithelial cells direct monocyte transepithelial migration upon influenza virus infection: impact of chemokines and adhesion molecules. *J Immunol* (2006) 177:1817–24. doi:10.4049/jimmunol.177.3.1817

35. Hammond ME, Lapointe GR, Feucht PH, Hilt S, Gallegos CA, Gordon CA, et al. IL-8 induces neutrophil chemotaxis predominantly via type I IL-8 receptors. *J Immunol* (1995) 155:1428–33.

36. Herold S, Gabrielli NM, Vadasz I. Novel concepts of acute lung injury and alveolar-capillary barrier dysfunction. *Am J Physiol Lung Cell Mol Physiol* (2013) 305:L665–81. doi:10.1152/ajplung.00232.2013

37. Bauer TT, Montón C, Torres A, Cabello H, Fillela X, Maldonado A, et al. Comparison of systemic cytokine levels in patients with acute respiratory distress syndrome, severe pneumonia, and controls. *Thorax* (2000) 55:46–52. doi:10.1136/thorax.55.1.46

38. Hoshino T, Okamoto M, Sakazaki Y, Kato S, Young HA, Aizawa H. Role of proinflammatory cytokines IL-18 and IL-1beta in bleomycin-induced lung injury in humans and mice. *Am J Respir Cell Mol Biol* (2009) 41:661–70. doi:10.1165/rcmb.2008-0182OC

39. Olman MA, White KE, Ware LB, Simmons WL, Benveniste EN, Zhu S, et al. Pulmonary edema fluid from patients with early lung injury stimulates fibroblast proliferation through IL-1β-induced IL-6 expression. *J Immunol* (2004) 172:2668–77. doi:10.4049/jimmunol.172.4.2668

40. Sordi R, Menezes-de-Lima O, Della-Justina AM, Rezende E, Assreuy J. Pneumonia-induced sepsis in mice: temporal study of inflammatory and cardiovascular parameters. *Int J Exp Pathol* (2013) 94:144–55. doi:10.1111/iep.12016

41. Herold S, Tabar TS, Janssen H, Hoegner K, Cabanski M, Lewe-Schlosser P, et al. Exudate macrophages attenuate lung injury by the release of IL-1 receptor antagonist in Gram-negative pneumonia. *Am J Respir Crit Care Med* (2011) 183:1380–90. doi:10.1164/rccm.201009-1431OC

42. Lee YM, Hybertson BM, Cho HG, Terada LS, Cho O, Repine AJ, et al. Platelet-activating factor contributes to acute lung leak in rats given interleukin-1 intratracheally. *Am J Physiol Lung Cell Mol Physiol* (2000) 279:L75–80.

43. Roux J, Kawakatsu H, Gartland B, Pespeni M, Sheppard D, Matthay MA, et al. Interleukin-1β decreases expression of the epithelial sodium channel α-subunit in alveolar epithelial cells via a p38 MAPK-dependent signaling pathway. *J Biol Chem* (2005) 280:18579–89. doi:10.1074/jbc.M410561200

44. Yang H, Ko HJ, Yang JY, Kim JJ, Seo SU, Park SG, et al. Interleukin-1 promotes coagulation, which is necessary for protective immunity in the lung against *Streptococcus pneumoniae* infection. *J Infect Dis* (2013) 207:50–60. doi:10.1093/infdis/jis651

45. Bastarache JA, Wang L, Geiser T, Wang Z, Albertine KH, Matthay MA, et al. The alveolar epithelium can initiate the extrinsic coagulation cascade through expression of tissue factor. *Thorax* (2007) 62:608–16. doi:10.1136/thx.2006.063305

46. Idell S. Coagulation, fibrinolysis, and fibrin deposition in acute lung injury. *Crit Care Med* (2003) 31:S213–20. doi:10.1097/01.CCM.0000057846.21303.AB

47. Vadász I, Morty RE, Olschewski A, Königshoff M, Kohstall MG, Ghofrani HA, et al. Thrombin impairs alveolar fluid clearance by promoting endocytosis of Na+,K+-ATPase. *Am J Respir Cell Mol Biol* (2005) 33:343–54. doi:10.1165/rcmb.2004-0407OC

48. Kurdowska A, Miller EJ, Noble JM, Baughman RP, Matthay MA, Brelsford WG, et al. Anti-IL-8 autoantibodies in alveolar fluid from patients with the adult respiratory distress syndrome. *J Immunol* (1996) 157:2699–706.

49. Pease J, Sabroe I. The role of interleukin-8 and its receptor in inflammatory lung disease: implications for therapy. *Am J Respir Med* (2002) 1:19–25. doi:10.1007/BF03257159

50. Goodman RB, Strieter RM, Martin DP, Steinberg KP, Milberg JA, Maunder RJ, et al. Inflammatory cytokines in patients with persistence of the acute respiratory distress syndrome. *Am J Respir Crit Care Med* (1996) 154:602–11. doi:10.1164/ajrccm.154.3.8810593

51. Chen Z, Shao X, Dou X, Zhang X, Wang Y, Zhu C, et al. Role of the *Mycoplasma pneumoniae*/interleukin-8/neutrophil axis in the pathogenesis of pneumonia. *PLoS One* (2016) 11:e0146377. doi:10.1371/journal.pone.0146377

52. Chang YJ, Liu CY, Chiang BL, Chao YC, Chen CC. Induction of IL-8 release in lung cells via activator protein-1 by recombinant baculovirus displaying severe acute respiratory syndrome-coronavirus spike proteins: identification of two functional regions. *J Immunol* (2004) 173:7602–14. doi:10.4049/jimmunol.173.12.7602

53. Redondo E, Gazquez A, Vadillo S, Garcia A, Franco A, Masot AJ. Induction of interleukin-8 and interleukin-12 in neonatal ovine lung following experimental inoculation of bovine respiratory syncytial virus. *J Comp Pathol* (2014) 150:434–48. doi:10.1016/j.jcpa.2013.08.002

54. Roux J, McNicholas CM, Carles M, Goolaerts A, Houseman BT, Dickinson DA, et al. IL-8 inhibits cAMP-stimulated alveolar epithelial fluid transport via a GRK2/PI3K-dependent mechanism. *FASEB J* (2013) 27:1095–106. doi:10.1096/fj.12-219295

55. Shull MM, Ormsby I, Kier AB, Pawlowski S, Diebold RJ, Yin M, et al. Targeted disruption of the mouse transforming growth factor-beta 1 gene results in multifocal inflammatory disease. *Nature* (1992) 359:693–9. doi:10.1038/359693a0

56. Gong D, Shi W, Yi SJ, Chen H, Groffen J, Heisterkamp N. TGFbeta signaling plays a critical role in promoting alternative macrophage activation. *BMC Immunol* (2012) 13:31. doi:10.1186/1471-2172-13-31

57. Pittet JF, Griffiths MJ, Geiser T, Kaminski N, Dalton SL, Huang X, et al. TGF-beta is a critical mediator of acute lung injury. *J Clin Invest* (2001) 107:1537–44. doi:10.1172/JCI11963

58. Frank J, Roux J, Kawakatsu H, Su G, Dagenais A, Berthiaume Y, et al. Transforming growth factor-beta1 decreases expression of the epithelial sodium channel alphaENaC and alveolar epithelial vectorial sodium and fluid transport via an ERK1/2-dependent mechanism. *J Biol Chem* (2003) 278:43939–50. doi:10.1074/jbc.M304882200

59. Peters DM, Vadasz I, Wujak L, Wygrecka M, Olschewski A, Becker C, et al. TGF-beta directs trafficking of the epithelial sodium channel ENaC which has implications for ion and fluid transport in acute lung injury. *Proc Natl Acad Sci U S A* (2014) 111:E374–83. doi:10.1073/pnas.1306798111

60. Wujak LA, Becker S, Seeger W, Morty RE. TGF-β regulates Na,K-ATPase activity by changing the regulatory subunit stoichiometry of the Na, K-ATPase complex. *FASEB J* (2011) 25(Suppl 1039.9). Available from: http://www.fasebj.org/content/25/1_Supplement/1039.9

61. Wujak ŁA, Blume A, Baloğlu E, Wygrecka M, Wygowski J, Herold S, et al. FXYD1 negatively regulates Na(+)/K(+)-ATPase activity in lung alveolar epithelial cells. *Respir Physiol Neurobiol* (2016) 220:54–61. doi:10.1016/j.resp.2015.09.008

62. Budinger GRS, Chandel NS, Donnelly HK, Eisenbart J, Oberoi M, Jain M. Active transforming growth factor-β1 activates the procollagen I promoter in patients with acute lung injury. *Intensive Care Med* (2005) 31:121–8. doi:10.1007/s00134-004-2503-2

63. Neill DR, Fernandes VE, Wisby L, Haynes AR, Ferreira DM, Laher A, et al. T regulatory cells control susceptibility to invasive pneumococcal pneumonia in mice. *PLoS Pathog* (2012) 8:e1002660. doi:10.1371/journal.ppat.1002660

64. Schultz-Cherry S, Hinshaw VS. Influenza virus neuraminidase activates latent transforming growth factor beta. *J Virol* (1996) 70:8624–9.

65. Li N, Ren A, Wang X, Fan X, Zhao Y, Gao GF, et al. Influenza viral neuraminidase primes bacterial coinfection through TGF-beta-mediated expression of host cell receptors. *Proc Natl Acad Sci U S A* (2015) 112:238–43. doi:10.1073/pnas.1414422112

66. Rynda-Apple A, Robinson KM, Alcorn JF. Influenza and bacterial superinfection: illuminating the immunologic mechanisms of disease. *Infect Immun* (2015) 83:3764–70. doi:10.1128/IAI.00298-15

67. Hogner K, Wolff T, Pleschka S, Plog S, Gruber AD, Kalinke U, et al. Macrophage-expressed IFN-beta contributes to apoptotic alveolar epithelial cell injury in severe influenza virus pneumonia. *PLoS Pathog* (2013) 9:e1003188. doi:10.1371/journal.ppat.1003188

68. Kirshner JR, Karpova AY, Kops M, Howley PM. Identification of TRAIL as an interferon regulatory factor 3 transcriptional target. *J Virol* (2005) 79:9320–4. doi:10.1128/JVI.79.14.9320-9324.2005

69. Herold S, Steinmueller M, von Wulffen W, Cakarova L, Pinto R, Pleschka S, et al. Lung epithelial apoptosis in influenza virus pneumonia: the role of macrophage-expressed TNF-related apoptosis-inducing ligand. *J Exp Med* (2008) 205:3065–77. doi:10.1084/jem.20080201

70. Ellis GT, Davidson S, Crotta S, Branzk N, Papayannopoulos V, Wack A. TRAIL+ monocytes and monocyte-related cells cause lung damage and thereby increase susceptibility to influenza-*Streptococcus pneumoniae* coinfection. *EMBO Rep* (2015) 16:1203–18. doi:10.15252/embr.201540473

71. Coutinho-Silva R, Ojcius DM. Role of extracellular nucleotides in the immune response against intracellular bacteria and protozoan parasites. *Microbes Infect* (2012) 14:1271–7. doi:10.1016/j.micinf.2012.05.009

72. Savio LE, Coutinho-Silva R. Purinergic signaling in infection and autoimmune disease. *Biomed J* (2016) 39:304–5. doi:10.1016/j.bj.2016.09.002

73. Blaug S, Rymer J, Jalickee S, Miller SS. P2 purinoceptors regulate calcium-activated chloride and fluid transport in 31EG4 mammary epithelia. *Am J Physiol Cell Physiol* (2003) 284:C897–909. doi:10.1152/ajpcell.00238.2002

74. Pochynyuk O, Bugaj V, Vandewalle A, Stockand JD. Purinergic control of apical plasma membrane PI(4,5)P2 levels sets ENaC activity in principal cells. *Am J Physiol Renal Physiol* (2008) 294:F38–46. doi:10.1152/ajprenal.00403.2007

75. Wolk KE, Lazarowski ER, Traylor ZP, Yu EN, Jewell NA, Durbin RK, et al. Influenza A virus inhibits alveolar fluid clearance in BALB/c mice. *Am J Respir Crit Care Med* (2008) 178:969–76. doi:10.1164/rccm.200803-455OC

76. Aeffner F, Woods PS, Davis IC. Ecto-5'-nucleotidase CD73 modulates the innate immune response to influenza infection but is not required for development of influenza-induced acute lung injury. *Am J Physiol Lung Cell Mol Physiol* (2015) 309:L1313–22. doi:10.1152/ajplung.00130.2015

77. Akaike T, Noguchi Y, Ijiri S, Setoguchi K, Suga M, Zheng YM, et al. Pathogenesis of influenza virus-induced pneumonia: involvement of both nitric oxide and oxygen radicals. *Proc Natl Acad Sci U S A* (1996) 93:2448–53. doi:10.1073/pnas.93.6.2448

78. Nielsen VG, Baird MS, Chen LAN, Matalon S. DETANONOate, a nitric oxide donor, decreases amiloride-sensitive alveolar fluid clearance in rabbits. *Am J Respir Crit Care Med* (2000) 161:1154–60. doi:10.1164/ajrccm.161.4.9907033

79. Youssef JA, Thibeault DW, Rezaiekhaligh MH, Mabry SM, Norberg MI, Truog WE. Influence of inhaled nitric oxide and hyperoxia on Na, K-ATPase expression and lung edema in newborn piglets. *Neonatology* (1999) 75:199–209. doi:10.1159/000014096

80. Matthay MA, Su X. Pulmonary barriers to pneumonia and sepsis. *Nat Med* (2007) 13:780–1. doi:10.1038/nm0707-780

81. Nguyen M, Pace AJ, Koller BH. Mice lacking NKCC1 are protected from development of bacteremia and hypothermic sepsis secondary to bacterial pneumonia. *J Exp Med* (2007) 204:1383–93. doi:10.1084/jem.20061205

82. Nathan C, Cars O. Antibiotic resistance – problems, progress, and prospects. *N Engl J Med* (2014) 371:1761–3. doi:10.1056/NEJMp1408040

83. Pendleton JN, Gorman SP, Gilmore BF. Clinical relevance of the ESKAPE pathogens. *Expert Rev Anti Infect Ther* (2013) 11:297–308. doi:10.1586/eri.13.12

84. Blackwell TS, Stecenko AA, Christman JW. Dysregulated NF-κB activation in cystic fibrosis: evidence for a primary inflammatory disorder. *Am J Physiol Lung Cell Mol Physiol* (2001) 281:L69–70.

85. Su X, Looney MR, Su H, Lee JW, Song Y, Matthay MA. Role of CFTR expressed by neutrophils in modulating acute lung inflammation and injury in mice. *Inflamm Res* (2011) 60:619–32. doi:10.1007/s00011-011-0313-x

86. Nieto-Torres JL, DeDiego ML, Verdiá-Báguena C, Jimenez-Guardeño JM, Regla-Nava JA, Fernandez-Delgado R, et al. Severe acute respiratory syndrome coronavirus envelope protein ion channel activity promotes virus fitness and pathogenesis. *PLoS Pathog* (2014) 10:e1004077. doi:10.1371/journal.ppat.1004077

87. Triantafilou K, Triantafilou M. Ion flux in the lung: virus-induced inflammasome activation. *Trends Microbiol* (2014) 22:580–8. doi:10.1016/j.tim.2014.06.002

88. Mizgerd JP. Lung infection – a public health priority. *PLoS Med* (2006) 3:e76. doi:10.1371/journal.pmed.0030076

89. Graham RL, Donaldson EF, Baric RS. A decade after SARS: strategies for controlling emerging coronaviruses. *Nat Rev Microbiol* (2013) 11:836–48. doi:10.1038/nrmicro3143

90. Zhu H, Webby R, Lam TT, Smith DK, Peiris JS, Guan Y. History of Swine influenza viruses in Asia. *Curr Top Microbiol Immunol* (2013) 370:57–68. doi:10.1007/82_2011_179

91. Zumla A, Memish ZA, Maeurer M, Bates M, Mwaba P, Al-Tawfiq JA, et al. Emerging novel and antimicrobial-resistant respiratory tract infections: new drug development and therapeutic options. *Lancet Infect Dis* (2014) 14:1136–49. doi:10.1016/S1473-3099(14)70828-X

92. Gonzales JN, Lucas R, Verin AD. The acute respiratory distress syndrome: mechanisms and perspective therapeutic approaches. *Austin J Vasc Med* (2015) 2:1009.

93. Tzotzos S, Fischer B, Fischer H, Pietschmann H, Lucas R, Dupré G, et al. AP301, a synthetic peptide mimicking the lectin-like domain of TNF, enhances amiloride-sensitive Na(+) current in primary dog, pig and rat alveolar type II cells. *Pulm Pharmacol Ther* (2013) 26:356–63. doi:10.1016/j.pupt.2012.12.011

94. Hartmann EK, Boehme S, Duenges B, Bentley A, Klein KU, Kwiecien R, et al. An inhaled tumor necrosis factor-alpha-derived TIP peptide improves the pulmonary function in experimental lung injury. *Acta Anaesthesiol Scand* (2013) 57:334–41. doi:10.1111/aas.12034

95. Krenn K, Croize A, Klein KU, Böhme S, Markstaller K, Ullrich R, et al. Oral inhalation of AP301 peptide activates pulmonary oedema clearance: initial results from a phase IIa clinical trial in mechanically ventilated ICU patients. *Eur Respir J* (2014) 44:1386.

96. Fang X, Neyrinck AP, Matthay MA, Lee JW. Allogeneic human mesenchymal stem cells restore epithelial protein permeability in cultured human alveolar type II cells by secretion of angiopoietin-1. *J Biol Chem* (2010) 285:26211–22. doi:10.1074/jbc.M110.119917

97. Mutlu GM, Dumasius V, Burhop J, McShane PJ, Meng FJ, Welch L, et al. Upregulation of alveolar epithelial active Na+ transport is dependent on beta2-adrenergic receptor signaling. *Circ Res* (2004) 94:1091–100. doi:10.1161/01.RES.0000125623.56442.20

98. Mutlu GM, Factor P. Alveolar epithelial beta2-adrenergic receptors. *Am J Respir Cell Mol Biol* (2008) 38:127–34. doi:10.1165/rcmb.2007-0198TR

99. Gao Smith F, Perkins GD, Gates S, Young D, McAuley DF, Tunnicliffe W, et al. Effect of intravenous beta-2 agonist treatment on clinical outcomes in acute respiratory distress syndrome (BALTI-2): a multicentre, randomised controlled trial. *Lancet* (2012) 379:229–35. doi:10.1016/S0140-6736(11)61623-1

100. National Heart, Lung, and Blood Institute Acute Respiratory Distress Syndrome(ARDS)Clinical Trials Network, Matthay MA, Brower RG, Carson S, Douglas IS, Eisner M, et al. Randomized, placebo-controlled clinical trial of an aerosolized beta(2)-agonist for treatment of acute lung injury. *Am J Respir Crit Care Med* (2011) 184:561–8. doi:10.1164/rccm.201012-2090OC

101. Chiarella SE, Soberanes S, Urich D, Morales-Nebreda L, Nigdelioglu R, Green D, et al. Beta(2)-Adrenergic agonists augment air pollution-induced IL-6 release and thrombosis. *J Clin Invest* (2014) 124:2935–46. doi:10.1172/JCI75157

102. Barquin N, Ciccolella DE, Ridge KM, Sznajder JI. Dexamethasone upregulates the Na-K-ATPase in rat alveolar epithelial cells. *Am J Physiol* (1997) 273:L825–30.

103. Itani OA, Auerbach SD, Husted RF, Volk KA, Ageloff S, Knepper MA, et al. Glucocorticoid-stimulated lung epithelial Na(+) transport is associated with regulated ENaC and sgk1 expression. *Am J Physiol Lung Cell Mol Physiol* (2002) 282:L631–41. doi:10.1152/ajplung.00085.2001

104. Nakamura K, Stokes JB, McCray PB Jr. Endogenous and exogenous glucocorticoid regulation of ENaC mRNA expression in developing kidney and lung. *Am J Physiol Cell Physiol* (2002) 283:C762–72. doi:10.1152/ajpcell.00029.2002

105. Heremans H, Dillen C, Groenen M, Matthys P, Billiau A. Role of interferon-gamma and nitric oxide in pulmonary edema and death induced by lipopolysaccharide. *Am J Respir Crit Care Med* (2000) 161:110–7. doi:10.1164/ajrccm.161.1.9902089

4

TNF Lectin-Like Domain Restores Epithelial Sodium Channel Function in Frameshift Mutants Associated with Pseudohypoaldosteronism Type 1B

Anita Willam[1,2]*, Mohammed Aufy[1], Susan Tzotzos[2], Dina El-Malazi[1], Franziska Poser[1], Alina Wagner[1], Birgit Unterköfler[1], Didja Gurmani[1], David Martan[1], Shahid Muhammad Iqbal[1], Bernhard Fischer[2], Hendrik Fischer[2], Helmut Pietschmann[2], Istvan Czikora[3], Rudolf Lucas[3], Rosa Lemmens-Gruber[1] and Waheed Shabbir[1,2]

[1] Department of Pharmacology and Toxicology, University of Vienna, Vienna, Austria, [2] APEPTICO GmbH, Vienna, Austria,
[3] Vascular Biology Center, Medical College of Georgia, Augusta University, Augusta, GA, United States

*Correspondence:
Anita Willam
anita.willam@univie.ac.at

Previous *in vitro* studies have indicated that tumor necrosis factor (TNF) activates amiloride-sensitive epithelial sodium channel (ENaC) current through its lectin-like (TIP) domain, since cyclic peptides mimicking the TIP domain (e.g., solnatide), showed ENaC-activating properties. In the current study, the effects of TNF and solnatide on individual ENaC subunits or ENaC carrying mutated glycosylation sites in the α-ENaC subunit were compared, revealing a similar mode of action for TNF and solnatide and corroborating the previous assumption that the lectin-like domain of TNF is the relevant molecular structure for ENaC activation. Accordingly, TNF enhanced ENaC current by increasing open probability of the glycosylated channel, position N511 in the α-ENaC subunit being identified as the most important glycosylation site. TNF significantly increased Na$^+$ current through ENaC comprising only the pore forming subunits α or δ, was less active in ENaC comprising only β-subunits, and showed no effect on ENaC comprising γ-subunits. TNF did not increase the membrane abundance of ENaC subunits to the extent observed with solnatide. Since the α-subunit is believed to play a prominent role in the ENaC current activating effect of TNF and TIP, we investigated whether TNF and solnatide can enhance $\alpha\beta\gamma$-ENaC current in α-ENaC loss-of-function frameshift mutants. The efficacy of solnatide has been already proven in pathological conditions involving ENaC in phase II clinical trials. The frameshift mutations αI68fs, αT169fs, αP197fs, αE272fs, αF435fs, αR438fs, αY447fs, αR448fs, αS452fs, and αT482fs have been reported to cause pseudohypoaldosteronism type 1B (PHA1B), a rare, life-threatening, salt-wasting disease, which hitherto has been treated only symptomatically. In a heterologous expression system, all frameshift mutants showed significantly reduced amiloride-sensitive whole-cell current compared to wild type $\alpha\beta\gamma$-ENaC, whereas membrane abundance varied between mutants. Solnatide restored function in α-ENaC frameshift mutants to current density levels of wild type ENaC or higher despite their lacking a binding site for solnatide, previously located to the region between TM2 and the C-terminus of the α-subunit. TNF similarly restored current density to wild type levels in the mutant αR448fs. Activation of βγ-ENaC may contribute to this moderate current enhancement, but whatever the mechanism, experimental data indicate that solnatide could be a new strategy to treat PHA1B.

Keywords: lectin-like domain of tumor necrosis factor, TIP peptides, solnatide (AP301), amiloride-sensitive epithelial sodium channel, pseudohypoaldosteronism type 1B

INTRODUCTION

Tumor necrosis factor (TNF) is a mammalian inflammatory cytokine, which exerts a plethora of effects primarily aimed at defending the host against invading pathogens. Apart from mediating its activities through cross-linking with specific receptors on the surface of mammalian cells (1), TNF participates in innate immune functions through a lectin-like (TIP) domain, spatially distinct from the TNF-receptor binding site (2–4). The lectin-like domain of TNF recognizes and interacts with specific oligosaccharide moieties, in particular N,N'-diacetylchitobiose (5). TNF is crucially involved in the control of *Trypanosoma brucei brucei* and *T. cruzei* infections, through the trypanolytic effect triggered by interaction of its lectin-like domain with the N-linked N,N'-diacetylchitobiose core of the variant surface glycoproteins (VSG) of these organisms (1, 2, 6–14). Another effect of the TNF TIP domain observed in early work was the amiloride-sensitive increase in membrane conductance in microvascular endothelial cells (MVECs) (4) and alveolar epithelial cells (15), an effect which we now know is due to activation of the amiloride-sensitive epithelial sodium channel (ENaC) (16). The potential physiological role of the lectin-like domain of TNF in resolution of alveolar edema has been demonstrated in various rodent models of flooded lungs (15, 17, 18). Furthermore, transgenic mice expressing a mutated TNF lectin-like domain are more prone to develop lung edema than their wild-type (WT) counterparts when challenged with the bacterial toxin pneumolysin (PLY) (19).

The synthetic, cyclic, 17-residue peptide, solnatide, mimics the lectin-like domain (TIP) of human TNF (2). Like TNF, TIP peptide can influence regulation of alveolar fluid balance. Solnatide has been shown to activate fluid reabsorption in *in situ* and *in vivo* flooded rat lung models (18) and a mouse version the TIP peptide, mTIP, decreased pulmonary edema in isolated, endotoxin-injured rabbit lung (20). Moreover, solnatide, instilled intratracheally into rats prior to lung transplantation, significantly improved lung function, indicating its use as a potential therapy for ischemia reperfusion injury associated with lung transplantation (21). Inhalation of nebulized solnatide in a porcine bronchoalveolar lavage (BAL) model of acute lung injury (ALI) resulted in an increased PaO_2/FiO_2 ratio and reduced extravascular lung water index (EVLWI) (22). More recently, solnatide demonstrated profound therapeutic activity in a rat model of pulmonary edema induced by acute hypobaric hypoxia and exercise (23).

Solnatide activates both endogenously and heterologously expressed ENaC by increasing the open state probability, P_o, of the channel (16, 24, 25). The oligosaccharide-binding property of the TIP domain of TNF plays an important role in the mechanism by which TNF and solnatide interact with and activate

ENaC, although the exact nature of this interaction is not yet understood. Elimination of the Na^+ current-enhancing effect of solnatide following PNGase F-mediated deglycosylation of A549 and H441 cells or of HEK-293 cells heterologously expressing human ENaC suggested that TIP interacts with carbohydrate groups on the extracellular loop of ENaC subunits (16, 19). Proof of the importance of interaction with glycosylated residues in the extracellular loop of ENaC for TIP potentiation of Na^+ current was obtained from studies with heterologously expressed ENaC in which the five Asn glycosylation sites in the extracellular loop of alpha ENaC had been removed, singly or multiply, by mutation to Gln (26).

The current-potentiating effect of solnatide not only manifests itself in channel kinetics but also in abundance of ENaC subunits at the membrane. We have observed a temporary increase in abundance of α-, β-, γ-, and δ-ENaC 5 and 10 min after prior exposure of HEK-293 cells transiently expressing ENaC to solnatide, but after 1 h, levels return to those seen in the absence of solnatide (16, 26). The solnatide-induced increase in membrane abundance of pore-forming α- and δ-ENaC subunits is significant statistically whereas that of β- and γ-ENaC subunits only slight (26).

In this study, we explore the mechanism of TIP activation of ENaC in electrophysiological and Western blotting experiments using TNF and solnatide. Direct interaction of TNF with ENaC has hitherto not been reported, and so its physiological role in alveolar liquid clearance (ALC) during lung inflammation has been largely inferred from numerous studies with solnatide. A recent study, which sought to determine the precise mechanism by which solnatide stimulated Na^+ uptake in the presence or absence of PLY, demonstrated that TIP activates ENaC through binding to the carboxyl-terminal domain of the α subunit (19). In the present study, we investigated how native TNF affects Na^+ current and membrane abundance of ENaC subunits in cells heterologously expressing WT hENaC and mutant hENaC and compared and contrasted these observations to our findings with solnatide.

Surprisingly, solnatide rescues the loss-of-function phenotype in ENaC mutants carrying mutations at conserved positions in α-, β-, and γ-ENaC known to cause pseudohypoaldosteronism type 1B (PHA1B), restoring current levels in these mutant ENaC-expressing cells to WT levels or even higher (27). PHA1B is a very rare inherited disease caused by mutations in the genes encoding the α (SCNN1A), β (SCNN1B), or γ (SCNN1G), subunit of ENaC, resulting in defective transepithelial sodium transport (28). PHA1B usually manifests itself in the neonatal period with life-threatening salt loss, hyperkalemia, acidosis, and elevated aldosterone levels due to end-organ resistance to aldosterone.

Patients suffering from PHA1B are at risk from life-threatening, salt-losing crises, combined with severe hyperkalemia and dehydration throughout their entire lives (29, 30). There is as yet no definitive treatment for PHA1B other than supportive management aimed to reduce sodium wasting and hyperkalemia and to restore water–electrolyte and acid–base balance.

In the work reported here, we investigate whether α-ENaC frameshift mutants known to cause PHA1B are also rescued by solnatide, even though they lack the carboxyl-terminal domain of α-ENaC previously postulated to be the site of interaction of solnatide with ENaC (19, 31).

MATERIALS AND METHODS

Cell Culture
Human alveolar epithelial A549 cells (ATCC no. CCL-185) in passages 80–97 and human embryonic kidney HEK-293 cells (ATCC no. CRL-1573) in passages 3–25 were seeded in Dulbecco's modified Eagle medium/F12 nutrient mixture Ham plus L-glutamine (DMEM/F-12; Gibco™ by Life Technologies, LifeTech Austria), supplemented with 10% fetal bovine serum (FBS; Gibco™ by Life Technologies, LifeTech Austria) and 1% penicillin–streptomycin (Sigma-Aldrich, Vienna, Austria). Cells were maintained at 37°C with 5% CO_2 in a humidified incubator.

Molecular Biological Methods
cDNAs encoding α-, β-, and γ-hENaC were a kind gift from Dr. Peter M. Snyder (University of Iowa, Carver College of Medicine, Iowa City, USA). cDNA-encoding δ-hENaC was a kind gift from Dr. Mike Althaus (Justus-Liebig University, Giessen, Germany).

Site-Directed Mutagenesis
Point mutations of α-, β-, γ- and δ-hENaC and PHA1B frameshift mutations of α-hENaC were prepared with the QuikChange Lightning Site-Directed Mutagenesis Kit (Agilent Technologies, CA, USA). Mutagenic primers were designed individually with the Primer Design Program provided on the producer's website or for the frameshift mutations the same base changes as reported in patients (see **Table 2**) were performed. Primers were ordered from Sigma-Aldrich, Vienna, Austria.

Mutant strand synthesis, digestion of template, and transformation were performed according to the manufacturer's protocol, and plasmid DNA was extracted from *Escherichia coli* (*E. coli*) cells using the GeneJET Plasmid Miniprep Kit (Thermo Scientific, Loughborough, UK). The mutant DNA was checked by sequencing from LGC Genomics GmbH, Berlin, Germany.

Larger amounts of DNA were provided by amplifying WT or mutant α-, β-, γ-, or δ-hENaC in DH5α competent cells (Invitrogen by Thermo Fisher Scientific, CA, USA) and then extracting DNA using the Plasmid Midi Kit (QIAGEN GmbH, Hilden, Germany).

Transfection
HEK-293 cells were transfected 1 day after cell seeding using X-tremeGENE HP DNA transfection reagent (Roche Diagnostics, Mannheim, Germany) according to the manufacturer's protocol. A set of WT or mutant αβγ- or δβγ-hENaC, or α-, β-, γ-, or δ-hENaC alone was used, and the ratio of DNA to transfection reagent was 1:3. The expression was highest 48–72 h after transfection.

Cell Surface Biotinylation and Western Blotting
Cell surface biotinylation was performed as previously described (26). In brief, A549 cells or transiently transfected HEK-293 cells were grown in 10 cm dishes in 37°C, 5% CO_2 incubator in DMEM medium supplemented with 5% FBS. Cells were treated with 40 nM TNF or 200 nM solnatide for 5, 10, or 30 min when 90% confluency had been reached. Medium was aspirated, and then cells were washed twice with 10 ml ice-cold phosphate-buffered saline (PBS), covered with 2.5 mg EZ-Link Sulfo-NHS-SS-Biotin (Thermo Scientific, Rockford, USA), dissolved in 10 ml ice-cold PBS, and incubated at 4°C with gentle agitation for 30 min. Fifty milliliters of quenching solution were added to cells; then cells were scraped in solution and transferred to fresh 50 ml tube. Cell suspension was centrifuged at $500 \times g$ for 3 min. Supernatant was discarded, and 5 ml of Tris-buffered saline (TBS) was added to the cell pellet. The cell pellet was resuspended and centrifuged at $500 \times g$ for 3 min. Supernatant was discarded and cell pellet was resuspended in lysis buffer containing protease inhibitor cocktail (10 µM pepstatin A, 10 µM phenylmethylsulfonyl fluoride, and 10 µM leupeptin) and transferred to fresh 1.5 ml centrifuge tube. Cell pellet was then homogenized on ice by ultrasonication using 1 s bursts and incubated on ice for at least 30 min. Intact cells and nuclei were pelleted by centrifugation at $10,000 \times g$ for 2 min under cooling conditions. Pellet was then discarded and supernatant was transferred to fresh tube, incubated overnight with 0.5 ml NeutrAvidin Agarose under gentle rotation at 4°C and centrifuged at $500 \times g$ for 5 min under cooling conditions. Supernatant was then discarded and the pellet washed twice with 200 µl lysis buffer. The biotinylated proteins were eluted with 100 µl sodium dodecyl sulfate (SDS) sample buffer (62.5 mM Tris, pH 6.8, 1% SDS, 10% glycerine, 50 mM dithiothreitol) containing 10 µM E64 at 65°C for 10 min. Sample was then centrifuged at $500 \times g$ for 2 min. Pellet was discarded and supernatant subjected to protein electrophoresis and immunoblotting. The biotinylated proteins were separated under reducing conditions by SDS-PAGE using 7.5% SDS gel along with prestained protein marker (cat. #12949 from Cell Signaling). Proteins were then transferred onto a nitrocellulose membrane (UltraCruz™ 0.45 mm, Santa Cruz Biotechnology, TX, USA) by semi-dry blotting at 25 V for 30 min. Unspecific binding sites were blocked by incubating the membrane overnight at 4°C with 3% FBS in PBS supplemented with 0.02% sodium azide. Membrane was then incubated for 90 min with primary antibody (anti-α-hENaC, anti-δ-hENaC, and anti-β-actin from Sigma Aldrich; anti-β- and anti-γ-hENaC from Santa Cruz Biotechnology). Membrane was washed 5× with 10 ml PBS containing 0.1% Tween-20 (PBST), and corresponding horseradish peroxidase-conjugated secondary antibodies (Santa Cruz Biotechnology) were applied. After 90-min incubation, membrane was washed 3× with PBST and once with PBS. Enhanced chemiluminescence (ECL) substrate (Amersham

ECL Plus Western Blotting Detection Reagent, GE Healthcare, Vienna, Austria) was used for visualization. Following incubation for 2 min, membranes were exposed to X-ray films (Amersham Hyperfilm ECL, GE Healthcare). Exposed films were scanned and quantified using ImageJ (NIH, MD, USA).

Electrophysiology

Electrophysiological experiments were performed as described in detail by Shabbir et al. (16). Briefly, effects of TNF and solnatide on WT and mutated hENaC were studied on transfected HEK-293 cells at room temperature (19–22°C) 24–48 h after plating. Currents were recorded with the patch clamp method in the whole-cell mode. The chamber contained 1 ml of the bath solution of the following composition (in mM): 145 NaCl, 2.7 KCl, 1.8 CaCl$_2$, 2 MgCl$_2$, 5.5 glucose, and 10 HEPES, adjusted to pH 7.4 with 1 M NaOH solution. Micropipettes were pulled from thin-walled borosilicate glass capillaries (Harvard Apparatus, Holliston, MA, USA) with a DMZ Zeitz Puller to obtain electrode resistances ranging from 2 to 5 MΩ. The pipette solution contained (in millimolars): 135 potassium methane sulfonate, 10 KCl, 6 NaCl, 1 Mg$_2$ATP, 2 Na$_3$ATP, 10 HEPES, and 0.5 EGTA, adjusted to pH 7.2 with 1 M KOH solution. Chemicals for pipette and bathing solutions were supplied by Sigma-Aldrich (Vienna, Austria). Electrophysiological measurements were carried out with an Axopatch 200B patch clamp amplifier (Axon Instruments, CA, USA). Capacity transients were canceled, and series resistance was compensated. Whole-cell currents were filtered at 5 kHz and sampled at 10 kHz. Data acquisition and storage were processed directly to a PC equipped with pCLAMP 10.2 software (Axon Instruments, CA, USA). After GΩ-seal formation, the equilibration period of 5 min was followed by control recordings at a holding potential of −100 mV. Then, aliquots of a stock solution, which was prepared with distilled water, were cumulatively added into the bath solution. The wash-in phase lasted about 1–5 min. After steady-state had been reached, the same experimental protocol was applied for each concentration of TNF and solnatide as well as during control recordings.

Statistical Analysis

Data were analyzed with OriginPro 2017 (OriginLab, Northampton, MA, USA) and figures were edited with CorelDRAW X7 (Corel Corporation, Ottawa, ON, Canada). Data are represented as mean ± SEM of at least three independent biological replicates/experiments. Significant differences of two independent values were evaluated by unpaired Student's t-test. Whereas one-way ANOVA followed by Tukey's *post hoc* test was used when groups of data were compared with each other. The type of statistical test is indicated in the figure legends. In case no specific test is mentioned, ANOVA was performed.

Test Compounds

Tumor necrosis factor (CAS Registry Number 94948-59-1, Sigma-Aldrich, Austria) and the TNF lectin-like domain derived peptide solnatide, also known as AP301 and called TIP peptide [CAS Registry Number: 259206-53-6; CA Index Name: L-cysteine, L-cysteinylglycyl-L-glutaminyl-L-arginyl-L-.alpha.-glutamyl-L-threonyl-L-prolyl-L-.alpha.-glutamylglycyl-L-alanyl-L-.alpha.-glutamyl-L-alanyl-L-lysyl-L-prolyl-L-tryptophyl-L-tyrosyl-, cyclic (1.fwdarw.17)-disulfide], with the amino acid sequence CGQRETPEGAEAKPWYC were tested for their ability to activate wild-type and mutant ENaC. Synthesis and description of solnatide is reported in detail by Hazemi et al. (24).

RESULTS

Electrophysiological TNF–ENaC Interaction

In a recent study by Czikora et al. (19) the authors postulated for the first time a direct interaction between the cytokine TNF and the amiloride-sensitive sodium ion channel in a multiple step manner, starting with the interaction with glycosylated membrane components, followed by caveolae-dependent uptake and finally binding to the carboxyl-terminal domain of the α-subunit. This mode of action would suggest a physiological role of the lectin-like domain of TNF in ALC. However, in Czikora's study, using a cyclic peptide which mimics the lectin-like domain of TNF, it was not demonstrated directly that native TNF can also activate ENaC *via* these proposed mechanisms.

In previous experiments with A549 cells that endogenously express α-, β-, γ-, and δ-subunits, we could demonstrate a current activating effect by both TNF as well as the TIP peptide solnatide (24), and this increase in current by TNF (**Figure 1**) and solnatide (16) was confirmed in heterologously expressed αβγ-ENaC and individual ENaC subunits. The onset of action

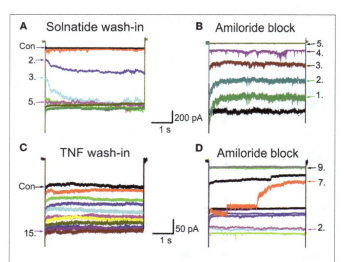

FIGURE 1 | Original traces of wild-type (WT) epithelial sodium channel (ENaC) showing solnatide and tumor necrosis factor (TNF) wash-in and amiloride block. The control whole-cell current (Con; untreated) of HEK-293 cells transiently transfected with WT αβγ-ENaC. Each set of traces represents current measured when cells were clamped at −100 mV, using 20 s pulse intervals. Pulse numbers are indicated to show the time course of wash-in and amiloride block. **(A)** Typical 200 nM solnatide wash-in; 5th pulse showed the steady-state level. **(B)** Typical 10 μM amiloride block of 200 nM solnatide-induced current; 5th pulse showed full block of inward sodium current. **(C)** Typical 20 nM TNF wash-in; 15th pulse showed the steady-state level. **(D)** Typical 10 μM amiloride block of 20 nM TNF-induced current; 9th pulse showed full block of inward sodium current.

TNF and Membrane Abundance of ENaC

In A549 cells (**Figure 2B**), as well as in heterologously expressed α- and δ-ENaC, treatment with 40 nM TNF caused a significant, transient increase in membrane abundance of α- and δ-subunits after 10 min ($p < 0.01$, $n = 4$), while the increase of the β- and γ-subunit was not significant. The increased expression of α- and δ-subunits returned to control values after 30 min (**Figure 2B**). These results confirm data obtained in presence of solnatide (26) with the only difference that for TNF a longer incubation time of 10 min was needed to observe an increase in membrane expression of α- and δ-subunits. Furthermore, our data with TNF on the membrane expression level also underline the importance of the N-linked glycosylation sites for the interaction of the cytokine with the ion channel. WT and single or quintuple (αM5) α-subunit mutants (N232Q, N293Q, N312Q, N397Q, N511Q) were transfected along with βγ-hENaC in HEK-293 cells. Expression levels of αN232Q mutant in presence of TNF were comparable to WT, whereas in αN511Q and α-ENaC lacking all five glycosylation sites an increase of membrane abundance of α-ENaC by 40 nM TNF was inhibited (**Figure 2A**). These results indicate that in the α-subunit, position N511 plays a prominent role in the interaction of TNF with ENaC (**Figure 2A**). As Czikora et al. (19) postulated that the carboxyl terminal of α-hENaC is essential for the interaction with the lectin-like domain of TNF, we deleted the carboxyl-terminal domain by introducing stop codons at L576 in α-hENaC to generate αL576X, as well as in the δ-subunit at position D522 to create δD522X. In these mutants, no increase in membrane abundance could be observed in presence of TNF (**Figure 3**), which again confirms the data with solnatide (26).

α-ENaC Frameshift Mutations

Unexpectedly, solnatide rescues the loss-of-function phenotype in ENaC mutants (27) carrying mutations at conserved positions in α-, β-, and γ-ENaC known to cause PHA1B. Since the α-subunit is supposed to play a prominent role in the ENaC current activation by TNF and TIP peptide, we investigated whether TNF and solnatide can also enhance αβγ-ENaC current in α-ENaC loss-of-function frameshift mutants, i.e., αI68fs, αT169fs, αP197fs, αE272fs, αF435fs, αR438fs, αY447fs, αR448fs, αS452fs, and αT482fs (**Table 2**), which have been reported to cause PHA1B. These frameshift mutants lack the carboxyl-terminal domain of α-ENaC previously postulated

was slower with TNF compared to solnatide and was blocked by 10 μM amiloride within a few pulses (**Figure 1**). Therefore, as a next step, we studied the effect of native TNF on hENaC in more detail.

To study single subunits and mutant ENaC HEK-293 cells were used, as no mRNA encoding ENaC subunits has been found in untransfected HEK-293 cells indicating no endogenous expression of ENaC (40). Only cells with a clear amiloride response and with significantly higher current than non-transfected (16) and mock-transfected (27) HEK-293 cells were used for data analysis. In αβγ-ENaC heterologously expressed in HEK-293 cells, TNF enhanced amiloride-sensitive sodium current with approximately 8-fold higher potency (EC$_{50}$: 6.7 ± 2.1 nM) than solnatide (EC$_{50}$: 54.7 ± 2.2 nM), and TNF was even about 13-fold more effective than solnatide in α- and δ-ENaC subunits (**Table 1**). Notably, however, the maximal steady-state current level of the TNF-activated current in αβγ-ENaC was significantly ($p < 0.001$, $n = 7$) lower than that of solnatide-induced current (**Table 1**). The main targets of TNF were the pore-forming subunits α- and δ-ENaC, similar to what has been shown previously for solnatide (16) (**Table 1**). Interestingly, compared to solnatide, the current-activating effect of TNF was more pronounced in the individual subunits, but without statistically significant difference. The weakest current increase by TNF was found in the γ-subunit, so that no reliable EC$_{50}$ value could be estimated.

In A549 cells single channel open probability, mean open time, number and duration of bursts were significantly increased by TNF and solnatide without affecting conductivity of the channel, and this increase was completely abolished in PNGase F pretreated cells (16). To verify which of the putative N-linked glycosylation sites participate in binding of TNF to the extracellular loop we generated single N (asparagine) to Q (glutamine) mutants in the human α-subunit at each potential glycosylation site (N232, N293, N312, N397, N511) and co-expressed these mutated α-subunits in HEK-293 cells along with βγ-subunits. Similar to solnatide, but less pronounced, we could show that each N-glycan was involved in TNF-induced increase in current with position αN511 being the most important glycosylation site. For comparison, the maximal TNF-induced current of 162.5 ± 7.5 pA in αβγ-ENaC ($n = 7$) was significantly lower in αN232Qβγ-ENaC with 84.7 ± 8.8 pA ($p < 0.001$, $n = 5$), and attenuation of TNF-induced current was most pronounced in the mutant αN511Qβγ-ENaC with 50.7 ± 5.3 pA ($p < 0.001$, $n = 4$).

TABLE 1 | Comparison of the effect of tumor necrosis factor (TNF) and solnatide on amiloride-sensitive Na⁺ current.

hENaC subunit(s)	Amiloride-sensitive control current (pA)	Maximal induced current (pA)		EC$_{50}$ (nM)	
		Tumor necrosis factor (TNF) ($n = 5$)	Solnatide[a]	TNF ($n = 5$)	Solnatide[a]
αβγ	75.8 ± 4.5	162.5 ± 7.5***	953.2 ± 11.5	6.7 ± 2.1***	54.7 ± 2.2
α	55.3 ± 5.5	48.1 ± 5.0***	11.3 ± 6.2	4.2 ± 1.9***	57.8 ± 3.4
β	11.5 ± 3.7	18.5 ± 5.5	n.d.	18.8 ± 2.9	n.d.
γ	14.0 ± 5.1	8.0 ± 3.3	n.d.	n.d.	n.d.
δ	60.6 ± 2.5	27.8 ± 2.1***	15.6 ± 7.9	5.0 ± 0.3***	63.5 ± 9.9

[a]Data from Ref. (16).

***$p < 0.001$, t-test, significant difference between maximal TNF- and solnatide-induced current and significant difference between EC$_{50}$ values for TNF and solnatide, respectively.

n.d., no detectable current.

Values are given as mean ± S.E.

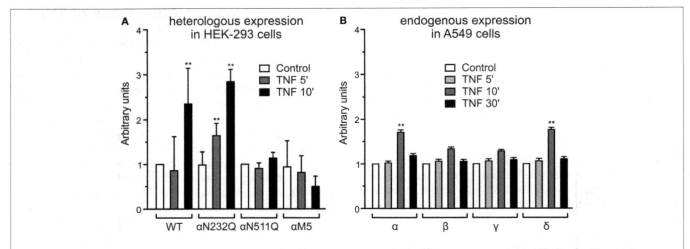

FIGURE 2 | Effect of tumor necrosis factor (TNF) on membrane abundance of N-linked glycosylation site mutations in the extracellular loop of α-epithelial sodium channel (ENaC) and of single subunits of ENaC. (A) A complex of wild-type (WT) αβγ- or single αN232Q and αN511Q mutants as well as quintuple α-ENaC mutant (N232Q, N293Q, N312Q, N397Q, N511Q) combined with WT βγ-ENaC was heterologously expressed in HEK-293 cells, untreated (control) or treated with 40 nM TNF for 5 or 10 min. Biotinylated surface proteins were analyzed using Western blot; the expression of α-ENaC was normalized compared to β-actin and set in relation to WT control (=1). Significant differences are indicated, **$p < 0.01$ ($n = 3$). **(B)** Biotinylated surface proteins from A549 cells untreated or after 5, 10, or 30 min treatment with 40 nM TNF, heterologously expressing αβγδ-ENaC, were analyzed with anti-α-, β-, γ-, or δ-ENaC antibodies. The expression was normalized to β-actin and set in relation to its respective control. Significant differences are indicated, **$p < 0.01$ ($n = 3$).

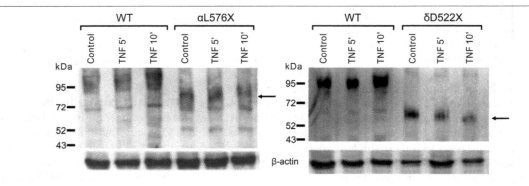

FIGURE 3 | Effect of tumor necrosis factor (TNF) on membrane abundance of αL576X and δD522X mutants. Mutant αL576X (left blot) or δD522X (right blot) was co-expressed with wild-type (WT) βγ-hENaC in HEK-293 cells. WT αβγ- or δβγ-epithelial sodium channel (ENaC) was used as reference. Cells were treated with 40 nM TNF for 5 or 10 min, as indicated, or untreated (control). Biotinylated surface proteins were blotted and visualized with anti-α-ENaC (left blot) or anti-δ-ENaC (right blot) antibodies. WT α- and δ-ENaC show a band at about 95 kDa, whereas the truncated mutants are shorter (the relevant bands are indicated by arrows). A representative blot out of three independent biological replicates is shown in each case.

to be the site of interaction of solnatide with ENaC (19, 31). Apart from αI68fs all studied frameshift mutants originate in the extracellular loop of α-ENaC predominantly clustering in the thumb. Worth mentioning, all described frameshift mutations have the WT sequence before the mutation and some random amino acids after the mutations, until a stop codon occurs. The theoretical total length of the truncated proteins is indicated in **Table 2**.

Solnatide Restores Amiloride-Sensitive Sodium Current in Frameshift Mutations of α-ENaC

To determine whether TNF and solnatide not only activate Na⁺ current in WT αβγ-ENaC but also in PHA1B-causing α-ENaC frameshift mutations, experiments were performed by transfecting mutant α-ENaC together with WT βγ-subunits into HEK-293 cells. The macroscopic amiloride-sensitive Na⁺ currents of all investigated α-ENaC frameshift PHA1B mutants were significantly ($p < 0.001$, for number of experiments see **Table 3**) decreased compared to WT control level (**Figure 4A**). Remarkably, solnatide was able to activate the reduced current in all studied frameshift mutants up to or even higher than WT control current in absence of solnatide (**Figure 4B**), even though these mutants lack the carboxyl-terminal domain of α-ENaC previously postulated to be the site of interaction of solnatide with ENaC (19, 31). A maximum level of concentration-dependent current activation was reached at 200 nM with EC_{50} values as

TABLE 2 | Total protein length and affected regions of α-frameshift mutations that are verified to occur in PHA1B patients.

Mutant (protein)	Truncated protein length (AA)	Affected region	Domain location in homology model of mouse α-ENaC (32)	Mutation in patient (DNA)	First published in
αI68fs	142	Exon 2 cytoplasmic	Intracellular	203delTC	(33)
αT169fs	203	Exon 3 extracellular loop	Finger	505delAC	(34)
αP197fs	204	Exon 3 extracellular loop	Finger	587-588insC	(35)
αE272fs	309	Exon 4 extracellular loop	Finger	814-815insG	(36)
αF435fs	480	Exon 8 extracellular loop	Thumb	1305delC	(34)
αR438fs	480	Exon 8 extracellular loop	Thumb	1311delG	(36)
αY447fs	458	Exon 8 extracellular loop	Thumb	1340insT	(37)
αR448fs	459	Exon 8 extracellular loop	Thumb	1342-1343insTACA	(35)
αS452fs	480	Exon 8 extracellular loop	Thumb	1356delC	(38)
αT482fs	495	Exon 10 extracellular loop	Palm	1449delC	(39)

TABLE 3 | EC$_{50}$ values of pseudohypoaldosteronism type 1B frameshift mutants for solnatide.

Construct	EC$_{50}$	n
Wild-type (WT)	54.7 ± 2.2	11
αI68fs	73.4 ± 13.4	9
αT169fs	58.3 ± 5.2	9
αP197fs	84.0 ± 4.9***	5
αE272fs	75.6 ± 5.4***	5
αF435fs	64.6 ± 8.7	7
αR438fs	56.6 ± 8.0	7
αY447fs	57.2 ± 4.8	7
αR448fs	50.8 ± 2.4	3
αS452fs	68.5 ± 4.1**	5
αT482fs	50.8 ± 5.5	5

*Significant difference compared to WT was calculated with the unpaired Student's t-test, **p < 0.01, ***p < 0.001.*

indicated in **Table 3**. TNF was also able to activate current in mutant ENaC; in case of αR448fs (**Figure 5**) up to WT control current without treatment (compare with **Figure 4**). Similar to WT ENaC the maximal TNF-induced current is lower than the solnatide-induced current in αR448fs mutant (compare **Figure 5** and **Table 1**), but the approximately 3.5-fold increase (TNF-induced/amiloride-sensitive current) in mutant ENaC exceeds the 2-fold current activation in WT ENaC after treatment with TNF. Mutant solnatide (T6A, E8A, E11A), which had no current-activating effect on WT ENaC (24), also had no effect on PHA1B mutants αF435fs and αR448fs.

Varied Effect of Solnatide on Membrane Abundance of α-ENaC Frameshift Mutants

To study α-ENaC protein abundance in plasma membrane cell surface, biotinylation of HEK-293 cells transiently transfected with WT or different PHA1B mutants was followed by SDS-PAGE and immunoblotting. Expression of frameshift mutants varied markedly. For example, expression of αF435fs, αY447fs, αR448fs, and αT482fs was highly significantly ($p < 0.001$, $n = 4$), and αP197fs was significantly ($p < 0.01$, $n = 4$) increased compared to WT. Notably, expression of the two mutants αF435fs and αT482fs was strikingly increased although the amiloride-sensitive Na$^+$ current was significantly ($p < 0.001$, $n = 7$ and $p < 0.001$, $n = 5$, respectively) attenuated (**Figure 4A**). Expression of αR438fs and

αS452fs was comparable to WT ENaC, whereas expression of αI68fs, αT169fs, and αE272fs was significantly ($p < 0.001$, $n = 4$) decreased compared to expression of WT ENaC. Treatment of HEK-293 cells expressing WT or mutant frameshift α-ENaC with solnatide led to a transient and significant increase in membrane abundance of α-ENaC (**Table 4**).

Deglycosylation of α-ENaC Frameshift Mutations

We have previously shown that glycosylation of the extracellular loop of ENaC is one of the prerequisites of solnatide-induced ENaC activation (26). To validate the role of glycosylation in TNF- and solnatide-induced amiloride-sensitive Na$^+$ current activation in frameshift mutants, cell surface expression and patch-clamp experiments were performed following PNGase F treatment of αR448fsβγ as an example. As shown in **Figure 5**, no current could be induced by TNF or solnatide in αR448fs ($n = 3$) mutants when preincubated with PNGase F.

Taken together, these results indicate that frameshift mutation αR448fsβγ requires glycosylation of extracellular sites of ENaC for solnatide and TNF-induced activation of amiloride-sensitive sodium current.

For studies on the role of glycosylation in expression, the two mutants, αR448fs and αT482fs, were chosen, because they showed a marked increase in membrane expression in presence of solnatide. As illustrated in **Figures 6** and **7**, the solnatide induced increase in membrane abundance was completely abolished in deglycosylated mutants.

Role of β- and γ-ENaC in α-ENaC Frameshift Mutations

Lucas et al. (31) identified positions V567, E568, and E571 in the α-subunit as the crucial sites for binding of the lectin-like domain of TNF. They generated alanine replacement mutants in this region of α-ENaC and examined its interaction with the TIP peptide. In triple V567A/E568A/E571A and double V567A/E568A mutants, they found reduced binding capacity of the TIP peptide. Despite the absence of these relevant binding sites in our studied α-frameshift mutants, solnatide caused a significant current increase. As solnatide showed a small current increase in WT βγ-ENaC, we created alanine mutants (βM2γM2) in equivalent residues of β(E539A, E542A)- and γ(E548A, E551A)-ENaC. E539 and E542 in β-ENaC and E548 and E551 in γ-ENaC

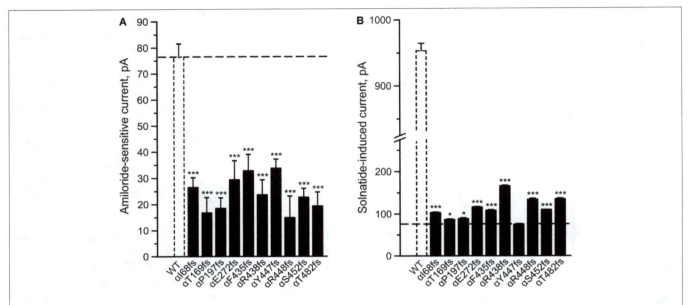

FIGURE 4 | Amiloride-sensitive sodium current and solnatide-induced current in pseudohypoaldosteronism type 1B (PHA1B) frameshift mutants. Wild-type (WT) or mutant α-epithelial sodium channel (ENaC) was co-expressed with βγ subunits in HEK-293 cells. Cells were patched in the whole-cell mode, and the inward current was elicited at −100 mV. The 10 μM amiloride-sensitive current (A) and 200 nM solnatide-induced current (B) of 10 frameshift mutations in α-ENaC associated with PHA1B (black bars) are shown in relation to WT (white, broken bar). For comparison the amiloride-sensitive current of WT αβγ-ENaC is indicated as broken line. Significant difference compared to WT control was calculated using one-way ANOVA followed by Tukey's post hoc test, *$p < 0.05$, ***$p < 0.001$ ($n = 3–11$).

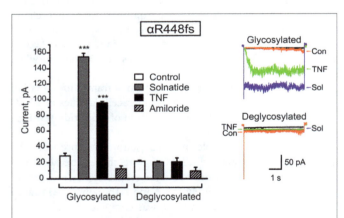

FIGURE 5 | Deglycosylation of R448fs with PNGase F abolished both solnatide- and tumor necrosis factor (TNF)-induced activation. Mean values of 200 nM solnatide- and 20 nM TNF-induced inward currents in control (glycosylated) and 100 units PNGase F treated (deglycosylated) αR448fsβγ (left), ***$p < 0.001$ compared with control as determined by unpaired Student's t-test, $n = 3$. Typical solnatide- and TNF-induced current traces of αR448fsβγ in control and PNGase F (100 U) treated transiently transfected HEK-293 cells. For comparison, original traces from separate solnatide and TNF experiments are superimposed (right).

TABLE 4 | Effect of solnatide on membrane abundance of α-epithelial sodium channel frameshift mutations.

Mutation	Control	Solnatide 5 min	Solnatide 10 min
Wild-type	1	1.48 ± 0.12***	1.40 ± 0.09***
αI68fs	0.15 ± 0.06	0.25 ± 0.07*	0.32 ± 0.11**
αT169fs	0.54 ± 0.06	0.80 ± 0.03***	0.46 ± 0.09
αP197fs	1.18 ± 0.05	1.33 ± 0.07**	0.48 ± 0.09***
αE272fs	0.35 ± 0.06	0.72 ± 0.03***	0.64 ± 0.05***
αF435fs	2.37 ± 0.15	3.71 ± 0.20***	2.82 ± 0.17**
αR438fs	0.90 ± 0.07	1.39 ± 0.14***	0.87 ± 0.10
αY447fs	1.27 ± 0.10	1.57 ± 0.13***	1.89 ± 0.16***
αR448fs	1.32 ± 0.10	5.88 ± 0.32***	1.30 ± 0.12
αS452fs	1.11 ± 0.25	1.36 ± 0.11***	1.94 ± 0.08***
αT482fs	4.67 ± 0.27	6.23 ± 0.24***	4.58 ± 0.30

*$p < 0.05$, **$p < 0.01$, ***$p < 0.001$, significant difference from respective control values (one-way ANOVA, Tukey's post hoc test).

are homologous to E568 and E571 in the α-subunit, whereas the V567 residue of α-ENaC is I538 in β-ENaC and I547 in γ-ENaC. Solnatide, however, still increased the amiloride-sensitive sodium current in these mutants, which implies that these regions in β- and γ-ENaC do not play any role in the current-activating effect of α-frameshift mutations.

DISCUSSION

We have previously shown that the synthetic cyclic peptide solnatide, which mimics the lectin-like domain of TNF, requires one of the two pore-forming α- and δ-ENaC subunits to induce its maximum amiloride-sensitive sodium current-activating effect (16). Loss-of-function mutations in ENaC genes translate into the salt-wasting genetic disease PHA1B (33, 41). We have also shown that loss-of-function point mutations of ENaC found in PHA1B patients conduct significantly low current when transfected along with WT β- and γ-subunits (27). Remarkably, amiloride-sensitive

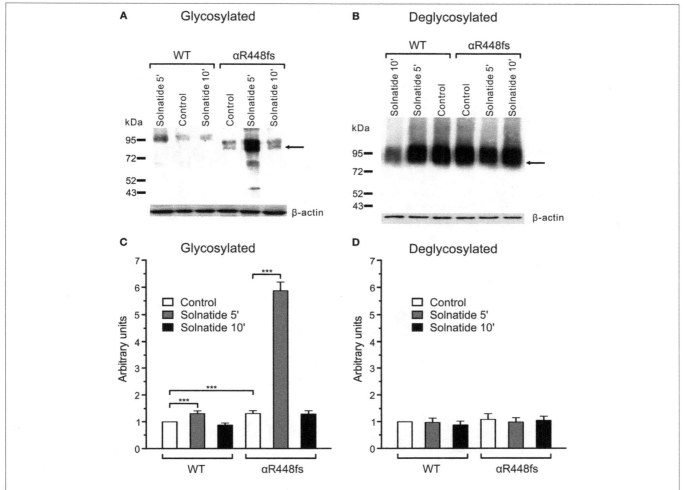

FIGURE 6 | **Effect of solnatide on the membrane abundance of αR448fs without and with PNGase F treatment.** Biotinylated surface proteins of HEK-293 cells heterologously expressing WT αβγ-epithelial sodium channel (ENaC) or αR448fsβγ-ENaC treated with 200 nM solnatide at indicated time points and/or 100 units PNGase F were blotted and analyzed with anti-α-ENaC antibody. One representative blot out of four independent biological replicates is shown before [(A); glycosylated] and after PNGase F treatment [(B); deglycosylated]. Wild-type (WT) α-ENaC shows a band at about 95 kDa and for mutant α-ENaC the protein band, which was used for quantification is indicated by arrows. α-ENaC expression was normalized to β-actin and set in relation to WT control (= 1). The membrane abundance of glycosylated αR448fs-ENaC is highly increased after 5 min of solnatide treatment (C), whereas after PNGase F treatment no differences can be observed [(D); deglycosylated]. Significant differences are indicated, ***$p < 0.001$ ($n = 4$).

currents were restored to WT control levels by solnatide and its congener, AP318 (27). In the present study, experiments were performed to elucidate the effect of the TNF lectin-like domain, both as an integral part of the TNF molecule as well as represented by solnatide, on PHA1B frameshift mutations.

Lectin-Mediated Activation of ENaC by TNF

The mechanism of TNF-induced ion channel modulation has been intensively studied and, in particular, TNF in combination with other cytokines could drive a pathological condition to a more aggressive state (42, 43). However, as a possible therapeutic molecule, the machinery of TNF-induced activation of ion channels is still largely unknown (44). TNF exhibits a dual role of action in pathological conditions; specifically, TNF has been shown to contribute to the pathogenesis and development of pulmonary edema, through binding to TNF receptors and consequent initiation of the inflammatory cascade. However, some studies have demonstrated surprisingly that TNF can also promote alveolar fluid reabsorption *in vivo* and *in vitro*, a protective effect mediated by the lectin-like domain of the cytokine, which is spatially distinct from the TNF-receptor binding sites (45).

The current-enhancing effect of TNF on different ion channels including ENaC has been documented (15, 46). We have previously shown that solnatide, mimicking the lectin-like domain of TNF, can activate WT ENaC channels (16, 24, 26), as well as ENaC carrying PHA1B-causing mutations (27). In the present study, our data provide evidence for a mechanism of lectin-like domain-mediated, TNF-induced activation of ENaC carrying PHA1B-causing frameshift mutations. Our data demonstrate that TNF has to bind to ENaC glycosylation

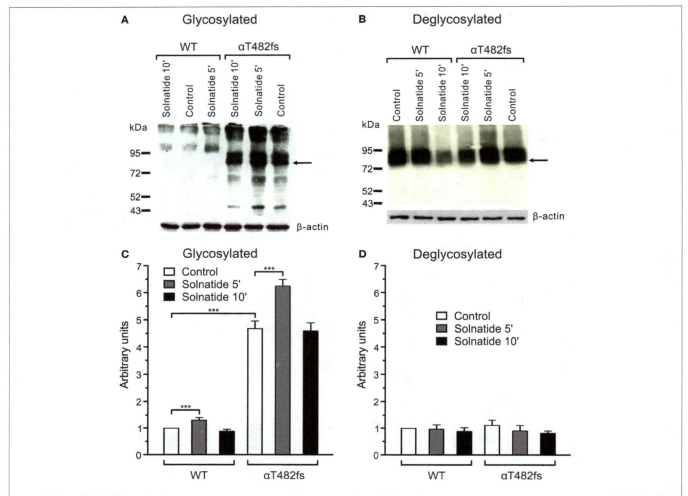

FIGURE 7 | **Effect of solnatide on the membrane abundance of αT482fs without and with PNGase F treatment.** Biotinylated surface proteins of HEK-293 cells heterologously expressing wild-type (WT) αβγ-epithelial sodium channel (ENaC) or αT482fsβγ-ENaC treated with 200 nM solnatide at indicated time points and/or 100 units PNGase F were blotted and analyzed with anti-α-ENaC antibody. One representative blot out of four independent biological replicates is shown before [(A); glycosylated] and after PNGase F treatment [(B); deglycosylated]. WT α-ENaC shows a band at about 95 kDa and for mutant α-ENaC the protein band which was used for quantification is indicated by arrows. α-ENaC expression was normalized to β-actin and set in relation to WT control (=1). The membrane abundance of glycosylated αT482fs-ENaC is already increased without solnatide (control) compared to WT and even more after 5 min of solnatide treatment (C), whereas after PNGase F treatment no differences can be observed [(D); deglycosylated]. Significant differences are indicated, ***$p < 0.001$ ($n = 4$).

sites of the extracellular loop through its lectin-like domain in order to exert its ENaC-activating effect as well as to increase translocation of newly synthesized channels to the plasma membrane. Notably, one TNF molecule, which exists as a stable homotrimer (47) contains three lectin-like domains which make the TNF a highly potent activator of ENaC compared to solnatide (a single lectin-like domain mimicking molecule); see EC_{50} values in **Table 1**. In contrast, the maximal stimulatory effect of solnatide was greater and was reached more rapidly after ~2-min exposure, compared to that of TNF, which was reached after ~5 min (**Figure 1**). The maximum induced current for solnatide was 953.2 ± 11.5 pA compared to 162.5 ± 7.5 pA induced by TNF (**Table 1**). The reason for slower time course of activation and smaller current induced by TNF could be that TNF is a bulkier, larger molecule (the mature TNF trimer has a molecular mass of approximately 52 kD) than solnatide (17-mer cyclic peptide, molecular mass 1.9 kD) and hence occupies more space around the extracellular loop of ENaC, around which in comparison more molecules of solnatide could be accommodated and simultaneously engage with glycosylation or other sites of interaction.

An alternative interpretation of slower TNF time course of activation of ENaC compared to solnatide could be that TNF and solnatide interact with both the extracellular and intracellular domains of ENaC; the time required to activate ENaC would simply reflect the necessity of TNF and solnatide to penetrate the plasma membrane. Binding of the triad of lectin-like domains at the tip of the native TNF homotrimer to glycosylation sites on the ENaC heterooligomer might hinder further folding and subsequent penetration of the TNF molecule across the plasma membrane. We have previously shown that solnatide required αβγ-ENaC or δβγ-ENaC to show its maximum stimulatory effect (16). To our surprise, in single subunit experiments, TNF-induced current was higher than solnatide-induced current (**Table 1**).

Direct interaction of TNF with ENaC has hitherto not been reported and so its physiological role in improving ALC during lung inflammation has been largely inferred from numerous studies with solnatide and other TIP peptides (18, 20–23). A recent study which sought to determine the precise mechanism by which solnatide stimulated Na⁺ uptake in the presence or absence of PLY, demonstrated that TIP activates ENaC through binding to the carboxyl-terminal domain of the α-subunit (19). Using heterologously expressed WT ENaC we show in the present study that native TNF enhances Na⁺ current, although the maximum TNF-activated current is less than with solnatide.

Tumor necrosis factor, like solnatide, also requires the intracellular carboxyl-terminal region of α- or δ-ENaC to exert its effect of bringing about an increase in membrane abundance of the respective subunits (**Figure 3**). Thus, with the mutants αL576Xβγ-ENaC and δD522Xβγ-ENaC, which lack the region between TM2 and the carboxyl terminus of α- or δ-hENaC, respectively, the increase in membrane abundance seen with WT α- or δ-ENaC was not observed (**Figure 3**). These data are in agreement with our previously published reports (19, 26, 31) that the carboxyl-terminal domain of α- or δ-ENaC is an essential motif for TNF lectin-like domain induced activation of the channel.

The possibility exists that TNF binds to the cell membrane surrounding or in the vicinity of oligomeric ENaC in a general, non-specific manner, thereby altering the disposition of ENaC in the bilayer and resulting in a conformation with a higher P_o. Such an affect would still be amiloride-sensitive if the amiloride-binding sites in ENaC subunits were intact and accessible and would be eliminated by addition of amiloride. A precedent for such non-specific membrane insertion of TNF at low pH has been documented (48). Specifically, a role has been suggested for residues in the lectin-like domain of TNF in membrane insertion. The lectin-like domain occupies residues Cys101-Glu116 of human TNF (2), located in triplicate in the highly flexible loop region at the apex of the bell-shaped native TNF trimer (49). Trp114, the first-ordered residue after the apical flexible loop (47), is buried at pH 7.4 but could readily become exposed to an aqueous milieu upon protonation of nearby residues (e.g., Glu116, a salt-bridge participant), resulting in increased surface hydrophobicity and a tendency for insertion into the lipid bilayer by hydrophobic interactions (48). Moreover, membrane penetration has been shown to stabilize the low pH conformation of TNF, and membrane inserted TNF exhibits a native trimeric structure (48). The corresponding bulky, hydrophobic region of TIP peptides (Trp15 in solnatide) has been shown to be one of the essential characteristic features required for the Na⁺ current-potentiating effect of these peptides (24). In the case of solnatide, the cyclic peptide is totally exposed to the aqueous environment leading one to question whether Trp15 would similarly lend to the peptide the tendency for membrane insertion by hydrophobic interaction. Earlier studies with artificial lysosomes, however, could produce no evidence of direct membrane interaction of this TIP peptide (50), leading the authors to conclude that interaction of the TIP domain *via* an ion channel or other membrane protein was required for its current-potentiating effect.

Restoration of ENaC Current in Frameshift Mutants by TNF and Solnatide

Previously it has been shown that frameshift mutations in pacemaker channels (*HCN4*) do produce a functional channel, which shows normal intracellular trafficking and membrane integration, when transfected in mammalian cells (51), whereas in the case of the cardiac sodium channel (*SCN5A*), a complete loss-of-function phenotype was reported (52).

Computational and site-directed mutagenesis approaches have shown that the lectin-like domain of TNF and solnatide, the synthetic peptide which mimics it, exert their ENaC-activating effect through binding with glycosylation sites of extracellular loops of ENaC (26, 53). Because solnatide has been shown to directly bind with glycosylation sites of ENaC, we treated αR448fsβγ-ENaC with PNGase F prior to testing in a patch clamp assay with solnatide and TNF. Convincingly, neither TNF nor solnatide potentiated amiloride-sensitive current in αR448fsβγ-ENaC following PNGase F treatment, contrary to the activation observed without prior PNGase F treatment (**Figure 5**). PNGase F treatment also abolished the increase in membrane abundance observed with mutants αR448fs and αT482fs in the presence of solnatide (**Figures 6** and **7**). These results indicate and are consistent with our previous results that glycosylation sites on

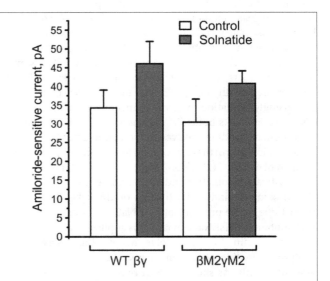

FIGURE 8 | βE539AE542AγE548AE551A mutants (βM2γM2) did not affect the solnatide-induced activation of βγ-epithelial sodium channel (ENaC). HEK-293 cells transiently transfected with wild-type (WT) βγ- or mutant βM2γM2-ENaC were patched in the whole-cell mode. The inward current at −100 mV was measured in absence (control) and presence of 200 nM solnatide and the 10 µM amiloride-sensitive current was calculated. E539 and E542 in β-ENaC and E548 and E551 in γ-ENaC are homologous to the postulated solnatide-binding sites (V567, E568 and E571 in α-ENaC (31), but solnatide was still able to activate βM2γM2-ENaC (not significant) to an equal extent as WT βγ-ENaC (n = 3).

the extracellular loop of ENaC are essential for solnatide-induced activation of ENaC (16, 26).

All the frameshift mutants described in the current work lack the amiloride-binding site of the α-subunit, located in TM2, but retain amiloride-binding sites in the co-expressed WT β- and γ-subunits. The amiloride-binding site of α-ENaC is at S556, the position corresponding to Gly439 in ASIC1 (54) and located in the middle of TM2. Amiloride-binding sites occur at equivalent positions in the β- and γ-ENaC subunits (54, 55). The amiloride sensitivity shown by the PHA1B frameshift mutants described in the present work must therefore be due to amiloride binding to sites in the β- and γ-subunits.

In the present study we analyzed frameshift mutations of α-ENaC which produce a truncated ENaC α-subunit. We found that these frameshift mutants can generate amiloride-sensitive current, but it is significantly lower than WT ENaC (**Figure 4A**). Remarkably, solnatide restored the amiloride-sensitive current in all these frameshift mutants to WT or higher levels (**Figure 4B**). As shown in **Table 2**, these mutants generate a truncated α-ENaC of different lengths ranging from 142 (I68fs) to 495 (T482fs) amino acid residues. The αI68fs mutation results in production of a truncated α-subunit comprising a polypeptide chain of 142 amino acid residues, of which residues 1–67 are WT and 68–142 are non-native due to the shift in the reading frame of the mRNA transcript by two nucleotide positions. Analysis of the 142 mutant amino acid sequence with the TMPred bioinformatics tool for prediction of membrane-spanning regions, failed to detect any TM regions, whereas in WT α-hENaC, TM1 is located between residues F86-F110 by sequence comparison with the ENaC homolog, ASIC1 (56). The 142-residue polypeptide resulting from the αI68fs mutation is unlikely to penetrate the membrane, but may associate intracellularly with β- and γ-subunits and thus be detectable in the biotinylated membrane protein fraction.

Previous work of others had shown that the PHA1B mutant αI68fs conducts 0.1% current compared with WT when co-expressed with rat βγ-ENaC in *Xenopus* oocytes (57). Surprisingly, solnatide induced a current increase in αI68fsβγ-ENaC, which lacks both TM regions and all hitherto known or hypothesized binding motifs for solnatide activation, namely: glycosylation sites in the extracellular loop (26), carboxyl-terminal domain of α-ENaC (19); V567 and E568 in TM2, residues found to be critical for solnatide and TNF binding (31).

The solnatide-induced activation of αI68fsβγ-ENaC could be in part due to the presence of βγ-ENaC subunits co-transfected with mutant αI68fsENaC. In fact, this applies to all the frameshift mutants examined here. To solve this puzzling discrepancy, we analyzed solnatide activation of ENaC comprising the β- and γ-subunits only. As shown in **Figure 8**, solnatide could activate the inward sodium current through βγ-ENaC channels to a level comparable to that observed for αI68fsβγ-ENaC (**Figure 4B**). These data indicate and are in agreement with our previously published results (16), namely that solnatide can activate βγ-ENaC marginally. Solnatide has been shown to activate ENaC by binding critical residues located in TM2 of α-hENaC (31). Lucas et al. (31) found that double (V567A,E568A) and triple (V567A, E568A, E571A) α-ENaC mutants showed reduced binding capacity to solnatide and TNF, resulting in an abolition of the

increase in P_o usually observed with WT ENaC in the presence of solnatide, although membrane expression was the same as WT. To explore the possibility that the observed potentiation of Na⁺ current in the αI68fsβγ-ENaC mutant could be due to binding of solnatide or TNF to residues of βγ-ENaC equivalent to E568 and E571, two of the three residues in TM2 of α-ENaC studied by Lucas et al. (31), we generated point mutations of β-ENaC: E539A, E542A and γ-ENaC: E548, E551 (**Figure 8**). A small increase in the amiloride-sensitive Na⁺ current was still observed with βE539A, E542A, γE548A, E551A-ENaC in the presence of solnatide (**Figure 8**). These results indicate that some other mechanism is responsible for solnatide-induced potentiation of the Na⁺ current, albeit small, in these βγ-ENaC TM2 mutants, which lack α-ENaC and therefore the crucial residues V567A, E568A in TM2, as well as residues in β- and γ-ENaC, E539, E542 and E548, E551, respectively, equivalent to E568 and E571 in α-ENaC. Such a mechanism could explain the Na⁺ current-potentiating effect of solnatide on the αI68fsβγ-ENaC and the other frameshift mutants examined in the present study.

Langloh et al. (58) also studied the effects of mutating residues in TM2 of α-hENaC, but unlike the alanine mutants described above, they mutated highly conserved glutamic acid residues to arginine, E568R, E571R, and D575R, thus reversing the charge at these important positions in TM2. Whole-cell amiloride-sensitive current recorded from oocytes injected with the α-ENaC mutants along with WT β- and γ-ENaC, was low compared with the WT channel, but plasma membrane abundance of the mutant channels was the same as that of WT. The mutations decreased channel conductance but did not affect Na⁺:K⁺ permeability.

Results of earlier experiments conducted by our group with mutants αL576Xβγ-ENaC and δD522Xβγ-ENaC, which lack the region between TM2 and the carboxyl terminus of α- or δ-hENaC (26), had indicated a residual albeit non-significant increase in the amiloride-sensitive current in the presence of solnatide. A channel lacking all carboxyl termini, namely αL576XβD546XγD556X, showed an even slighter, non-significant increase of current after treatment with solnatide in preliminary experiments. This small increase was not seen in the case of αL576Xβγ-ENaC and δD522Xβγ-ENaC in which the glycosylation sites in the extracellular loop had been removed by mutation (26). Thus, apart from the requirement for an intact carboxyl-terminal region in the α-subunit, some other unknown glycosylation-mediated mechanisms seem to play a minor role in TIP activation of ENaC.

A striking feature of the frameshift mutations examined in this work is their non-random distribution in the 3D molecular structure of the α-ENaC subunit. Specifically, of the 10 reported mutations in the current report, five (50%) are located in the thumb domain (**Table 2**) according to the domain nomenclature established for the ENaC homolog, ASIC1 (56). Of the remaining mutations, three are located in the finger domain, one in the palm domain, and one intracellularly. Another α-ENaC frameshift mutation causing PHA1B previously investigated by our group, S243fs (27, 39), is located in the finger domain. Although we cannot purport to have investigated all known PHA1B mutations (some of which have not been reported in the literature), there does seem to be a trend for the thumb domain of α-ENaC to manifest only frameshift mutations, since all PHA1B-causing mutations so far located to the thumb domain of α-ENaC are frameshift mutations (unpublished findings) translated from exon 8 of the mRNA transcript. All frameshift mutations result in truncated polypeptide chains that contain the α-ENaC amino terminal native sequence preceding the mutation followed by a sequence of non-native residues of varying length, depending on the position of the mutation and length of the out-of-frame mRNA before a stop codon is encountered (**Table 2**). At the gene level, a mutational hotspot resulting in insertion or deletion of nucleotide base pairs might be the cause of such clustering of mutations in exon 8. The results presented here suggest that at the protein level, since α-subunits are detected by surface biotinylation, a channel with severely reduced Na^+ conducting capacity is produced, apparently comprised of truncated α-subunit and full-length wild-type β- and γ-subunits. Alternatively, truncated polypeptide chains are trafficked to the membrane, but Na^+ conducting channels, albeit of severely compromised activity, are assembled from β- and γ-subunits only.

The effect of solnatide on increasing membrane abundance in the frameshift mutants was extremely varied and no trend could be discerned, other than that the effect is transient with a peak around 5−10 min of exposure to solnatide, suggesting that solnatide exerts its effect by increasing trafficking of mutant α-ENaC to the membrane. Some mutants, specifically αF435fs and αT482fs, were characterized by a markedly increased membrane abundance of the truncated subunit compared to WT ENaC in the absence of solnatide, the membrane abundance increasing even further following exposure to solnatide (**Table 4**). All frameshift mutants described here lack the "PPxY" and "YXXΦ" motifs located in the intracellular carboxyl-terminal region and required for ubiquitination and endocytosis (59, 60), and in the absence of which, mutant subunits would accumulate at the cell surface. This could explain the significantly higher abundance in the membrane of some of the frameshift mutants compared to WT ENaC. The increase in abundance of mutant subunits compared to WT does not seem to correlate with higher amiloride-sensitive current either without or in the presence of solnatide (**Figure 4, Table 4**), suggesting that these mutant subunits are mostly dysfunctional proteins. Nevertheless, mutant subunits do increase in abundance in response to solnatide and this effect, combined with the increase in P_o brought about by the lectin-like domain interacting with mutant α-subunits and possibly with WT β- and γ-subunits results in solnatide rescuing these PHA1B frameshift mutants and restoring amiloride-sensitive Na^+ current to physiological levels.

Concluding Remarks

The results presented here validate the use of TIP peptides as experimental models for the TNF lectin-like domain, previously assumed in numerous studies (19, 21, 31, 45, 61). Although the PHA1B frameshift mutants investigated in the present study lack features shown in earlier studies to be critical for TNF lectin-like domain interaction with ENaC, the fact that solnatide potentiates amiloride-sensitive Na^+ current to physiological levels, rescuing the mutants, indicates that some additional glycosylation-dependent mechanism, possibly involving β- and γ-ENaC, contributes to the solnatide-induced amiloride-sensitive Na^+ current. Consequently, as we previously reported for point mutations causing PHA1B (27), TIP peptides would seem to be good candidates for lead compounds in the drug development process for treatment of this life-threatening hereditary disease caused by loss-of-function mutations in ENaC.

AUTHOR CONTRIBUTIONS

AW gave substantial contribution to the design of the work, performed experiments, analyzed and interpreted data, and drafted the work. MA performed experiments, analyzed and interpreted data, and drafted the work. ST gave substantial contributions to the conception and design of the work, interpretation of data, and drafted the work. DEM, FP, and SI performed electrophysiological experiments, analyzed data, and drafted the work. ALW, BU, DG, and DM performed Western blot experiments, analyzed data, and drafted the work. BF, HF, and HP gave contribution to the conception of the work and revised it critically. IC and RL interpreted data and revised the work critically for important intellectual content. RL-G gave substantial contribution to the conception and design of the work, interpretation of data, and drafted the work. WS gave substantial contribution to the design of the work, performed experiments, analyzed data, and drafted the work. All the authors approved the version to be published and agree to be accountable for the content of the work.

REFERENCES

1. Truyens C, Torrico F, Lucas R, De Baetselier P, Buurman WA, Carlier Y. The endogenous balance of soluble tumor necrosis factor receptors and tumor necrosis factor modulates cachexia and mortality in mice acutely infected with *Trypanosoma cruzi. Infect Immun* (1999) 67:5579–86.
2. Lucas R, Magez S, De Leys R, Fransen L, Scheerlinck JP, Rampelberg M, et al. Mapping the lectin-like activity of tumor necrosis factor. *Science* (1994) 263:814–7. doi:10.1126/science.8303299
3. Olson EJ, Standing JE, Griego-Harper N, Hoffman OA, Limper AH. Fungal beta-glucan interacts with vitronectin and stimulates tumor

necrosis factor alpha release from macrophages. *Infect Immun* (1996) 64:3548–54.
4. Hribar M, Bloc A, van der Goot FG, Fransen L, De Baetselier P, Grau GE, et al. The lectin-like domain of tumor necrosis factor-alpha increases membrane conductance in microvascular endothelial cells and peritoneal macrophages. *Eur J Immunol* (1999) 29:3105–11.
5. Sherblom AP, Decker JM, Muchmore AV. The lectin-like interaction between recombinant tumor necrosis factor and uromodulin. *J Biol Chem* (1988) 263:5418–24.
6. Tarleton RL. Tumour necrosis factor (cachectin) production during experimental Chagas' disease. *Clin Exp Immunol* (1988) 73:186–90.

7. Muñoz-Fernández MA, Fernández MA, Fresno M. Activation of human macrophages for the killing of intracellular *Trypanosoma cruzi* by TNF-alpha and IFN-gamma through a nitric oxide-dependent mechanism. *Immunol Lett* (1992) 33:35–40. doi:10.1016/0165-2478(92)90090-B

8. Magez S, Lucas R, Darji A, Songa EB, Hamers R, De Baetselier P. Murine tumour necrosis factor plays a protective role during the initial phase of the experimental infection with *Trypanosoma brucei brucei*. *Parasite Immunol* (1993) 15:635–41. doi:10.1111/j.1365-3024.1993.tb00577.x

9. Lucas R, Magez S, Songa B, Darji A, Hamers R, de Baetselier P. A role for TNF during African trypanosomiasis: involvement in parasite control, immunosuppression and pathology. *Res Immunol* (1993) 144:370–6. doi:10.1016/S0923-2494(93)80082-A

10. Lima EC, Garcia I, Vicentelli MH, Vassalli P, Minoprio P. Evidence for a protective role of tumor necrosis factor in the acute phase of *Trypanosoma cruzi* infection in mice. *Infect Immun* (1997) 65:457–65.

11. Magez S, Geuskens M, Beschin A, del Favero H, Verschueren H, Lucas R, et al. Specific uptake of tumor necrosis factor-alpha is involved in growth control of *Trypanosoma brucei*. *J Cell Biol* (1997) 137:715–27. doi:10.1083/jcb.137.3.715

12. Lucas R, Garcia I, Donati YR, Hribar M, Mandriota SJ, Giroud C, et al. Both TNF receptors are required for direct TNF-mediated cytotoxicity in microvascular endothelial cells. *Eur J Immunol* (1998) 28:3577–86.

13. Magez S, Radwanska M, Beschin A, Sekikawa K, De Baetselier P. Tumor necrosis factor alpha is a key mediator in the regulation of experimental *Trypanosoma brucei* infections. *Infect Immun* (1999) 67:3128–32.

14. Beschin A, Bilej M, Brys L, Torreele E, Lucas R, Magez S, et al. Convergent evolution of cytokines. *Nature* (1999) 400:627–8. doi:10.1038/23164

15. Fukuda N, Jayr C, Lazrak A, Wang Y, Lucas R, Matalon S, et al. Mechanisms of TNF-alpha stimulation of amiloride-sensitive sodium transport across alveolar epithelium. *Am J Physiol Lung Cell Mol Physiol* (2001) 280:L1258–65.

16. Shabbir W, Scherbaum-Hazemi P, Tzotzos S, Fischer B, Fischer H, Pietschmann H, et al. Mechanism of action of novel lung edema therapeutic AP301 by activation of the epithelial sodium channel. *Mol Pharmacol* (2013) 84:899–910. doi:10.1124/mol.113.089409

17. Elia N, Tapponnier M, Matthay MA, Hamacher J, Pache JC, Brundler MA, et al. Functional identification of the alveolar edema reabsorption activity of murine tumor necrosis factor-alpha. *Am J Respir Crit Care Med* (2003) 168:1043–50. doi:10.1164/rccm.200206-618OC

18. Braun C, Hamacher J, Morel DR, Wendel A, Lucas R. Dichotomal role of TNF in experimental pulmonary edema reabsorption. *J Immunol* (2005) 175:3402–8. doi:10.4049/jimmunol.175.5.3402

19. Czikora I, Alli A, Bao HF, Kaftan D, Sridhar S, Apell HJ, et al. A novel TNF-mediated mechanism of direct epithelial sodium channel activation. *Am J Respir Crit Care Med* (2014) 190:522–32. doi:10.1164/rccm.201405-0833OC

20. Vadász I, Schermuly RT, Ghofrani HA, Rummel S, Wehner S, Mühldorfer I, et al. The lectin-like domain of tumor necrosis factor-alpha improves alveolar fluid balance in injured isolated rabbit lungs. *Crit Care Med* (2008) 36:1543–50. doi:10.1097/CCM.0b013e31816f485e

21. Hamacher J, Stammberger U, Roux J, Kumar S, Yang G, Xiong C, et al. The lectin-like domain of tumor necrosis factor improves lung function after rat lung transplantation – potential role for a reduction in reactive oxygen species generation. *Crit Care Med* (2010) 38:871–8. doi:10.1097/CCM.0b013e3181cdf725

22. Hartmann EK, Boehme S, Duenges B, Bentley A, Klein KU, Kwiecien R, et al. An inhaled tumor necrosis factor-alpha-derived TIP peptide improves the pulmonary function in experimental lung injury. *Acta Anaesthesiol Scand* (2013) 57:334–41. doi:10.1111/aas.12034

23. Zhou Q, Wang D, Liu Y, Yang X, Lucas R, Fischer B. Solnatide demonstrates profound therapeutic activity in a rat model of pulmonary edema induced by acute hypobaric hypoxia and exercise. *Chest* (2016) 151:658–67. doi:10.1016/j.chest.2016.10.030

24. Hazemi P, Tzotzos SJ, Fischer B, Andavan GS, Fischer H, Pietschmann H, et al. Essential structural features of TNF-α lectin-like domain derived peptides for activation of amiloride-sensitive sodium current in A549 cells. *J Med Chem* (2010) 53:8021–9. doi:10.1021/jm100767p

25. Tzotzos S, Fischer B, Fischer H, Pietschmann H, Lucas R, Dupré G, et al. AP301, a synthetic peptide mimicking the lectin-like domain of TNF, enhances amiloride-sensitive Na(+) current in primary dog, pig and rat alveolar type II cells. *Pulm Pharmacol Ther* (2013) 26:356–63. doi:10.1016/j.pupt.2012.12.011

26. Shabbir W, Tzotzos S, Bedak M, Aufy M, Willam A, Kraihammer M, et al. Glycosylation-dependent activation of epithelial sodium channel by solnatide. *Biochem Pharmacol* (2015) 98:740–53. doi:10.1016/j.bcp.2015.08.003

27. Willam A, Aufy M, Tzotzos S, Evanzin H, Chytracek S, Geppert S, et al. Restoration of epithelial sodium channel function by synthetic peptides in pseudohypoaldosteronism type 1B mutants. *Front Pharmacol* (2017) 8:85. doi:10.3389/fphar.2017.00085

28. Hanukoglu A, Edelheit O, Shriki Y, Gizewska M, Dascal N, Hanukoglu I. Renin-aldosterone response, urinary Na/K ratio and growth in pseudohypoaldosteronism patients with mutations in epithelial sodium channel (ENaC) subunit genes. *J Steroid Biochem Mol Biol* (2008) 111(3–5):268–74. doi:10.1016/j.jsbmb.2008.06.013

29. Zennaro MC, Lombès M. Mineralocorticoid resistance. *Trends Endocrinol Metab* (2004) 15(6):264–70. doi:10.1016/j.tem.2004.06.003

30. Riepe FG. Clinical and molecular features of type 1 pseudohypoaldosteronism. *Horm Res* (2009) 72:1–9. doi:10.1159/000224334

31. Lucas R, Yue Q, Alli A, Duke BJ, Al-Khalili O, Thai TL, et al. The lectin-like domain of TNF increases ENaC open probability through a novel site at the interface between the second transmembrane and C-terminal domains of the α subunit. *J Biol Chem* (2016) 291:23440–51. doi:10.1074/jbc.M116.718163

32. Kashlan OB, Adelman JL, Okumura S, Blobner BM, Zuzek Z, Hughey RP, et al. Constraint-based, homology model of the extracellular domain of the epithelial Na+ channel α subunit reveals a mechanism of channel activation by proteases. *J Biol Chem* (2011) 286:649–60. doi:10.1074/jbc.M110.167098

33. Chang SS, Grunder S, Hanukoglu A, Rösler A, Mathew PM, Hanukoglu I, et al. Mutations in subunits of the epithelial sodium channel cause salt wasting with hyperkalaemic acidosis, pseudohypoaldosteronism type 1. *Nat Genet* (1996) 12:248–53. doi:10.1038/ng0396-248

34. Kerem E, Bistritzer T, Hanukoglu A, Hofmann T, Zhou Z, Bennett W, et al. Pulmonary epithelial sodium-channel dysfunction and excess airway liquid in pseudohypoaldosteronism. *N Engl J Med* (1999) 341:156–62. doi:10.1056/NEJM199907153410304

35. Welzel M, Akin L, Büscher A, Güran T, Hauffa BP, Högler W, et al. Five novel mutations in the SCNN1A gene causing autosomal recessive pseudohypoaldosteronism type 1. *Eur J Endocrinol* (2013) 168:707–15. doi:10.1530/EJE-12-1000

36. Wang J, Yu T, Yin L, Li J, Yu L, Shen Y, et al. Novel mutations in the SCNN1A gene causing Pseudohypoaldosteronism type 1. *PLoS One* (2013) 8:e65676. doi:10.1371/journal.pone.0065676

37. Saxena A, Hanukoglu I, Saxena D, Thompson RJ, Gardiner RM, Hanukoglu A, et al. Novel mutations responsible for autosomal recessive multisystem pseudohypoaldosteronism and sequence variants in epithelial sodium channel alpha-, beta-, and gamma-subunit genes. *J Clin Endocrinol Metab* (2002) 87:3344–50. doi:10.1210/jcem.87.7.8674

38. Edelheit O, Hanukoglu I, Gizewska M, Kandemir N, Tenenbaum-Rakover Y, Yurdakök M, et al. Novel mutations in epithelial sodium channel (ENaC) subunit genes and phenotypic expression of multisystem pseudohypoaldosteronism. *Clin Endocrinol (Oxf)* (2005) 62:547–53. doi:10.1111/j.1365-2265.2005.02255.x

39. Schaedel C, Marthinsen L, Kristoffersson AC, Kornfält R, Nilsson KO, Orlenius B, et al. Lung symptoms in pseudohypoaldosteronism type 1 are associated with deficiency of the alpha-subunit of the epithelial sodium channel. *J Pediatr* (1999) 135:739–45. doi:10.1016/S0022-3476(99)70094-6

40. Ruffieux-Daidié D, Poirot O, Boulkroun S, Verrey F, Kellenberger S, Staub O. Deubiquitylation regulates activation and proteolytic cleavage of ENaC. *J Am Soc Nephrol* (2008) 19(11):2170–80. doi:10.1681/ASN.2007101130

41. Gründer S, Firsov D, Chang SS, Jaeger NF, Gautschi I, Schild L, et al. A mutation causing pseudohypoaldosteronism type 1 identifies a conserved glycine that is involved in the gating of the epithelial sodium channel. *EMBO J* (1997) 16:899–907. doi:10.1093/emboj/16.5.899

42. Théâtre E, Bours V, Oury C. A P2X ion channel-triggered NF-kappaB pathway enhances TNF-alpha-induced IL-8 expression in airway epithelial cells. *Am J Respir Cell Mol Biol* (2009) 41:705–13. doi:10.1165/rcmb.2008-0452OC

43. Khalil M, Babes A, Lakra R, Forsch S, Reeh PW, Wirtz S, et al. Transient receptor potential melastatin 8 ion channel in macrophages modulates colitis through a balance-shift in TNF-alpha and interleukin-10 production. *Mucosal Immunol* (2016) 9:1500–13. doi:10.1038/mi.2016.16

44. Wilson MR, Wakabayashi K, Bertok S, Oakley CM, Patel BV, O'Dea KP, et al. Inhibition of TNF receptor p55 by a domain antibody attenuates the initial phase of acid-induced lung injury in mice. *Front Immunol* (2017) 8:128. doi:10.3389/fimmu.2017.00128

45. Yang G, Hamacher J, Gorshkov B, White R, Sridhar S, Verin A, et al. The dual role of TNF in pulmonary edema. *J Cardiovasc Dis Res* (2010) 1:29–36. doi:10.4103/0975-3583.59983

46. Chen X, Pang RP, Shen KF, Zimmermann M, Xin WJ, Li YY, et al. TNF-α enhances the currents of voltage gated sodium channels in uninjured dorsal root ganglion neurons following motor nerve injury. *Exp Neurol* (2011) 227:279–86. doi:10.1016/j.expneurol.2010.11.017

47. Sprang SR, Eck MJ. The 3D structure of TNF. In: Beutler B, editor. *Tumor Necrosis Factors: The Molecules and Their Emerging Role in Medicine.* New York: Raven (1992). p. 11–32.

48. Baldwin RL, Stolowitz ML, Hood L, Wisnieski BJ. Structural changes of tumor necrosis factor alpha associated with membrane insertion and channel formation. *Proc Natl Acad Sci U S A* (1996) 93:1021–6. doi:10.1073/pnas.93.3.1021

49. Eck MJ, Sprang SR. The structure of tumor necrosis factor-alpha at 2.6 A resolution. Implications for receptor binding. *J Biol Chem* (1989) 264:17595–605.

50. Van der Goot FG, Pugin J, Hribar M, Fransen L, Dunant Y, De Baetselier P, et al. Membrane interaction of TNF is not sufficient to trigger increase in membrane conductance in mammalian cells. *FEBS Lett* (1999) 460:107–11. doi:10.1016/S0014-5793(99)01294-6

51. Schulze-Bahr E, Neu A, Friederich P, Kaupp UB, Breithardt G, Pongs O, et al. Pacemaker channel dysfunction in a patient with sinus node disease. *J Clin Invest* (2003) 111:1537–45. doi:10.1172/JCI16387

52. Kawakami H, Aiba T, Yamada T, Okayama H, Kazatani Y, Konishi K, et al. Variable phenotype expression with a frameshift mutation of the cardiac sodium channel gene *SCN5A. J Arrhythm* (2013) 29:291–5. doi:10.1016/j.joa.2013.04.005

53. Dulebo A, Ettrich R, Lucas R, Kaftan D. A computational study of the oligosaccharide binding sites in the lectin-like domain of Tumor Necrosis Factor and the TNF-derived TIP peptide. *Curr Pharm Des* (2012) 18:4236–43. doi:10.2174/138161212802430549

54. Schild L, Schneeberger E, Gautschi I, Firsov D. Identification of amino acid residues in the alpha, beta, and gamma subunits of the epithelial sodium channel (ENaC) involved in amiloride block and ion permeation. *J Gen Physiol* (1997) 109:15–26. doi:10.1085/jgp.109.1.15

55. Kellenberger S, Gautschi I, Schild L. An external site controls closing of the epithelial Na$^+$ channel ENaC. *J Physiol* (2002) 543:413–24. doi:10.1113/jphysiol.2002.022020

56. Jasti J, Furukawa H, Gonzales EB, Gouaux E. Structure of acid-sensing ion channel 1 at 1.9 A resolution and low pH. *Nature* (2007) 449:316–23. doi:10.1038/nature06163

57. Bonny O, Rossier BC. Disturbances of Na/K balance: pseudohypoaldosteronism revisited. *J Am Soc Nephrol* (2002) 13:2399–414. doi:10.1097/01.ASN.0000028641.59030.B2

58. Langloh AL, Berdiev B, Ji HL, Keyser K, Stanton BA, Benos DJ. Charged residues in the M2 region of alpha-hENaC play a role in channel conductance. *Am J Physiol Cell Physiol* (2000) 278:C277–91.

59. Wiemuth D, Ke Y, Rohlfs M, McDonald FJ. Epithelial sodium channel (ENaC) is multi-ubiquitinated at the cell surface. *Biochem J* (2007) 405:147–55. doi:10.1042/BJ20060747

60. Bobby R, Medini K, Neudecker P, Lee TV, Brimble MA, McDonald FJ, et al. Structure and dynamics of human Nedd4-1 WW3 in complex with the αENaC PY motif. *Biochim Biophys Acta* (2013) 1834:1632–41. doi:10.1016/j.bbapap.2013.04.031

61. Xiong C, Yang G, Kumar S, Aggarwal S, Leustik M, Snead C, et al. The lectin-like domain of TNF protects from listeriolysin-induced hyperpermeability in human pulmonary microvascular endothelial cells – a crucial role for protein kinase C-alpha inhibition. *Vascul Pharmacol* (2010) 52:207–13. doi:10.1016/j.vph.2009.12.010

Cytokine-Regulation of Na⁺-K⁺-Cl⁻ Cotransporter 1 and Cystic Fibrosis Transmembrane Conductance Regulator—Potential Role in Pulmonary Inflammation and Edema Formation

Sarah Weidenfeld[1,2] and Wolfgang M. Kuebler[1,2,3]*

[1] Keenan Research Centre for Biomedical Science, St. Michael's Hospital, Toronto, ON, Canada, [2] Institute of Physiology, Charité-Universitätsmedizin Berlin, Berlin, Germany, [3] Department of Surgery and Physiology, University of Toronto, Toronto, ON, Canada

*Correspondence:
Wolfgang M. Kuebler
wolfgang.kuebler@charite.de

Pulmonary edema, a major complication of lung injury and inflammation, is defined as accumulation of extravascular fluid in the lungs leading to impaired diffusion of respiratory gases. Lung fluid balance across the alveolar epithelial barrier protects the distal airspace from excess fluid accumulation and is mainly regulated by active sodium transport and Cl^- absorption. Increased hydrostatic pressure as seen in cardiogenic edema or increased vascular permeability as present in inflammatory lung diseases such as the acute respiratory distress syndrome (ARDS) causes a reversal of transepithelial fluid transport resulting in the formation of pulmonary edema. The basolateral expressed Na^+-K^+-$2Cl^-$ cotransporter 1 (NKCC1) and the apical Cl^- channel cystic fibrosis transmembrane conductance regulator (CFTR) are considered to be critically involved in the pathogenesis of pulmonary edema and have also been implicated in the inflammatory response in ARDS. Expression and function of both NKCC1 and CFTR can be modulated by released cytokines; however, the relevance of this modulation in the context of ARDS and pulmonary edema is so far unclear. Here, we review the existing literature on the regulation of NKCC1 and CFTR by cytokines, and—based on the known involvement of NKCC1 and CFTR in lung edema and inflammation—speculate on the role of cytokine-dependent NKCC1/CFTR regulation for the pathogenesis and potential treatment of pulmonary inflammation and edema formation.

Keywords: lung inflammation, pulmonary edema, CFTR, NKCC1, cytokines

INTRODUCTION

Pulmonary edema, defined as excessive fluid accumulation in the interstitial and air spaces of the lungs, is a life-threatening condition leading to impaired gas exchange and respiratory failure. Depending on the underlying cause, pulmonary edema is distinguished into two types; hydrostatic and permeability-type edema. The most common form of hydrostatic edema is cardiogenic edema which occurs as major complication of left-sided heart failure and is characterized by increased transcapillary hydrostatic pressure gradients between pulmonary vasculature and interstitial space resulting in interstitial lung edema and flooding of the alveoli with protein-poor fluid. Permeability-type lung edema, also referred to as non-cardiogenic pulmonary edema, is defined by an exudation of protein-rich fluid into the alveoli and develops characteristically in the process of inflammatory lung diseases such as the acute respiratory distress syndrome (ARDS) (1, 2). Two processes are critical for the accumulation of protein-rich fluid in the alveolar space: (1) the disruption of endothelial and epithelial barriers leading to increased vascular permeability and (2) the dysregulated expression or impaired function of ion channels in alveolar epithelial cells limiting fluid removal from the distal airspaces. As such, repair of the epithelial cell barrier and effective clearance of fluid from air spaces are essential prerequisites for resolution of pulmonary edema.

Several transporters (specified in the Section "Fluid Transport of Alveolar Epithelium"), expressed on alveolar type I (ATI) and type II (ATII) cells, are involved in active transport of salt and water through the epithelial barrier leading to alveolar fluid clearance (AFC). AFC is impaired in more than 80% of ARDS patients and associated with increased morbidity and mortality (3). Therefore, manipulation of alveolar fluid transport could represent a suitable therapeutically target. However, molecular mechanism resulting in impaired epithelial fluid transport remains unclear. Inflammatory responses involving upregulation of pro-inflammatory cytokines including interleukin-1β (IL-1β), IL-8, tumor necrosis factor-α (TNF-α), and transforming growth factor-β (TGF-β) and their accumulation in BALF and edema fluid are a critical hallmark of ARDS (4–7). In addition to their role in immune responses, these pro-inflammatory mediators are considered to inhibit alveolar fluid transport by regulation of sodium and chloride transporter (7). However, present understandings of mechanisms by which cytokines regulate ion transport are far from complete, with previous work having focused on the regulation of Na^+ transport via epithelial Na^+ channel (ENaC) and the Na^+/K^+-ATPase. In this review, we propose that cytokine-dependent regulation of Na^+-K^+-$2Cl^-$ cotransporter 1 (NKCC1) and Cl^- channel cystic fibrosis transmembrane conductance regulator (CFTR) may play a critical role in lung edema formation and pulmonary inflammation. To this end, we first outline the general principles of alveolar fluid transport and the role of inflammatory cytokines in lung edema formation, then focus specifically on the role of NKCC1 and CFTR in pulmonary edema and inflammation, and their regulation by cytokines, and finally conclude by proposing a critical role for cytokine-dependent regulation of NKCC1 and CFTR as a novel concept in the pathogenesis of pulmonary edema.

REGULATION OF ACTIVE SALT AND WATER TRANSPORT AND EDEMA FORMATION

Fluid Transport of Alveolar Epithelium

The alveolar epithelium forms a tight barrier between vasculature and air-filled compartment to control movement of protein and fluid under physiological conditions. It comprises ATI cells, which are responsible for gas exchange across the alveolo-capillary barrier, and ATII cells that fulfill several functions, most notably production and release of surfactant (8).

In the intact lung, AFC constantly moves fluid from the alveolar space across the epithelial barrier into the interstitial space. Na^+ is actively absorbed on the apical side of alveolar epithelial cells, which is mediated by several sodium channels (**Figure 1**), most notably the amiloride-sensitive ENaC (9), the sodium glucose transporter (SGLT) (10, 11) and the sodium-coupled neutral amino acid transporter (SNAT) (12–14). On the basolateral surface, Na^+ extrusion to the interstitial space is driven through the Na^+-K^+-ATPase (8) and the Na^+/H^+ antiporter (15). For electroneutrality and osmotic balance, Cl^- and water follow the electrochemical gradient partly paracellularly and partly through aquaporins (specifically aquaporin 5) (16) and chloride channels, predominantly CFTR (17). Although it was thought that channels and transporter are primarily expressed in ATII cells, recent data demonstrated that ATI cells contain ENaC, CFTR, and the Na^+-K^+-ATPase suggesting a role for ATI cells in alveolar fluid transport (9, 18).

In response to lung injury and inflammation, the epithelial barrier becomes disrupted leading to increased influx of protein-rich fluid and formation of pulmonary edema (**Figure 1**). Furthermore, the physiological protection provided by active salt and water transport is attenuated, resulting in impaired AFC in patients with both cardiogenic (19) and permeability-type (3) lung edema. On top of that, AFC may reverse into active alveolar fluid secretion (AFS), thus promoting rather than resolving edema formation. Recently, work from our group identified basolateral NKCC1 and apical-expressed CFTR as critical for the reversal of an absorptive into a secretory alveolar epithelium by driving Cl^- secretion (20). Specifically, we could show that an acute increase in left atrial pressure decreases amiloride-sensitive Na^+ uptake across the alveolar epithelium and concomitantly stimulates Na^+ and Cl^- uptake via basolateral NKCC1 and Cl^- secretion into the alveolar space via apical CFTR, thus effectively reversing Na^+-driven AFC into Cl^- driven AFS. Importantly, inhibition of CFTR and NKCC1 improved AFC and attenuated edema formation. In line with this concept, previous studies have reported similar beneficial effects of NKCC inhibition on edema formation in different organs in that bumetanide reduced cerebral edema formation in response to ischemia (21) and furosemide improved fluid balance and reduced pulmonary edema in ARDS patients (22). Although these effects have traditionally been attributed to diuretic effects of non-specific NKCC inhibitors, improvement of respiratory function by furosemide in lung edema precedes the onset of diuresis (23, 24), suggesting alternative mechanisms such as NKCC/CFTR-mediated AFS in edema formation.

Pro-Inflammatory Cytokines in Lung Edema Formation

During early stages of injury, the lung is the site of acute inflammatory processes with excessive transepithelial neutrophil migration and continuous release and activation of pro-inflammatory mediators. Pro-inflammatory cytokines, produced by circulating

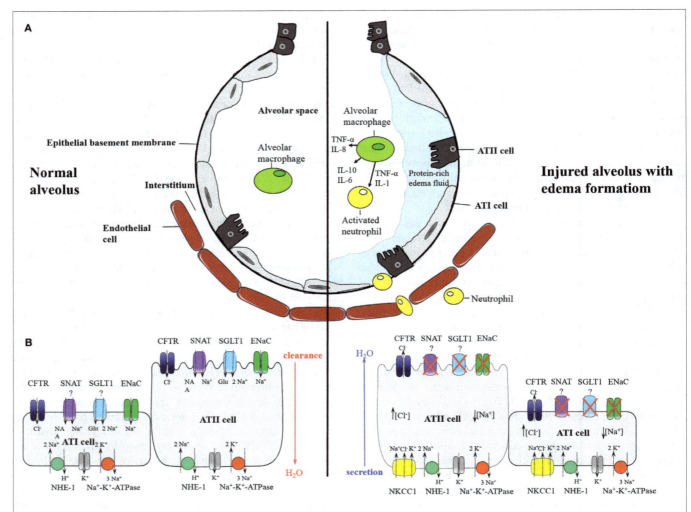

FIGURE 1 | (A) Schematic model of the normal alveolus (left) and the injured alveolus (right) with edema formation in inflammatory lung disease. In pulmonary inflammation, the epithelial and endothelial barrier become disrupted leading to influx of protein-rich edema fluid and migration of neutrophils from the vasculature into the alveolar space. In the air space, alveolar macrophages secrete proinflammatory cytokines that stimulate chemotaxis and activate neutrophils which in turn produce and release further cytokines. (B) Distribution of epithelial ion transporter and proposed mechanism of alveolar fluid clearance (AFC) (left) and secretion (right). In alveolar type II and presumably also type I cells, AFC is mediated through apical Na⁺ entry by sodium channels like epithelial Na⁺ channel (ENac), sodium-coupled amino acid transporter (SNATs), and sodium glucose transporter (SGLT). Basolateral extrusion is driven by Na⁺-K⁺-ATPase and sodium hydrogen exchanger (NHE). Water and Cl⁻ follow for electroneutrality. In pulmonary edema, ENaC and probably other sodium transporter are inhibited generating a gradient for Na⁺ influx via basolateral NKCC1. Cl⁻ enters in cotransport with Na⁺, and exits along an electrochemical gradient on the apical side through CFTR, resulting in Cl⁻-driven fluid secretion and formation of lung edema.

monocytes, alveolar macrophages, and neutrophils, promote recruitment and activation of additional immune cells and inflammatory molecules. A variety of cytokines and growth factors can be detected in BALF and edema fluid of ARDS patients including TNF-α, IL-1β, IL-8, and TGF-β1 (5, 6, 25, 26). These cytokines have been implicated to play a crucial role in the pathophysiology of pulmonary edema formation.

A critical involvement of TNF-α in edema formation has been documented in a series of experimental and clinical studies, which have previously been reviewed in detail (27). In brief, TNF-α reduces the expression of ENaC mRNA in alveolar epithelial cells and thereby decreases amiloride-sensitive sodium uptake (28). However, there is also evidence for a protective effect of TNF-α in pulmonary edema formation, as demonstrated by Borjesson and colleagues who identified in a rat model of intestinal ischemia-reperfusion, a TNF-α-dependent stimulation of AFC in the early phase of injury (29). Similarly, a TNF-dependent and amiloride-sensitive increase in alveolar fluid resorption was detected in a rat model of *Pseudomonas aeruginosa* pneumonia (30).

Inhibition of growth factor TGF-β1 protects wild-type mice from pulmonary edema in a bleomycin-induced lung injury model (31). An increased TGF-β1 activity in distal airways has been shown to promote edema by reducing alveolar epithelial sodium uptake and AFC. This effect of TGF-β1 is considered to be dependent on activation of the MAPK-ERK1/2 pathway resulting in decreased expression of ENaC mRNA (32). A similar effect has been described for IL-1β, which was shown to reduce ENaC expression through p38–MAPK-dependent inhibition of ENaC promoter activity (33). In contrast, an *in vitro* study reported an IL-1β-mediated increase in epithelial repair induced by edema fluid (34).

The chemotactic mediator IL-8 promotes edema formation by blocking AFC (35). Accordingly, inhibition of IL-8 significantly diminishes edema caused by smoke inhalation, acid aspiration, or ischemia-reperfusion injury (36–38).

Overall, there is evidence that cytokines are important regulators of active ion transport and AFC. However, exact regulation of ion channels by inflammatory cytokines may be a complex phenomenon with functional effects depending on temporal and spatial profiles, interdependence between various cytokines, and the presence (*in vivo* situation) or absence (*in vitro* assays) of immune cells. Detailed dissection of these scenarios poses a considerable challenge in terms of both resources and appropriate assays, yet would provide an invaluable platform for a better understanding of the complex crosstalk between inflammation and ion channel activity in a wide range of pulmonary and systemic inflammatory diseases.

CFTR AND NKCC1 IN INFLAMMATORY LUNG DISEASE AND PULMONARY EDEMA

Na⁺-K⁺-Cl⁻ Cotransporter

The Na-K-Cl cotransporter (NKCC) mediates active electroneutral uptake of one Na^+ and K^+ with 2 Cl^- molecules along an inwardly directed electrochemical gradient for Na^+ and Cl^-. Of the two known isoforms, NKCC1 and NKCC2, NKCC1 is found on the basolateral side on epithelial and endothelial cells in several organs, including the alveolar epithelium. In contrast, apically expressed NKCC2 is only present in the kidney epithelium (39). Both isoforms are sensitive to loop diuretics like bumetanide and furosemide, which inhibit ion translocation (40).

To maintain cell shape and integrity during active salt and water secretion, activation of NKCC1 is strictly regulated. Activity of NKCC1 can be induced through hyperosmotic stress (41), low intracellular Na^+ level, increase in intracellular cAMP, or changes in cell shape, and depends on direct phosphorylation by Ste20-related proline/alanine-rich kinase (SPAK) and oxidative stress responsive kinases (OSR1) (42).

Cystic Fibrosis Transmembrane Conductance Regulator (CFTR)

CFTR, which has been identified as the mutated gene in cystic fibrosis patients (43), is considered an atypical ATP-binding cassette (ABC) transporter which is activated by phosphorylation and ATP hydrolysis (44). It permits bidirectional transport of Cl^- anion depending on the electrochemical gradient. CFTR is expressed on apical membranes of epithelial cells in distal airways and alveolar epithelium, where it mediates Cl^- transport to maintain alveolar fluid homeostasis (45). CFTR expression and activation depends on intracellular cAMP or cGMP, which activate PKA and cGKII (46) leading to upregulation of CFTR expression and phosphorylation (47, 48).

Expression of NKCC1 and CFTR in Inflammatory Lung Diseases

NKCC1 and CFTR are both involved in a variety of biological processes ranging from ion transport to regulation of macrophage activation and modulation of cytokine production (49–52). Of relevance for this review, NKCC1 and CFTR have also been implicated in pulmonary inflammatory processes.

NKCC1 is upregulated in response to Gram-negative bacterial toxins like lipopolysaccharide (LPS) in the lung and kidney (53). Whether this enhanced NKCC1 gene expression is, however, mediated directly by LPS binding to its receptor inducing intracellular signaling or via released inflammatory cytokines like TNF-α after LPS stimulation remains to be elucidated.

Nguyen and colleagues (54) proposed a role for NKCC1 in inflammatory processes in response to *Klebsiella pneumoniae* infection. Mice lacking NKCC1 were protected from bacteremia and lethal sepsis after infection and showed decreased vascular permeability. The number of migrated neutrophils in the air space was increased leading to a reduced number of *K. pneumoniae* in the lung of NKCC1-deficient mice. A potential mechanism that may explain the involvement of NKCC1 in edema formation and neutrophil transmigration was proposed by Matthay and Su (55), who speculated that expression of NKCC1 in endothelial and epithelial cells might be upregulated by inflammatory molecules in response to bacterial infections; however, this hypothesis still awaits functional validation, and regulatory pathways involved remain to be clarified. Along similar lines, a study by Andrade and colleagues reported upregulated NKCC1 expression along with downregulated ENaC in response to *Leptospirosis* infection, a model of sepsis leading to edema formation and ARDS (56). The authors proposed a regulation of transporter expression via JNK and NF-κB pathways during leptospirosis-induced pulmonary edema, yet exact signaling cascades remain unclear.

CFTR is considered an important modulator of inflammatory responses in the lung. Absence of a functional CFTR leads to chronic pulmonary inflammation, as seen in cystic fibrosis patients (57). In a murine model of cerebral and uterine *Chlamydia trachomatis* infection, CFTR mRNA and protein were shown to be upregulated causing increased tissue fluid accumulation and edema formation (58). The authors hypothesized that increased CFTR expression and abnormal fluid accumulation upon *C. trachomatis* infection may depend on increased cytokine release. In pulmonary epithelial cells, CFTR functions as receptor for *P. aeruginosa* internalization leading to CFTR translocation into lipid rafts (59) and NF-κB mediated expression of IL-1β (60). However, the role of CFTR in lung injury and edema formation may be more complex. In a CF mouse model using CFTR-deficient animals, Bruscia and colleagues (61) demonstrated an enhanced pulmonary inflammatory response with elevated cytokine levels in response to chronic LPS exposure. Similarly, Su and coworkers (51) reported aggravated inflammatory cytokine release and edema formation following LPS challenge in mice bearing the human functional CFTR mutation, F508del-CF, or in mice treated with a pharmacological CFTR inhibitor. Importantly, subsequent chimeric experiments in wild-type mice reconstituted with F508del neutrophils or bone marrow, respectively, revealed that pro-inflammatory, pro-edematous effect of functional CF inhibition was attributable to the lack of CFTR on immune cells, specifically neutrophils, rather than epithelial or other parenchymal cells (51). Hence, CFTR may promote both pro-and anti-edematous effects in inflammatory lung disease depending on its site of expression.

Taken together, functional concepts involving NKCC1 and CFTR in fluid transport and edema formation (**Figure 1A**) in combination with data demonstrating differential regulation of NKCC1 and CFTR in lung injury that coincides with edema formation point toward a critical role for CFTR and NKCC1 in infection-induced pulmonary edema. While molecular mechanisms underlying the regulation of NKCC1 and CFTR by infectious pathogens remain to be elucidated, it is tempting to speculate on a critical role for inflammatory cytokines as putative mediators in the regulation of these channels. As discussed in the following section, multifunctional cytokines like TNF-α, IL-1β, and IL-8 are particularly attractive candidates as key regulators of NKCC1 and CFTR.

Regulation of NKCC1 and CFTR by Cytokines

Various signaling pathways have been suggested to play a role in NKCC1 activation and expression including WNK, MAP kinase/ERK, p38, and JNK pathways (62–64). Notably, these pathways are also known to be stimulated by cytokines and growth factors like TNF-α and TGF-β, which activate intracellular p38 and JNK pathways (65, 66). In pulmonary inflammation, cytokines may bind to receptors on alveolar epithelial cells and induce intracellular pathways resulting in activation of NKCC1, yet, direct evidence for such an effect in the intact, inflamed lung is presently outstanding. Consistent with this notion, however, NKCC1 mRNA and protein levels were found to be selectively upregulated by TNF-α and IL-1β in endothelial and epithelial cells (53, 67). Conversely, inhibition of TNF-α and IL-1β by hypertonicity was found to be beneficial in cerebral edema, and the functional role of TNF-α and IL-1β in the regulation of NKCC1 expression was validated *in vitro*, leading the authors to propose that TNF-α and IL-1β may directly upregulate NKCC1 expression via JNK- and p38-dependent pathways (67).

For CFTR, the interplay between inflammatory cytokines and channel expression/activity is even more complex. As such, IL-8 has been shown to indirectly regulate activity and biosynthesis of CFTR through inhibition of the β_2-adrenergic receptor (AR) pathway (35) and subsequent phosphorylation of CFTR via cAMP-mediated PKA activation, which is considered to be essential for AFC (68). Downregulation of $\beta2$-AR in ATII cells by IL-8 blocked fluid transport across the alveolar epithelium via inhibition of CFTR phosphorylation and expression (35). Likewise, TGF-β has been proposed to diminish cAMP-driven chloride transport in colonic epithelia via inhibition of CFTR mRNA expression and protein synthesis (69). In 2007, Lee and colleagues (7) investigated the effect of edema fluid on transporter

expression in alveolar epithelial cells and showed that cytokine-containing edema fluid decreases expression and activation of CFTR leading to decreased AFC. However, incubation with individual cytokines alone did not alter CFTR expression, suggesting a complex regulatory mechanism.

Other studies, reported an upregulation of CFTR mRNA and protein by IL-1β (70–72). The NF-κB-pathway has been identified to be involved in the IL-1β-dependent increase in CFTR expression (70). In agreement with this effect, CTFR-dependent AFS has been shown to be stimulated by IL-1β and TNF-α in airway submucosal glands via cAMP-dependent activation of PKA (73).

Contradictions in CFTR regulatory processes and its involvement in fluid transport and edema formation may result from differences in expressed transport system in various cell types, and such heterogeneity may also be present in the pulmonary epithelium. Recently, it has been proposed that the distal airways might be comprised of secreting areas, located in the contra-luminal regions of the pleats, and absorbing areas in the folds (74). Secretion and absorption of fluid is considered to occur simultaneously and independently maintaining the required level of airway surface liquid. Regulation of transporter expression may also vary in these areas. NKCC1 has been found to be abundantly expressed in the pleats of distal airways and less in the folds (75). No change in CFTR expression was detected in different areas (75), which is not surprising assuming CFTR is involved in fluid secretion and absorption. In lung injury, impaired alveolar fluid transport might be triggered by cytokine-mediated differential expression of ion channels including NKCC1 and CFTR that may putatively result in an increased expression and/or activation of NKCC1 and CFTR in secretory epithelia and an inhibition of channels in absorptive areas (**Figure 2**). While largely speculative at this stage, this hypothetical concept of a spatially (and potentially temporally) differential regulation of ion channels involved in fluid absorption and secretion by inflammatory cytokines highlights the need for expanded research in this fascinating field. An in-depth understanding of changes in ion and fluid flux and their regulation may provide for optimized targets for edema resolution in acute inflammatory lung disease.

CONCLUSION

Acute respiratory distress syndrome with edema formation is a serious complication in critically ill patients. Resolution of edema needs strategies to restore epithelial barrier function and improve AFC. Formation of pulmonary edema in inflammatory lung diseases is caused by the loss of endothelial and epithelial barrier and impaired fluid and ion transport across the alveolar epithelium. Pro-inflammatory cytokines like TNF-α, TGF-$\beta1$, and IL-1β, which are released and activated in the early phase of lung inflammation, may regulate expression and activity of ion channels involved in fluid transport including NKCC1 and CFTR. Regulation of NKCC1 and CFTR is, however, complex, with discrepant results potentially depending on time profile, cell type, and co-stimulation by different cytokines resulting in a distinct multi-dimensional response that favors AFS while impairing AFC. Manipulation of expression and activity of NKCC1 and

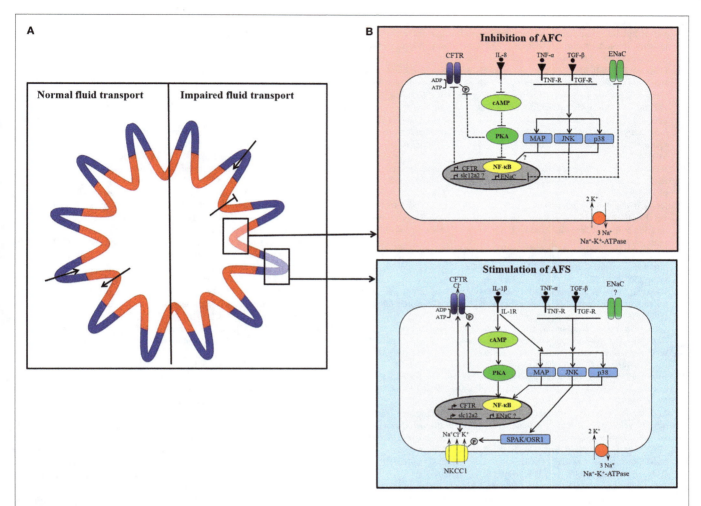

FIGURE 2 | (A) Proposed model of organization of small airways. In lung epithelium, independent groups of cells simultaneously secrete and absorb to maintain fluid homeostasis. Under normal conditions, cells located in the pleats secrete fluid (blue) and cells located around the folds concurrently absorb secreted fluid (red). In lung injury, fluid transport in absorptive areas may be blocked while fluid secretion stays intact or increases. **(B)** Simplified, hypothetical concept of differential cytokine-dependent regulation of ion transporter in absorptive (red) and secretory (blue) areas in inflammatory lung disease. In apsorptive areas, AFC is impaired presumably through cytokine-mediated inhibition of CFTR and epithelial Na+ channel (ENaC). Proinflammatory cytokines [tumor necrosis factor-α (TNF-α), transforming growth factor-β (TGF-β), interleukin1β (IL-1β)] bind to their receptor inducing intracellular signaling cascades of MAP-kinases, JNK, p38, which prevent expression of ENaC. IL-8 blocks CFTR expression and activation by inhibition of cAMP/PKA pathway. In secretory areas, fluid secretion is stimulated by cytokines. Receptor binding of IL-1β, TNF-α, and TGF-β induces intracellular signaling pathways leading to activation and expression of CFTR and NKCC1.

CFTR might serve as therapeutic target in inflammatory lung diseases with edema formation.

AUTHOR CONTRIBUTIONS

Both authors, SW and WK, meet the following four criteria of authorship: 1. Substantial contributions to the conception or design of the work. 2. Drafting the work and revising it critically for important intellectual content. 3. Final approval of the version to be published; 4. Agreement to be accountable for all aspects of the work in ensuring that questions related to the accuracy or integrity of any part of the work are appropriately investigated and resolved.

REFERENCES

1. Ware LB, Matthay MA. Acute pulmonary edema. *N Engl J Med* (2005) 353:2788–96. doi:10.1056/NEJMcp052699
2. Murray JF. Pulmonary edema: pathophysiology and diagnosis. *Int J Tuberc Lung Dis* (2011) 15:155–60, i.
3. Ware LB, Matthay MA. Alveolar fluid clearance is impaired in the majority of patients with acute lung injury and the acute respiratory distress syndrome. *Am J Respir Crit Care Med* (2001) 163:1376–83. doi:10.1164/ajrccm.163.6.2004035
4. Ware LB, Matthay MA. The acute respiratory distress syndrome. *N Engl J Med* (2000) 342:1334–49. doi:10.1056/NEJM200005043421806

5. Pugin J, Verghese G, Widmer MC, Matthay MA. The alveolar space is the site of intense inflammatory and profibrotic reactions in the early phase of acute respiratory distress syndrome. *Crit Care Med* (1999) 27:304–12. doi:10.1097/00003246-199902000-00036

6. Olman MA, White KE, Ware LB, Simmons WL, Benveniste EN, Zhu S, et al. Pulmonary edema fluid from patients with early lung injury stimulates fibroblast proliferation through IL-1 induced IL-6 expression. *J Immunol* (2004) 172:2668–77. doi:10.4049/jimmunol.172.4.2668

7. Lee JW, Fang X, Dolganov G, Fremont RD, Bastarache JA, Ware LB, et al. Acute lung injury edema fluid decreases net fluid transport across human alveolar epithelial type II cells. *J Biol Chem* (2007) 282:24109–19. doi:10.1074/jbc.M700821200

8. Matthay MA, Folkesson HG, Clerici C. Lung epithelial fluid transport and the resolution of pulmonary edema. *Physiol Rev* (2002) 82:569–600. doi:10.1152/physrev.00003.2002

9. Johnson MD, Bao H-F, Helms MN, Chen X-J, Tigue Z, Jain L, et al. Functional ion channels in pulmonary alveolar type I cells support a role for type I cells in lung ion transport. *Proc Natl Acad Sci U S A* (2006) 103:4964–9. doi:10.1073/pnas.0600855103

10. de Prost N, Saumon G. Glucose transport in the lung and its role in liquid movement. *Respir Physiol Neurobiol* (2007) 159:331–7. doi:10.1016/j.resp.2007.02.014

11. Basset G, Crone C, Saumon G. Fluid absorption by rat lung in situ: pathways for sodium entry in the luminal membrane of alveolar epithelium. *J Physiol* (1987) 384:325–45. doi:10.1113/jphysiol.1987.sp016457

12. Clerici C, Soler P, Saumon G. Sodium-dependent phosphate and alanine transports but sodium-independent hexose transport in type II alveolar epithelial cells in primary culture. *Biochim Biophys Acta* (1991) 1063:27–35. doi:10.1016/0005-2736(91)90349-D

13. Brown SE, Kim KJ, Goodman BE, Wells JR, Crandall ED. Sodium-amino acid cotransport by type II alveolar epithelial cells. *J Appl Physiol* (1985) 59:1616–22.

14. Michaut P, Planes C, Escoubet B, Clement A, Amiel C, Clerici C. Rat lung alveolar type II cell line maintains sodium transport characteristics of primary culture. *J Cell Physiol* (1996) 169:78–86. doi:10.1002/(SICI)1097-4652(199610)169:1<78:AID-JCP8>3.0.CO;2-B

15. Nord EP, Brown SE, Crandall ED. Characterization of Na$^+$-H$^+$ antiport in type II alveolar epithelial cells. *Am J Physiol* (1987) 252:C490–8.

16. Dobbs LG, Gonzalez R, Matthay MA, Carter EP, Allen L, Verkman AS. Highly water-permeable type I alveolar epithelial cells confer high water permeability between the airspace and vasculature in rat lung. *Proc Natl Acad Sci U S A* (1998) 95:2991–6. doi:10.1073/pnas.95.6.2991

17. Sartori C, Matthay MA. Alveolar epithelial fluid transport in acute lung injury: new insights. *Eur Respir J* (2002) 20:1299–313. doi:10.1183/09031936.02.00401602

18. Ridge KM, Olivera WG, Saldias F, Azzam Z, Horowitz S, Rutschman DH, et al. Alveolar type 1 cells express the alpha2 Na,K-ATPase, which contributes to lung liquid clearance. *Circ Res* (2003) 92:453–60. doi:10.1161/01.RES.0000059414.10360.F2

19. Verghese GM, Ware LB, Matthay BA, Matthay MA. Alveolar epithelial fluid transport and the resolution of clinically severe hydrostatic pulmonary edema. *J Appl Physiol* (1999) 87:1301–12.

20. Solymosi EA, Kaestle-Gembardt SM, Vadász I, Wang L, Neye N, Chupin CJA, et al. Chloride transport-driven alveolar fluid secretion is a major contributor to cardiogenic lung edema. *Proc Natl Acad Sci U S A* (2013) 110:E2308–16. doi:10.1073/pnas.1216382110

21. O'Donnell ME, Tran L, Lam TI, Liu XB, Anderson SE. Bumetanide inhibition of the blood-brain barrier Na-K-Cl cotransporter reduces edema formation in the rat middle cerebral artery occlusion model of stroke. *J Cereb Blood Flow Metab* (2004) 24:1046–56. doi:10.1097/01.WCB.0000130867.32663.90

22. National Heart, Lung, and Blood Institute Acute Respiratory Distress Syndrome (ARDS) Clinical Trials Network, Wiedemann HP, Clinic C, Wheeler AP, Bernard GR, University V, et al. Comparison of two fluid-management strategies in acute lung injury. *N Engl J Med* (2006) 354:2564–75. doi:10.1056/NEJMoa062200

23. Biddle TL, Yu PN. Effect of furosemide on hemodynamics and lung water in acute pulmonary edema secondary to myocardial infarction. *Am J Cardiol* (1979) 43:86–90. doi:10.1016/0002-9149(79)90049-3

24. Ali J, Chernicki W, Wood LD. Effect of furosemide in canine low-pressure pulmonary edema. *J Clin Invest* (1979) 64:1494–504. doi:10.1172/JCI109608

25. Miller EJ, Cohen AB, Matthay MA. Increased interleukin-8 concentrations in the pulmonary edema fluid of patients with acute respiratory distress syndrome from sepsis. *Crit Care Med* (1996) 24:1448–54. doi:10.1097/00003246-199609000-00004

26. Kubo K, Hanaoka M, Hayano T, Miyahara T, Hachiya T, Hayasaka M, et al. Inflammatory cytokines in BAL fluid and pulmonary hemodynamics in high-altitude pulmonary edema. *Respir Physiol* (1998) 111:301–10. doi:10.1016/S0034-5687(98)00006-1

27. Yang G, Hamacher J, Gorshkov B, White R, Sridhar S, Verin A, et al. The dual role of TNF in pulmonary edema. *J Cardiovasc Dis Res* (2010) 1:29–36. doi:10.4103/0975-3583.59983

28. Dagenais A, Fréchette R, Yamagata Y, Yamagata T, Carmel J-F, Clermont M-E, et al. Downregulation of ENaC activity and expression by TNF-α in alveolar epithelial cells. *Am J Physiol Lung Cell Mol Physiol* (2004) 286:L301–11. doi:10.1152/ajplung.00326.2002

29. Börjesson A, Norlin A, Wang X, Andersson R, Folkesson HG. TNF-alpha stimulates alveolar liquid clearance during intestinal ischemia-reperfusion in rats. *Am J Physiol Lung Cell Mol Physiol* (2000) 278:L3–12.

30. Rezaiguia S, Garat C, Delclaux C, Meignan M, Fleury J, Legrand P, et al. Acute bacterial pneumonia in rats increases alveolar epithelial fluid clearance by a tumor necrosis factor-alpha–dependent mechanism. *J Clin Invest* (1997) 99:325–35. doi:10.1172/JCI119161

31. Pittet JF, Griffiths MJ, Geiser T, Kaminski N, Dalton SL, Huang X, et al. TGF-beta is a critical mediator of acute lung injury. *J Clin Invest* (2001) 107:1537–44. doi:10.1172/JCI11963

32. Frank J, Roux J, Kawakatsu H, Su G, Dagenais A, Berthiaume Y, et al. Transforming growth factor-β1 decreases expression of the epithelial sodium channel αENaC and alveolar epithelial vectorial sodium and fluid transport via an ERK1/2-dependent mechanism. *J Biol Chem* (2003) 278:43939–50. doi:10.1074/jbc.M304882200

33. Roux J, Kawakatsu H, Gartland B, Pespeni M, Sheppard D, Matthay MA, et al. Interleukin-1β decreases expression of the epithelial sodium channel α-subunit in alveolar epithelial cells via a p38 MAPK-dependent signaling pathway. *J Biol Chem* (2005) 280:18579–89. doi:10.1074/jbc.M410561200

34. Geiser T, Atabai K, Jarreau PH, Ware LB, Pugin J, Matthay MA. Pulmonary edema fluid from patients with acute lung injury augments in vitro alveolar epithelial repair by an IL-1beta-dependent mechanism. *Am J Respir Crit Care Med* (2001) 163:1384–8. doi:10.1164/ajrccm.163.6.2006131

35. Roux J, McNicholas CM, Carles M, Goolaerts A, Houseman BT, Dickinson DA, et al. IL-8 inhibits cAMP-stimulated alveolar epithelial fluid transport via a GRK2/PI3K-dependent mechanism. *FASEB J* (2013) 27:1095–106. doi:10.1096/fj.12-219295

36. De Perrot M, Sekine Y, Fischer S, Waddell TK, Mcrae K, Liu M, et al. Interleukin-8 release during early reperfusion predicts graft function in human lung transplantation. *Am J Respir Crit Care Med* (2002) 165:211–5. doi:10.1164/rccm2011151

37. Laffon M, Pittet JF, Modelska K, Matthay MA, Young DM. Interleukin-8 mediates injury from smoke inhalation to both the lung endothelial and the alveolar epithelial barriers in rabbits. *Am J Respir Crit Care Med* (1999) 160:1443–9. doi:10.1164/ajrccm.160.5.9901097

38. Modelska K, Pittet JF, Folkesson HG, Broaddus VC, Matthay MA. Acid-induced lung injury: protective effect of anti-interleukin-8 pretreatment on alveolar epithelial barrier function in rabbits. *Am J Respir Crit Care Med* (1999) 160:1450–6. doi:10.1164/ajrccm.160.5.9901096

39. Payne JA, Xu JC, Haas M, Lytle CY, Ward D, Forbush B. Primary structure, functional expression, and chromosomal localization of the bumetanide-sensitive Na-K-Cl cotransporter in human colon. *J Biol Chem* (1995) 270:17977–85. doi:10.1074/jbc.270.30.17977

40. Russell JM. Sodium-potassium-chloride cotransport. *Physiol Rev* (2000) 80:211–76.

41. Liedtke CM, Cole TS. Activation of NKCC1 by hyperosmotic stress in human tracheal epithelial cells involves PKC-delta and ERK. *Biochim Biophys Acta* (2002) 1589:77–88. doi:10.1016/S0167-4889(01)00189-6

42. Hannemann A, Flatman PW. Phosphorylation and transport in the Na-K-2Cl cotransporters, NKCC1 and NKCC2A, compared in HEK-293 cells. *PLoS One* (2011) 6:e17992. doi:10.1371/journal.pone.0017992

43. Zeitlin PL, Crawfordt I, Lut L, Woel S, Cohen ME, Donowitz M, et al. CFTR protein expression in primary and cultured epithelia (cystic fibrosis transmembrane conductance regulator/chloride channel). *Cell Biol* (1992) 89:344–7.

44. Riordan JR. Assembly of functional CFTR chloride channels. *Annu Rev Physiol* (2005) 67:701–18. doi:10.1146/annurev.physiol.67.032003.154107

45. Jiang X, Ingbar DH, O'Grady SM. Adrenergic stimulation of Na$^+$ transport across alveolar epithelial cells involves activation of apical Cl channels. *Am J Physiol* (1998) 275:C1610–20.

46. Hofmann F, Ammendola A, Schlossmann J. Rising behind NO: cGMP-dependent protein kinases. *J Cell Sci* (2000) 113:1671–6.

47. Sood R, Bear C, Auerbach W, Reyes E, Jensen T, Kartner N, et al. Regulation of CFTR expression and function during differentiation of intestinal epithelial cells. *EMBO J* (1992) 11:2487–94.

48. Frizzell RA, Hanrahan JW. Physiology of epithelial chloride and fluid secretion. *Cold Spring Harb Perspect Med* (2012) 2:a009563. doi:10.1101/cshperspect.a009563

49. Haas M, Forbush B. The Na-K-Cl cotransporter of secretory epithelia. *Annu Rev Physiol* (2000) 62:515–34. doi:10.1146/annurev.physiol.62.1.515

50. Gao Z, Su X. CFTR regulates acute inflammatory responses in macrophages. *QJM* (2015) 108:951–8. doi:10.1093/qjmed/hcv067

51. Su X, Looney MR, Su H, Lee JW, Song Y, Matthay MA. Role of CFTR expressed by neutrophils in modulating acute lung inflammation and injury in mice. *Inflamm Res* (2011) 60:619–32. doi:10.1007/s00011-011-0313-x

52. Rubin BK. CFTR is a modulator of airway inflammation. *Am J Physiol Lung Cell Mol Physiol* (2007) 292:L381–2. doi:10.1152/ajplung.00375.2006

53. Topper JN, Wasserman SM, Anderson KR, Cai J, Falb D, Gimbrone MA. Expression of the bumetanide-sensitive Na-K-Cl cotransporter BSC2 is differentially regulated by fluid mechanical and inflammatory cytokine stimuli in vascular endothelium. *J Clin Invest* (1997) 99:2941–9. doi:10.1172/JCI119489

54. Nguyen M, Pace AJ, Koller BH. Mice lacking NKCC1 are protected from development of bacteremia and hypothermic sepsis secondary to bacterial pneumonia. *J Exp Med* (2007) 204:1383–93. doi:10.1084/jem.20061205

55. Matthay MA, Su X. Pulmonary barriers to pneumonia and sepsis. *Nat Med* (2007) 13:780–1. doi:10.1038/nm0707-780

56. Andrade L, Rodrigues AC Jr, Sanches TR, Souza RB, Seguro AC. Leptospirosis leads to dysregulation of sodium transporters in the kidney and lung. *Am J Physiol Renal Physiol* (2007) 292:F586–92. doi:10.1152/ajprenal.00102.2006

57. Terheggen-Lagro SW, Rijkers GT, van der Ent CK. The role of airway epithelium and blood neutrophils in the inflammatory response in cystic fibrosis. *J Cyst Fibros* (2005) 4:15–23. doi:10.1016/j.jcf.2005.05.007

58. Ajonuma LC, He Q, Sheung Chan PK, Yu Ng EH, Fok KL, Yan Wong CH, et al. Involvement of cystic fibrosis transmembrane conductance regulator in infection-induced edema. *Cell Biol Int* (2008) 32:801–6. doi:10.1016/j.cellbi.2008.03.010

59. Kowalski MP, Pier GB. Localization of cystic fibrosis transmembrane conductance regulator to lipid rafts of epithelial cells is required for *Pseudomonas aeruginosa*-induced cellular activation. *J Immunol* (2004) 172:418–25. doi:10.4049/jimmunol.172.1.418

60. Reiniger N, Lee MM, Coleman FT, Ray C, Golan DE, Pier GB. Resistance to *Pseudomonas aeruginosa* chronic lung infection requires cystic fibrosis transmembrane conductance regulator-modulated interleukin-1 (IL-1) release and signaling through the IL-1 receptor. *Infect Immun* (2007) 75:1598–608. doi:10.1128/IAI.01980-06

61. Bruscia E, Zhang PX, Barone C, Scholte B, Homer RJ, Krause D, et al. Increased susceptibility of cftr$^{-/-}$ mice to LPS-induced lung remodeling. *Am J Physiol Lung Cell Mol Physiol* (2016) 310(8):L711–9. doi:10.1152/ajplung.00284.2015

62. Bachmann O, Wüchner K, Rossmann H, Leipziger J, Osikowska B, Colledge WH, et al. Expression and regulation of the Na$^+$-K$^+$-2Cl cotransporter NKCC1 in the normal and CFTR-deficient murine colon. *J Physiol* (2003) 549:525–36. doi:10.1113/jphysiol.2002.030205

63. Hoorn EJ, Nelson JH, McCormick JA, Ellison DH. The WNK kinase network regulating sodium, potassium, and blood pressure. *J Am Soc Nephrol* (2011) 22:605–14. doi:10.1681/ASN.2010080827

64. Jaggi AS, Kaur A, Bali A, Singh N. Expanding spectrum of sodium potassium chloride co-transporters in the pathophysiology of diseases. *Curr Neuropharmacol* (2015) 13:369–88. doi:10.2174/1570159X13666150205130359

65. Clark AR, Dean JL, Saklatvala J. The p38 MAPK pathway mediates both antiinflammatory and proinflammatory processes: comment on the article by Damjanov and the editorial by Genovese. *Arthritis Rheum* (2009) 60:3513–4. doi:10.1002/art.24919

66. Johnson GL, Lapadat R, Johnson GL, Lapadat R, Lapadat R. Mitogen-activated protein kinase pathways mediated by ERK, JNK, and p38 protein kinases. *Science* (2002) 298:1911–2. doi:10.1126/science.1072682

67. Huang LQ, Zhu GF, Deng YY, Jiang WQ, Fang M, Chen CB, et al. Hypertonic saline alleviates cerebral edema by inhibiting microglia-derived TNF-α and IL-1β-induced Na-K-Cl cotransporter up-regulation. *J Neuroinflammation* (2014) 11:102. doi:10.1186/1742-2094-11-102

68. O'Grady SM, Lee SY. Chloride and potassium channel function in alveolar epithelial cells. *Am J Physiol Lung Cell Mol Physiol* (2003) 284:L689–700. doi:10.1152/ajplung.00256.2002

69. Howe KL, Wang A, Hunter MM, Stanton BA, McKay DM. TGF-beta down-regulation of the CFTR: a means to limit epithelial chloride secretion. *Exp Cell Res* (2004) 298:473–84. doi:10.1016/j.yexcr.2004.04.026

70. Brouillard F, Bouthier M, Leclerc T, Clement A, Baudouin-Legros M, Edelman A. NF-kB mediates up-regulation of CFTR gene expression in Calu-3 cells by interleukin-1beta. *J Biol Chem* (2001) 276:9486–91. doi:10.1074/jbc.M006636200

71. Cafferata EG, González-Guerrico AM, Giordano L, Pivetta OH, Santa-Coloma TA. Interleukin-1 beta regulates CFTR expression in human intestinal T84 cells. *Biochim Biophys Acta* (2000) 1500:241–8. doi:10.1016/S0925-4439(99)00105-2

72. Cafferata EG, Guerrico AM, Pivetta OH, Santa-Coloma TA. NF-kappaB activation is involved in regulation of cystic fibrosis transmembrane conductance regulator (CFTR) by interleukin-1beta. *J Biol Chem* (2001) 276:15441–4. doi:10.1074/jbc.M010061200

73. Baniak N, Luan X, Grunow A, Machen TE, Ianowski JP. The cytokines interleukin-1β and tumor necrosis factor-α stimulate CFTR-mediated fluid secretion by swine airway submucosal glands. *Am J Physiol Lung Cell Mol Physiol* (2012) 303:L327–33. doi:10.1152/ajplung.00058.2012

74. Shamsuddin AKM, Quinton PM. Surface fluid absorption and secretion in small airways. *J Physiol* (2012) 5901515:3561–74. doi:10.1113/jphysiol.2012.230714

75. Flores-Delgado G, Lytle C, Quinton PM. Site of fluid secretion in small airways. *Am J Respir Cell Mol Biol* (2016) 54:312–8. doi:10.1165/rcmb.2015-0238RC

6

Alveolar Fluid Clearance in Pathologically Relevant Conditions: *In Vitro* and *In Vivo* Models of Acute Respiratory Distress Syndrome

Laura A. Huppert[1] and Michael A. Matthay[2]*

[1] *Department of Medicine, University of California, San Francisco, CA, USA,* [2] *Departments of Medicine and Anesthesia, UCSF School of Medicine, Cardiovascular Research Institute, San Francisco, CA, USA*

*Correspondence:
Michael A. Matthay
michael.matthay@ucsf.edu

Critically ill patients with respiratory failure from acute respiratory distress syndrome (ARDS) have reduced ability to clear alveolar edema fluid. This reduction in alveolar fluid clearance (AFC) contributes to the morbidity and mortality in ARDS. Thus, it is important to understand why AFC is reduced in ARDS in order to design targeted therapies. In this review, we highlight experiments that have advanced our understanding of ARDS pathogenesis, with particular reference to the alveolar epithelium. First, we review how vectorial ion transport drives the clearance of alveolar edema fluid in the uninjured lung. Next, we describe how alveolar edema fluid is less effectively cleared in lungs affected by ARDS and describe selected *in vitro* and *in vivo* experiments that have elucidated some of the molecular mechanisms responsible for the reduced AFC. Finally, we describe one potential therapy that targets this pathway: bone marrow-derived mesenchymal stem (stromal) cells (MSCs). Based on preclinical studies, MSCs enhance AFC and promote the resolution of pulmonary edema and thus may offer a promising cell-based therapy for ARDS.

Keywords: acute respiratory distress syndrome, alveolar fluid clearance, mesenchymal stem (stromal) cells, pulmonary edema, vectorial ion transport

INTRODUCTION

Pulmonary edema is the abnormal accumulation of fluid in the interstitium and air spaces of the lungs, which leads to impaired gas exchange and respiratory failure. Pulmonary edema can develop from increased pulmonary vascular pressure from left heart failure (cardiogenic pulmonary edema) (1) or from lung parenchymal damage from increased endothelial and epithelial permeability (non-cardiogenic pulmonary edema) (2). In both cases, the mechanism for the resolution of alveolar edema is the same: active ion transport across the alveolar epithelium creates an osmotic gradient that drives alveolar fluid clearance (AFC) (3). In the presence of acute lung endothelial and epithelial injury, there is complexity in describing the forces responsible for lung fluid clearance, meaning removal of edema from the lung itself. Net AFC does depend on an intact epithelial barrier that can transport ions from the apical to the basolateral surface and create a mini-osmotic gradient for alveolar fluid absorption. If transvascular fluid flux is increased across lung endothelium from increased pressure or increased permeability, then the rate of AFC will be reduced. Also, net lung fluid clearance will be less. Lung lymphatics do remove edema fluid in either hydrostatic or increased permeability lung edema, but they cannot entirely compensate for an increase in transvascular fluid flux or impaired AFC.

Acute respiratory distress syndrome (ARDS) is a syndrome of acute respiratory failure caused by non-cardiogenic pulmonary edema. The most common cause of ARDS is bacterial or viral pneumonia (4). Sepsis due to non-pulmonary sources, trauma, aspiration, pancreatitis, transfusion reactions, and drug reactions can also lead to ARDS (4). Criteria for the diagnosis of ARDS have changed over time, but the current definition includes arterial hypoxemia with PaO_2/FiO_2 ratio less than 300 mmHg, bilateral radiographic opacities, without evidence of that is not fully explained by cardiac failure or fluid overload (5). The mortality of ARDS is approximately 25–40% (6), and treatment remains primarily supportive with lung protective ventilation and a fluid conservative strategy (7).

Because ARDS has a broad clinical phenotype, it has been challenging to translate cell and animal studies to pharmacologic therapies that reduce human morbidity and mortality. Nonetheless, *in vitro* and *in vivo* studies have produced important insights about the pathogenesis of this condition, paving the way for targeted therapeutics. This review will focus on: (1) mechanisms that mediate the clearance of pulmonary edema in the uninjured lung, (2) why AFC is reduced in ARDS, resulting in the accumulation of pulmonary edema fluid, and (3) one potential treatment for ARDS with a cell-based therapy that may accelerate the rate of AFC.

PULMONARY EDEMA FLUID CLEARANCE IN THE UNINJURED LUNG

Before discussing AFC in ARDS, it is first important to review how pulmonary edema fluid is cleared in the uninjured lung. In the uninjured lung, vectorial ion transport across the alveolar epithelial cells creates an osmotic gradient that drives fluid from the airspaces into the lung interstitum (**Figure 1**). It was initially thought that alveolar epithelial type II cells were the primary cell responsible for vectorial ion transport, but subsequent studies demonstrated an important role for type I cells as well (8). The transport of sodium ions is the most important driver for the generation of the osmotic gradient: sodium is transported through the sodium channel (ENaC) on the apical surface and then by the Na/K ATPase on the basolateral surface into the lung microcirculation (9, 10). Knockout of the alpha-subunit of ENaC in mice resulted in the inability to remove lung fluid at birth with subsequent respiratory failure and death (9). In addition, non-selective cation channels, cyclic nucleotide-gated channels, and the cystic fibrosis transmembrane conductance regulator chloride channel also contribute to the creation of the osmotic gradient (3, 11). Aquaporins facilitate the movement of water across the epithelial surface, but are not required for fluid transport (12).

This system of active ion-driven alveolar fluid reabsorption is the primary mechanism that removes alveolar edema fluid under both physiologic and pathological conditions (9, 13, 14). However, in the setting of ARDS, the capacity to remove alveolar edema fluid is reduced, which is termed impaired AFC. A reduction in the rate of AFC in ARDS correlates with decreased

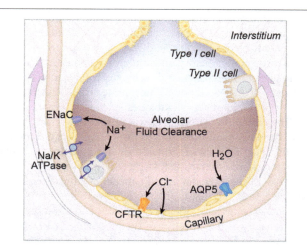

FIGURE 1 | Alveolar fluid clearance pathways. Shown are the interstitial, capillary, and alveolar compartments, with pulmonary edema fluid in the alveolus. Both type I (yellow) and type II (orange) alveolar cells are involved in transepithelial ion transport. Sodium (Na^+) is transported across the apical side of the type I and type II cells through the epithelial sodium channel (ENaC), and then across the basolateral side *via* the sodium/potassium ATPase pump (Na/K-ATPase). Chloride (Cl^-) is transported *via* the cystic fibrosis transmembrane conductance regulator (CFTR) channel or by a paracellular route. Additional cation channels also transport ions across the alveolar epithelium (not shown). This vectorial ion transport creates an osmotic gradient that drives the clearance of fluid. Specifically, water (H_2O) moves down the osmotic gradient through aquaporin channels, such as aquaporin 5 (AQP5) or *via* an intracellular route (not shown).

survival (15, 16). Therefore, it is critical to better understand why AFC is reduced in ARDS to better understand the pathogenesis of this condition.

PULMONARY EDEMA FLUID CLEARANCE IN ARDS

Multiple mechanisms explain why AFC is reduced in ARDS. First, both hypoxia and hypercapnia impair AFC. ENaC transcription and trafficking is downregulated and Na/K-ATPase functions less efficiently under states of low oxygen or high carbon dioxide, in part, because reactive oxygen species trigger endocytosis and cell necrosis (17–19). Therefore, supplemental oxygen and correction of hypercapnia can enhance the resolution of alveolar edema (17).

Second, biomechanical stress can reduce AFC. High tidal volumes and elevated airway pressures injure the alveolar epithelium, inducing cell death and inflammation, which reduces AFC (20). If pulmonary hydrostatic pressures are elevated, the rate of AFC is also reduced. These findings help explain the success of lung protective ventilation strategies and conservative fluid strategies in reducing the morbidity and mortality of ARDS (21, 22).

Third, ARDS pulmonary edema fluid contains high levels of pro-inflammatory cytokines including IL-1β, IL-8, TNFα, and TGFβ1 (23–25). Under controlled conditions, this inflammatory response is important for pathogen clearance. However, when excessive levels of cytokines are present, they instead can cause alveolar injury and decreased AFC (26–29). Moreover, once the epithelial barrier is breeched and alveolar fluid is released, components of the alveolar fluid may be recognized to induce downstream inflammatory and immune responses (30). There are no current therapies that directly target this pathway in the treatment of ARDS, although lung protective ventilation itself reduces pro-inflammatory cytokines such as IL-6 and IL-8 (4, 31). The remainder of this review will summarize our current understanding of alveolar ion transport in ARDS based on pathologically relevant *in vitro* and *in vivo* models, and discuss one potential new therapy that targets this pathway.

In 2006, Fang et al. developed a model of a polarized human alveolar type II cell that facilitated *in vitro* studies of AFC (32) (**Figure 2**). Using this model, Lee et al. found that transepithelial fluid transport is less effective in the presence of ARDS edema fluid and found that there are increased levels of cytokines and decreased levels of ion transport proteins in the presence of ARDS edema fluid compared to a plasma control (33). These data support the hypothesis that cytokine expression is increased in alveolar epithelium during ARDS, resulting in a decreased expression of alveolar ion channels and accumulation of alveolar edema fluid. In addition, the inflammatory edema fluid can also cause alveolar cell injury and necrosis, resulting in altered epithelial tight junctions (34, 35). The loss of tight junctions can negate the osmotic gradient, offsetting the effects of vectorial ion transport.

Subsequent *in vivo* studies expanded upon these findings and demonstrated that net AFC was reduced under clinically relevant pathologic conditions in animal models. In sheep, live *Pseudomonas aeruginosa* decreased AFC at both 4 and 24 h, an effect, which was associated with decreased AFC (36). In a mouse model of influenza pneumonia, the authors demonstrated that there was decreased AFC due to inhibition of the ENaC epithelial

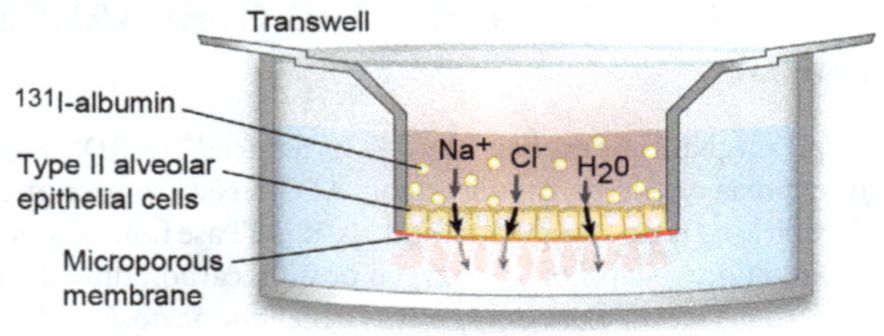

FIGURE 2 | *In vitro* model of polarized human alveolar type II epithelial cells. In 2006, Fang et al. developed an *in vitro* model of the polarized human alveolar epithelial surface, which has been used in multiple subsequent studies of alveolar fluid clearance (AFC) (32). To create this model, type II alveolar epithelial cells are isolated from human donor lungs and cultured on a collagen-I coated 24-well plate where they formed tight monolayers. Pulmonary edema fluid (pink), which contains water (H_2O), sodium ions (Na^+), chloride ions (Cl^-), as well as other ions and proteins, is mixed with ^{131}I-albumin (yellow circles) and introduced to the apical compartment. Pulmonary edema fluid is able to cross the alveolar cell monolayer, but ^{131}I-albumin cannot cross, so it is possible to calculate AFC by measuring the change in ^{131}I-albumin concentration between the apical and basal compartments.

sodium channel (37). These and other studies confirmed that AFC is reduced in lung injury through decreased efficiency of alveolar ion channels as well as altered permeability of the normally tight alveolar epithelium.

MESENCHYMAL STEM (STROMAL) CELLS (MSCs) AS A PROMISING THERAPY FOR ARDS

The laboratory-based investigations described above significantly advanced our understanding of ARDS pathophysiology, paving the way for targeted molecular therapies to improve the clinical treatment of patients with ARDS. MSCs are one such promising new cell-based therapy, which we will discuss in this section.

Mesenchymal stem (stromal) cells are bone marrow-derived cells that can differentiate *in vitro* into chondrocytes, osteoblasts, and adipocytes, although they do not have true stem cell properties *in vivo* (38). MSCs secrete paracrine factors that can decrease inflammation and enhance endothelial and epithelial repair (39). Several groups are studying the therapeutic potential of MSCs in sepsis (40, 41), diabetes (42), myocardial infarction (43), hepatic failure (44), and acute renal failure (45, 46). It was hypothesized that MSCs might also be beneficial in the treatment of ARDS.

To test this hypothesis, several groups studied whether MSCs could reduce the severity of lung, kidney, and brain injury in pre-clinical models (47). In 2007, Gupta et al. reported that treatment with MSCs improved survival and reduced pulmonary edema in *Escherichia coli* endotoxin-induced lung injury in mice (48). Subsequent studies showed that MSCs attenuated lung injury in mice and in *ex vivo* human lungs injured with live bacteria (49, 50). MSCs also enhance bacterial clearance and improve survival in mouse and rat models of sepsis (41, 51), and they have beneficial effects in ventilator-induced acute lung injury (52). Based on this preclinical data, phase 1 and 2 clinical trials are currently testing MSCs as a therapy for ARDS (53).

Given the potential therapeutic benefit of MSCs in the treatment of ARDS, it is important to understand their mechanism of action and several possible mechanisms have been implicated to date. In 2010, Fang et al. used SiRNA knockdown of paracrine soluble factors in the setting of MSC treatment *in vitro* in cultured human type 2 cells and found that angiopoietin-1 secretion was partially responsible for the beneficial effect of MSCs (54). Subsequent studies suggested that interleukin-1 receptor antagonist and growth factors such as keratinocyte growth (KGF) factor may also be involved in this process (52). KGF can upregulate AFC in *ex vivo* human lungs injured by endotoxin (55). A 2015 study demonstrated that lipoxin A4, a pro-resolving lipid mediator, is upregulated in the presence of MSCs, suggesting that this molecule may be important for MSC-mediated resolution of lung injury (56). Other studies indicated that the therapeutic effects of MSCs may also mediate the release of microvesicles, which are involved in cell–cell communication (57) or due to mitochondrial transfer (58). Thus, several mechanisms may explain MSC-mediated resolution of lung injury, and further studies are needed to fully characterize this process.

DISCUSSION

The importance of alveolar ion transport in AFC has been established, but further work is needed to better characterize this process. For example, type I alveolar cells participate in apical–basolateral fluid transport (8, 59), but there is no suitable cell culture model for type I cells so the physiology of these cells is not as well understood. In addition, sodium transport has been well characterized, but the contribution of transport of other ions is not as clear. Future experiments are needed to clarify the role of type I versus type II alveolar cells and the roles of additional ion channels in alveolar fluid transport.

The in vitro and in vivo models of ARDS have enhanced our understanding of ARDS pathophysiology. Not only are these models useful for the study of ARDS but measurements of AFC and paracellular permeability can also be used to better understand other pulmonary conditions. For example, Chan et al. (60) compared the extent to which avian influenza A (H5N1) virus and seasonal influenza A (H1N1) virus impair AFC and protein permeability using the transwell model first used in the ARDS models (60). The authors found that avian influenza A (H5N1) virus causes a more severe reduction in alveolar protein transport than the seasonal influenza A (H1N1) virus, mimicking its greater clinical severity. Future work can use these models to better understand how AFC is affected in other pulmonary pathologies as well.

Preliminary preclinical experiments have suggested that MSCs promote the resolution of alveolar edema fluid. It is possible that MSCs act directly on alveolar ion channels via cell–cell interactions or indirectly via paracrine factors; future experiments are needed to clarify their mechanism of action in the lung. If MSCs indeed promote AFC, they may serve as a promising cell-based therapy for ARDS.

SUMMARY

In this review, we have discussed how vectorial ion channels in alveolar epithelium generate an osmotic gradient that drives AFC in both physiologic and pathologic conditions. Both AFC and paracellular permeability can be measured using in vitro and in vivo models of ARDS, and these studies indicate that vectorial ion transport is less effective in injured lungs than in uninjured lungs. Recent studies suggest that MSCs interact with alveolar epithelium and ion channels to increase AFC and thus may serve as a promising treatment for ARDS.

AUTHOR CONTRIBUTIONS

LH and MM composed this mini-review manuscript together. LH is the first author.

ACKNOWLEDGMENTS

This work was supported by National Heart, Lung, and Blood Institute (NHLBIR37HL51856 and NHLBIU01HL1230004). The authors thank Diana Lim for creating the figures for this article.

REFERENCES

1. Staub NC. The pathogenesis of pulmonary edema. *Prog Cardiovasc Dis* (1980) 23(1):53–80. doi:10.1016/0033-0620(80)90005-5
2. Staub NC. Pulmonary edema due to increased microvascular permeability. *Annu Rev Med* (1981) 32(1):291–312. doi:10.1146/annurev.me.32.020181. 001451
3. Matthay MA, Folkesson HG, Clerici C. Lung epithelial fluid transport and the resolution of pulmonary edema. *Physiol Rev* (2002) 82(3):569–600. doi:10.1152/physrev.00003.2002
4. Matthay MA, Ware LB, Zimmerman GA. The acute respiratory distress syndrome. *J Clin Invest* (2012) 122(8):2731–40. doi:10.1172/JCI60331
5. Ferguson ND, Fan E, Camporota L, Antonelli M, Anzueto A, Beale R, et al. The Berlin definition of ARDS: an expanded rationale, justification, and supplementary material. *Intensive Care Med* (2012) 38(10):1573–85. doi:10.1007/s00134-012-2682-1
6. Rubenfeld GD, Caldwell E, Peabody E, Weaver J, Martin DP, Neff M, et al. Incidence and outcomes of acute lung injury. *N Engl J Med* (2005) 353(16):1685–93. doi:10.1056/NEJMoa050333
7. The Acute Respiratory Distress Syndrome Network. Ventilation with lower tidal volumes as compared with traditional tidal volumes for acute lung injury and the acute respiratory distress syndrome. *N Engl J Med* (2000) 342:1301–8. doi:10.1056/NEJM200005043421801
8. Johnson MD, Widdicombe JH, Allen L, Barbry P, Dobbs LG. Alveolar epithelial type I cells contain transport proteins and transport sodium, supporting an active role for type I cells in regulation of lung liquid homeostasis. *Proc Natl Acad Sci U S A* (2002) 99(4):1966–71. doi:10.1073/pnas.042689399
9. Canessa CM, Schild L, Buell G, Thorens B, Gautschi I, Horisberger JD, et al. Amiloride-sensitive epithelial Na+ channel is made of three homologous subunits. *Nature* (1994) 367(6462):463–7. doi:10.1038/367463a0
10. Matalon S, O'Brodovich H. Sodium channels in alveolar epithelial cells: molecular characterization, biophysical properties, and physiological

significance. *Annu Rev Physiol* (1999) 61(1):627–61. doi:10.1146/annurev.physiol.61.1.627
11. Fang X, Fukuda N, Barbry P, Sartori C, Verkman AS, Matthay MA. Novel role for CFTR in fluid absorption from the distal airspaces of the lung. *J Gen Physiol* (2002) 119(2):199–208. doi:10.1085/jgp.119.2.199
12. Verkman AS, Matthay MA, Song Y. Aquaporin water channels and lung physiology. *Am J Physiol Lung Cell Mol Physiol* (2000) 278(5):L867–79.
13. Eaton DC, Chen J, Ramosevac S, Matalon S, Jain L. Regulation of Na+ channels in lung alveolar type II epithelial cells. *Proc Am Thorac Soc* (2004) 1(1):10–6. doi:10.1513/pats.2306008
14. Mutlu GM, Sznajder JI. Mechanisms of pulmonary edema clearance. *Am J Physiol Lung Cell Mol Physiol* (2005) 289(5):L685–95. doi:10.1152/ajplung.00247.2005
15. Matthay MA, Wiener-Kronish JP. Intact epithelial barrier function is critical for the resolution of alveolar edema in humans. *Am Rev Respir Dis* (1990) 142(6,1):1250–7. doi:10.1164/ajrccm/142.6_Pt_1.1250
16. Ware LB, Matthay MA. Alveolar fluid clearance is impaired in the majority of patients with acute lung injury and the acute respiratory distress syndrome. *Am J Respir Crit Care Med* (2001) 163(6):1376–83. doi:10.1164/ajrccm.163.6.2004035
17. Vivona ML, Matthay M, Chabaud MB, Friedlander G, Clerici C. Hypoxia reduces alveolar epithelial sodium and fluid transport in rats: reversal by β-adrenergic agonist treatment. *Am J Respir Cell Mol Biol* (2001) 25(5):554–61. doi:10.1165/ajrcmb.25.5.4420
18. Vadász I, Raviv S, Sznajder JI. Alveolar epithelium and Na, K-ATPase in acute lung injury. *Intensive Care Med* (2007) 33(7):1243–51. doi:10.1007/s00134-007-0661-8
19. Briva A, Vadász I, Lecuona E, Welch LC, Chen J, Dada LA, et al. High CO2 levels impair alveolar epithelial function independently of pH. *PLoS One* (2007) 2(11):e1238. doi:10.1371/journal.pone.0001238
20. Frank JA, Gutierrez JA, Jones KD, Allen L, Dobbs L, Matthay MA. Low tidal volume reduces epithelial and endothelial injury in acid-injured rat lungs.

Am J Respir Crit Care Med (2002) 165(2):242–9. doi:10.1164/ajrccm.165.2. 2108087

21. Amato MBP, Barbas CSV, Medeiros DM, Laffey JG, Engelberts D, Kavanagh BP. Ventilation with lower tidal volumes as compared with traditional tidal volumes for acute lung injury. *N Engl J Med* (2000) 343(2000):812–4. doi:10.1056/NEJM200009143431113

22. Schuller D, Schuster DP. Fluid-management strategies in acute lung injury. *N Engl J Med* (2006) 355(11):1175. doi:10.1056/NEJMc061857

23. Pugin J, Verghese G, Widmer MC, Matthay MA. The alveolar space is the site of intense inflammatory and profibrotic reactions in the early phase of acute respiratory distress syndrome. *Crit Care Med* (1999) 27(2):304–12. doi:10.1097/00003246-199902000-00036

24. Olman MA, White KE, Ware LB, Simmons WL, Benveniste EN, Zhu S, et al. Pulmonary edema fluid from patients with early lung injury stimulates fibroblast proliferation through IL-1β-induced IL-6 expression. *J Immunol* (2004) 172(4):2668–77. doi:10.4049/jimmunol.172.4.2668

25. Ware LB, Matthay MA. The acute respiratory distress syndrome. *N Engl J Med* (2000) 342(18):1334–49. doi:10.1056/NEJM200005043421806

26. Fukuda N, Jayr C, Lazrak A, Wang Y, Lucas R, Matalon S, et al. Mechanisms of TNF-α stimulation of amiloride-sensitive sodium transport across alveolar epithelium. *Am J Physiol Lung Cell Mol Physiol* (2001) 280(6):L1258–65.

27. Elia N, Tapponnier M, Matthay MA, Hamacher J, Pache JC, Bründler MA, et al. Functional identification of the alveolar edema reabsorption activity of murine tumor necrosis factor-α. *Am J Respir Crit Care Med* (2003) 168(9):1043–50. doi:10.1164/rccm.200206-618OC

28. Dagenais A, Fréchette R, Yamagata Y, Yamagata T, Carmel JF, Clermont ME, et al. Downregulation of ENaC activity and expression by TNF-α in alveolar epithelial cells. *Am J Physiol Lung Cell Mol Physiol* (2004) 286(2):L301–11. doi:10.1152/ajplung.00326.2002

29. Roux J, Kawakatsu H, Gartland B, Pespeni M, Sheppard D, Matthay MA, et al. Interleukin-1β decreases expression of the epithelial sodium channel α-subunit in alveolar epithelial cells via a p38 MAPK-dependent signaling pathway. *J Biol Chem* (2005) 280(19):18579–89. doi:10.1074/jbc. M410561200

30. Hung CF, Mittelsteadt KL, Brauer R, McKinney BL, Hallstrand TS, Parks WC, et al. Lung pericyte-like cells are functional immune sentinel cells. *Am J Physiol Lung Cell Mol Physiol* (2017) 10:ajlung.00349.2016. doi:10.1152/ajplung.00349.2016

31. Parsons PE, Eisner MD, Thompson BT, Matthay MA, Ancukiewicz M, Bernard GR, et al. Lower tidal volume ventilation and plasma cytokine markers of inflammation in patients with acute lung injury. *Crit Care Med* (2005) 33(1):1–6. doi:10.1097/01.CCM.0000149854.61192.DC

32. Fang X, Song Y, Hirsch J, Galietta LJ, Pedemonte N, Zemans RL, et al. Contribution of CFTR to apical-basolateral fluid transport in cultured human alveolar epithelial type II cells. *Am J Physiol Lung Cell Mol Physiol* (2006) 290(2):L242–9. doi:10.1152/ajplung.00178.2005

33. Lee JW, Fang X, Dolganov G, Fremont RD, Bastarache JA, Ware LB, et al. Acute lung injury edema fluid decreases net fluid transport across human alveolar epithelial type II cells. *J Biol Chem* (2007) 282(33):24109–19. doi:10.1074/jbc. M700821200

34. Zemans RL, Colgan SP, Downey GP. Transepithelial migration of neutrophils: mechanisms and implications for acute lung injury. *Am J Respir Cell Mol Biol* (2009) 40(5):519–35. doi:10.1165/rcmb.2008-0348TR

35. Calfee CS, Matthay MA. Clinical immunology: culprits with evolutionary ties. *Nature* (2010) 464(7285):41–2. doi:10.1038/464041a

36. Kurahashi K, Kajikawa O, Sawa T, Ohara M, Gropper MA, Frank DW, et al. Pathogenesis of septic shock in *Pseudomonas aeruginosa* pneumonia. *J Clin Invest* (1999) 104(6):743–50. doi:10.1172/JCI7124

37. Chen XJ, Seth S, Yue G, Kamat P, Compans RW, Guidot D, et al. Influenza virus inhibits ENaC and lung fluid clearance. *Am J Physiol Lung Cell Mol Physiol* (2004) 287(2):L366–73. doi:10.1152/ajplung.00011.2004

38. Friedenstein AJ, Petrakova KV, Kurolesova AI, Frolova GP. Hetertrohic transplants of bone marrow. *Transplantation* (1968) 6(2):230–47. doi:10.1097/00007890-196803000-00009

39. Parekkadan B, Milwid JM. Mesenchymal stem cells as therapeutics. *Annu Rev Biomed Eng* (2010) 12:87. doi:10.1146/annurev-bioeng-070909-105309

40. Németh K, Leelahavanichkul A, Yuen PS, Mayer B, Parmelee A, Doi K, et al. Bone marrow stromal cells attenuate sepsis via prostaglandin E2-dependent reprogramming of host macrophages to increase their interleukin-10 production. *Nat Med* (2009) 15(1):42–9. doi:10.1038/nm.1905

41. Mei SH, Haitsma JJ, Dos Santos CC, Deng Y, Lai PF, Slutsky AS, et al. Mesenchymal stem cells reduce inflammation while enhancing bacterial clearance and improving survival in sepsis. *Am J Respir Crit Care Med* (2010) 182(8):1047–57. doi:10.1164/rccm.201001-0010OC

42. Lee RH, Seo MJ, Reger RL, Spees JL, Pulin AA, Olson SD, et al. Multipotent stromal cells from human marrow home to and promote repair of pancreatic islets and renal glomeruli in diabetic NOD/scid mice. *Proc Natl Acad Sci U S A* (2006) 103(46):17438–43. doi:10.1073/pnas.0608249103

43. Li TS, Hayashi M, Ito H, Furutani A, Murata T, Matsuzaki M, et al. Regeneration of infarcted myocardium by intramyocardial implantation of ex vivo transforming growth factor-β-preprogrammed bone marrow stem cells. *Circulation* (2005) 111(19):2438–45. doi:10.1161/01.CIR.0000167553.49133.81

44. Parekkadan B, Van Poll D, Suganuma K, Carter EA, Berthiaume F, Tilles AW, et al. Mesenchymal stem cell-derived molecules reverse fulminant hepatic failure. *PLoS One* (2007) 2(9):e941. doi:10.1371/journal.pone.0000941

45. Tögel F, Hu Z, Weiss K, Isaac J, Lange C, Westenfelder C. Administered mesenchymal stem cells protect against ischemic acute renal failure through differentiation-independent mechanisms. *Am J Physiol Renal Physiol* (2005) 289(1):F31–42. doi:10.1152/ajprenal.00007.2005

46. Ullah I, Subbarao RB, Rho GJ. Human mesenchymal stem cells-current trends and future prospective. *Biosci Rep* (2015) 35(2):e00191. doi:10.1042/BSR20150025

47. Matthay MA, Pati S, Lee JW. Mesenchymal stem (stromal) cells: biology and preclinical evidence for therapeutic potential for organ dysfunction following trauma or sepsis. *Stem Cells* (2017) 35:316–24. doi:10.1002/stem.2551

48. Gupta N, Su X, Popov B, Lee JW, Serikov V, Matthay MA. Intrapulmonary delivery of bone marrow-derived mesenchymal stem cells improves survival and attenuates endotoxin-induced acute lung injury in mice. *J Immunol* (2007) 179(3):1855–63. doi:10.4049/jimmunol.179.3.1855

49. Gupta N, Krasnodembskaya A, Kapetanaki M, Mouded M, Tan X, Serikov V, et al. Mesenchymal stem cells enhance survival and bacterial clearance in murine *Escherichia coli* pneumonia. *Thorax* (2012) 67(6):533–9. doi:10.1136/thoraxjnl-2011-201176

50. Lee JW, Krasnodembskaya A, McKenna DH, Song Y, Abbott J, Matthay MA. Therapeutic effects of human mesenchymal stem cells in ex vivo human lungs injured with live bacteria. *Am J Respir Crit Care Med* (2013) 187(7):751–60. doi:10.1164/rccm.201206-0990OC

51. Devaney J, Horie S, Masterson C, Elliman S, Barry F, O'Brien T, et al. Human mesenchymal stromal cells decrease the severity of acute lung injury induced by E. coli in the rat. *Thorax* (2015) 70(7):625–35. doi:10.1136/thoraxjnl-2015-206813

52. Walter J, Ware LB, Matthay MA. Mesenchymal stem cells: mechanisms of potential therapeutic benefit in ARDS and sepsis. *Lancet Respir Med* (2014) 2(12):1016–26. doi:10.1016/S2213-2600(14)70217-6

53. Wilson JG, Liu KD, Zhuo H, Caballero L, McMillan M, Fang X, et al. Mesenchymal stem (stromal) cells for treatment of ARDS: a phase 1 clinical trial. *Lancet Respir Med* (2015) 3(1):24–32. doi:10.1016/S2213-2600(14)70291-7

54. Fang X, Neyrinck AP, Matthay MA, Lee JW. Allogeneic human mesenchymal stem cells restore epithelial protein permeability in cultured human alveolar type II cells by secretion of angiopoietin-1. *J Biol Chem* (2010) 285(34):26211–22. doi:10.1074/jbc.M110.119917

55. Lee JW, Fang X, Gupta N, Serikov V, Matthay MA. Allogeneic human mesenchymal stem cells for treatment of E. coli endotoxin-induced acute lung injury in the ex vivo perfused human lung. *Proc Natl Acad Sci U S A* (2009) 106(38):16357–62. doi:10.1073/pnas.0907996106

56. Fang X, Abbott J, Cheng L, Colby JK, Lee JW, Levy BD, et al. Human mesenchymal stem (stromal) cells promote the resolution of acute lung injury in part through lipoxin A4. *J Immunol* (2015) 195(3):875–81. doi:10.4049/jimmunol.1500244

57. Zhu YG, Feng XM, Abbott J, Fang XH, Hao Q, Monsel A, et al. Human mesenchymal stem cell microvesicles for treatment of *Escherichia coli* endotoxin-induced acute lung injury in mice. *Stem Cells* (2014) 32(1):116–25. doi:10.1002/stem.1504

58. Islam MN, Das SR, Emin MT, Wei M, Sun L, Westphalen K, et al. Mitochondrial transfer from bone-marrow-derived stromal cells to pulmonary

alveoli protects against acute lung injury. *Nat Med* (2012) 18(5):759–65. doi:10.1038/nm.2736

59. Ridge KM, Olivera WG, Saldias F, Azzam Z, Horowitz S, Rutschman DH, et al. Alveolar type 1 cells express the $\alpha 2$ Na, K-ATPase, which contributes to lung liquid clearance. *Circ Res* (2003) 92(4):453–60. doi:10.1161/01.RES.0000059414.10360.F2

60. Chan MC, Kuok DI, Leung CY, Hui KP, Valkenburg SA, Lau EH, et al. Human mesenchymal stromal cells reduce influenza A H5N1-associated acute lung injury in vitro and in vivo. *Proc Natl Acad Sci U S A* (2016) 113(13):3621–6. doi:10.1073/pnas.1601911113

Inhibition of the NOD-Like Receptor Protein 3 Inflammasome is Protective in Juvenile Influenza A Virus Infection

Bria M. Coates[1,2]*, Kelly L. Staricha[1], Nandini Ravindran[1], Clarissa M. Koch[3], Yuan Cheng[3], Jennifer M. Davis[3], Dale K. Shumaker[3] and Karen M. Ridge[3,4]

[1] Department of Pediatrics, Feinberg School of Medicine, Northwestern University, Chicago, IL, United States, [2] Ann & Robert H. Lurie Children's Hospital of Chicago, Chicago, IL, United States, [3] Department of Medicine, Feinberg School of Medicine, Northwestern University, Chicago, IL, United States, [4] Department of Cell and Molecular Biology, Feinberg School of Medicine, Northwestern University, Chicago, IL, United States

*Correspondence:
Bria M. Coates
b-coates@northwestern.edu

Influenza A virus (IAV) is a significant cause of life-threatening lower respiratory tract infections in children. Antiviral therapy is the mainstay of treatment, but its effectiveness in this age group has been questioned. In addition, damage inflicted on the lungs by the immune response to the virus may be as important to the development of severe lung injury during IAV infection as the cytotoxic effects of the virus itself. A crucial step in the immune response to IAV is activation of the NOD-like receptor protein 3 (NLRP3) inflammasome and the subsequent secretion of the inflammatory cytokines, interleukin-1β (IL-1β), and interleukin-18 (IL-18). The IAV matrix 2 proton channel (M2) has been shown to be an important activator of the NLRP3 inflammasome during IAV infection. We sought to interrupt this ion channel-mediated activation of the NLRP3 inflammasome through inhibition of NLRP3 or the cytokine downstream from its activation, IL-1β. Using our juvenile mouse model of IAV infection, we show that inhibition of the NLRP3 inflammasome with the small molecule inhibitor, MCC950, beginning 3 days after infection with IAV, improves survival in juvenile mice. Treatment with MCC950 reduces NLRP3 levels in lung homogenates, decreases IL-18 secretion into the alveolar space, and inhibits NLRP3 inflammasome activation in alveolar macrophages. Importantly, inhibition of the NLRP3 inflammasome with MCC950 does not impair viral clearance. In contrast, inhibition of IL-1β signaling with the IL-1 receptor antagonist, anakinra, is insufficient to protect juvenile mice from IAV. Our findings suggest that targeting the NLRP3 inflammasome in juvenile IAV infection may improve disease outcomes in this age group.

Keywords: children, influenza, inflammasome, inflammation, MCC950, acute lung injury

INTRODUCTION

Influenza A virus (IAV) is a significant respiratory pathogen in the pediatric age group. Despite widespread vaccination efforts, ~80 per 100,000 children in the United States are hospitalized each year with seasonal IAV (1), and up to 24% of hospitalizations require intensive care unit admission for life-threatening disease (2). Underlying medical conditions increase the risk of severe IAV infection, but a considerable amount of morbidity and mortality occurs in healthy children. The effectiveness of antiviral drugs, which target IAV proteins, is hindered by the need to administer them early in the course of infection and the increasing resistance of seasonal IAV to these compounds (3). Consequently, therapy for children with severe IAV infection largely consists of supportive care. Hence, there is an urgent need to develop new therapeutic strategies to reduce the fatal pathology observed in children hospitalized with severe IAV infection.

The host immune response to IAV plays an important role in reducing morbidity and mortality as well as promoting viral clearance. However, IAV infections in pediatric patients can be associated with aberrant or dysregulated cytokine and cellular inflammatory responses [reviewed in Ref. (4)]. Among the potentially injurious cytokines produced during IAV infection are interleukin-1β (IL-1β) and interleukin-18 (IL-18), which are secreted following activation of the NOD-like receptor family pyrin domain containing 3 (NLRP3) inflammasome. The NLRP3 inflammasome is tightly regulated, requiring two signals for activation. Signal 1 occurs through pathogen detection by pattern recognition receptors that act through the transcription factor, NF-κB, to increase the expression of pro-IL-1β, as well as inflammasome components, including NLRP3 and pro-caspase-1. A second signal is then required for NRLP3 inflammasome complex assembly and activation. Several IAV-specific products have been identified as potent Signal 2 activators, including IAV viral RNA and IAV matrix 2 (M2) protein (5–7). The IAV M2 protein, a proton channel involved in viral replication (8), has been shown to activate the NLRP3 inflammasome in an IAV strain-independent manner (7). In bone marrow derived macrophages primed with lipopolysaccharide, which activates Signal 1, lentivirus expression of the M2 protein from a number of seasonal and pandemic strains of IAV resulted in IL-1β secretion. The IAV M2 protein activates the inflammasome by promoting proton efflux following M2 localization to the acidified Golgi apparatus. Inhibition of M2 protein function *via* the introduction of M2 mutants, or the use of amantadine or rimantadine, which block movement of protons through the M2 channel, has also been shown to inhibit IL-1β maturation and secretion (7). Unfortunately, the development of resistance to these medications has diminished their efficacy in the treatment of seasonal IAV, and they are no longer considered standard of care in the United States.

The role of NLRP3 inflammasome in IAV infection was first explored in mice deficient in its three components, NLRP3, caspase-1, or ASC. Decreased survival was consistently seen in mice lacking caspase-1 or ASC when challenged with IAV (9–11). However, the role of the NLRP3 protein itself appeared to be dependent on the inoculating dose of IAV, as NLRP3 deficiency did not impact mortality when a low dose of IAV was used (11), but did lead to worse survival after infection with higher doses (9, 10). The authors reasoned that the increased mortality seen in mice deficient in NLRP3 inflammasome components was due to impaired viral clearance, as viral titers remained elevated late in infection (9, 11). Conversely, more recent studies have demonstrated that excessive NLRP3 inflammasome activity can contribute to IAV-induced lung injury and death (6, 12). Therefore, NLRP3 inflammasome activity must be carefully controlled to achieve IAV clearance without causing unnecessary damage to surrounding tissues. This pathway may be of particular importance in the pathogenesis of severe IAV infection in

children (4, 13). Therefore, using our mouse model of pediatric IAV infection, which has been shown to mimic human disease, we investigated how modulation of the inflammatory response might change outcomes in life-threatening IAV infection. Using a small molecule inhibitor of the NLRP3 inflammasome (MCC950) and an antagonist of the receptor for IL-1β (anakinra), we found that inhibition of the NLRP3 inflammasome could ameliorate life-threatening IAV infection in juvenile mice, but inhibition of IL-1β signaling alone could not.

MATERIALS AND METHODS

Animals
129S wild-type mice were provided by Jackson Laboratories and bred in house. Mice were provided with food and water *ad libitum*, maintained on a 14 h light, 10 h dark cycle, and handled according to the National Institutes of Health guidelines. All procedures complied with federal guidelines and were approved by The Institutional Animal Care and Use Committee at Northwestern University.

Virus
Influenza virus strain A/WSN/1933 (WSN) was grown for 48 h at 37.5°C and 50% humidity in the allantoic cavities of 10- to 11-day-old fertile chicken eggs. Viral titers were measured by plaque assay in Madin–Darby canine kidney (MDCK) epithelial cells. Virus aliquots were stored in liquid nitrogen, and freeze/thaw cycles were avoided.

In Vitro Influenza Virus Infection of THP-1 Cells
THP-1 cells were plated in 6-well plates at a density of 0.5×10^6 per well. They were differentiated with phorbol myristate acetate (5 nM) for 48 h and cultured in complete RPMI medium for 72 h. Cells were infected with IAV WSN at a multiplicity of infection (MOI) of 1, 2, or 3 for 2 h. Cells were then washed with phosphate-buffered saline (PBS) and cultured in complete RPMI medium for 24 h. The cell-free supernatant was collected for ELISA. For drug-therapy experiments, differentiated THP-1 cells were treated with MCC950 (1 μM, Adipogen), anakinra (0.5 μg/mL, Kineret™), or vehicle control (PBS) for 1 h. Immediately after the drug treatment, cells were infected with IAV WSN (MOI 2) for 2 h. The infected cells were washed with PBS and cultured in complete RPMI medium containing MCC950 (1 μM), anakinra (0.5 μg/mL), or vehicle control for 24 h. The cell-free supernatant was collected for ELISA. ELISA was done for IL-1β (eBioscience, San Diego, CA, USA) and Caspase-1 (R&D Systems, Minneapolis, MN, USA).

Cell Imaging
Human THP-1 monocytes were plated on sterilized 18CIR-1 coverglasses in a 12-well plate at a density of 0.25–0.5 million cells per well and differentiated. Cells were then treated with an MOI of 2 of IAV for 24 h and probed for active caspase-1 by means of FAM-YVAD-FMK (FAM-FLICA caspase-1 assay kit #97, ImmunoChemistry, Bloomington, MN, USA) according to the

manufacturer's instructions. Nuclei were labeled with Hoechst 33342, and then cells were fixed in 2.7% paraformaldehyde for 5 min at room temperature. Images were acquired by means of a Nikon A1R laser scanning confocal microscope.

In Vivo Influenza Virus Infection

Juvenile (4-week-old) mice were anesthetized with isoflurane and infected intratracheally with WSN [12.5 plaque forming units (PFU) in 50 µL PBS] or an equal volume of PBS.

Inflammasome Inhibition *In Vivo*

MCC950 (Adipogen) reconstituted in sterile PBS was administered intraperitoneally in juvenile mice at a dose of 10 mg/kg daily beginning on day 3 postinfection (p.i.) until tissue harvest, death, or recovery. Anakinra (Kineret™) was administered intraperitoneally in juvenile mice at a dose of 100 mg/kg on day 3 p.i. until tissue harvest, death, or recovery.

Bronchoalveolar Lavage Fluid (BALF) Harvest

A 20-gauge angiocatheter was ligated into the trachea, and the lungs were lavaged twice with sterile PBS (700 µL). The lavage fluid was centrifuged at 1,000 g for 10 min. The pellet was resuspended, and the cells were counted using the Invitrogen Countess Automated Cell Counter (Invitrogen, Grand Island, NY, USA). Protein levels in the supernatant were measured by Bradford Assay (BioRad), and cytokine levels were measured using ELISA. Interleukin (IL)-18 was measured using the mouse IL-18 ELISA Kit (MBL International Corporation, Woburn, MA, USA) according to the manufacturer's instructions. Interleukin-6 (IL-6) was measured using the mouse IL-6 Ready-Set-GO ELISA Kits (eBioscience, San Diego, CA, USA). Interferon (IFN)-α was measured using the mouse IFN Alpha ELISA Kit (PBL Assay Science, Piscataway, NJ, USA).

Wet-to-Dry Weight Ratios

Mice were anesthetized and lungs were surgically removed *en bloc*. Lungs were weighed in a tared container. The lungs were then dried at 45°C in a Speed-Vac SC100 evaporator (Thermo Scientific, Waltham, MA, USA) until a constant weight was obtained, and the wet-to-dry weight ratio was calculated.

Histology

Mice were anesthetized and lungs were perfused *via* the right ventricle with 10 mL HBSS with calcium and magnesium. A 22-gauge angiocatheter was sutured into the trachea, heart and lungs were removed en bloc, and then lungs were inflated with 0.7 mL of 4% paraformaldehyde at a pressure not exceeding 16 cm H_2O. Tissue was fixed in 4% paraformaldehyde overnight at 4°C, then processed, embedded in paraffin, sectioned, and stained with hematoxylin and eosin (H&E). Images were acquired by means of a TissueGnostics automated slide imaging system (TissueGnostics, Vienna, Austria).

Lung Harvest and Homogenization

For plaque assay, lungs were homogenized in PBS (20 µL/mg lung). For western blot, lungs were homogenized in RIPA buffer with protease inhibitor (20 mM Tris–HCl, 150 mM NaCl, 1% Triton X-100, 0.1% SDS, Roche complete ULTRA Tablet). Homogenized lungs were centrifuged at 1,000 g. The supernatant was frozen at 80°C.

Western Blot

The presence of indicated proteins in lung homogenates from day 7 p.i. was assessed by western blotting using the following antibodies: NLRP3 (Adipogen), Caspase-1 (14F468) (Santa Cruz sc-56036), ASC (Adipogen), IL-18 (Biovision, 5180R-10), and Actin (Santa Cruz).

Flow Cytometry for Intracellular Staining of NLRP3 Inflammasome Components

Mice were anesthetized and lungs were perfused *via* the right ventricle with 10 mL HBSS with Ca^{2+} and Mg^{2+}. The lung lobes were removed and inflated with enzyme solution (5 mL of 0.2 mg/mL DNase I and 2 mg/mL Collagenase D in HBSS with Ca^{2+} and Mg^{2+}) using a 30G needle. The tissue was minced and then processed in GentleMACS dissociator (Miltenyi) according to the manufacturer's instructions. Processed lungs were passed through a 40 µm cell strainer, and red blood cells were lysed with BD Pharm Lyse (BD Biosciences, San Jose, CA, USA). Remaining cells were counted with a Countess Cell Counter (Invitrogen, Grand Island, NY, USA). CD45 microbeads were added, and cells were eluted according to the Miltenyi manufacturer's instructions. Cells were stained with viability dye Aqua (Invitrogen) and stained with a mixture of fluorochrome-conjugated antibodies (see **Table 1** for lists of fluorochromes, antibodies, manufacturers, and clones). Data were acquired on a BD LSR II flow cytometer using BD FACSDiva software (BD Biosciences), and data analyses were performed with FlowJo software (TreeStar, Ashland, OR, USA). Cell populations were identified using sequential gating strategy, and the percentage of cells in the live/singlets gate was multiplied by the number of live cells to obtain an absolute live-cell count. The expression of activation markers is presented as median fluorescence intensity (MFI).

TABLE 1 | Fluorochrome-conjugated antibodies used for flow cytometry.

Fluorochrome	Antibody	Manufacturer	Clone
FITC	CD45	eBioscience	30-F11
PerCPCy5.5	MHCII	BioLegend	M5/114.15.2
eFluor450	CD11b	eBioscience	M1/70
Alexa700	Ly6G	BD Pharmingen	1A8
APCCy7	Ly6C	eBioscience	HK1.4
PE	CD64	BioLegend	X54-5/7.1
PECF594	Siglec F	BD Horizon	E50-2440
PECy7	CD11c	BD Pharmingen	HL3

Additional antibodies used for intracellular staining:

Fluorochrome	Antibody	Manufacturer
APC	mNLRP3/NALP3	R&D
Biotin	Caspase-1	NOVUS
APC	Streptavidin	eBioscience

Plaque Assay

Confluent monolayers of MDCK cells were infected with stock virus or lung homogenate serially diluted in 1% bovine serum albumin Dulbecco's Modified Eagle Medium (DMEM) for 2 h at 37°C. Plates were washed with PBS and an overlay of 50% 2× Replacement Media (2× DMEM, 0.12 M NaHCO₃, 2% Penn-Strep, and 1% HEPES), 50% avecil (2.35%), and N-acetyl trypsin (1.5 µg/mL) remained on the cells for 72 h at 37°C. Overlay was removed, and the monolayers were then stained with Naphthalene Blue-Black and plaques counted.

Statistical Analysis

Data are expressed as means ± SD. Differences between two groups were assessed by using a Student's t-test. Differences between three or more groups were assessed using one-way analysis of variance with a Bonferroni multiple comparisons test. Values of $P < 0.05$ were considered to be significant. The log rank test was used in the analysis of the Kaplan–Meier curve. All analyses were performed using GraphPad Prism software version 6.0 for Windows (GraphPad Software, San Diego, CA, USA).

RESULTS

MCC950 and Anakinra Decrease NLRP3 Inflammasome Activity *In Vitro* in Macrophages Infected with IAV

MCC950 is a small molecule inhibitor of the NLRP3 inflammasome. Although its exact mechanism of action is unknown, it has been shown to be specific to NLRP3 and to prevent the activation of caspase-1 and the maturation and secretion of IL-1β and IL-18 in response to multiple NLRP3 inflammasome stimuli (14–16). Anakinra is a synthetic version of the naturally occurring IL-1β receptor antagonist. It prevents the downstream signaling of the IL-1β receptor. We tested the ability of MCC950 and anakinra to inhibit the NLRP3 inflammasome *in vitro*.

To determine the IAV inoculation dose necessary for NLRP3 inflammasome activation, we infected THP-1 cells (a human monocyte cell line derived from a 1-year-old patient) with IAV at an MOI of 1, 2, and 3 for 24 h. As shown in **Figures 1A,B**, there was a dose dependent increase in caspase-1 and IL-1β levels in the supernatant from IAV-infected macrophage cells. Based on these results we chose to test the ability of MCC950 and anakinra to inhibit NLRP3 inflammasome activation in response IAV at an MOI of 2.

THP-1 cells were pretreated with MCC950 (1 µM) or anakinra (0.5 µg/mL) and then infected with IAV (A/WSN/2009) at an MOI of 2. As shown in **Figures 1C,D**, cells infected with IAV had a robust increase in caspase-1 and IL-1β in the supernatant. In contrast, when the cells were treated with the NLRP3 inhibitor, MCC950, or the IL-1β receptor antagonist, anakinra, detection of caspase-1 and IL-1β during IAV infection was greatly reduced. Caspase-1 activation was also assessed using a specific fluorescent probe, FAM-YVAD-FMK (17). Cells infected with IAV showed robust caspase-1 activation following treatment with IAV, with caspase-1 forming aggregates throughout the cytoplasm. However, caspase-1 activation was severely reduced in cells treated with MCC950 prior to IAV infection. No caspase-1 activation was observed in uninfected THP-1 cells (**Figure 1E**).

MCC950 Improves Survival of Juvenile Mice Infected with IAV

The induction of IL-1β by IAV has been shown to be NLRP3 inflammasome dependent (8–10). We assessed the ability of MCC950 to prevent NLRP3 inflammasome activation and alter the young host's inflammatory response to IAV infection. Juvenile mice were infected with IAV [A/WSN/2009 12.5 PFU intratracheal (i.t.)] to achieve infection of the lower respiratory tract. Starting on day 3 p.i., we administered MCC950 [10 mg/kg intraperitoneal (i.p.), once daily (q.d.)] or an equal volume of vehicle control (i.p., q.d.) until recovery or death. We observed that the median survival of IAV-infected, vehicle-treated juvenile mice was day 11 p.i, with only 18% of PBS-treated mice surviving infection (**Figure 2A**). In contrast, 75% of IAV-infected, MCC950-treated juvenile mice were alive on day 11 p.i. IAV infection is typically associated with significant weight loss, which was observed in both IAV-infected, PBS-treated and IAV-infected, MCC950-treated mice. Importantly, the majority of the IAV-infected, MCC950-treated mice began to regain weight between days 8 and 9 p.i. (**Figure 2B**). Surviving IAV-infected, MCC950-treated juvenile mice exhibited coat ruffling, febrile shaking, and mild lethargy, but the majority of animals recovered. At 7 days p.i., indices of lung injury were not different between IAV-infected, PBS-treated and IAV-infected, MCC950-treated mice. Both groups displayed elevated levels of cellular infiltration (**Figure 2C**) and protein leakage (**Figure 2D**) into the BALF, and both groups had increased wet-to-dry weight ratios (**Figure 2E**). In accordance with this, histological examination of IAV-infected, PBS-treated and IAV-infected, MCC950-treated mice on day 7 p.i. demonstrated a similar degree of lung injury at this time point (**Figures 2F,G**).

MCC950 Inhibits the NLRP3 Inflammasome in Juvenile Lungs

We next sought to compare NLRP3 inflammasome activation in IAV-infected, PBS-treated and IAV-infected, MCC950-treated juvenile mice. IL-18 was elevated in the BALF from IAV-infected, PBS-treated mice, but was significantly attenuated in IAV-infected, MCC950-treated mice (**Figure 3A**). Importantly, the IAV-induced increase in NLRP3 protein expression observed in PBS-treated mice was absent in MCC950-treated mice (**Figure 3B**). Additional western blot analysis of inflammasome components in lung homogenates showed a similar increase in ASC in response to IAV infection in both PBS-treated and MCC950-treated mice (**Figure 3C**). Mature caspase-1 was increased in the BALF from IAV-infected, PBS-treated mice, compared to uninfected controls (**Figure 3D**). In contrast, caspase-1 secretion was inhibited in IAV-infected, MCC950-treated mice (**Figure 3D**). IL-6 and tumor necrosis-α (TNF-α), which are inflammatory cytokines that are not dependent on NLRP3 inflammasome activation, were not different between the two treatment groups (**Figures 3E,F**).

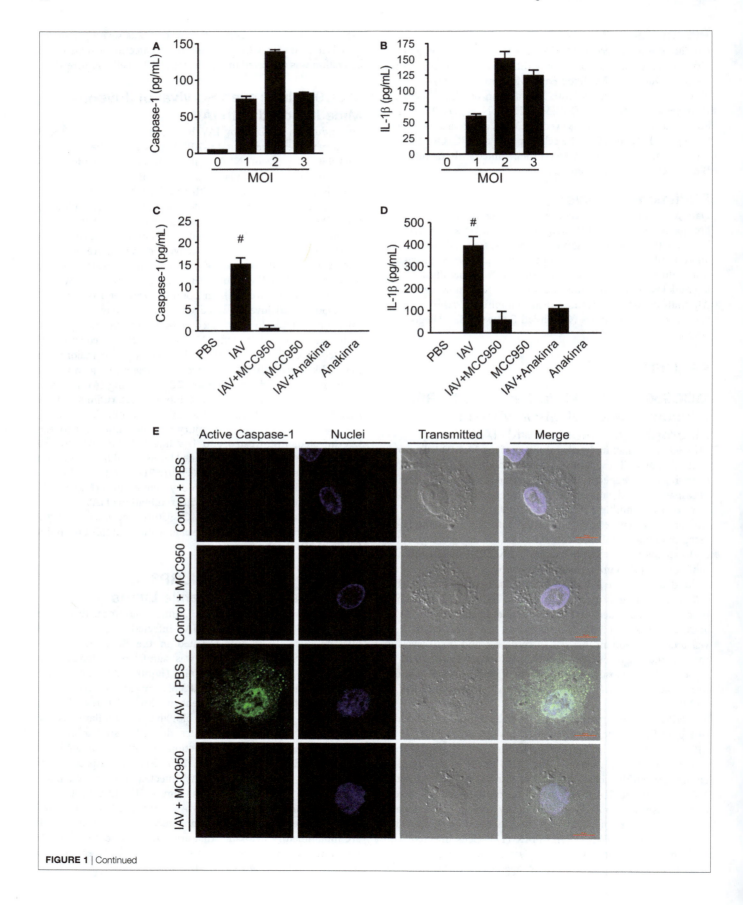

FIGURE 1 | Continued

FIGURE 1 | Continued
MCC950 and anakinra inhibit influenza A virus (IAV)-induced NOD-like receptor protein 3 inflammasome activation in THP-1 macrophages. Differentiated human THP-1 macrophages were infected with IAV (WSN) at a multiplicity of infection (MOI) of 1, 2, or 3 for 2 h. Infected cells were cultured for 24 h, and supernatant was evaluated by ELISA for **(A)** caspase-1 or **(B)** interleukin-1β (IL-1β). Differentiated human THP-1 macrophages were treated with MCC950, anakinra, or vehicle control. Cells were either infected with IAV (WSN, MOI 2) for 2 h or sham infected and treated with drug therapy alone. Cells were then washed and cultured in media containing MCC950, anakinra, or vehicle control. Supernatant was collected 24 h after IAV infection and evaluated by ELISA for **(C)** caspase-1 or **(D)** IL-1β. # indicates significant elevation over all other conditions. **(E)** MCC590-treated or vehicle-treated cells were fixed 24 h following IAV infection (WSN MOI 2) and fluorescently labeled to show active caspase-1 (green) and nuclei (blue). Scale bars, 10 μm.

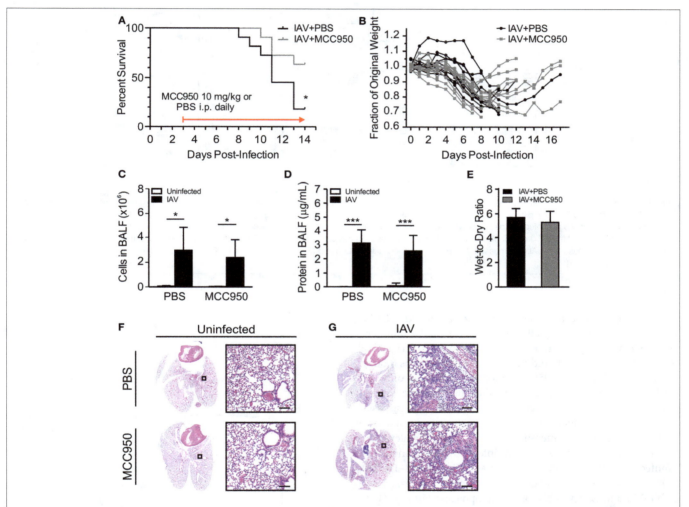

FIGURE 2 | MCC950 improves survival in juvenile mice infected with influenza A virus (IAV). Juvenile mice were infected with IAV [WSN 12.5 plaque forming units (PFU) intratracheal] and treated with MCC950 [10 mg/kg intraperitoneal (i.p.) daily] or phosphate-buffered saline (PBS) control beginning on day 3 postinfection (p.i.). **(A)** Mortality. **(B)** Weight loss. Bronchoalveolar lavage fluid (BALF) or whole lungs were collected from IAV-infected, MCC950-treated mice and IAV-infected, PBS-treated mice 7 days p.i. **(C)** Total number of cells in BALF. **(D)** Protein in BALF. **(E)** Wet-to-dry weight ratio. *$p < 0.05$, ***$p < 0.001$. **(F,G)** Hematoxylin and eosin stained lung sections from juvenile mice 7 days p.i. with 12.5 PFU of IAV and treatment with 10 mg/kg MCC950 or PBS control. Images shown are representative of three mice for each condition. Scale bars, 100 μm.

MCC950 Does Not Prevent Monocyte Recruitment to the Lungs but Does Inhibit NLRP3 Inflammasome Activation in Alveolar Macrophages

Macrophages are a main source of NLRP3 inflammasome activation during IAV infection (18). To investigate the impact of MCC950 treatment on NLRP3 inflammasome activation in these cells, we isolated alveolar macrophages (CD45+, CD64+, CD11c+, Siglec F+) and monocyte-derived cells (CD45+, CD11b+, Ly6C+, CD64+) from the lungs of IAV-infected, PBS-treated and IAV-infected, MCC950-treated mice using 10-color flow cytometry (19). In addition, we assessed the expression levels of NLRP3, caspase-1, and IL-1β with intracellular staining.

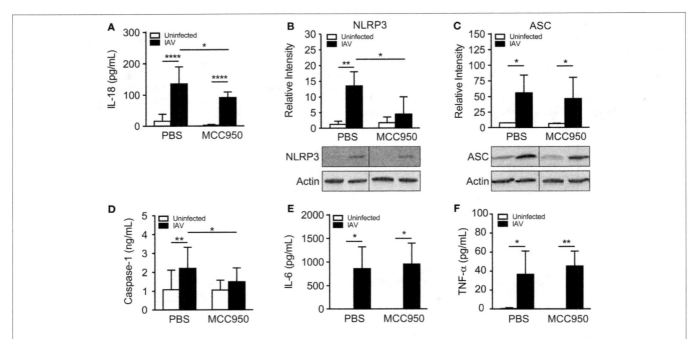

FIGURE 3 | MCC950 treatment decreases NOD-like receptor protein 3 (NLRP3) inflammasome activation in juvenile influenza A virus (IAV) infection. Juvenile mice were infected with IAV (WSN 12.5 plaque forming unit intratracheal) and treated with MCC950 (10 mg/kg intraperitoneal daily) or phosphate-buffered saline (PBS) control beginning on day 3 postinfection (p.i.). Bronchoalveolar lavage fluid (BALF) or whole lungs were collected from IAV-infected, MCC950-treated mice and IAV-infected, PBS-treated mice 7 days p.i. (A) Interleukin-18 (IL-18) in BALF as measured by ELISA. (B,C) NLRP3 and ASC in lung homogenates as measured by Western blot. (D) Caspase-1 in BALF as measured by ELISA. (E) Interleukin-6 (IL-6) and (F) tumor necrosis-α (TNF-α) in BALF as measured by ELISA. $*p < 0.05$, $**p < 0.01$, $****p < 0.0001$.

IAV infection caused an influx of monocyte-derived cells into the lungs. When analyzing all CD45+ cells, a similar number of alveolar macrophages (**Figure 4A**) and monocyte-derived cells (data not shown) were found in both treatment groups on day 7 p.i. To determine if MCC950 inhibited the expression of NLRP3 in these cells, we examined the median fluorescence intensity (MFI) of the inflammasome components, NLRP3 and caspase-1, and the product of its activation, IL-1β. All components of the NLRP3 inflammasome measured were significantly elevated in the alveolar macrophages of IAV-infected mice compared to uninfected controls (data not shown and **Figures 4B–D**). IAV-infected, MCC950-treated mice had significantly decreased levels of NLRP3 and IL-1β in alveolar macrophages (**Figures 4C,D**). These results are consistent with our finding that IAV-infected, MCC950-treated mice had decreased levels of NLRP3 in homogenized lungs as measured by Western blot, and IL-18 in BALF as measured by ELISA (see **Figure 3**).

MCC950 Does Not Impact Type I Interferon Production or Viral Clearance in Juvenile IAV Infection

Interferon-α (IFN-α) is a type I interferon secreted in response to viral infection to control viral replication and prevent propagation of the infection to neighboring cells. Mice infected with IAV, as well as mice treated with MCC950, had an increase in IFN-α levels on day 7 p.i. (**Figure 5A**). Consistent with this, viral

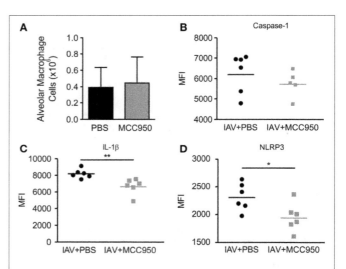

FIGURE 4 | MCC950 treatment decreases NOD-like receptor protein 3 (NLRP3) inflammasome activation in alveolar macrophages in juvenile mice infected with influenza A virus (IAV). Juvenile mice were infected with IAV (WSN 12.5 plaque forming unit intratracheal) and treated with MCC950 (10 mg/kg intraperitoneal daily) or phosphate-buffered saline (PBS) control beginning on day 3 postinfection (p.i.). Lungs were harvested 7 days p.i. and evaluated by flow cytometry for NLRP3 inflammasome activation using intracellular staining. (A) Number of alveolar macrophages in lung homogenates. (B–D) Median fluorescence intensity (MFI) of caspase-1, interleukin-1β (IL-1β), and NLRP3 in alveolar macrophages. $*p < 0.05$, $**p < 0.01$.

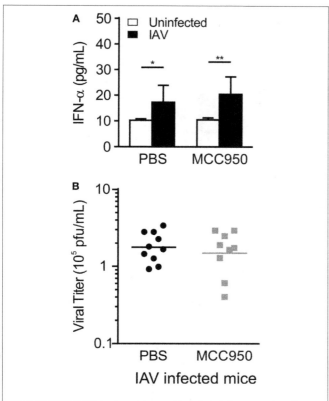

FIGURE 5 | MCC950 treatment does not impair viral clearance. Juvenile mice were infected with influenza A virus (IAV) (WSN 12.5 plaque forming unit intratracheal) and treated with MCC950 (10 mg/kg intraperitoneal daily) or phosphate-buffered saline (PBS) control beginning on day 3 postinfection (p.i.). Bronchoalveolar lavage fluid (BALF) or whole lungs were collected from IAV-infected, MCC950-treated mice and IAV-infected, PBS-treated mice 7 days p.i. (A) Interferon-α (IFN-α) in BALF as measured by ELISA. (B) Viral titer in lung homogenates was measured by plaque assay. *$p < 0.05$, **$p < 0.01$.

titers in the lung homogenates of IAV-infected, PBS-treated and IAV-infected, MCC950-treated mice as measured by plaque assay were equal (**Figure 5B**).

Anakinra Does Not Protect Juvenile Mice from IAV Infection

NOD-like receptor protein 3-dependent production of IL-1β and IL-18 may have downstream consequences with regard to IAV-induced inflammation and disease. IL-1β and IL-18 bind their cell-surface receptors (IL-1R and IL-18R, respectively) expressed on a range of cell types to induce potent NF-κB-dependent secondary cytokine production (20, 21). Importantly, lack of IL-1R resulted in reduced lung immunopathology following H1N1 infection, suggesting that IL-1R signaling may increase damage to the lung (22). Anakinra competes for the IL-1 receptor and blocks the actions of IL-1β. We investigated the impact of anakinra treatment on survival in IAV-infected juvenile mice. Juvenile mice were infected with IAV (A/WSN/2009 12.5 PFU i.t.) and anakinra (100 mg/kg i.p.) or an equal volume of vehicle control was administered i.p., q.d. beginning on day 3 p.i. and continuing until recovery or death. There was no statistically significant difference in the survival of IAV-infected mice treated with anakinra compared to those given vehicle control (**Figure 6A**). Initiating anakinra therapy on day 2 p.i. or day 4 p.i. also did not improve survival (data not shown). Measurement of protein leakage, IL-18, and IL-6 in BALF failed to show a difference between anakinra and control-treated mice on day 7 p.i. (**Figures 6B–D**). IFN-α secretion was not impacted by anakinra therapy, either, and viral titers from lung homogenates were equal in IAV-infected anakinra-treated mice, and IAV-infected PBS control-treated mice (**Figures 6E,F**). Finally, a similar degree of lung injury was seen on histological examination of IAV-infected, PBS-treated and IAV-infected, anakinra-treated mice on day 7 p.i. (**Figure 6G**).

DISCUSSION

The host response to IAV can exacerbate the morbidity associated with IAV infection (4, 23, 24). It is well established that the NLRP3 inflammasome is a major component of the host response to IAV (6). It is activated by the influenza M2 proton channel and results in the production of the potent inflammatory cytokines, IL-1β and IL-18 (7). While pathogen clearance and host survival depend on adequate activation of the innate immune system, an excessive inflammatory response to infection can be harmful to the young host. The NLRP3 inflammasome is protective in lethal mouse models of IAV infection (9–11). Loss of NLRP3, ASC, or caspase-1 in mice leads to decreased IL-1β and IL-18 secretion and increases mortality from IAV. Alternatively, excessive inflammasome activation may decrease survival by exacerbating the lung injury seen in lethal IAV infection (6). Therefore, inflammasome signaling must be tightly controlled to promote eradication of the virus while limiting collateral damage to the host. In severe IAV infection, this balance is not achieved, making the NLRP3 inflammasome an attractive therapeutic target. Early modulation of its activity may not only limit the production of injurious inflammatory cytokines, but also prevent the pyroptotic cell death and the ensuing tissue destruction caused by activated caspase-1. Thus, the identification of small molecule inhibitors of the NLRP3 inflammasome offers considerable therapeutic promise. To establish the optimal degree of NLRP3 inflammasome activation during IAV infection, we sought to modulate NLRP3 inflammasome signaling, with the goal of protecting juvenile mice from IAV-induced lung injury. We investigated the efficacy of MCC950, a potent inhibitor of NLRP3, as well as anakinra, a known inhibitor of the IL-1β pathway *via* IL-1 receptor.

MCC950 has been shown to be a specific NLRP3 inhibitor and to be protective in multiple models of injurious NLRP3 inflammasome activation (14–16). It can be given by oral, intravenous, and i.p. routes and is effective at doses ranging from 4 to 20 mg/kg in mouse models of autoimmune disease (experimental autoimmune encephalitis) (14), diseases of constitutive NLRP3 activation (cryopyrin-associated periodic syndrome) (14), and disorders in which NLRP3 has been shown to play an important role [including cardiac infarction (25) and non-alcoholic steatohepatitis (26)]. *In vitro* treatment of IAV-infected THP-1 macrophages with MCC950 confirmed that IAV-induced NLRP3 inflammasome

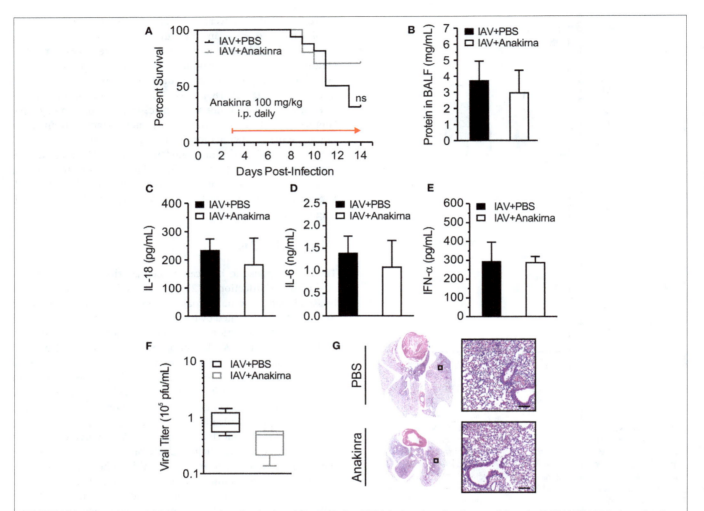

FIGURE 6 | Anakinra treatment does not protect juvenile mice from influenza A virus (IAV) infection. Juvenile mice were infected with IAV (WSN 12.5 plaque forming unit intratracheal) and treated with anakinra [100 mg/kg intraperitoneal (i.p.) daily] or vehicle control beginning on day 3 postinfection (p.i.). **(A)** Mortality. **(B)** Protein in bronchoalveolar lavage fluid (BALF) on day 7 p.i. **(C–E)** Interleukin-18 (IL-18), interleukin-6 (IL-6), and interferon-α (IFN-α) in BALF on day 7 p.i. as measured by ELISA. **(F)** Viral titer on day 7 p.i. was measured by plaque assay. **(G)** Hematoxylin and eosin stained lung sections from juvenile mice 7 days p.i. with IAV and treatment with anakinra or phosphate-buffered saline (PBS) control. Images shown are representative of three mice for each condition. Scale bars, 100 μm.

activation is effectively inhibited with this molecule. Interestingly, treatment of IAV-infected cells with the IL-1β receptor antagonist, anakinra, did not just block downstream signaling from the IL-1β receptor. It also appeared to inhibit NLRP3 inflammasome activation, as demonstrated by decreased caspase-1 and IL-1β in the supernatant from IAV-infected, anakinra-treated cells. Although anakinra classically targets IL-1β signaling by blocking the interaction of IL-1β with its receptor, it has also been shown to bind to and inhibit caspase-1, which likely explains our finding of NLRP3 inflammasome inhibition in IAV-infected cells treated with anakinra (27, 28). Consequently, we hypothesized that both MCC950 and anakinra had the potential to protect juvenile mice from IAV-induced NLRP3 inflammasome activation and lung injury.

Juvenile mice treated with MCC950 beginning 3 days p.i. were protected from IAV-induced mortality. We chose this timing for the initiation of therapy because this likely corresponds to when children infected with IAV develop symptoms and seek medical attention. The protection from IAV-induced mortality was associated with a decreased amount of NLRP3 in the lung homogenates, and decreased IL-18 levels in the BALF, from IAV-infected, MCC950-treated mice compared to IAV-infected, vehicle-treated mice, indicating that inhibition of the NLRP3 inflammasome was achieved. However, this protection from IAV-induced mortality was not associated with a decrease in traditional markers of lung injury, including cellular infiltration and protein leakage into the alveolar space. Since MCC950 therapy did not prevent IAV-induced lung injury on day 7 p.i., this suggests that MCC950 treatment improved survival by either halting disease progression or enhancing recovery. When CD45+ cells from IAV-infected mice were examined with intracellular staining, the greatest impact of NLRP3 inflammasome inhibition was found in alveolar macrophages. In these cells, MCC950 treatment decreased NLRP3 and IL-1β levels. As alveolar macrophages can promote alveolar epithelial cell repair (24), the switch from an inflammatory to an anti-inflammatory phenotype in alveolar macrophages may play an important role in recovery from IAV. We reason that inhibiting the NLRP3 inflammasome in this cell population may have played a key role in the beneficial effects of MCC950 therapy.

Other groups have shown varying degrees of protection from IAV (12) or the IAV virulence factor PB1-F2 (29) using MCC950 in murine models of adult IAV. Tate et al. were able to delay death from two different strains of IAV (A/PR/8/34 and HKx31) by a few days with MCC950 (5 mg/kg intranasal) treatment. Notably, timing of initiation of MCC950 therapy was important in their model, with early administration of the drug on day 1 p.i. harmful, and late administration after day 3 beneficial. This could be consistent with our proposal that NLRP3 inflammasome inhibition is important for recovery from IAV infection, rather than prevention of IAV-induced lung injury. However, evaluation of lung injury was not performed in their study. They were able to demonstrate prevention of immune cell infiltration into the lungs and decreased cytokine production, including IL-1β, IL-18, TNF-α, and IL-6, in BALF and serum. In our model of juvenile IAV infection, we did not see the same inhibition of immune cell recruitment to the lungs with MCC950 therapy (10 mg/kg i.p.). We also did not see the same suppression of IL-6 or TNF-α production. However, we were not surprised by this finding because these cytokines are not dependent on NLRP3 inflammasome activation. Importantly, we did see evidence of NLRP3 inflammasome inhibition in the resident alveolar macrophages, and decreased IL-18 in BALF, which may have contributed to the increased survival we found in mice treated with MCC950. Differences in our models may explain the disparate findings regarding cellular recruitment and cytokine suppression, highlighting the importance of the microenvironment when modulating the immune response to a pathogen. We administered the drug i.p. instead of intranasal to avoid repeated exposure to anesthesia, but these two delivery methods could result in different concentrations of the drug in the alveolar space. In addition, the half-life of the drug may be altered by delivery method, potentially limiting its efficacy. Perhaps more importantly, we used juvenile mice, which may have a propensity for worse disease (4, 30, 31). Innate immune signaling has been shown to be vary widely depending on age, making age-relevant models critical when studying inflammatory diseases (32–38).

Genetic deletion of NLRP3 inflammasome components leads to worse outcomes in IAV infection (9–11). This argues that abolishment of NLRP3 inflammasome signaling during IAV infection is harmful and that early NLRP3 inflammasome activation is necessary for controlling the infection and viral clearance. The finding from Tate et al. that early inhibition of NLRP3 with MCC950 increases mortality from IAV infection is consistent with this (12). In contrast, late inhibition was protective, which supports our finding that MCC950 treatment beginning 3 days p.i. improved survival in juvenile mice infected with IAV. The sensitivity of the outcome of NLRP3 modulation to timing and degree of inhibition is not unique to IAV infection, but a common theme in inflammatory responses to pathogens, where inadequate inflammation impairs pathogen clearance, but excessive inflammation causes collateral tissue damage and enhanced injury. This emphasizes the need for careful characterization of optimal treatment strategies in clinically relevant, age appropriate, models.

In contrast to our results from MCC950 treatment, anakinra treatment of IAV-infected juvenile mice did not show protection from IAV-induced mortality or lung injury. Despite achieving NLRP3 inflammasome suppression *in vitro*, anakinra therapy did not effectively decrease NLRP3 inflammasome activation or IL-18 secretion into the alveolar space in our *in vivo* model of juvenile IAV infection. Therefore, it was not surprising that we could not demonstrate protection from IAV with anakinra treatment. Instead, it suggests that once daily dosing with i.p. delivery was not sufficient to achieve caspase-1 inhibition. Alternatively, it argues that isolated IL-1 receptor antagonism is insufficient to protect juvenile mice from IAV infection because it leaves IL-18 signaling intact. There is one report of anakinra therapy (100 μg/mouse, intravenous, daily from day 2 to 6 p.i.) improving survival in IAV infection in adult mice (A/PR/8/34) (39), but only mortality was evaluated. Differences in our model, especially the age of the mice, may explain the discrepancy in our findings.

Influenza A virus is a source of significant morbidity and mortality in children, but current therapies are limited to early antiviral treatment and supportive care. There is considerable need for new strategies to improve outcomes in pediatric IAV infection, and the use of juvenile models to test these strategies is critical. Targeting the NLRP3 inflammasome may be beneficial in juvenile IAV infection and does not appear to impact viral clearance. Better understanding of how NLRP3 inflammasome inhibition improves mortality in juvenile IAV infection, and identification of the optimal timing and method of NLRP3 inflammasome inhibition in juvenile IAV infection, deserve further study.

ETHICS STATEMENT

This study was carried out in accordance with United States federal guidelines and was approved by The Institutional Animal Care and Use Committee at Northwestern University.

AUTHOR CONTRIBUTIONS

BC contributed to all aspects of this manuscript including experimental design, conduction of experiments, interpretation of data, and manuscript preparation. NR, YC, JD, and DS contributed to the conduction of the experiments, interpretation of data, and manuscript preparation. KS and CK contributed to experimental design, conduction of experiments, interpretation of data, and manuscript preparation. KR contributed to experimental design, interpretation of data, and manuscript preparation.

ACKNOWLEDGMENTS

Histology services were provided by the Northwestern University Research Histology and Phenotyping Laboratory, which is supported by NCI P30-CA060553 awarded to the Robert H. Lurie Comprehensive Cancer Center. Imaging work was performed at the Northwestern University Center for Advanced Microscopy, generously supported by NCI CCSG P30-CA060553 awarded

to the Robert H. Lurie Comprehensive Cancer Center. Flow cytometry was supported by the Northwestern University—Flow Cytometry Core Facility (Cancer Center Support Grant NCI CA060553).

REFERENCES

1. Rolfes MA, Foppa IM, Garg S, Flannery B, Brammer L, Singleton JA, et al. *Estimated Influenza Illnesses, Medical Visits, Hospitalizations, and Deaths Averted by Vaccination in the United States.* (2016). Available from: https://www.cdc.gov/flu/about/disease/2015-16.htm
2. Morgan CI, Hobson MJ, Seger B, Rice MA, Staat MA, Wheeler DS. 2009 pandemic influenza A (H1N1) in critically ill children in Cincinnati, Ohio. *Pediatr Criti Care Med* (2012) 13:e140–4. doi:10.1097/PCC.0b013e318228845f
3. Jefferson T, Jones MA, Doshi P, Del Mar CB, Hama R, Thompson MJ, et al. Neuraminidase inhibitors for preventing and treating influenza in healthy adults and children. *Cochrane Database Syst Rev* (2014) 4:CD008965. doi:10.1002/14651858.CD008965.pub4
4. Coates BM, Staricha KL, Wiese KM, Ridge KM. Influenza A virus infection, innate immunity, and childhood. *JAMA Pediatr* (2015) 169(10):956–63. doi:10.1001/jamapediatrics.2015.1387
5. Chakrabarti A, Banerjee S, Franchi L, Loo Y-M, Gale M, Núñez G, et al. RNase L activates the NLRP3 inflammasome during viral infections. *Cell Host Microbe* (2015) 17:466–77. doi:10.1016/j.chom.2015.02.010
6. McAuley JL, Tate MD, MacKenzie-Kludas CJ, Pinar A, Zeng W, Stutz A, et al. Activation of the NLRP3 inflammasome by IAV virulence protein PB1-F2 contributes to severe pathophysiology and disease. *PLoS Pathog* (2013) 9:e1003392. doi:10.1371/journal.ppat.1003392
7. Ichinohe T, Pang IK, Iwasaki A. Influenza virus activates inflammasomes via its intracellular M2 ion channel. *Nat Immunol* (2010) 11:404–10. doi:10.1038/ni.1861
8. Pinto LH, Lamb RA. The M2 proton channels of influenza A and B viruses. *J Biol Chem* (2006) 281:8997–9000. doi:10.1074/jbc.R500020200
9. Allen IC, Scull MA, Moore CB, Holl EK, McElvania-TeKippe E, Taxman DJ, et al. The NLRP3 inflammasome mediates in vivo innate immunity to influenza A virus through recognition of viral RNA. *Immunity* (2009) 30:556–65. doi:10.1016/j.immuni.2009.02.005
10. Thomas PG, Dash P, Aldridge JR, Ellebedy AH, Reynolds C, Funk AJ, et al. The intracellular sensor NLRP3 mediates key innate and healing responses to influenza A virus via the regulation of caspase-1. *Immunity* (2009) 30:566–75. doi:10.1016/j.immuni.2009.02.006
11. Ichinohe T, Lee HK, Ogura Y, Flavell R, Iwasaki A. Inflammasome recognition of influenza virus is essential for adaptive immune responses. *J Exp Med* (2009) 206:79–87. doi:10.1084/jem.20081667
12. Tate MD, Ong JDH, Dowling JK, McAuley JL, Robertson AB, Latz E, et al. Reassessing the role of the NLRP3 inflammasome during pathogenic influenza A virus infection via temporal inhibition. *Sci Rep* (2016) 6:27912. doi:10.1038/srep27912
13. Oshansky CM, Gartland AJ, Wong S-S, Jeevan T, Wang D, Roddam PL, et al. Mucosal immune responses predict clinical outcomes during influenza infection independently of age and viral load. *Am J Respir Crit Care Med* (2014) 189:449–62. doi:10.1164/rccm.201309-1616OC
14. Coll RC, Robertson AAB, Chae JJ, Higgins SC, Muñoz-Planillo R, Inserra MC, et al. A small-molecule inhibitor of the NLRP3 inflammasome for the treatment of inflammatory diseases. *Nat Med* (2015) 21:248–55. doi:10.1038/nm.3806
15. Primiano MJ, Lefker BA, Bowman MR, Bree AG, Hubeau C, Bonin PD, et al. Efficacy and pharmacology of the NLRP3 inflammasome inhibitor CP-456,773 (CRID3) in murine models of dermal and pulmonary inflammation. *J Immunol* (2016) 197:2421–33. doi:10.4049/jimmunol.1600035
16. Shao B-Z, Xu Z-Q, Han B-Z, Su D-F, Liu C. NLRP3 inflammasome and its inhibitors: a review. *Front Pharmacol* (2015) 6:262. doi:10.3389/fphar.2015.00262

17. Santos dos G, Rogel MR, Baker MA, Troken JR, Urich D, Morales-Nebreda L, et al. Vimentin regulates activation of the NLRP3 inflammasome. *Nat Commun* (2015) 6:6574. doi:10.1038/ncomms7574
18. Kanneganti T-D, Body-Malapel M, Amer A, Park J-H, Whitfield J, Franchi L, et al. Critical role for cryopyrin/Nalp3 in activation of caspase-1 in response to viral infection and double-stranded RNA. *J Biol Chem* (2006) 281:36560–8. doi:10.1074/jbc.M607594200
19. Misharin AV, Morales-Nebreda L, Mutlu GM, Budinger GRS, Perlman H. Flow cytometric analysis of macrophages and dendritic cell subsets in the mouse lung. *Am J Respir Cell Mol Biol* (2013) 49:503–10. doi:10.1165/rcmb.2013-0086MA
20. Weber A, Wasiliew P, Kracht M. Interleukin-1 (IL-1) pathway. *Sci Signal* (2010) 3:cm1. doi:10.1126/scisignal.3105cm1
21. Guo H, Callaway JB, Ting JP-Y. Inflammasomes: mechanism of action, role in disease, and therapeutics. *Nat Med* (2015) 21:677–87. doi:10.1038/nm.3893
22. Schmitz N, Kurrer M, Bachmann MF, Kopf M. Interleukin-1 is responsible for acute lung immunopathology but increases survival of respiratory influenza virus infection. *J Virol* (2005) 79:6441–8. doi:10.1128/JVI.79.10.6441-6448.2005
23. van de Sandt CE, Kreijtz JHCM, Rimmelzwaan GF. Evasion of influenza A viruses from innate and adaptive immune responses. *Viruses* (2012) 4:1438–76. doi:10.3390/v4091438
24. Herold S, Becker C, Ridge KM, Budinger GRS. Influenza virus-induced lung injury: pathogenesis and implications for treatment. *Eur Respir J* (2015) 45:1463–78. doi:10.1183/09031936.00186214
25. van Hout GPJ, Bosch L, Ellenbroek GHJM, de Haan JJ, van Solinge WW, Cooper MA, et al. The selective NLRP3-inflammasome inhibitor MCC950 reduces infarct size and preserves cardiac function in a pig model of myocardial infarction. *Eur Heart J* (2017) 38(11):828–36. doi:10.1093/eurheartj/ehw247
26. Mridha AR, Wree A, Robertson AAB, Yeh MM, Johnson CD, Van Rooyen DM, et al. NLRP3 inflammasome blockade reduces liver inflammation and fibrosis in experimental NASH in mice. *J Hepatol* (2017) 66(5):1037–46. doi:10.1016/j.jhep.2017.01.022
27. Abbate A, Salloum FN, Vecile E, Das A, Hoke NN, Straino S, et al. Anakinra, a recombinant human interleukin-1 receptor antagonist, inhibits apoptosis in experimental acute myocardial infarction. *Circulation* (2008) 117:2670–83. doi:10.1161/CIRCULATIONAHA.107.740233
28. Iannitti RG, Napolioni V, Oikonomou V, De Luca A, Galosi C, Pariano M, et al. IL-1 receptor antagonist ameliorates inflammasome-dependent inflammation in murine and human cystic fibrosis. *Nat Commun* (2016) 7:10791. doi:10.1038/ncomms10791
29. Pinar A, Dowling JK, Bitto NJ, Robertson AAB, Latz E, Stewart CR, et al. PB1-F2 peptide derived from avian influenza A virus H7N9 induces inflammation via activation of the NLRP3 inflammasome. *J Biol Chem* (2017) 292:826–36. doi:10.1074/jbc.M116.756379
30. Yasui H, Kiyoshima J, Hori T. Reduction of influenza virus titer and protection against influenza virus infection in infant mice fed *Lactobacillus casei* Shirota. *Clin Diagn Lab Immunol* (2004) 11:675–9. doi:10.1128/CDLI.11.4.675-679.2004
31. Sun S, Zhao G, Xiao W, Hu J, Guo Y, Yu H, et al. Age-related sensitivity and pathological differences in infections by 2009 pandemic influenza A (H1N1) virus. *Virol J* (2011) 8:52. doi:10.1186/1743-422X-8-52
32. Corbett NP, Blimkie D, Ho KC, Cai B, Sutherland DP, Kallos A, et al. Ontogeny of toll-like receptor mediated cytokine responses of human blood mononuclear cells. *PLoS One* (2010) 5:e15041. doi:10.1371/journal.pone.0015041

33. Prendergast AJ, Klenerman P, Goulder PJR. The impact of differential antiviral immunity in children and adults. *Nat Rev Immunol* (2012) 12:636–48. doi:10.1038/nri3277

34. Philbin VJ, Levy O. Developmental biology of the innate immune response: implications for neonatal and infant vaccine development. *Pediatr Res* (2009) 65:98R–105R. doi:10.1203/PDR.0b013e31819f195d

35. Burl S, Townend J, Njie-Jobe J, Cox M, Adetifa UJ, Touray E, et al. Age-dependent maturation of toll-like receptor-mediated cytokine responses in Gambian infants. *PLoS One* (2011) 6:e18185. doi:10.1371/journal.pone.0018185

36. Levy O. Innate immunity of the human newborn: distinct cytokine responses to LPS and other toll-like receptor agonists. *J Endotoxin Res* (2005) 11:113–6. doi:10.1179/096805105X37376

37. Belderbos ME, van Bleek GM, Levy O, Blanken MO, Houben ML, Schuijff L, et al. Skewed pattern of toll-like receptor 4-mediated cytokine production in human neonatal blood: low LPS-induced IL-12p70 and high IL-10 persist throughout the first month of life. *Clin Immunol* (2009) 133:228–37. doi:10.1016/j.clim.2009.07.003

38. Kollmann TR, Crabtree J, Rein-Weston A, Blimkie D, Thommai F, Wang XY, et al. Neonatal innate TLR-mediated responses are distinct from those of adults. *J Immunol* (2009) 183:7150–60. doi:10.4049/jimmunol.0901481

39. Shirey KA, Lai W, Patel MC, Pletneva LM, Pang C, Kurt-Jones E, et al. Novel strategies for targeting innate immune responses to influenza. *Mucosal Immunol* (2016) 9:1173–82. doi:10.1038/mi.2015.141

Epithelial Sodium Channel-α Mediates the Protective Effect of the TNF-Derived TIP Peptide in Pneumolysin-Induced Endothelial Barrier Dysfunction

Istvan Czikora[1]*, Abdel A. Alli[2,3], Supriya Sridhar[1], Michael A. Matthay[4], Helena Pillich[5], Martina Hudel[5], Besim Berisha[5], Boris Gorshkov[1], Maritza J. Romero[1,6], Joyce Gonzales[7], Guangyu Wu[6], Yuqing Huo[1,7], Yunchao Su[6], Alexander D. Verin[1,7], David Fulton[1,6], Trinad Chakraborty[5], Douglas C. Eaton[8] and Rudolf Lucas[1,6,7]*

[1] Vascular Biology Center, Medical College of Georgia, Augusta University, Augusta, GA, United States, [2] Department of Physiology and Functional Genomics, University of Florida College of Medicine, Gainesville, FL, United States, [3] Division of Nephrology, Hypertension, and Renal Transplantation, Department of Medicine, University of Florida College of Medicine, Gainesville, FL, United States, [4] Cardiovascular Research Institute, UCSF, San Francisco, CA, United States, [5] Institute for Medical Microbiology, Justus-Liebig University, Giessen, Germany, [6] Department of Pharmacology and Toxicology, Medical College of Georgia, Augusta University, Augusta, GA, United States, [7] Department of Medicine, Medical College of Georgia, Augusta University, Augusta, GA, United States, [8] Department of Physiology, Emory University School of Medicine, Atlanta, GA, United States

*Correspondence:
Rudolf Lucas
rlucas@augusta.edu;
Istvan Czikora
iczikora@augusta.edu

Background: *Streptococcus pneumoniae* is a major etiologic agent of bacterial pneumonia. Autolysis and antibiotic-mediated lysis of pneumococci induce release of the pore-forming toxin, pneumolysin (PLY), their major virulence factor, which is a prominent cause of acute lung injury. PLY inhibits alveolar liquid clearance and severely compromises alveolar–capillary barrier function, leading to permeability edema associated with pneumonia. As a consequence, alveolar flooding occurs, which can precipitate lethal hypoxemia by impairing gas exchange. The α subunit of the epithelial sodium channel (ENaC) is crucial for promoting Na^+ reabsorption across Na^+-transporting epithelia. However, it is not known if human lung microvascular endothelial cells (HL-MVEC) also express ENaC-α and whether this subunit is involved in the regulation of their barrier function.

Methods: The presence of α, β, and γ subunits of ENaC and protein phosphorylation status in HL-MVEC were assessed in western blotting. The role of ENaC-α in monolayer resistance of HL-MVEC was examined by depletion of this subunit by specific siRNA and by employing the TNF-derived TIP peptide, a specific activator that directly binds to ENaC-α.

Results: HL-MVEC express all three subunits of ENaC, as well as acid-sensing ion channel 1a (ASIC1a), which has the capacity to form hybrid non-selective cation channels with ENaC-α. Both TIP peptide, which specifically binds to ENaC-α, and the specific ASIC1a activator MitTx significantly strengthened barrier function in PLY-treated HL-MVEC. ENaC-α depletion significantly increased sensitivity to PLY-induced hyperpermeability and in addition, blunted the protective effect of both the TIP peptide and MitTx, indicating an important role for ENaC-α and for hybrid NSC channels in barrier function of HL-MVEC. TIP peptide blunted PLY-induced phosphorylation of both calmodulin-dependent kinase II (CaMKII) and of its substrate, the actin-binding protein filamin A (FLN-A), requiring the expression of both ENaC-α and ASIC1a. Since non-phosphorylated FLN-A promotes ENaC channel open probability and blunts stress fiber formation, modulation of this activity represents an attractive target for the protective actions of ENaC-α in both barrier function and liquid clearance.

Conclusion: Our results in cultured endothelial cells demonstrate a previously unrecognized role for ENaC-α in strengthening capillary barrier function that may apply to the human lung. Strategies aiming to activate endothelial NSC channels that contain ENaC-α should be further investigated as a novel approach to improve barrier function in the capillary endothelium during pneumonia.

Keywords: epithelial sodium channel, non-selective cation channel, TNF, pneumonia, pneumolysin, endothelial barrier function

INTRODUCTION

Pulmonary permeability edema is a life-threatening complication of severe pneumonia and acute respiratory distress syndrome (ARDS), characterized by impaired alveolar liquid clearance (ALC) and alveolar–capillary hyperpermeability (1). Antibiotic treatment of patients infected with *Streptococcus pneumoniae* significantly reduces bacterial load, but it can also cause massive release of bacterial toxins in the lung compartment (2). The 53-kDa pneumococcal pore-forming virulence factor pneumolysin (PLY) was shown to be an important mediator of permeability edema, due to its capacity to impair both endothelial (3, 4) and epithelial barrier function (5). Although pneumococci release sufficient amounts of PLY to perforate the host cell plasma membrane, this does not necessarily cause immediate cell death, since membrane segments harboring toxin-induced pores can be either internalized or eliminated by microvesicle shedding. Dysregulation of cellular homeostasis secondary to transient pore formation/elimination is likely responsible for the damaging actions of PLY (6). To date, no proven treatment exists for increased pulmonary permeability edema, apart from ventilation strategies. Hence, the search for novel therapeutic agents that have the ability to restore both endothelial barrier function and ALC capacity is warranted.

Apart from impairing barrier function, PLY has also been shown to decrease the activity of the epithelial sodium channel (ENaC) (7), which is expressed on the apical side of alveolar epithelial cells and which, together with the basolaterally expressed Na^+–K^+-ATPase (8, 9), represents the primary mediator of Na^+ uptake and liquid clearance in the alveolar compartment. In its native form, ENaC consists of three subunits, α, β, and γ (10, 11), but also a fourth δ subunit has been described, which can substitute for the α subunit (12). ENaC activity is defined as the product of its surface expression N, which is at least partially determined by Nedd-4-2-dependent ubiquitination (13) and its open probability Po, the latter of which is significantly increased by the formation of a complex comprised of ENaC subunits with MARCKS and PIP_2 (14). In order to be fully functional, ENaC

has to interact with the actin cytoskeleton and in particular with the actin-binding protein, filamin A (FLN-A) (15).

We recently demonstrated that the 17 residue circular TIP peptide (sequence: CGQRETPEGAEAKPWYC), which mimics the lectin-like domain of TNF, directly binds to two domains within the crucial α subunit of ENaC (16–18). The TIP peptide, through binding to residues Val567 and Glu568 increases the channel's open probability time by promoting complex formation between human ENaC-α and MARCKS (18). In addition, the peptide augments ENaC-α surface expression in PLY-treated H441 cells, by means of reducing the subunit's ubiquitination (18). This activity requires the presence of N-glycosylated Asn residues in the extracellular loop of the subunit (17). The presence of the TIP peptide has been shown to increase ALC and to ameliorate acute lung injury *in vivo* in several species (16, 19–23). The TIP peptide is well tolerated, and no significant side effects have been reported upon inhalation in healthy male volunteers (24). The TIP peptide is emerging as a potential therapeutic candidate for improving lung function. Data from two phase IIa clinical trials with inhalation of TIP peptide (a.k.a. AP301 and solnatide) in acute lung injury patients, the majority of which had severe pneumonia, and another trial in patients with primary graft dysfunction upon lung transplantation (www.ClinicalTrials.gov, Identifier NCT01627613 and NCT02095626, respectively) document efficacy. Both of these pathologies are characterized by capillary endothelial dysfunction.

Although originally thought to mainly constitute the rate-limiting entry step in Na^+ reabsorption across lung, kidney, and colon epithelia, it has become clear in recent years that ENaC may also play an important role in the vasculature. In large vessels, ENaC is expressed in both endothelial and vascular smooth muscle cell compartments, where it operates as a mechano-sensitive channel, exposed to varying rates of blood flow and laminar shear stress (25). In contrast to large vessels, the presence or role of ENaC in the microvasculature, such as in the capillaries in the lung, remains understudied and represents the primary focus of this study. The TIP peptide was shown to increase Na^+ uptake in pulmonary microvascular endothelial cells (26) and to restore impaired endothelial barrier function in the presence of the pore-forming toxins PLY and listeriolysin-O (3, 27).

In view of the previously observed protective activities of the TNF-derived TIP peptide on capillary barrier function in the presence of bacterial toxins, in this study, we investigated the role of its binding partner—ENaC-α—in microvascular endothelial cell barrier function. Our objective was to identify those common signaling molecules modified by bacterial toxins that are involved in both endothelial barrier impairment and ENaC dysfunction.

MATERIALS AND METHODS

Cells

Human lung microvascular endothelial cells (HL-MVEC) were grown in complete EBM-2 medium (Lonza, Walkersville, MD, USA) at 37°C and 5% CO_2. Experiments with PLY were performed in serum-free medium, since the toxin's activity is neutralized by cholesterol.

PLY Purification

Pneumolysin was purified from a recombinant *Listeria innocua* 6a strain expressing LPS-free PLY. The batch of PLY used in this study had a specific activity of 1.25×10^7 hemolytic units per milligram.

Biochemicals

Rabbit polyclonal anti-ENaC-α (59), β (60), and γ (2102) antibodies were generated in the laboratory of D.C.E (14), anti-human FLN-A, anti-human phospho-FLN-A, anti-human CaMKII, anti-human phospho-CaMKII, and anti-Actin HRP were from Cell Signaling Technology (Danvers, MA, USA). Rabbit anti-human ENaC-α was from Novus Biologicals (Littleton, CO, USA), a rabbit anti-human ASIC1 for IP was from EMD Millipore (Temecula, CA, USA), and a rabbit anti-hASIC1 antibody for WB was a kind gift from Dr. John Wemmie, University of Iowa. Goat anti-rabbit secondary antibodies conjugated to HRP were from Cell Signaling Technology (Danvers, MA, USA). MitTx was purchased from Alomone (Jerusalem, Israel), CaMKII inhibitor XII was from EMD Millipore (Billerica, MA, USA), and the TIP peptide was custom-ordered and purchased from AMBIOPHARM (North-Augusta, SC, USA).

Depletion of ENaC-α or Acid-Sensing Ion Channel 1a (ASIC1a) in HL-MVEC

Human lung microvascular endothelial cells were treated with a pool of target-specific 19–25 nt siRNAs designed to knock down either ENaC-α conducting subunit or ASIC1a gene expression, and non-specific, non-targeting siRNA were obtained from Ambion (Grand Island, NY, USA). All siRNA's were received in lyophilized form. HL-MVEC were transfected at 70–80% confluence with 50–75 nM final concentration of siRNA using siPORT™ Amine transfection reagent (Ambion, Life Technologies, Grand Island, NY, USA) and used for further experiments at 48 h post transfection.

Immunoprecipitation

Human lung microvascular endothelial cells were grown in 60-mm culture flasks and were washed with PBS, scraped, and lysed in 400 µl of 20 mM Tris–HCl, pH 7.4 buffer containing 0.15 M NaCl, 1% non-idet P-40, 2 mM EDTA, as well as protease inhibitors. Lysates were incubated with empty beads in order to remove the non-specific binding partners (preclearing step) and subsequently with ASIC1 antibody for 1 h at 4°C. The mixture of the antibody and the precleared whole cell lysate was then incubated with agarose G magnetic beads overnight at 4°C, followed by three washing steps with PBS containing 2% BSA and eluted in 150 µl of Laemmli buffer. The resulting supernatants were analyzed by western blotting with ENaC-α antibody.

Immunoblotting Procedure

Immediately after treatment, HL-MVEC were washed twice with ice-cold PBS and lysed with RIPA buffer containing a phosphatase and a protease inhibitor mixture. After centrifugation, clear supernatants were mixed with SDS sample buffer and boiled for 5 min. Protein extracts were separated on SDS/PAGE, transferred to a nitrocellulose membrane, incubated with primary antibodies, and subsequently after washing with HRP-conjugated secondary Ab. Immunoreactive proteins were visualized with Clarity solution (Bio-Rad, Hercules, CA, USA) and were then captured using ChemiDoc system (Bio-Rad). The relative intensity of each protein band was quantified using the ImageLab software (Bio-Rad).

NanoPro Technology

Immediately after treatment, cells were washed and lysed with buffers from ProteinSimple (Santa Clara, CA, USA) as described previously (28). Preparation of cell lysates for size-based assay, using the Peggy system, was performed as described by the manufacturer (ProteinSimple).

Measurement of Transendothelial Electrical Resistance

Transendothelial electrical resistance in HL-MVEC monolayers [electrical cell-substrate impedance sensing (ECIS) system 1600R; Applied Biophysics, Troy, NY, USA] was measured as described previously (3).

Statistical Analysis

All experimental data are presented as mean ± SD. Control samples and those obtained upon various stimuli were compared by unpaired Student's *t*-test. For multiple group comparisons, one-way ANOVA was used. Also, $p < 0.05$ was considered statistically significant.

RESULTS

HL-MVEC Express All ENaC Subunits

We previously demonstrated, using whole cell voltage-clamped patch clamp, that TIP peptide increased amiloride-sensitive Na^+ currents in freshly isolated mouse MVEC (26). Here, we investigated whether HL-MVEC express the three ENaC subunits. Immunoblotting analysis revealed the presence of both uncleaved and mature ENaC-α, β, and γ subunits in human lung MVEC (**Figure 1**). The immunoreactive bands of ENaC-α at 95, 75, and 65 kDa represent different forms of the subunit, resulting from posttranslational modifications (e.g., glycosylation) and proteolytic processing.

ENaC-α Expression Strengthens Barrier Function in PLY-Treated HL-MVEC Monolayers

The association of ENaC with the cytoskeletal network at the apical membrane is required to help maintain its presence at this site and to prevent its removal by endocytosis (30, 31). It has not yet been investigated whether activation of the channel also affects endothelial barrier function. We therefore investigated whether ENaC expression in HL-MVEC monolayers affects barrier function, by depleting ENaC-α using specific siRNA, employing scrambled non-specific siRNA as a control. The efficacy of the siRNA-mediated depletion is shown in **Figure 2A**. As shown in **Figure 2B**, transfection with ENaC-α siRNA significantly reduced expression of ENaC-α in HL-MVEC, using the prominent 75 kDa band corresponding to the mature subunit for quantification. Depletion of ENaC-α significantly increased sensitivity of HL-MVEC to PLY at 30 min post addition of the toxin (**Figure 2C**). This was measured as normalized monolayer resistance, using ECIS (ECIS1600R, Applied Biophysics, Troy, NY, USA), in cells treated with 60 ng/ml PLY for 30 min. Silencing of ENaC-α did not affect basal barrier function (data not shown). The protective action of the TIP peptide (50 μg/ml) in PLY-induced barrier dysfunction, which we reported previously (3) and which was also observed in the presence of scrambled siRNA, was eliminated after depleting ENaC-α (**Figure 2C**). These results suggest an important role for ENaC-α in restoring capillary barrier function in the face of PLY challenge.

ENaC-α Stimulation Blunts PLY-Induced CaMKII Activation and FLN-A Phosphorylation

Apart from its role in endothelial barrier function demonstrated above, ENaC-α has also been shown to be crucial for ALC (32), since mice lacking the subunit die shortly after birth with flooded lungs. ALC is, in part, modulated by ENaC activity. As such, we wanted to identify an interacting partner that binds to ENaC-α and that regulates both barrier function and Na$^+$ uptake. The actin-binding protein FLN-A, in its non-phosphorylated form, is a prominent regulator of endothelial barrier function, since it prevents stress fiber formation (33). FLN-A directly associates with ENaC subunits and promotes their association with the chaperone protein MARCKS, thereby inducing complex formation of the channel with PIP$_2$ (15). This complex formation is crucial for regulating the open probability of ENaC (14). Increased intracellular Ca^{2+} levels mobilize calmodulin, which in turn activates calmodulin-dependent kinase II (CaMKII), which then

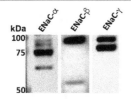

FIGURE 1 | Representative western blot of basal expression of α, β, and γ epithelial sodium channel (ENaC) subunits in human lung microvascular endothelial cells. The immunoreactive bands at 95, 75, and 65 kDa are different forms of the subunits resulting from posttranslational modifications (e.g., glycosylation) and proteolytic processing. We previously confirmed the identity of similar bands excised from Coomassie stained gels after immunoprecipitation using the ENaC-α 59 and ENaC-β 60 antibodies and then performing LC/MS. We further corroborated the specificity of these antibodies by performing competition experiments using the recombinant fusion proteins that were used as the immunogens to generate the ENaC-α 59 and ENaC-β 60 antibodies (14). The characterization of the ENaC-γ 2102 antibody was described elsewhere (29). Although these ENaC antibodies cross-react with mouse, rat, and human species, we do expect there to be some variations in the previously reported sizes of the bands for ENaC expressed in the kidneys and, as shown here, in the lungs. These variations might be due to differences in proteases within the kidneys and lungs that cleave ENaC.

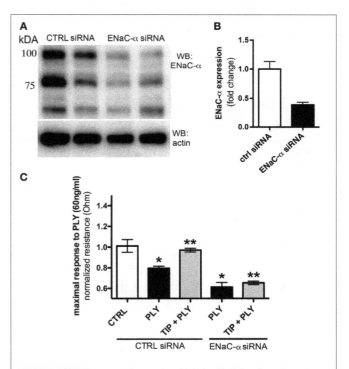

FIGURE 2 | **(A)** Representative western blot of epithelial sodium channel (ENaC)-α expression in human lung microvascular endothelial cells (HL-MVEC), transfected with either scrambled siRNA (control) or ENaC-α siRNA. **(B)** Efficacy of siRNA-mediated depletion of ENaC-α, relative protein expression in HL-MVEC. **(C)** Transendothelial resistance (measured in electrical cell-substrate impedance sensing 1600R) in HL-MVEC, transfected with scrambled siRNA or ENaC-α siRNA and treated for 30 min with 60 ng/ml of PLY (corresponding with the maximal drop in resistance), in the presence or absence of TIP peptide (*$p < 0.05$ versus ctrl, **$p < 0.05$ versus PLY).

phosphorylates its substrate, FLN-A (15, 33). Phosphorylated FLN-A blunts the association of ENaC with MARCKS, and impairs ENaC activity (15).

Pneumolysin (100 or 200 ng/ml) induces FLN-A phosphorylation from as early as 15 min and persisting for at least 60 min (**Figure 3A**). TIP peptide (50 µg/ml), as well as the CaMKII inhibitor XII (1mM) inhibits FLN-A phosphorylation induced by PLY (60 ng/ml) (**Figures 3B,C**). As shown in **Figure 4A**, PLY-treatment (90 ng/ml) induces CaMKII activation in HL-MVEC within 10 min. Thus, both PLY-induced phosphorylation of FLN-A and CaMKII can be partially inhibited by the TIP peptide or by a CaMKII inhibitor (**Figures 3A,B and 4A,B**). Taken together, these data indicate that PLY, whose deleterious actions on barrier function in HL-MVEC monolayers are at least partially dependent on promoting Ca^{2+} influx (3), has the capacity to activate CaMKII, which in turn increases phosphorylation of FLN-A. TIP peptide binding to ENaC-α at least partially blunts these events.

The Hybrid ENaC-α/ASIC1a Non-Selective Cation Channel Mediates Barrier Protection from PLY

In order to address the apparent discrepancy between our results with the TIP peptide, which improves barrier function in HL-MVEC, and results obtained by others demonstrating that aldosterone-induced activation of ENaC leads to stiffening in large vessel endothelial cells (34), we investigated the potential implication of other, non-selective cation channels (NSC) in the ability of the TIP peptide to preserve barrier function in PLY-treated HL-MVEC monolayers. Indeed, ENaC-α is not only a subunit of ENaC but also a component of hybrid NSC channels, where it forms a complex with the ASIC1a subunit (35–37). These hybrid NSC channels, when expressed in type 2 alveolar epithelial cells, were recently shown to contribute significantly to ALC (37).

MitTx (20 nM), an activator of ASIC1a and of NSC (38, 39), significantly reduced PLY-mediated (60 ng/ml) barrier dysfunction in HL-MVEC, to the same extent as the TIP peptide (50 µg/ml) (**Figure 5A**). siRNA-mediated depletion of ENaC-α abrogated the protective effect of both MitTx and TIP peptide in PLY-treated HL-MVEC monolayers (**Figure 5A**). Moreover, siRNA-mediated depletion of ASIC1a, which is expressed in HL-MVEC (**Figure 5D**) abrogated the inhibitory effect of the TIP peptide on PLY-induced FLN-A phosphorylation (**Figures 5B,C**). Of note, PLY induced significantly higher FLN-A phosphorylation in cells lacking ASIC1a (**Figure 5B**). These results indicate that NSC channels at least partially

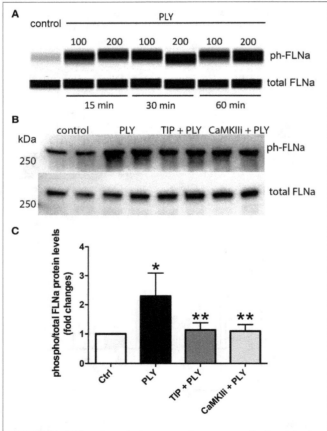

FIGURE 3 | **(A)** Time-dependent representative nanopro technology-based western blot of PLY-induced filamin A (FLN-A) phosphorylation in human lung microvascular endothelial cells (HL-MVEC) (100 and 200 ng/ml), as described (28). **(B)** Representative western blot. **(C)** Quantification of phospho- over total protein ratio of PLY (60 ng/ml)-mediated FLN-A phosphorylation in HL-MVEC after 20 min. Cells were either pretreated with TIP peptide (50 µg/ml) or the CaMKII inhibitor (1 mM) for 15 min. Values are presented as means ± SD of three independent experiments in duplicates (*$p < 0.05$ versus ctrl, **$p < 0.05$ versus PLY).

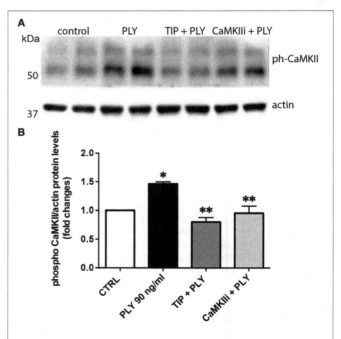

FIGURE 4 | **(A)** Representative western blot and **(B)** quantification of phospho-CaMKII over actin ratio of PLY (90 ng/ml)-mediated CaMKII activation in human lung microvascular endothelial cells after 20 min. Cells were either pretreated with TIP peptide (50 µg/ml) or the CaMKII inhibitor XII (1 mM) for 15 min. Values are presented as means ± SD of three independent experiments in duplicates (*$p < 0.05$ versus ctrl, **$p < 0.05$ versus PLY).

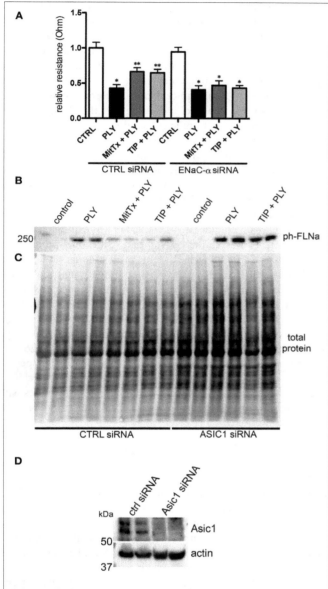

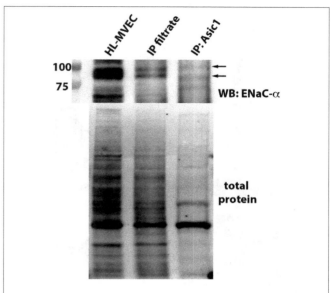

FIGURE 5 | **(A)** Transendothelial resistance (measured in electrical cell-substrate impedance sensing 1600R) in human lung microvascular endothelial cells (HL-MVEC), transfected with scrambled siRNA or epithelial sodium channel (ENaC)-α siRNA and treated for 30 min with 60 ng/ml of PLY, in the presence or absence of TIP peptide (50 µg/ml) or MitTx (20 nM) ($n = 3$, SEM) (*$p < 0.05$ versus ctrl, **$p < 0.05$ versus PLY). **(B)** Representative western blot and quantification of phospho- over total protein ratio of PLY (60 ng/ml)-mediated filamin A (FLN-A) phosphorylation in HL-MVEC after 20 min. Cells were either pretreated with TIP peptide (50 µg/ml) or MitTx (20 nM) for 15 min. **(C)** Representative stain-free blot showing total protein transferred to the nitrocellulose membrane. **(D)** siRNA-mediated acid-sensing ion channel 1a (ASIC1a) silencing in HL-MVEC.

mediate barrier protection against PLY in HL-MVEC and that both ENaC-α and ASIC1a subunits are crucial for this activity. To confirm this interaction, we performed a co-IP experiment using ASIC1a antibody as bait. We detected two bands corresponding to uncleaved (95 kDa) and mature (around 75 kDa) ENaC-α in the immunoprecipates (**Figure 6**).

FIGURE 6 | Representative immunoprecipitation experiment assessing binding of epithelial sodium channel (ENaC)-α (indicated by arrows) to native ASIC1 in human lung microvascular endothelial cells (HL-MVEC) and representative stain-free blot showing the total protein transferred to the nitrocellulose membrane before the co-IP experiment (whole HL-MVEC lysate—first lane), the filtrate after the co-IP (second lane), and the eluent (eluted from the ASIC1 antibody-decorated magnetic beads—third lane).

DISCUSSION

Decreased lung capillary barrier function represents one of the major complications of severe pneumonia and ARDS and promotes the development of permeability edema. Upon autolysis or antibiotic-induced lysis, the G+ pathogen *S. pneumoniae*, the main etiological agent of community acquired pneumonia in the US, releases the cholesterol-binding and pore-forming toxin PLY.

Pneumolysin-induced Ca^{2+}-influx, which is blunted by lanthanum chloride, is crucial for the ability of the toxin to induce hyperpermeability in human lung MVEC (3). PLY reduces endothelial barrier function in part by means of activating protein kinase C-α, which in turn impairs NO generation by endothelial nitric oxide synthase (eNOS) (3, 4), which was shown to be required for basal barrier function (40). Increased Ca^{2+} influx can also mobilize calmodulin, which activates CaMKII. Activated CaMKII phosphorylates the actin-binding protein FLN-A. Although the non-phosphorylated form of FLN-A prevents stress fiber formation, increased Ca^{2+} influx promotes the shift to its phosphorylated form, which is incapable of supporting barrier integrity (15).

Apart from preventing stress fiber formation, FLN-A also promotes the interaction between the chaperone protein MARCKS and ENaC subunits (15), which in turn increases the open probability time of the channel. As summarized in **Figure 7**, our findings suggest that ENaC-α, as a subunit of NSC, can be activated by the TIP peptide, whereas the ASIC1a subunit of NSC is activated by MitTx. Both of these mechanisms of NSC activation promote barrier protection, by means of reducing PLY-induced activation of CaMKII, FLN-A phosphorylation, and finally lung capillary barrier dysfunction, respectively. A role for ENaC-α in epidermal barrier protection

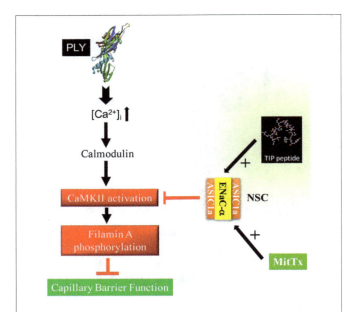

FIGURE 7 | Proposed sequence of events in the role of epithelial sodium channel (ENaC)-α in barrier protection in pneumolysin (PLY)-treated human lung microvascular endothelial cells. PLY, upon pore formation, increases Ca²⁺-influx (3), which in turn mobilizes calmodulin. Calmodulin activates CaMKII, which in turn phosphorylates its substrate filamin A (FLN-A) (15). Phosphorylated FLN-A promotes stress fiber formation and increases capillary permeability. Activation of NSC, by either TIP peptide (binding to ENaC-α) or MitTx [binding to acid-sensing ion channel 1a (ASIC1a)], abrogates PLY-mediated CaMKII activation and protects as such from PLY-induced hyperpermeability.

was shown previously (41). Of note, a recent study demonstrated that both the β1 subunit of the Na⁺–K⁺-ATPase as well as the α subunit of ENaC strengthen capillary endothelial barrier function in mice in the presence of LPS (42). These data together with those presented here suggest an important role for ENaC-α in protecting endothelial barrier function in the presence of bacterial toxins.

Our results with the TNF-derived TIP peptide, which directly binds to ENaC-α and which has the capacity to increase both expression and open probability of ENaC in the presence of PLY, are in sharp contrast to the suggested role of ENaC in aldosterone-induced vascular stiffening and eNOS dysfunction in large vessel endothelial cells (34). Although it cannot be excluded that aldosterone, apart from activating ENaC also activates other pathways possible leading to endothelial dysfunction (43), and that large vessel endothelial cells, as investigated in the Kusche-Vihrog studies, are phenotypically different from microvascular endothelial cells, our results indicate that ENaC-α participates in barrier strengthening in HL-MVEC at least partially in the context of a complex different from classical ENaC.

Acid-sensing ion channels represent a family of proteins activated upon extracellular acidification (35). Although primarily found in neurons, ASIC1 expression was also demonstrated in type 2 alveolar epithelial cells, where they play an important role in vectorial Na⁺ transport-mediated ALC (37), as well as in cerebral arteries (44) and in pulmonary arterial smooth muscle cells (45). We demonstrate here that human pulmonary microvascular endothelial cells also express ASIC1a. MitTx, an ASIC1 and NSC activator, which does not interact with ENaC, strengthens barrier function in PLY-treated HL-MVEC. However, the protective effects of MitTx are blunted in cells in which ENaC-α was depleted, indicating that its actions are not mediated by the typical ASIC1a channel complex, but rather by an ASIC1a/ENaC-α hybrid. Moreover, the inhibitory effect of the TIP peptide on PLY-induced FLN-A phosphorylation is abrogated in cells in which ASIC1a was depleted, indicating that the classical ENaC channel complex is not sufficient to mediate its effect. These results indicate that, rather than the classical ASIC1a and ENaC channels, a hybrid NSC channel, consisting of both ASIC1a and ENaC-α, is likely to mainly mediate the protective effects of both the TIP peptide and MitTx in lung capillary endothelial cells. This mechanism could be especially relevant in conditions of acidification, as can be found during bacterial pneumonia. Acidification of exhaled breath condensate in ventilated acute lung injury and ARDS patients was shown to correlate with local pulmonary inflammation (46). As such, it seems plausible that under these conditions, ASCIC1a, as well as NSC can be activated.

In conclusion, our data indicate that the barrier protective effect of ENaC-α in PLY-treated HL-MVEC monolayers is at least partially mediated by NSC channels in these cells. As such, the TIP peptide, which has the capacity to activate both ALC across alveolar epithelium and endothelial barrier function in the presence of bacterial toxins, could represent a therapeutically promising candidate to tackle pulmonary permeability edema associated with bacterial pneumonia. *In vivo* studies will be needed to further test this mechanism under pathologically relevant conditions.

AUTHOR CONTRIBUTIONS

Conception or design of the work: IC, AAA, MM, DF, TC, DE, and RL; acquisition, analysis, or interpretation of data: IC, SS, BG, HP, MH, BB, MR, and JG: drafting the work: IC and RL; revising it critically for important intellectual content: AAA, MR, GW, YH, YS, AV, DF, and DE. All authors approved the final version of the manuscript and agreed to be accountable for all aspects of the work in ensuring that questions related to the accuracy or integrity of any part of the work are appropriately investigated and resolved.

ACKNOWLEDGMENTS

The authors thank Dr. Wemmie, University of Iowa, for the kind gift of anti-ASIC1a antibodies and Dr. Hummler-Beermann, University of Lausanne, for helpful discussions.

FUNDING

This work was supported by PO1 grant HL101902 from the NHLBI (to AV and DF) and in part by K01 DK099617 (to AAA), Extramural Success Award from the Vice President for Research at Augusta University (to RL), AHA Scientist Development Grant 17SDG33680024 (to IC), as well as by SFB grant TR-84 "Innate Immunity of the Lung" from the German Research Foundation (DFG) (to HP and TC). The work was also supported by ADA grant #1-16-IBS-196 (to RL, AV, and DF) and NHLBI grant HL51856 (to MAM). RL is a Mercator Fellow of the DFG.

REFERENCES

1. Matthay MA, Ware LB, Zimmerman GA. The acute respiratory distress syndrome. *J Clin Invest* (2012) 122(8):2731–40. doi:10.1172/JCI60331
2. Anderson R, Steel HC, Cockeran R, von Gottberg A, de Gouveia L, Klugman KP, et al. Comparison of the effects of macrolides, amoxicillin, ceftriaxone, doxycycline, tobramycin and fluoroquinolones, on the production of pneumolysin by *Streptococcus pneumoniae in vitro*. *J Antimicrob Chemother* (2007) 60(5):1155–8. doi:10.1093/jac/dkm338
3. Lucas R, Yang G, Gorshkov BA, Zemskov EA, Sridhar S, Umapathy NS, et al. Protein kinase C-α and arginase I mediate pneumolysin-induced pulmonary endothelial hyperpermeability. *Am J Respir Cell Mol Biol* (2012) 47(4):445–53. doi:10.1165/rcmb.2011-0332OC
4. Chen F, Kumar S, Yu Y, Aggarwal S, Gross C, Wang Y, et al. PKC-dependent phosphorylation of eNOS at T495 regulates eNOS coupling and endothelial barrier function in response to G$^+$-toxins. *PLoS One* (2014) 9(7):e99823. doi:10.1371/journal.pone.0099823
5. Statt S, Ruan JW, Hung LY, Chang CY, Huang CT, Lim JH, et al. Statin-conferred enhanced cellular resistance against bacterial pore-forming toxins in airway epithelial cells. *Am J Respir Cell Mol Biol* (2015) 53(5):689–702. doi:10.1165/rcmb.2014-0391OC
6. Wolfmeier H, Radecke J, Schoenauer R, Koeffel R, Babiychuk VS, Drücker P, et al. Active release of pneumolysin prepores and pores by mammalian cells undergoing a *Streptococcus pneumoniae* attack. *Biochim Biophys Acta* (2016) 1860(11 Pt A):2498–509. doi:10.1016/j.bbagen.2016.07.022
7. Lucas R, Sridhar S, Rick FG, Gorshkov B, Umapathy NS, Yang G, et al. Agonist of growth hormone-releasing hormone reduces pneumolysin-induced pulmonary permeability edema. *Proc Natl Acad Sci U S A* (2012) 109(6):2084–9. doi:10.1073/pnas.1121075109
8. Vadász I, Raviv S, Sznajder JI. Alveolar epithelium and Na,K-ATPase in acute lung injury. *Intensive Care Med* (2007) 33(7):1243–51. doi:10.1007/s00134-007-0661-8
9. Azzam ZS, Sznajder JI. Lung edema clearance: relevance to patients with lung injury. *Rambam Maimonides Med J* (2015) 6(3):e0025. doi:10.5041/RMMJ.10210
10. Eaton DC, Helms MN, Koval M, Bao HF, Jain L. The contribution of epithelial sodium channels to alveolar function in health and disease. *Annu Rev Physiol* (2009) 71:403–23. doi:10.1146/annurev.physiol.010908.163250
11. Kashlan OB, Kleyman TR. Epithelial Na$^+$ channel regulation by cytoplasmic and extracellular factors. *Exp Cell Res* (2012) 318(9):1011–9. doi:10.1016/j.yexcr.2012.02.024
12. Ji HL, Zhao RZ, Chen ZX, Shetty S, Idell S, Matalon S. δ ENaC: a novel divergent amiloride-inhibitable sodium channel. *Am J Physiol Lung Cell Mol Physiol* (2012) 303(12):L1013–26. doi:10.1152/ajplung.00206.2012
13. Snyder PM. Down-regulating destruction: phosphorylation regulates the E3 ubiquitin ligase Nedd4-2. *Sci Signal* (2009) 2(79):e41. doi:10.1126/scisignal.279pe41
14. Alli AA, Bao HF, Alli AA, Aldrugh Y, Song JZ, Ma HP, et al. Phosphatidylinositol phosphate-dependent regulation of *Xenopus* ENaC by MARCKS protein. *Am J Physiol Renal Physiol* (2012) 303(6):F800–11. doi:10.1152/ajprenal.00703.2011
15. Alli AA, Bao HF, Liu BC, Yu L, Aldrugh S, Montgomery DS, et al. Calmodulin and CaMKII modulate ENaC activity by regulating the association of MARCKS and the cytoskeleton with the apical membrane. *Am J Physiol Renal Physiol* (2015) 309(5):F456–63. doi:10.1152/ajprenal.00631.2014
16. Czikora I, Alli A, Bao HF, Kaftan D, Apell HJ, White R, et al. A novel TNF-mediated mechanism of direct epithelial sodium channel activation. *Am J Respir Crit Care Med* (2014) 190(5):522–32. doi:10.1164/rccm.201405-0833OC
17. Shabbir W, Tzotzos S, Bedak M, Aufy M, Willam A, Kraihammer M, et al. Glycosylation-dependent activation of epithelial sodium channel by solnatide. *Biochem Pharmacol* (2015) 98(4):740–53. doi:10.1016/j.bcp.2015.08.003
18. Lucas R, Yue Q, Alli A, Duke BJ, Thai TL, Hamacher J, et al. The lectin-like domain of TNF increases ENaC open probability through a novel site at the interface between the second transmembrane and C-terminal domains of the α-subunit. *J Biol Chem* (2016) 291(45):23440–51. doi:10.1074/jbc.M116.718163
19. Vadász I, Schermuly RT, Ghofrani HA, Rummel S, Wehner S, Mühldorfer I, et al. The lectin-like domain of tumor necrosis factor-alpha improves alveolar fluid balance in injured isolated rabbit lungs. *Crit Care Med* (2008) 36(5):1543–50. doi:10.1097/CCM.0b013e31816f485e
20. Braun C, Hamacher J, Morel D, Wendel A, Lucas R. Dichotomal role of TNF in experimental pulmonary edema reabsorption. *J Immunol* (2005) 175(5):3402–8. doi:10.4049/jimmunol.175.5.3402
21. Elia N, Tapponnier M, Matthay MA, Hamacher J, Pache JC, Bründler MA, et al. Identification of the alveolar edema reabsorption activity of murine tumor necrosis factor. *Am J Respir Crit Care Med* (2003) 168:1043–50. doi:10.1164/rccm.200206-618OC
22. Hamacher J, Stammberger U, Roux J, Kumar S, Yang G, Xiong C, et al. The lectin-like domain of TNF improves lung function after rat lung transplantation – potential role for a reduction in reactive oxygen species generation. *Crit Care Med* (2010) 38(3):871–8. doi:10.1097/CCM.0b013e3181cdf725
23. Hartmann EK, Boehme S, Duenges B, Bentley A, Klein KU, Kwiecien R, et al. An inhaled tumor necrosis factor-alpha-derived TIP peptide improves the pulmonary function in experimental lung injury. *Acta Anaesthesiol Scand* (2013) 57(3):334–41. doi:10.1111/aas.12034
24. Schwameis R, Eder S, Pietschmann H, Fischer B, Mascher H, Tzotzos S, et al. A FIM study to assess safety and exposure of inhaled single doses of AP301-A specific ENaC channel activator for the treatment of acute lung injury. *J Clin Pharmacol* (2014) 54(3):341–50. doi:10.1002/jcph.203
25. Kusche-Vihrog K, Jeggle P, Oberleithner H. The role of ENaC in vascular endothelium. *Pflugers Arch* (2014) 466(5):851–9. doi:10.1007/s00424-013-1356-3
26. Hribar M, Bloc A, van der Goot FG, Fransen L, De Baetselier P, Grau GE, et al. The lectin-like domain of tumor necrosis factor-alpha increases membrane conductance in microvascular endothelial cells and peritoneal macrophages. *Eur J Immunol* (1999) 29(10):3105–11. doi:10.1002/(SICI)1521-4141(199910)29:10<3105::AID-IMMU3105>3.3.CO;2-1
27. Xiong C, Yang G, Kumar S, Aggarwal S, Leustik M, Snead C, et al. The lectin-like domain of TNF protects from Listeriolysin-induced hyperpermeability in human pulmonary microvascular endothelial cells – a crucial role for protein kinase C-alpha inhibition. *Vascul Pharmacol* (2010) 52(5–6):207–13. doi:10.1016/j.vph.2009.12.010
28. Loose M, Hudel M, Zimmer K-P, Garcia E, Hammerschmidt S, Lucas R, et al. Pneumococcal hydrogen peroxide induced stress signalling regulates inflammatory genes. *J Infect Dis* (2015) 211(2):306–16. doi:10.1093/infdis/jiu428
29. Malik B, Schlanger L, Al-Khalili O, Bao HF, Yue G, Price SR, et al. ENaC degradation in A6 cells by the ubiquitin-proteosome proteolytic pathway. *J Biol Chem* (2001) 276:12903–10. doi:10.1074/jbc.M010626200
30. Reifenberger MS, Yu L, Bao HF, Duke BJ, Liu BC, Ma HP, et al. Cytochalasin E alters the cytoskeleton and decreases ENaC activity in *Xenopus* 2F3 cells. *Am J Physiol Renal Physiol* (2014) 307:F86–95. doi:10.1152/ajprenal.00251.2013
31. Cantiello HF, Stow JL, Prat AG, Ausiello DA. Actin filaments regulate epithelial Na$^+$ channel activity. *Am J Physiol Cell Physiol* (1991) 261:C882–8.
32. Hummler E, Barker P, Gatzy J, Beermann F, Verdumo C, Schmidt A, et al. Early death due to defective neonatal lung liquid clearance in α-ENaC-deficient mice. *Nat Genet* (1996) 12(3):325–38. doi:10.1038/ng0396-325
33. Borbiev T, Verin AD, Shi S, Liu F, Garcia JG. Regulation of endothelial cell barrier function by calcium/calmodulin-dependent protein kinase II. *Am J Physiol Lung Cell Mol Physiol* (2001) 280(5):L983–90.
34. Jeggle P, Callies C, Tarjus A, Fassot C, Fels J, Oberleithner H, et al. Epithelial sodium channel stiffens the vascular endothelium in vitro and in Liddle mice. *Hypertension* (2013) 61(5):1053–9. doi:10.1161/HYPERTENSIONAHA.111.199455
35. Waldmann R, Champigny G, Lingueglia E, De Weille JR, Heurteaux C, Lazdunski M. H(+)-gated cation channels. *Ann N Y Acad Sci* (1999) 868:67–76. doi:10.1111/j.1749-6632.1999.tb11274.x
36. Meltzer RH, Kapoor N, Qadri YJ, Anderson SJ, Fuller CM, Benos DJ. Heteromeric assembly of acid-sensitive ion channel and epithelial sodium channel subunits. *J Biol Chem* (2007) 282(35):25548–59. doi:10.1074/jbc.M703825200
37. Trac PT, Thai TL, Linck V, Zou L, Greenlee MM, Yue Q, et al. Alveolar non-selective channels are ASIC1a/α-ENaC channels and contribute to AFC. *Am J Physiol Lung Cell Mol Physiol* (2017) 312:L797–811. doi:10.1152/ajplung.00379.2016
38. Bohlen CJ, Chesler AT, Sharif-Naeini R, Medzihradszky KF, Zhou S, King D, et al. A heteromeric Texas coral snake toxin targets acid-sensing ion channels to produce pain. *Nature* (2011) 479(7373):410–4. doi:10.1038/nature10607

39. Baron A, Diochot S, Salinas M, Deval E, Noël J, Lingueglia E. Venom toxins in the exploration of molecular, physiological and pathophysiological functions of acid-sensing ion channels. *Toxicon* (2013) 75:187–204. doi:10.1016/j.toxicon.2013.04.008

40. Predescu D, Predescu S, Shimizu J, Miyawaki-Shimizu K, Malik AB. Constitutive eNOS-derived nitric oxide is a determinant of endothelial junctional integrity. *Am J Physiol Lung Cell Mol Physiol* (2005) 289(3):L371–81. doi:10.1152/ajplung.00175.2004

41. Charles RP, Guitard M, Leyvraz C, Breiden B, Haftek M, Haftek-Terreau Z, et al. Postnatal requirement of the epithelial sodium channel for maintenance of epidermal barrier function. *J Biol Chem* (2008) 283(5):2622–30. doi:10.1074/jbc.M708829200

42. Lin X, Barravecchia M, Kothari P, Young JL, Dean DA. β1-Na(+),K(+)-ATPase gene therapy upregulates tight junctions to rescue lipopolysaccharide-induced acute lung injury. *Gene Ther* (2016) 23(6):489–99. doi:10.1038/gt.2016.19

43. Chrissobolis S. Vascular consequences of aldosterone excess and mineralocorticoid receptor antagonism. *Curr Hypertens Rev* (2017) 13:46–56. doi:10.2174/1573402113666170228151402

44. Lin LH, Jin J, Nashelsky MB, Talman WT. Acid-sensing ion channel 1 and nitric oxide synthase are in adjacent layers in the wall of rat and human cerebral arteries. *J Chem Neuroanat* (2014) 6(1–62):161–8. doi:10.1016/j.jchemneu.2014.10.002

45. Nitta CH, Osmond DA, Herbert LM, Beasley BF, Resta TC, Walker BR, et al. Role of ASIC1 in the development of chronic hypoxia-induced pulmonary hypertension. *Am J Physiol Heart Circ Physiol* (2014) 306(1):H41–52. doi:10.1152/ajpheart.00269.2013

46. Gessner C, Hammerschmidt S, Kuhn H, Seyfarth HJ, Sack U, Engelmann L, et al. Exhaled breath condensate acidification in acute lung injury. *Respir Med* (2003) 97(11):1188–94. doi:10.1016/S0954-6111(03)00225-7

FXYD5 is an Essential Mediator of the Inflammatory Response during Lung Injury

Patricia L. Brazee[1], Pritin N. Soni[1], Elmira Tokhtaeva[2,3], Natalia Magnani[1], Alex Yemelyanov[1], Harris R. Perlman[4], Karen M. Ridge[1], Jacob I. Sznajder[1], Olga Vagin[2,3†] and Laura A. Dada[1*†]

[1] Pulmonary and Critical Care Division, Feinberg School of Medicine, Northwestern University, Chicago, IL, United States, [2] Department of Physiology, David Geffen School of Medicine, UCLA, Los Angeles, CA, United States, [3] Veterans Administration Greater Los Angeles Healthcare System, Los Angeles, CA, United States, [4] Division of Rheumatology, Feinberg School of Medicine, Northwestern University, Chicago, IL, United States

*Correspondence:
Laura A. Dada
lauradada@northwestern.edu

†These authors have contributed equally to this work.

The alveolar epithelium secretes cytokines and chemokines that recruit immune cells to the lungs, which is essential for fighting infections but in excess can promote lung injury. Overexpression of FXYD5, a tissue-specific regulator of the Na,K-ATPase, in mice, impairs the alveolo-epithelial barrier, and FXYD5 overexpression in renal cells increases C-C chemokine ligand-2 (CCL2) secretion in response to lipopolysaccharide (LPS). The aim of this study was to determine whether FXYD5 contributes to the lung inflammation and injury. Exposure of alveolar epithelial cells (AEC) to LPS increased FXYD5 levels at the plasma membrane, and FXYD5 silencing prevented both the activation of NF-κB and the secretion of cytokines in response to LPS. Intratracheal instillation of LPS into mice increased FXYD5 levels in the lung. FXYD5 overexpression increased the recruitment of interstitial macrophages and classical monocytes to the lung in response to LPS. FXYD5 silencing decreased CCL2 levels, number of cells, and protein concentration in bronchoalveolar lavage fluid (BALF) after LPS treatment, indicating that FXYD5 is required for the NF-κB-stimulated epithelial production of CCL2, the influx of immune cells, and the increase in alveolo-epithelial permeability in response to LPS. Silencing of FXYD5 also prevented the activation of NF-κB and cytokine secretion in response to interferon α and TNF-α, suggesting that pro-inflammatory effects of FXYD5 are not limited to the LPS-induced pathway. Furthermore, in the absence of other stimuli, FXYD5 overexpression in AEC activated NF-κB and increased cytokine production, while FXYD5 overexpression in mice increased cytokine levels in BALF, indicating that FXYD5 is sufficient to induce the NF-κB-stimulated cytokine secretion by the alveolar epithelium. The FXYD5 overexpression also increased cell counts in BALF, which was prevented by silencing the CCL2 receptor (CCR2), or by treating mice with a CCR2-blocking antibody, confirming that FXYD5-induced CCL2 production leads to the recruitment of monocytes to the lung. Taken together, the data demonstrate that FXYD5 is a key contributor to inflammatory lung injury.

Keywords: alveolar epithelium, inflammation, FXYD5, acute lung injury, C-C chemokine ligand-2

INTRODUCTION

The alveolar epithelium not only is responsible for gas exchange but also acts as a physical and immunological barrier for all inhaled substances and microbial products. Alveolar epithelial cells (AEC) also contribute to innate immunity by secreting cytokines and chemokines, which recruit phagocytic myeloid cells and other inflammatory cells to the site of infection (1–3). During lung inflammation, the interaction of monocyte chemoattractant protein C-C chemokine ligand-2 (CCL2) secreted by AEC with its receptor, CC chemokine receptor 2 (CCR2), results in cellular recruitment to the lung. Present in a subset of peripheral monocytes, CCR2 serves as marker for classical monocyte inflammation (4–7). Recruitment of circulating monocytes to tissues is essential for effective control and clearance of infections, but if not controlled, it can become harmful, contributing to disease progression.

The alveolar epithelium is comprised of large flat type I alveolar (ATI) epithelial cells and cuboidal type II alveolar (ATII) epithelial cells. Both ATI and ATII cell types have important roles in airway surveillance through the initial recognition of microbial pathogens and bacterial toxins by various pattern recognition receptors (PRR) such as toll-like receptors (TLR) and nod-like receptors to activate the host defense (8). Lipopolysaccharide (LPS), a glycolipid of the outer membrane of Gram-negative bacteria is a major cause of morbidity and mortality in humans (9–11). Acute exposure to LPS increases cytokine release and disrupts the alveolo-capillary barrier, resulting in pulmonary edema and the recruitment of inflammatory cells into the lung (12–15). The response to LPS is initiated by interaction with TLR4 in association with the accessory proteins MD-2 and CD-14 (10, 16, 17). TLR4 is constitutively expressed in primary alveolar type II cells as well as in the adenocarcinoma cell line A549 (18). Exposure of lung epithelial cells to LPS leads to the activation of the NF-κB family of transcription factors, which in turn directs the expression of pro-inflammatory mediators (16, 19).

FXYD proteins, named after an invariant FXYD sequence, were first described as tissue-specific modulators of Na,K-ATPase activity (20–26). This family contains seven integral membrane proteins that interact with the Na,K-ATPase and regulate its function in a tissue-specific manner (27, 28). FXYD5, also known as dysadherin, is not only involved in the regulation of Na,K-ATPase activity (29, 30) but also acts as a tumorigenic protein when overexpressed (31, 32). Its expression is elevated in metastatic tumors, suggesting FXYD5 as an oncogenic marker (32–38). FXYD5 is also expressed in normal tissues, including the alveolar epithelium (24, 26, 29, 30, 39, 40). In cancer cells, CCL2 has been identified as a mediator of FXYD5 effects on cell migration (41). In these cells, FXYD5 has been shown to regulate CCL2 expression through the activation of the NF-κB signaling pathway.

Several publications have suggested a role of FXYD5 in the regulation of inflammation. In AEC, we have described that *in vivo* overexpression of FXYD5 impairs the interaction between Na,K-ATPase subunits in neighboring cells, disrupting the alveolar barrier (26), which might contribute to the recruitment of inflammatory cells into the alveolar compartment.

Also, overexpression of FXYD5 in normal kidney epithelial cells increases the inflammatory response to LPS in a tumor necrosis factor α (TNF-α) receptor-dependent manner and the levels of FXYD5 are increased in lungs after treatment of mice with LPS (30). Supporting a role for FXYD5 in inflammatory diseases, the expression levels of FXYD5 are elevated in the lungs of patients with acute lung injury (42). However, whether endogenous FXYD5 plays a role in the epithelial inflammatory response remains mostly unknown. Here, using *in vivo* and *in vitro* models, we investigated the mechanism by which the increase of FXYD5 in AEC contributes to lung inflammation and injury.

MATERIALS AND METHODS

Reagents
Chemical and cell culture reagents were purchased from Sigma-Aldrich or Corning Life Sciences unless stated otherwise. LPS from Escherichia coli 0111:B4 was from Sigma-Aldrich.

Cell Culture
Mouse lung epithelial MLE-12 and human epithelial A549 cells (ATCC) were grown and maintained as previously described (43, 44).

LPS-Induced Lung Inflammation and Injury Model
Mice were provided with food and water *ad libitum*, maintained on a 14-h-light–10-h-dark cycle, and handled according to National Institutes of Health guidelines and an experimental protocol approved by the Northwestern University Institutional Animal Care and Use Committee. C57BL/6 mice (10–12 weeks of age) were given intratracheal instillation of LPS (3 mg/kg body weight) for up to 24 h as we previously described (45). Bronchoalveolar lavage fluid (BALF) was obtained through a 20-gage angiocath ligated into the trachea through a tracheostomy (26). A total of 1-ml of PBS was instilled into the lungs and then aspirated three times. BALF was collected for cell counts, protein quantification, and cytokine determination as we previously described (30, 46). RNA was isolated from lung peripheral tissue using an RNeasy kit (QIAGEN) and reverse transcribed using qScript cDNA synthesis (Quanta Biosciences). Quantitative PCRs were set up using iQ SYBR Green Super mix (Bio Rad). Data were normalized to the abundance of L19 mRNA. The primers for FXYD5, CCL2, GAPDH, and L19 were: FXYD5 5′ CAT CCT ACA TTG AAC ATC CA 3′ and 5′ TGA GAC AAC TGC CTA CAC 3′; L19 5′ AGC CTG TGA CTG TCC ATT C 3′ and 5′ ATC CTC ATC CTT CTC ATC CAG 3′; CCL2 5′ CCT GTC ATG CTT CTG GGC CTG C 3′ and 5′ GGG GCG TTA ACT GCA TCT GGC TG 3′; and GAPDH 5′ AAC TTT GGC ATT GTG GAA GGG CTC 3′ and 5′ TGG AAG AGT GGG AGT TGC TGT TGA 3′. Proteins were determined in cell lysates or total membranes as we previously described (26, 43).

Lentivirus Instillation
To knock down mouse FXYD5 protein *in vivo* in lung, we generated the VSVG pseudotyped lentiviruses (10^9–10^{10} TU/ml) expressing

FXYD5 is an Essential Mediator of the Inflammatory Response during Lung Injury

mouse FXYD5 shRNA and non-silencing shRNA as control (47, 48) (provided by DNA/RNA Delivery Core, SDRC, Northwestern University, Chicago, IL, USA). For lentivirus packaging, 293T packaging cells (Gene Hunter Corporation) were transiently transfected using Transit-2020 reagent (Mirus) with the following vectors: second generation packaging vectors psPAX2 and pMD2.G (Addgene) and third generation lentiviral expression vector pLKO (Sigma). The pLKO vectors used encoded two specific shRNAs against mouse FXYD5 (Cat# TRCN0000079348, sense: CCTCCAAACTACACCAACTCA; and Cat# TRCN0000079352, sense: GTGCTGTTCATCACGGGAATT), and a non-silencing control shRNA (Cat# SHC002) (all from Sigma). FXYD5 shRNA and control non-silencing shRNA viruses were intratracheally instilled in mice in a volume of 50 µl. FXYD5 silencing was confirmed by RT-qPCR and Western blot analysis as described above.

Adenoviral Infection

$CCR2^{-/-}$ mice were purchased from Jackson Laboratories (49). WT C57BL/6 or $CCR2^{-/-}$ mice at 8–12 weeks of age were infected with Ad-mCherry-HA-FXYD5 (Ad-FXYD5; 1×10^9 plaque-forming units (pfu)/animal) in 50% surfactant vehicle as previously described (30, 50) and housed in a containment facility. After 72 h, BALF was collected and used as described above. Control adenovirus (Ad-Null) was purchased from Viraquest, Inc. Cells were infected with Ad-Null or Ad-FXYD5 20 pfu/cell as previously described (26).

Analysis of Cytokines and Chemokines

The concentration of CCL2/MCP-1 (Affymetrix), TNF-α (Affymetrix), and IL-6 (Life Technologies) in the BALF or cell culture supernatants were quantified by ELISA following the manufacturer's instructions.

In Vitro Treatment of AEC and siRNA Transfection

MLE-12 or A549 cells were transfected with 120 pmol of mouse or human FXYD5 siRNA duplex (final concentration 100 µM) (Santa Cruz Biotechnology), respectively, using Lipofectamine RNAiMAX (Invitrogen). A non-silencing negative control siRNA was purchased from Santa Cruz Biotechnology. Experiments were performed 24 h after transfection. Cells were starved for 2 h by incubation in culture media containing 2.5% fetal bovine serum and treated with LPS (100 ng/ml) for the indicated times. Supernatants were collected for cytokine analysis and cells were biotinylated by the membrane-impermeable biotinylation reagent where indicated; cells lysates, total membranes, or surface biotinylated proteins were isolated for SDS-PAGE and immunoblot analysis as previously described (26, 43). The following mouse monoclonal antibodies were used: HA (Biolegend clone 16B12 #901502; 1:1,000), pIKBα (Cell Signaling Technology #9246; 1:500), IKBα (Cell Signaling Technology #4814; 1:500), E-cadherin (E-cad) (BD Biosciences #610182, 1:2,500 dilution). The following polyclonal antibodies were used: FXYD5 (Sigma-Aldrich #HPA010817, 1:1,000 and M178 from Santa Cruz Biotechnology #98247, 1:200), and β-actin (Cell Signaling Technology #4967, 1:1,000). Immunoblots were quantified by

densitometry using Image J 1.46r (National Institutes of Health, Bethesda, MD). Where indicated, surface biotinylated proteins were treated with O-glycosidase and Neuraminidase Bundle according to the manufacturer's instructions (New England Biolabs, Inc.) prior to loading on SDS-PAGE as we previously described (26).

Interferon α (IFN-α, Biolegend) and TNF-α (Biolegend) were added to A549 cells for up to 24 and 2 h, respectively, as described for LPS treatment.

Flow Cytometry and Cell Sorting

Myeloid populations from whole lung were isolated and defined as previously described (51). Briefly, perfused lungs were inflated with digestion buffer (1 mg/ml of Collagenase D and 0.1 mg/ml DNase I, both from Roche) and coarsely minced with scissors before processing in C-tubes (Miltenyi) with a GentleMACS dissociator (Miltenyi), according to the manufacturer's instructions. Homogenate was passed through 40-µm nylon mesh to obtain a single-cell suspension and subjected to red blood cell lysis (BD Pharm Lyse, BD Biosciences). Live cells were counted using a Countess cell counter (Invitrogen) by trypan blue exclusion.

Cells were then stained with the following cocktail: CD45-FITC (eBioscience #11-0451-81, 0.1 µg/µl), MHCII-PerCPCy5.5 (Biolegend #107626, 0.01 µg/µl), Ly6C-eFluor450 (eBioscience #348-5932-80, 0.02 µg/µl), CD24-APC (eBioscience #317-0242-80, 0.01 µg/µl), Ly6G-Alexa700 (BD Bioscience #561236, 0.04 µg/µl), NK1.1-Alexa700 (BD Bioscience #560515, 0.06 µg/µl), CD11b-APCcy7 (Biolegend #101225, 0.02 µg/µl), CD64-PE (Biolegend #139303, 0.02 µg/µl), SiglecF-PECF594 (BD Bioscience #562757, 0.02 µg/µl), CD11c-PEcy7 (BD Bioscience #561022, 0.02 µg/µl). Multicolor flow cytometry was performed with an LSR Fortessa using DIVA software (BD Biosciences) and the following gating outlined below and in **Figure 5**. FlowJo software version 10.0.8 (FlowJo, LLC) was used for all compensation and data analysis.

After excluding doublets and dead cells, myeloid cells were identified using the pan-hematopoietic marker CD45 (51). As shown in **Figure 5**, the CD45$^+$ population was then separated into Ly6G/NK1.1$^-$ and Ly6G/NK1.1$^+$ populations using a shared channel to pull out NK cells (NK1.1$^+$ CD11b^{hi} CD24^{hi}) and neutrophils (Ly6G CD11b^{int} CD24^{int}). The Ly6G/NK1.1$^-$ population was further divided based on SiglecF and CD11c expression to identify alveolar macrophages (SiglecF^{hi} CD11c^{hi}) and eosinophils (SiglecF^{hi} CD11c^{low}). From the remaining SiglecF^{low} CD11c^{low} group, a CD11b^{hi} population was then selected and segregated based on MHCII expression. Within the MHCII^{low} cluster, cells could be defined as classical monocytes (Ly6C^{hi}) or non-classical monocytes (Ly6C^{low}). Alternatively, interstitial macrophages (IMs) were identified as MHCII^{hi} CD64^{hi} CD24^{low}.

Mouse ATII cells (mATII) were isolated and defined as previously described (52). Briefly, whole lung was subjected to enzymatic and manual digestion to obtain a single cell suspension. Cells were then stained with Epcam (eBioscience #17-5791-80, 0.1 µg/ml), CD45, CD31-PE (eBioscience #12-0311-81, 0.1 µg/ml), and MHCII-eFlour450 (eBioscience #48-5321-82, 0.1 µg/ml). mATII cells were identified as CD45$^-$ EpCAM$^+$, CD31$^-$ and sorted on a BD FACSAria 5-laser.

Fluorescent Staining and Confocal Microscopy

Isolated mATII cells were plated on glass-bottom dishes (MatTek corporation), fixed by incubation with 3.75% formaldehyde in PBS for 15 min at 37°C, and actin filaments were visualized using fluorescein phalloidin (Thermo Fisher Scientific) as described previously (53). Confocal microscopy images of mCherry-tagged FXYD5 and stained actin filaments were acquired using a Zeiss LSM 510 laser scanning confocal microscope and ZEN 2009 software (Carl Zeiss MicroImaging GmbH).

Anti-CCR2 Antibody Treatment

Mice were injected retro-orbitally with 6 µg/100 µl of anti-CCR2 monoclonal antibody (clone MC-21) in PBS (49) 48 h after adenoviral instillation. Mice were sacrificed after 24 h and BALF was obtained as described above.

Statistical Analysis

Data are expressed as mean ± SD. For comparisons between two groups, significance was evaluated by Student's t-test, and when more than two groups were compared, one-way ANOVA was used followed by the Dunnett's or Sidak test using GraphPad Prism 7.02 software.

RESULTS

The Increase in FXYD5 Is Required for the Secretion of Inflammatory Mediators by the AEC in Response to LPS

Alveolar epithelial cells produce the first wave of cytokines, which trigger local and systemic inflammatory responses (54). We have reported that overexpression of FXYD5 in normal kidney epithelial cells increases the inflammatory response to LPS (40) and that overexpression of FXYD5 in the mouse alveolar epithelium increases alveolar epithelial permeability (26). Moreover, treatment of mice with LPS increased the level of FXYD5 in lungs (30). However, whether endogenous FXYD5 plays a role in the generation of an alveolar epithelial inflammatory response to LPS has not been studied. To determine whether LPS modulates FXYD5 levels in AEC, MLE-12 cells were treated with LPS for up to 24 h and cell culture media, cell lysates, and surface biotinylated plasma membrane (PM) proteins were collected. In the PM fraction of MLE-12 cells, FXYD5 was detected as a 60–70 kDa band (**Figure 1A**), suggesting that the plasmalemma-located FXYD5 is heavily O-glycosylated in these cells similar to that found in A549 cells (26). An additional 25 kDa band was seen in MLE-12 cell lysates (not shown) that represents the intracellular immature unglycosylated or less glycosylated fraction of FXYD5. LPS time dependently increased PM level of FXYD5 in MLE-12 cells with a peak at 6 h (**Figure 1A**). CCL2, which is abundantly produced by ATII cells, plays an important role in the local regulation of inflammatory processes (55). As expected, treatment of MLE-12 cells for 6 h with LPS strongly stimulated CCL2 mRNA synthesis as well as the secretion of CCL2 and IL-6 into the culture media compared with untreated controls (**Figures 1B–D**). Silencing of FXYD5 in those cells with a specific siRNA prevented the LPS-stimulated

increase in the transcription of CCL2 and secretion of both cytokines as compared with a control siRNA (**Figures 1B–D**). In isolated primary mouse ATII, infection with lentivirus coding for specific shRNA FXYD5 prevented the LPS-stimulated increase in FXYD5 and CCL2 mRNA by 62 and 30%, respectively (**Figure 1E**).

Next, we investigated the signaling pathway by which the increase in FXYD5 regulates cytokine production. The dominant pathway triggered by PRR activation is the canonical NF-κB pathway. The NF-κB complex comprises IκB (inhibitor of NF-κB) bound to two proteins, p50 and p65; when not stimulated, the complex resides in the cytoplasm. Different stimuli lead to phosphorylation and degradation of IκB removing inhibitory effects and allowing the translocation of active NF-κB, the p50-p65 heterodimer, to the nuclei (56). Nuclear translocation triggers the expression of over 150 genes, including those encoding cytokines (57). We analyzed whether FXYD5 promotes the secretion of cytokines *via* the NF-κB signaling pathway by assessing the phosphorylation of one of IκB proteins, IκBα. In A549 cells, 6 h of LPS treatment led to an increase in FXYD5 at the PM similar to the one observed in MLE-12 (**Figure 1F**). A549 cells were transfected with siRNA specific for FXYD5, 24 h later stimulated with LPS for 6 h, and phosphorylation of IκBα was assessed in cell lysates. LPS treatment increased the IκBα phosphorylation, which was prevented by FXYD5 silencing (**Figure 1F**). Taken together, the results indicate that FXYD5 is required for the NF-κB-dependent secretion of inflammatory cytokines and chemokines induced by LPS, suggesting that FXYD5 is an important mediator of the pro-inflammatory response of AEC to LPS.

Increased FXYD5 Is Sufficient to Induce AEC Secretion of Inflammatory Mediators

Previous studies in breast cancer cells have demonstrated that FXYD5 knockdown decreases, while FXYD5 overexpression increases, both the NF-κB-responsive promoter activity and CCL2 production in cancer cells (41). To determine whether the increase in FXYD5 in AEC induces the NF-κB-dependent secretion of pro-inflammatory mediators, we infected cells with Ad-FXYD5, and 40 h after infection, determined the expression of FXYD5 (**Figure 2A**), phosphorylation of IκBα (**Figure 2B**), cellular levels of CCL2 mRNA (**Figure 2C**), and CCL2 and IL-6 levels in the culture media (**Figures 2D,E**). Expression of exogenous FXYD5 stimulated IκBα phosphorylation, the synthesis of CCL2 mRNA, and the release of CCL2 and IL-6 by AEC, suggesting that the increase in FXYD5 is sufficient to induce the inflammatory response in AEC.

Increased FXYD5 in AEC Contributes to the Inflammatory Response to LPS *In Vivo*

To determine whether FXYD5, which is abundantly expressed in ATII cells (26), contributes to the inflammatory response in LPS-induced acute lung injury, we performed intratracheal instillation of LPS into mice and measured FXYD5 mRNA and protein levels in lung peripheral tissue after 2, 4, 6, and 24 h. Administration of LPS time dependently increased the level of FXYD5 mRNA with a peak after 6 h of instillation (**Figure 3A**). In mouse lung peripheral tissue lysates, FXYD5 was detected by Western blot

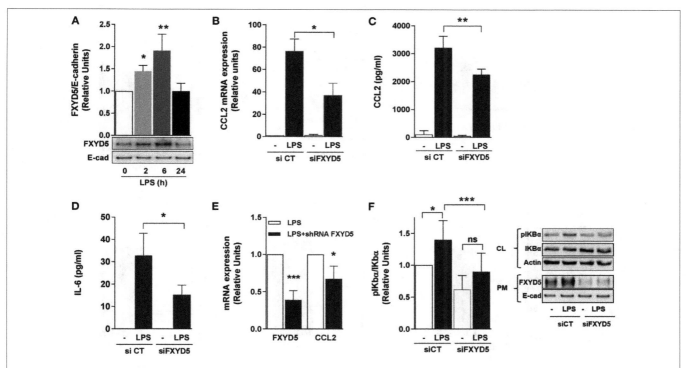

FIGURE 1 | **FXYD5 plays a role in LPS-induced inflammatory response by activating the NF-κB signaling pathway in alveolar epithelial cells.** **(A)** MLE-12 cells were treated with 100 ng/ml LPS for the indicated period of time, PM proteins were isolated after cell surface labeling with biotin and characterized by immunoblot with an anti-FXYD5 specific antibody. Densitometric quantification of immunoblots of FXYD5 in relation to E-cad is shown (n = 3). **(B)** MLE-12 were cells transfected with a FXYD5-specific siRNA and 24 h later treated with LPS for 6 h. CCL2 mRNA was measured by RT-qPCR n = 4. **(C,D)** MLE-12 cells were treated like in B, culture media was collected, and CCL2 **(C)** and IL-6 **(D)** were determined by ELISA (n = 5). **(E)** FXYD5 was silenced in isolated mATII cells with shFXYD5 for 72 h and then treated with LPS for 6 h. FXYD5 and CCL2 mRNA were measured by RT-qPCR (n = 3). **(F)** A549 cells were treated as in B and cell lysate (CL) and PM proteins were isolated after cell surface labeling with biotin. Densitometric quantification (left panel) of immunoblots (right panel) of pIκBα in relation to total IκBα is shown (n = 6). Values of PBS-treated controls were normalized to 1. Bars represent means ± SD. Statistical significance was analyzed by one way ANOVA and Dunnetts's **(A)** or Sidak's multiple comparison test **(B–D,F)** or Student's t-test **(E)**. *$p \leq 0.05$; **$p \leq 0.01$; ***$p \leq 0.001$; ns, non-significant.

in two bands, a major band at 60–70 kDa and a minor band at 25 kDa (**Figure 3B**). Only the 60–70 kDa fraction of FXYD5 is seen in surface biotinylated fraction in MLE-12 cells (**Figure 1B**), indicating that the 60–70 kDa in mouse lung lysates corresponds to the mature heavily glycosylated FXYD5 residing at the PM. LPS increased the abundance of both forms in a time-dependent manner. To assess whether the inflammatory response elicited by LPS in the lung is dependent on the presence of FXYD5, we silenced FXYD5 by instillation of lentiviral particles coding for shFXYD5, which decreased FXYD5 expression in the peripheral tissue by ~70% (**Figures 3C,D**). Treatment with LPS increased the concentration of proteins in the BALF (a measure of the permeability of the alveolo-capillary barrier) and total cell count in BALF (a measure of inflammatory cell recruitment to the lung) (**Figures 3E,F**). A decrease in FXYD5 in the lung peripheral tissue lowered the concentration of proteins in the BALF after LPS treatment as compared with control mice exposed to LPS (**Figure 3E**). Also, BALF from mice with silenced FXYD5 contained fewer inflammatory cells and reduced CCL2 after LPS treatment than that obtained from sh-control-treated mice (**Figures 3F,G**), suggesting that FXYD5 contributes to the LPS-induced production of CCL2 and the recruitment of inflammatory cells into the lung.

To determine whether the relationship between elevated FXYD5 and inflammation is causal, we studied the effects of intratracheal administration of an endotoxin-free adenoviral construct coding for mouse mCherry-HA-FXYD5 (Ad-FXYD5) or an empty adenovirus (Ad-Null) to mice (26). ATII cells from infected mice were isolated by flow-cytometry as CD45⁻ CD31⁻ Ep-Cam⁺ cells. The expression of exogenous FXYD5 in ATII cells was evident from the red fluorescence of the mCherry tag present in this construct (**Figure 4A**). Instillation of Ad-FXYD5 increased total cell number in BALF (**Figure 4B**) as compared with mice infected with Ad-Null. Moreover, in agreement with our *in vitro* data, FXYD5 overexpression in mice increased the levels of CCL2 mRNA (**Figure 4C**) and the secretion of CCL2, TNF-α, and IL-6 into the alveolar space (**Figures 4D–F**).

FXYD5 Induces the Recruitment of Different Subsets of Myeloid Cells to the Lung

Together, the results in **Figures 3** and **4** suggest that FXYD5 is required for LPS-induced cellular infiltration into the alveolar space. To evaluate whether the increased level of FXYD5 leads

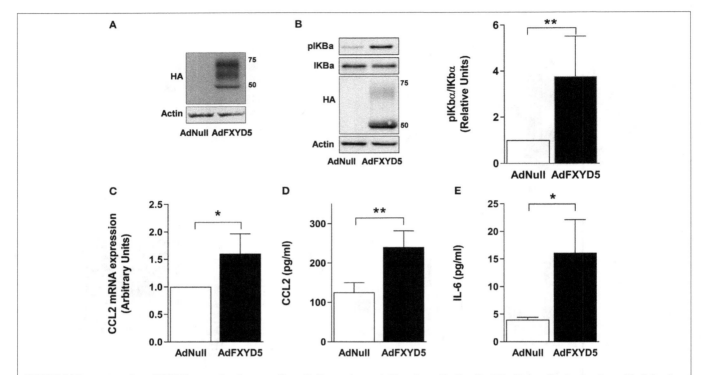

FIGURE 2 | **Overexpression of FXYD5 promotes the secretion of inflammatory cytokines by activating the NF-κB signaling in alveolar epithelial cells.** **(A)** MLE-12 cells were incubated with Ad-Null or Ad-FXYD5 as described in Section "Materials and Methods." The expression of FXYD5 was determined in the CL by Western blot with an HA antibody. **(B)** A549 cells were treated as in **(A)** and CL was isolated. Left panel: representative immunoblots. Right panel: densitometric quantification of pIκBα in relation to total IκBα. The expression of FXYD5 was determined with an HA antibody (n = 4). **(C)** MLE-12 cells were treated as in **(A)** and CCL2 mRNA was quantified by RT-qPCR (n = 3). **(D–E)** MLE-12 cells were treated as in **(A)**, culture media was collected, and CCL2, n = 5 **(D)** and IL-6, n = 5 **(E)** were determined by ELISA. Values of AdNull-treated controls were normalized to 1. Bars represent means ± SD. Statistical significance was analyzed by unpaired Student's t-test. *$p \leq 0.05$; **$p \leq 0.01$.

to enhanced recruitment of specific subcellular myeloid populations into the lung, mice were instilled with Ad-FXYD5 72 h prior to treatment with LPS for 24 h, and changes in leukocyte populations within the lung were analyzed by flow cytometry. After excluding doublets and dead cells, myeloid cells were identified using pan-hematopoietic marker CD45. Using the gating strategy described in the Section "Materials and Methods" and **Figure 5A**, no significant differences were detected in the recruitment of Ly6G+CD11b^{int}CD24^{int} neutrophils (**Figure 5B**), NK1.1+CD11b^{hi}CD24^{hi} NK cells (**Figure 5C**), or SiglecF^{hi}CD11c^{hi} alveolar macrophages (**Figure 5D**) while SiglecF^{hi}CD11c^{low} eosinophils (**Figure 5E**) were increased after infection with AdFXYD5. Additionally, we observed increased recruitment of CD11b^{hi}MHCII^{hi} IMs (**Figure 5F**) and CD11b^{hi} MHCII^{low}Ly6C^{hi} classical monocytes (**Figure 5G**) in the presence of higher levels of FXYD5 post-LPS challenge.

CCR2+ Classical Monocytes Are Involved in FXYD5-Mediated Inflammation

In mice, expression of Ly6C and CD11b identifies a subset of monocytes that expresses high levels of CCR2 (58). CCL2 and its receptor CCR2 are critical determinants for recruitment of monocytes to the lungs (4, 6, 59, 60), where they have key roles in amplifying lung injury by orchestrating an overly exuberant inflammatory response (1, 14, 61). To determine whether classical monocytes contribute to the FXYD5-induced inflammatory response, we infected mice with Ad-FXYD5 or Ad-Null, and 48 h after the infection depleted monocytes by the injection of an anti-CCR2 antibody. The presence of the antibody decreased the cellular infiltration into the lung, stimulated by infection with Ad-FXYD5 (**Figure 6A**). As an alternative approach, CCR2$^{-/-}$ mice, which lack CCR2, and WT mice were infected with Ad-FXYD5, and BALF was collected after 72 h. The absence of CCR2 decreased the cellular infiltrates in the lungs (**Figure 6B**), suggesting, again, that classical monocytes play a role in FXYD5-induced inflammation. The levels of CCL2 were significantly increased in the CCR2 KO infected with Ad-FXYD5 as compared with the WT-infected mouse (**Figure 6C**).

Taken together, the results demonstrate that the FXYD5 abundance in AEC is increased in response to LPS, and the prevention of this increase by silencing FXYD5 partially abolishes pro-inflammatory effects of LPS. The increased levels of FXYD5 activate the production of CCL2 by AEC, which, in turn, leads to the recruitment of CCR2+ monocytes cells into the alveolar spaces to worsen lung injury.

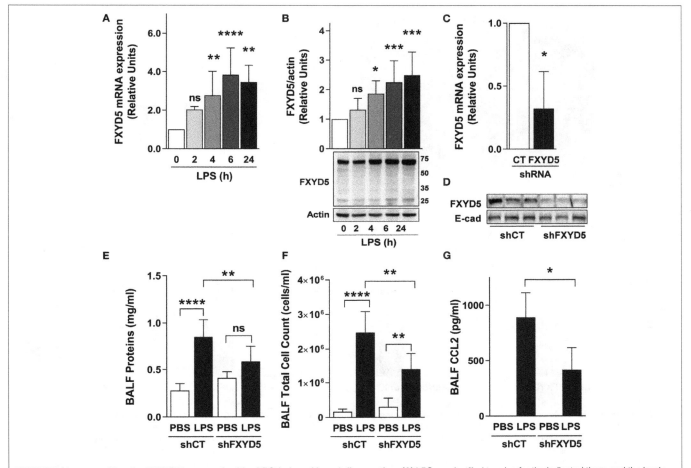

FIGURE 3 | **Increased levels of FXYD5 are required for LPS-induced lung inflammation.** (A) LPS was instilled to mice for the indicated times and the levels of FXYD5 mRNA were determined by RT-qPCR in lung peripheral tissue (n = 8). (B) Mice were treated as in A and FXYD5 was determined in lung peripheral tissue cell lysates by Western blot. Bars indicate densitometric quantification of plasma membrane FXYD5 (top band) in relation to actin (n = 8). (C,D) Control (CT) or shFXYD5 lentiviral constructs were instilled into mice. Silencing was assessed by measuring FXYD5 mRNA by RT-qPCR (C). n = 4 or protein abundance in lung peripheral tissue total membranes (D). Representative immunoblot showing the abundance of FXYD5, E-cadherin was used as a loading control n = 6. (E–G) Mice treated as in C were given LPS for 6 h and BALF was obtained. Proteins (E), total cells (F), and CCL2 (G) were determined as described in Section "Materials and Methods." Values of PBS-treated controls were normalized to 1. Bars represent means ± SD. Statistical significance was analyzed by one way ANOVA and Dunnetts's (A,B) unpaired Student's t-test (D) or Sidak's multiple comparison test (E,F). *$p \leq 0.05$; **$p \leq 0.01$; ***$p \leq 0.001$.

FXYD5 Is Required for NF-κB Activation Downstream of Several Cytokine Receptors

Since expression of exogenous FXYD5 induces the inflammatory response even in the absence of LPS, we studied whether FXYD5 contributes to pro-inflammatory pathways downstream of receptors other than TLR4. To address this question, we measured the activation of NF-κB and the production of cytokines after stimulating A549 cells in the presence or absence of FXYD5 with IFN-α (100 U/ml) or TNF-α (50 ng/ml). IFN-α signals through the type I interferon receptor (IFNAR) (62), while the effects of TNF-α are initiated by its binding to the ubiquitously expressed TNF receptor 1 (TNFR1) or to the TNF receptor 2 that is mainly expressed in lymphocytes and endothelial cells (63). Treatment with IFN-α induced the phosphorylation of IκBα that was detected after 15 min and reached its maximum after 1 h (**Figure 7A**). The knockdown of FXYD5 prevented the activation of NF-κB and significantly inhibited the increase in cytokine secretion in response to IFN-α (**Figures 7A–C**).

Treatment of epithelial cells with TNF-α led to the phosphorylation of IκB and a dramatic decrease in its total amount after 5 min of treatment (**Figure 7D**), suggesting a rapid degradation of IκBα in these conditions. The loss of IκBα was followed by its partial recovery after 1 and 2 h of treatment (**Figure 7D**), which is consistent with previously published data on rapid re-synthesis of IκBα after its TNF-α-induced degradation (64). FXYD5 silencing prevented the TNF-α-induced phosphorylation of IκBα and the concomitant production of IL-6 and CCL2 (**Figures 7E,F**). Collectively, these results suggest that FXYD5 is a required mediator of the inflammatory response in epithelial cells.

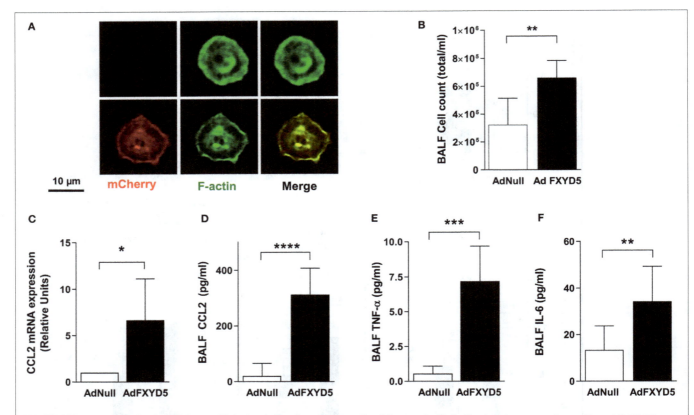

FIGURE 4 | **Increased levels of FXYD5 are sufficient to induce lung inflammation**. Mice were instilled with adenoviruses encoding m-Cherry-HA-FXYD5 (AdFXYD5) or an empty control (AdNull) and 72 h later ATII cells, BALF or lung peripheral tissue were isolated. **(A)** Confocal microscopy analyses of FACS-sorted mice ATII cells. Red m-cherry fluorescence reflects the expression of FXYD5. Green fluorescence shows actin filaments used to visualize cells. **(B)** Total cell count in BALF. **(C)** CCL2 mRNA was determined by RT-qPCR in lung peripheral tissue. **(D–F)** CCL2, TNF-α, and IL-6 were determined by ELISA in BALF. Values of Ad-Null-treated controls were normalized to 1. Bars represent means ± SD $n \leq 5$. Statistical significance was analyzed by unpaired Student's t-test. *$p \leq 0.05$; **$p \leq 0.01$; ***$p \leq 0.001$.

DISCUSSION

The respiratory epithelium is constantly exposed to invading particles and potential pathogens. In addition to creating a barrier for pathogens, AEC secrete inflammatory mediators that recruit innate and adaptive immune cells to the alveolar space (1, 4, 7, 65–68). The mechanisms regulating the extent of epithelial inflammatory responses to infection and tissue injury are not fully understood. The data presented here demonstrate that in AEC, FXYD5, acting upstream of NF-κB, is necessary and sufficient for the secretion of pro-inflammatory cytokines *in vivo* and *in vitro*. Under our experimental conditions, LPS rapidly increases FXYD5 in AEC resulting in the secretion of CCL2 and the recruitment of CCR2+ monocytes to the alveolar space. These monocytes, often referred as inflammatory monocytes, are responsible for the secretion of a large number of soluble mediators that regulate the activity of other inflammatory cells.

Lipopolysaccharide-induced acute lung injury is an animal model that replicates several key pathologic processes of acute respiratory distress syndrome, including cytokine release, inflammatory cell influx, and lung capillary permeability, which results in pulmonary edema (69). In our study, LPS stimulation of isolated mouse ATII cells, as well as mouse and human alveolar epithelial cell lines, resulted in a rapid and substantial increase in the secretion of several cytokines. These effects were prevented by silencing FXYD5 using different silencing RNA, which strongly suggests a role for FXYD5 in the production of inflammatory mediators by AEC. Moreover, acute overexpression of FXYD5 in AEC increased secretion of CCL2 and IL-6. In conjunction with our previous data showing that FXYD5 overexpression produces a disruptive effect on alveolar–epithelial barrier (26), these results suggest that FXYD5 impairs the integrity of the barrier not only by directly disrupting epithelial junctions formed by Na,K-ATPase β1 subunits (26) but also by secreting cytokines that recruit immune cells into alveolar spaces, which further enhance the impairment of alveolar–epithelial barrier.

In agreement with our previous report (30), we found that inhalation of LPS results in a time-dependent increase in FXYD5 expression in the lung. This increase temporally correlated with the secretion of cytokines into the BALF and recruitment of immune cells to the lung. Either after LPS instillation or FXYD5 overexpression, we observed that a significant portion of FXYD5 is localized at the PM and heavily O-glycosylated (26), which contrasts with previous studies that reported that in normal tissues, including the lung, FXYD5 is expressed only as a low molecular mass protein with no or very minimal glycosylation (24, 29).

FXYD5 is an Essential Mediator of the Inflammatory Response during Lung Injury

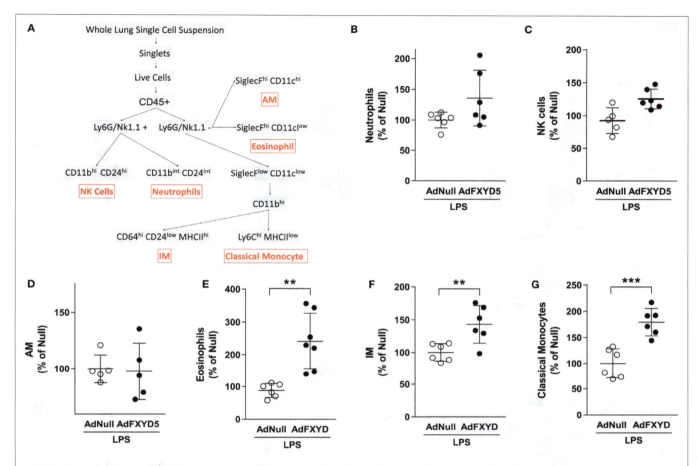

FIGURE 5 | FXYD5-induced changes in myeloid-cell subsets in mouse lungs during LPS-induced lung injury. (A) Gating strategy used to identify myeloid-cell subsets in the normal mouse lung. **(B–G)** Mice were instilled with Ad-FXYD5 or Ad-Null and treated with LPS for 12 h. Cells were isolated from enzymatically digested mouse lungs. Changes of myeloid-cell subsets in Ad-FXYD5-infected mice relative to Ad-Null-infected control identified as described in **(A)** are shown. Values of Ad-Null-treated controls were normalized to 100%. Values represent means ± SD $n = 6$. Differences between groups were compared using unpaired Student's t-test. $**p \leq 0.01$; $***p \leq 0.001$.

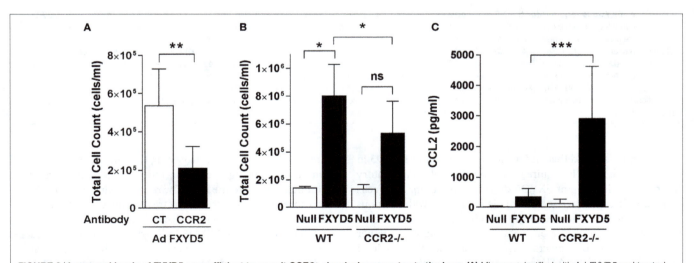

FIGURE 6 | Increased levels of FXYD5 are sufficient to recruit CCR2+ classical monocytes to the lung. (A) Mice were instilled with Ad-FXYD5 and treated with the anti-CCR2 antibody for 24 h prior to the measurements. Total cell count in BALF was determined ($n = 5$). **(B,C)** WT and CCR2$^{-/-}$ mice were instilled like in **(A)**. Total cell counts $n = 3$ **(B)** and CCL2 $n = 4$ **(C)** were determined in BALF. Values represent means ± SD. Differences between groups were compared using unpaired Student's t-test or one way ANOVA Sidak's multiple comparison test. $*p \leq 0.05$ $**p \leq 0.01$; $***p \leq 0.001$.

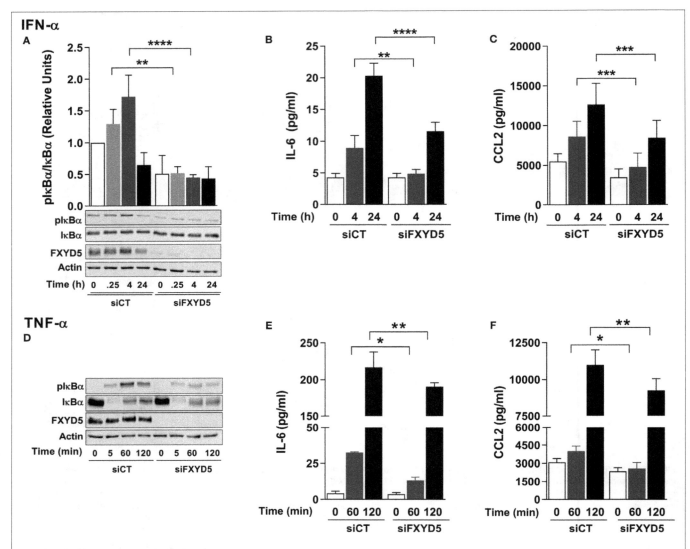

FIGURE 7 | FXYD5 is required for the NF-κB-mediated secretion of cytokines in response to IFN-α and TNF-α by alveolar epithelial cells. (A) A549 cells were transfected with a control (siCT) or FXYD5 specific (siFXYD5) siRNA, 24 h later treated with 100 U/ml IFN-α for the indicated period of time, and cell lysates were analyzed by immunoblot using specific antibodies as indicated. Bottom panel: representative immunoblots. Top panel: densitometric quantification of pIκBα in relation to total IκBα n = 4. (B,C) A549 cells were treated as in (A), culture media was collected, and IL-6 (B) and CCL2 (C) were determined by ELISA n = 3. (D). A549 cells were transfected with siCT or siFXYD5, 24 h later treated with 50 ng/ml TNF-α for the indicated period of time, and cell lysates were analyzed by immunoblot using specific antibodies as indicated. Representative immunoblots n = 4. (E,F) A549 cells were treated as in (D), culture media was collected, and IL-6 (E) and CCL2 (F) were determined by ELISA n = 4. Values of PBS-treated controls were normalized to 1. Bars represent means ± SD. Statistical significance was analyzed by one way ANOVA and Sidak's multiple comparison test. *$p \leq 0.05$; **$p \leq 0.01$; ***$p \leq 0.001$; ****$p \leq 0.0001$, ns, non-significant.

Moreover, we showed that endogenous expression of FXYD5 in the lung epithelium is required for the epithelial inflammatory response, as silencing of FXYD5 decreased the number of cells in BALF after LPS treatment. This is consistent with previous reports suggesting that leukocyte recruitment during bacterial infection is due to the response of the alveolar epithelium rather than resident alveolar macrophages (8) and that the profile of cytokines released by ATII cells determines specific leukocyte recruitment (70). The data presented here demonstrate that FXYD5 overexpression in the absence of LPS or other stimuli is sufficient to activate cytokine secretion in AEC and to increase the number of cells in BALF, suggesting that the increase in FXYD5 alone, by stimulating cytokine secretion, leads to the recruitment of immune cells into the lung. The recruitment of cells by FXYD5 overexpression was decreased by treating mice with the antibody against CCR2, and the same effect was observed in mice lacking CCR2, indicating that FXYD5-induced secretion of CCL2 causes chemotaxis of CCR2-positive monocytes to the alveolar spaces.

The overexpression of FXYD5 in conjunction with LPS treatment significantly increased the recruitment of interstitial and monocyte-derived macrophages to the lung. Tissue resident alveolar macrophages are the predominant immune cells found within the alveolar airspaces during steady-state conditions, while classical inflammatory Ly6C[hi] monocytes and IM represent a very low proportion of circulating white blood cells in an uninfected mouse and are rapidly recruited to sites of infection and inflammation (58, 71, 72). Upon stimulation, Ly6C[hi] monocytes exit the bone marrow in a CC-chemokine receptor 2 (CCR2)-dependent manner and are recruited to inflamed tissues (58). In agreement with our data, it has been described that IM expand more rapidly in response to foreign stimuli compared with alveolar macrophages as IM are preferentially replenished from blood monocytes (72) and CCR2[+] monocytes emigration from the bone marrow is normal during early-stage of bacterial infection of mice (58). In addition, overexpression of FXYD5 increased the recruitment of eosinophils to the lung in response to LPS. These data suggest that FXYD5 induces secretion of other cytokines/chemokines because CCL2 is not among the major chemoattractants of eosinophils such as IL-5, RANTES (CCL5), eotaxin, and others (73–76).

Further, we demonstrated that the presence of FXYD5 in AEC is required for NF-κB activation induced by LPS, TNF-α, or IFN-α as FXYD5 silencing prevented IκBα phosphorylation and reduced cytokine secretion in response to these stimuli. Moreover, overexpression of FXYD5 in the absence of any stimuli induced both IκBα phosphorylation and cytokine secretion. Taken together, these results indicate that FXYD5 is an important component of NF-κB signaling pathway. This conclusion is consistent with previously published data showing that FXYD5 overexpression in breast cancer cells induces the phosphorylation of AKT (38), which promotes the transcriptional activity of NF-κB-responsive promoter elements and increases levels of CCL2 mRNA (38, 41). Taken together, these data suggest that FXYD5 increases CCL2 transcription by inducing AKT-dependent activation of NF-κB signaling. In support of a role of an FXYD5/AKT dependent activation of NF-κB, binding of IFN-α to IFNAR activates PI3K *via* STAT5, which in turn, activates NF-κB (77–79). Activation of PI3K has been also described downstream of TLR4 and TNFR1 (80, 81). Our recent data in kidney cells, stably transfected with FXYD5, suggested that FXYD5 modulates NF-κB signaling by regulating the location of TNF-α receptor, TNFR1 (30). It is possible that the plasmalemma-located FXYD5, by interacting with the PM receptor complexes, modulates their association with other proteins as well as their location and mobility in the membrane. Such a possibility is consistent with the data showing that the efficiency of LPS/TLR4 signaling is affected by receptor mobility in the lipid bilayer that permits its clustering and binding to other proteins (82–85). However, considering significant differences in the composition of these receptor complexes as well as the fact that FXYD5 activates NF-κB even in the absence of other stimuli, a possibility that the intracellular forms of FXYD5 contribute to NF-κB signaling downstream of the PM receptors but upstream IκBα phosphorylation cannot be excluded. Taken together, our results suggest that the presence of FXYD5 in the alveolar epithelium is required for stimuli-induced pulmonary inflammation and injury. The deleterious effects of enhanced FXYD5 may be twofold: (1) the impairment of the function of the epithelial barrier through the disruption of adherens junctions (26) and (2), as shown here, the activation of the NF-κB pathway to recruit CCR2[+] monocytes and IMs.

In conclusion, FXYD5 is a pro-inflammatory protein, which activates NF-κB-dependent cytokine secretion and infiltration of immune cells to the alveolar spaces. A better understanding of the mechanism by which alveolar epithelial FXYD5 modulates the expression of CCL2 and other cytokines may help to develop new therapies for the treatment of pulmonary inflammation following exposure to various Gram-negative bacteria commonly found in hospital settings.

AUTHOR CONTRIBUTIONS

PB, PS, ET, AY, and NM performed experiments; PB assisted with the research design and data analysis; KR, HP, and JS provided reagents; PB, HP, KR, and JS discussed and edited the manuscript; OV and LD designed the research, performed experiments, analyzed data, and wrote the manuscript.

ACKNOWLEDGMENTS

This work was supported by the Northwestern University—Flow Cytometry Core Facility supported by Cancer Center Support Grant (NCI CA060553). Flow Cytometry Cell Sorting was performed on a BD FACSAria SORP system, purchased through the support of NIH 1S10OD011996-01.

REFERENCES

1. Herold S, Gabrielli NM, Vadasz I. Novel concepts of acute lung injury and alveolar-capillary barrier dysfunction. *Am J Physiol Lung Cell Mol Physiol* (2013) 305:L665–81. doi:10.1152/ajplung.00232.2013
2. Short KR, Kroeze EJ, Fouchier RA, Kuiken T. Pathogenesis of influenza-induced acute respiratory distress syndrome. *Lancet Infect Dis* (2014) 14:57–69. doi:10.1016/S1473-3099(13)70286-X
3. Brune K, Frank J, Schwingshackl A, Finigan J, Sidhaye VK. Pulmonary epithelial barrier function: some new players and mechanisms. *Am J Physiol Lung Cell Mol Physiol* (2015) 308:L731–45. doi:10.1152/ajplung.00309.2014
4. Maus U, Von Grote K, Kuziel WA, Mack M, Miller EJ, Cihak J, et al. The role of CC chemokine receptor 2 in alveolar monocyte and neutrophil immigration in intact mice. *Am J Respir Crit Care Med* (2002) 166:268–73. doi:10.1164/rccm.2112012

5. Rose CE Jr, Sung SS, Fu SM. Significant involvement of CCL2 (MCP-1) in inflammatory disorders of the lung. *Microcirculation* (2003) 10:273–88. doi:10.1038/sj.mn.7800193
6. Maus UA, Wellmann S, Hampl C, Kuziel WA, Srivastava M, Mack M, et al. CCR2-positive monocytes recruited to inflamed lungs downregulate local CCL2 chemokine levels. *Am J Physiol Lung Cell Mol Physiol* (2005) 288:L350–8. doi:10.1152/ajplung.00061.2004
7. Herold S, Von Wulffen W, Steinmueller M, Pleschka S, Kuziel WA, Mack M, et al. Alveolar epithelial cells direct monocyte transepithelial migration upon influenza virus infection: impact of chemokines and adhesion molecules. *J Immunol* (2006) 177:1817–24. doi:10.4049/jimmunol.177.3.1817
8. Thorley AJ, Grandolfo D, Lim E, Goldstraw P, Young A, Tetley TD. Innate immune responses to bacterial ligands in the peripheral human lung – role of alveolar epithelial TLR expression and signalling. *PLoS One* (2011) 6:e21827. doi:10.1371/journal.pone.0021827

9. Martin GS, Mannino DM, Eaton S, Moss M. The epidemiology of sepsis in the United States from 1979 through 2000. *N Engl J Med* (2003) 348:1546–54. doi:10.1056/NEJMoa022139

10. Guillot L, Medjane S, Le-Barillec K, Balloy V, Danel C, Chignard M, et al. Response of human pulmonary epithelial cells to lipopolysaccharide involves toll-like receptor 4 (TLR4)-dependent signaling pathways: evidence for an intracellular compartmentalization of TLR4. *J Biol Chem* (2004) 279:2712–8. doi:10.1074/jbc.M305790200

11. Sender V, Stamme C. Lung cell-specific modulation of LPS-induced TLR4 receptor and adaptor localization. *Commun Integr Biol* (2014) 7:e29053. doi:10.4161/cib.29053

12. Aderem A, Ulevitch RJ. Toll-like receptors in the induction of the innate immune response. *Nature* (2000) 406:782–7. doi:10.1038/35021228

13. Mutlu GM, Sznajder JI. Mechanisms of pulmonary edema clearance. *Am J Physiol Lung Cell Mol Physiol* (2005) 289:L685–95. doi:10.1152/ajplung.00247.2005

14. Dhaliwal K, Scholefield E, Ferenbach D, Gibbons M, Duffin R, Dorward DA, et al. Monocytes control second-phase neutrophil emigration in established lipopolysaccharide-induced murine lung injury. *Am J Respir Crit Care Med* (2012) 186:514–24. doi:10.1164/rccm.201112-2132OC

15. Do-Umehara HC, Chen C, Urich D, Zhou L, Qiu J, Jang S, et al. Suppression of inflammation and acute lung injury by Miz1 via repression of C/EBP-delta. *Nat Immunol* (2013) 14:461–9. doi:10.1038/ni.2566

16. Fitzgerald KA, Rowe DC, Barnes BJ, Caffrey DR, Visintin A, Latz E, et al. LPS-TLR4 signaling to IRF-3/7 and NF-kappaB involves the toll adapters TRAM and TRIF. *J Exp Med* (2003) 198:1043–55. doi:10.1084/jem.20031023

17. Lu YC, Yeh WC, Ohashi PS. LPS/TLR4 signal transduction pathway. *Cytokine* (2008) 42:145–51. doi:10.1016/j.cyto.2008.01.006

18. Schulz C, Farkas L, Wolf K, Kratzel K, Eissner G, Pfeifer M. Differences in LPS-induced activation of bronchial epithelial cells (BEAS-2B) and type II-like pneumocytes (A-549). *Scand J Immunol* (2002) 56:294–302. doi:10.1046/j.1365-3083.2002.01137.x

19. Skerrett SJ, Liggitt HD, Hajjar AM, Ernst RK, Miller SI, Wilson CB. Respiratory epithelial cells regulate lung inflammation in response to inhaled endotoxin. *Am J Physiol Lung Cell Mol Physiol* (2004) 287:L143–52. doi:10.1152/ajplung.00030.2004

20. Crambert G, Geering K. FXYD proteins: new tissue-specific regulators of the ubiquitous Na,K-ATPase. *Sci STKE* (2003) 2003:RE1. doi:10.1126/stke.2003.166.re1

21. Garty H, Karlish SJ. FXYD proteins: tissue-specific regulators of the Na,K-ATPase. *Semin Nephrol* (2005) 25:304–11. doi:10.1016/j.semnephrol.2005.03.005

22. Geering K. Function of FXYD proteins, regulators of Na, K-ATPase. *J Bioenerg Biomembr* (2005) 37:387–92. doi:10.1007/s10863-005-9476-x

23. Geering K. FXYD proteins: new regulators of Na-K-ATPase. *Am J Physiol Renal Physiol* (2006) 290:F241–50. doi:10.1152/ajprenal.00126.2005

24. Lubarski I, Karlish SJ, Garty H. Structural and functional interactions between FXYD5 and the Na+-K+-ATPase. *Am J Physiol Renal Physiol* (2007) 293:F1818–26. doi:10.1152/ajprenal.00367.2007

25. Miller TJ, Davis PB. FXYD5 modulates Na+ absorption and is increased in cystic fibrosis airway epithelia. *Am J Physiol Lung Cell Mol Physiol* (2008) 294:L654–64. doi:10.1152/ajplung.00430.2007

26. Tokhtaeva E, Sun H, Deiss-Yehiely N, Wen Y, Soni PN, Gabrielli NM, et al. The O-glycosylated ectodomain of FXYD5 impairs adhesion by disrupting cell-cell trans-dimerization of Na,K-ATPase beta1 subunits. *J Cell Sci* (2016) 129:2394–406. doi:10.1242/jcs.186148

27. Lindzen M, Aizman R, Lifshitz Y, Lubarski I, Karlish SJ, Garty H. Structure-function relations of interactions between Na,K-ATPase, the gamma subunit, and corticosteroid hormone-induced factor. *J Biol Chem* (2003) 278:18738–43. doi:10.1074/jbc.M213253200

28. Garty H, Karlish SJ. Role of FXYD proteins in ion transport. *Annu Rev Physiol* (2006) 68:431–59. doi:10.1146/annurev.physiol.68.040104.131852

29. Lubarski I, Asher C, Garty H. FXYD5 (dysadherin) regulates the paracellular permeability in cultured kidney collecting duct cells. *Am J Physiol Renal Physiol* (2011) 301:F1270–80. doi:10.1152/ajprenal.00142.2011

30. Lubarski-Gotliv I, Asher C, Dada LA, Garty H. FXYD5 protein has a pro-inflammatory role in epithelial cells. *J Biol Chem* (2016) 291:11072–82. doi:10.1074/jbc.M115.699041

31. Shimamura T, Sakamoto M, Ino Y, Sato Y, Shimada K, Kosuge T, et al. Dysadherin overexpression in pancreatic ductal adenocarcinoma reflects tumor aggressiveness: relationship to e-cadherin expression. *J Clin Oncol* (2003) 21:659–67. doi:10.1200/JCO.2003.06.179

32. Park JR, Kim RJ, Lee YK, Kim SR, Roh KJ, Oh SH, et al. Dysadherin can enhance tumorigenesis by conferring properties of stem-like cells to hepatocellular carcinoma cells. *J Hepatol* (2011) 54:122–31. doi:10.1016/j.jhep.2010.06.026

33. Ino Y, Gotoh M, Sakamoto M, Tsukagoshi K, Hirohashi S. Dysadherin, a cancer-associated cell membrane glycoprotein, down-regulates E-cadherin and promotes metastasis. *Proc Natl Acad Sci U S A* (2002) 99:365–70. doi:10.1073/pnas.012425299

34. Shimada Y, Yamasaki S, Hashimoto Y, Ito T, Kawamura J, Soma T, et al. Clinical significance of dysadherin expression in gastric cancer patients. *Clin Cancer Res* (2004) 10:2818–23. doi:10.1158/1078-0432.CCR-0633-03

35. Batistatou A, Peschos D, Tsanou H, Charalabopoulos A, Nakanishi Y, Hirohashi S, et al. In breast carcinoma dysadherin expression is correlated with invasiveness but not with E-cadherin. *Br J Cancer* (2007) 96:1404–8. doi:10.1038/sj.bjc.6603743

36. Mitselou A, Batistatou A, Nakanishi Y, Hirohashi S, Vougiouklakis T, Charalabopoulos K. Comparison of the dysadherin and E-cadherin expression in primary lung cancer and metastatic sites. *Histol Histopathol* (2010) 25:1257–67. doi:10.14670/HH-25.1257

37. Maehata Y, Hirahashi M, Aishima S, Kishimoto J, Hirohashi S, Yao T, et al. Significance of dysadherin and E-cadherin expression in differentiated-type gastric carcinoma with submucosal invasion. *Hum Pathol* (2011) 42:558–67. doi:10.1016/j.humpath.2010.08.016

38. Lee YK, Lee SY, Park JR, Kim RJ, Kim SR, Roh KJ, et al. Dysadherin expression promotes the motility and survival of human breast cancer cells by AKT activation. *Cancer Sci* (2012) 103:1280–9. doi:10.1111/j.1349-7006.2012.02302.x

39. Lubarski I, Pihakaski-Maunsbach K, Karlish SJ, Maunsbach AB, Garty H. Interaction with the Na,K-ATPase and tissue distribution of FXYD5 (related to ion channel). *J Biol Chem* (2005) 280:37717–24. doi:10.1074/jbc.M506397200

40. Lubarski Gotliv I. FXYD5: Na+/K+-ATPase regulator in health and disease. *Front Cell Dev Biol* (2016) 4:26. doi:10.3389/fcell.2016.00026

41. Nam JS, Kang MJ, Suchar AM, Shimamura T, Kohn EA, Michalowska AM, et al. Chemokine (C-C motif) ligand 2 mediates the prometastatic effect of dysadherin in human breast cancer cells. *Cancer Res* (2006) 66:7176–84. doi:10.1158/0008-5472.CAN-06-0825

42. Wujak LA, Blume A, Baloglu E, Wygrecka M, Wygowski J, Herold S, et al. FXYD1 negatively regulates Na(+)/K(+)-ATPase activity in lung alveolar epithelial cells. *Respir Physiol Neurobiol* (2016) 220:54–61. doi:10.1016/j.resp.2015.09.008

43. Dada LA, Chandel NS, Ridge KM, Pedemonte C, Bertorello AM, Sznajder JI. Hypoxia-induced endocytosis of Na,K-ATPase in alveolar epithelial cells is mediated by mitochondrial reactive oxygen species and PKC-z. *J Clin Invest* (2003) 111:1057–64. doi:10.1172/JCI16826

44. Kanter JA, Sun H, Chiu S, Decamp MM, Sporn PH, Sznajder JI, et al. Decreased CXCL12 is associated with impaired alveolar epithelial cell migration and poor lung healing after lung resection. *Surgery* (2015) 158:1073–80; discussion 1080–2. doi:10.1016/j.surg.2015.04.051

45. Zhang Q, Kuang H, Chen C, Yan J, Do-Umehara HC, Liu XY, et al. The kinase Jnk2 promotes stress-induced mitophagy by targeting the small mitochondrial form of the tumor suppressor ARF for degradation. *Nat Immunol* (2015) 16:458–66. doi:10.1038/ni0715-785b

46. Urich D, Eisenberg JL, Hamill KJ, Takawira D, Chiarella SE, Soberanes S, et al. Lung-specific loss of the laminin alpha3 subunit confers resistance to mechanical injury. *J Cell Sci* (2011) 124:2927–37. doi:10.1242/jcs.080911

47. Zufferey R, Dull T, Mandel RJ, Bukovsky A, Quiroz D, Naldini L, et al. Self-inactivating lentivirus vector for safe and efficient in vivo gene delivery. *J Virol* (1998) 72:9873–80.

48. Daugherty RL, Serebryannyy L, Yemelyanov A, Flozak AS, Yu HJ, Kosak ST, et al. alpha-Catenin is an inhibitor of transcription. *Proc Natl Acad Sci U S A* (2014) 111:5260–5. doi:10.1073/pnas.1308663111

49. Misharin AV, Cuda CM, Saber R, Turner JD, Gierut AK, Haines GK III, et al. Nonclassical Ly6C(-) monocytes drive the development of inflammatory arthritis in mice. *Cell Rep* (2014) 9:591–604. doi:10.1016/j.celrep.2014.09.032

50. Factor P, Saldias F, Ridge K, Dumasius V, Zabner J, Jaffe HA, et al. Augmentation of lung liquid clearance via adenovirus-mediated transfer of a Na,K-ATPase beta1 subunit gene. *J Clin Invest* (1998) 102:1421–30. doi:10.1172/JCI3214

51. Misharin AV, Morales-Nebreda L, Mutlu GM, Budinger GR, Perlman H. Flow cytometric analysis of macrophages and dendritic cell subsets in the mouse lung. *Am J Respir Cell Mol Biol* (2013) 49:503–10. doi:10.1165/rcmb.2013-0086MA

52. Peteranderl C, Morales-Nebreda L, Selvakumar B, Lecuona E, Vadasz I, Morty RE, et al. Macrophage-epithelial paracrine crosstalk inhibits lung edema clearance during influenza infection. *J Clin Invest* (2016) 126:1566–80. doi:10.1172/JCI83931

53. Vagin O, Tokhtaeva E, Sachs G. The role of the beta1 subunit of the Na,K-ATPase and its glycosylation in cell-cell adhesion. *J Biol Chem* (2006) 281:39573–87. doi:10.1074/jbc.M606507200

54. Sanders CJ, Doherty PC, Thomas PG. Respiratory epithelial cells in innate immunity to influenza virus infection. *Cell Tissue Res* (2011) 343(1):13–21. doi:10.1007/s00441-010-1043-z

55. Paine R III, Rolfe MW, Standiford TJ, Burdick MD, Rollins BJ, Strieter RM. MCP-1 expression by rat type II alveolar epithelial cells in primary culture. *J Immunol* (1993) 150:4561–70.

56. Hayden MS, Ghosh S. Innate sense of purpose for IKKbeta. *Proc Natl Acad Sci U S A* (2014) 111:17348–9. doi:10.1073/pnas.1419689111

57. Carayol N, Chen J, Yang F, Jin T, Jin L, States D, et al. A dominant function of IKK/NF-kappaB signaling in global lipopolysaccharide-induced gene expression. *J Biol Chem* (2006) 281:31142–51. doi:10.1074/jbc.M603417200

58. Shi C, Pamer EG. Monocyte recruitment during infection and inflammation. *Nat Rev Immunol* (2011) 11:762–74. doi:10.1038/nri3070

59. Kuziel WA, Morgan SJ, Dawson TC, Griffin S, Smithies O, Ley K, et al. Severe reduction in leukocyte adhesion and monocyte extravasation in mice deficient in CC chemokine receptor 2. *Proc Natl Acad Sci U S A* (1997) 94:12053–8. doi:10.1073/pnas.94.22.12053

60. Rosseau S, Hammerl P, Maus U, Walmrath HD, Schutte H, Grimminger F, et al. Phenotypic characterization of alveolar monocyte recruitment in acute respiratory distress syndrome. *Am J Physiol Lung Cell Mol Physiol* (2000) 279:L25–35.

61. Su X. Leading neutrophils to the alveoli: who is the guider? *Am J Respir Crit Care Med* (2012) 186:472–3. doi:10.1164/rccm.201207-1235ED

62. de Weerd NA, Samarajiwa SA, Hertzog PJ. Type I interferon receptors: biochemistry and biological functions. *J Biol Chem* (2007) 282:20053–7. doi:10.1074/jbc.R700006200

63. Walczak H. TNF and ubiquitin at the crossroads of gene activation, cell death, inflammation, and cancer. *Immunol Rev* (2011) 244:9–28. doi:10.1111/j.1600-065X.2011.01066.x

64. Beg AA, Finco TS, Nantermet PV, Baldwin AS Jr. Tumor necrosis factor and interleukin-1 lead to phosphorylation and loss of I kappa B alpha: a mechanism for NF-kappa B activation. *Mol Cell Biol* (1993) 13:3301–10. doi:10.1128/MCB.13.6.3301

65. Maus U, Huwe J, Ermert L, Ermert M, Seeger W, Lohmeyer J. Molecular pathways of monocyte emigration into the alveolar air space of intact mice. *Am J Respir Crit Care Med* (2002) 165:95–100. doi:10.1164/ajrccm.165.1.2106148

66. Chuquimia OD, Petursdottir DH, Rahman MJ, Hartl K, Singh M, Fernandez C. The role of alveolar epithelial cells in initiating and shaping pulmonary immune responses: communication between innate and adaptive immune systems. *PLoS One* (2012) 7:e32125. doi:10.1371/journal.pone.0032125

67. Chuquimia OD, Petursdottir DH, Periolo N, Fernandez C. Alveolar epithelial cells are critical in protection of the respiratory tract by secretion of factors able to modulate the activity of pulmonary macrophages and directly control bacterial growth. *Infect Immun* (2013) 81:381–9. doi:10.1128/IAI.00950-12

68. Stegemann-Koniszewski S, Jeron A, Gereke M, Geffers R, Kroger A, Gunzer M, et al. Alveolar type II epithelial cells contribute to the anti-influenza A virus response in the lung by integrating pathogen- and microenvironment-derived signals. *MBio* (2016) 7:e276–216. doi:10.1128/mBio.00276-16

69. Hakansson HF, Smailagic A, Brunmark C, Miller-Larsson A, Lal H. Altered lung function relates to inflammation in an acute LPS mouse model. *Pulm Pharmacol Ther* (2012) 25:399–406. doi:10.1016/j.pupt.2012.08.001

70. Thorley AJ, Ford PA, Giembycz MA, Goldstraw P, Young A, Tetley TD. Differential regulation of cytokine release and leukocyte migration by lipopolysaccharide-stimulated primary human lung alveolar type II epithelial cells and macrophages. *J Immunol* (2007) 178:463–73. doi:10.4049/jimmunol.178.1.463

71. Morales-Nebreda L, Misharin AV, Perlman H, Budinger GR. The heterogeneity of lung macrophages in the susceptibility to disease. *Eur Respir Rev* (2015) 24:505–9. doi:10.1183/16000617.0031-2015

72. Duan M, Hibbs ML, Chen W. The contributions of lung macrophage and monocyte heterogeneity to influenza pathogenesis. *Immunol Cell Biol* (2016) 95:225–35. doi:10.1038/icb.2016.97

73. Rosenberg HF, Dyer KD, Foster PS. Eosinophils: changing perspectives in health and disease. *Nat Rev Immunol* (2013) 13:9–22. doi:10.1038/nri3341

74. Felton JM, Lucas CD, Rossi AG, Dransfield I. Eosinophils in the lung – modulating apoptosis and efferocytosis in airway inflammation. *Front Immunol* (2014) 5:302. doi:10.3389/fimmu.2014.00302

75. Travers J, Rothenberg ME. Eosinophils in mucosal immune responses. *Mucosal Immunol* (2015) 8:464–75. doi:10.1038/mi.2015.2

76. Ravin KA, Loy M. The eosinophil in infection. *Clin Rev Allergy Immunol* (2016) 50:214–27. doi:10.1007/s12016-015-8525-4

77. Caraglia M, Vitale G, Marra M, Budillon A, Tagliaferri P, Abbruzzese A. Alpha-interferon and its effects on signalling pathways within cells. *Curr Protein Pept Sci* (2004) 5:475–85. doi:10.2174/1389203043379378

78. van Boxel-Dezaire AH, Rani MR, Stark GR. Complex modulation of cell type-specific signaling in response to type I interferons. *Immunity* (2006) 25:361–72. doi:10.1016/j.immuni.2006.08.014

79. Hervas-Stubbs S, Perez-Gracia JL, Rouzaut A, Sanmamed MF, Le Bon A, Melero I. Direct effects of type I interferons on cells of the immune system. *Clin Cancer Res* (2011) 17:2619–27. doi:10.1158/1078-0432.CCR-10-1114

80. Ha T, Liu L, Kelley J, Kao R, Williams D, Li C. Toll-like receptors: new players in myocardial ischemia/reperfusion injury. *Antioxid Redox Signal* (2011) 15:1875–93. doi:10.1089/ars.2010.3723

81. Sun H, Zhu X, Cai W, Qiu L. Hypaphorine attenuates lipopolysaccharide-induced endothelial inflammation via regulation of TLR4 and PPAR-gamma dependent on PI3K/Akt/mTOR signal pathway. *Int J Mol Sci* (2017) 18:844. doi:10.3390/ijms18040844

82. Palsson-McDermott EM, O'Neill LA. Signal transduction by the lipopolysaccharide receptor, toll-like receptor-4. *Immunology* (2004) 113:153–62. doi:10.1111/j.1365-2567.2004.01976.x

83. Freudenberg MA, Tchaptchet S, Keck S, Fejer G, Huber M, Schutze N, et al. Lipopolysaccharide sensing an important factor in the innate immune response to Gram-negative bacterial infections: benefits and hazards of LPS hypersensitivity. *Immunobiology* (2008) 213:193–203. doi:10.1016/j.imbio.2007.11.008

84. Tan Y, Kagan JC. A cross-disciplinary perspective on the innate immune responses to bacterial lipopolysaccharide. *Mol Cell* (2014) 54:212–23. doi:10.1016/j.molcel.2014.03.012

85. Tan Y, Kagan JC. Microbe-inducible trafficking pathways that control toll-like receptor signaling. *Traffic* (2017) 18:6–17. doi:10.1111/tra.12454

Hypercapnia Impairs ENaC Cell Surface Stability by Promoting Phosphorylation, Polyubiquitination and Endocytosis of β-ENaC in a Human Alveolar Epithelial Cell Line

Paulina Gwoździńska [1], Benno A. Buchbinder [1], Konstantin Mayer [1], Susanne Herold [1], Rory E. Morty [1,2], Werner Seeger [1,2] and István Vadász [1]*

[1] Department of Internal Medicine, Justus Liebig University, Universities of Giessen and Marburg Lung Center, German Center for Lung Research, Giessen, Germany, [2] Max Planck Institute for Heart and Lung Research, Bad Nauheim, Germany

*Correspondence:
István Vadász
istvan.vadasz@innere.med.
uni-giessen.de

Acute lung injury is associated with formation of pulmonary edema leading to impaired gas exchange. Patients with acute respiratory distress syndrome (ARDS) require mechanical ventilation to improve oxygenation; however, the use of relatively low tidal volumes (to minimize further injury of the lung) often leads to further accumulation of carbon dioxide (hypercapnia). Hypercapnia has been shown to impair alveolar fluid clearance (AFC), thereby causing retention of pulmonary edema, and may lead to worse outcomes; however, the underlying molecular mechanisms remain incompletely understood. AFC is critically dependent on the epithelial sodium channel (ENaC), which drives the vectorial transport of Na^+ across the alveolar epithelium. Thus, in the current study, we investigated the mechanisms by which hypercapnia effects ENaC cell surface stability in alveolar epithelial cells (AECs). Elevated CO_2 levels led to polyubiquitination of β-ENaC and subsequent endocytosis of the α/β-ENaC complex in AECs, which were prevented by silencing the E3 ubiquitin ligase, Nedd4-2. Hypercapnia-induced ubiquitination and cell surface retrieval of ENaC were critically dependent on phosphorylation of the Thr615 residue of β-ENaC, which was mediated by the extracellular signal-regulated kinase (ERK)1/2. Furthermore, activation of ERK1/2 led to subsequent activation of AMP-activated protein kinase (AMPK) and c-Jun N-terminal kinase (JNK)1/2 that in turn phosphorylated Nedd4-2 at the Thr899 residue. Importantly, mutation of Thr899 to Ala markedly inhibited the CO_2-induced polyubiquitination of β-ENaC and restored cell surface stability of the ENaC complex, highlighting the critical role of Nedd4-2 phosphorylation status in targeting ENaC. Collectively, our data suggest that elevated CO_2 levels promote activation of the ERK/AMPK/JNK axis in a human AEC line, in which ERK1/2 phosphorylates β-ENaC whereas JNK mediates phosphorylation of Nedd4-2, thereby facilitating the channel–ligase interaction. The hypercapnia-induced ENaC dysfunction may contribute to impaired alveolar edema clearance and thus, interfering with these molecular mechanisms may improve alveolar fluid balance and lead to better outcomes in patients with ARDS.

Keywords: carbon dioxide, epithelial sodium channel, sodium transport, ubiquitination, alveolar fluid clearance, alveolar epithelium, mitogen-activated protein kinase signaling

INTRODUCTION

Carbon dioxide (CO_2) is formed as a by-product of cellular respiration and is eliminated from the body during breathing (1). In respiratory disorders that are associated with alveolar hypoventilation, retention of CO_2 is often detected, which leads to elevated CO_2 concentrations in the blood, also known as hypercapnia (2). For example, patients with severe acute respiratory distress syndrome (ARDS) frequently present with hypercapnia, which may be enhanced due to mechanical ventilation with low tidal volumes to minimize further ventilator-induced injuries to the lung (3). It is increasingly evident that the alveolar epithelium is capable of sensing of elevated CO_2 levels, which initiate specific signaling signatures and alter the function of alveolar epithelial and other cells (2, 4). While some of these effects are anti-inflammatory, which may be beneficial in the context of excessive inflammation, others impair innate immunity, mitochondrial function, cellular repair, and alveolar epithelial barrier function, which are clearly detrimental in the setting of ARDS (5–10).

A fully functional alveolar epithelial barrier is crucial for maintaining optimal fluid balance and gas exchange in the lung (11, 12). In order to keep the alveolar space "dry," excess alveolar liquid is reabsorbed from the air space into the interstitium by a well-characterized active sodium transport process in which Na^+ enters the alveolar epithelial type I and type II cells through the apically located epithelial sodium channel (ENaC) and is subsequently pumped out basolaterally by the Na,K-ATPase. This creates a Na^+ gradient, which drives paracellular movement of water leading to its clearance from the alveolar space (11, 12). Importantly, it has been clearly demonstrated that in most patients with ARDS alveolar fluid clearance (AFC) is impaired and that those patients with ARDS and impaired AFC the mortality is significantly higher than in ARDS patients with normal AFC (13).

Other than in the alveolar epithelium, ENaC molecules are expressed in the apical surface of various tight epithelia including kidney, colon, and respiratory airways where ENaC is located along the entire length of motile cilia and regulate osmolarity of the periciliary fluid (14). ENaC usually consists of three subunits (α [or δ, depending on the species, tissue, and cell type], β, and γ) (15–17). A functional ENaC complex requires at least one α- or δ-subunit, whereas the β- and γ-subunits are necessary for proper trafficking and activity of the channel (15, 16, 18). In line with this notion, mice lacking α-ENaC are unable to clear lung fluid from the alveoli and die nearly immediately after birth (19). The significance of β-ENaC in the regulation of channel activity has been highlighted in transgenic mice overexpressing this subunit in the lung (20). In these animals, an increase in alveolar epithelial Na^+ uptake due to β-ENaC overexpression, probably by promoting trafficking of ENaC to the cell surface and enhancing channel activity, leads to lung dehydration and causes a CF-like phenotype. Cell surface abundance of ENaC is modified by the E3 ubiquitin ligase Nedd4-2, which by interaction with the PY motif, located at the C-termini of each subunit of the channel, promotes ubiquitination and subsequent clathrin-mediated endocytosis of the channel (21–23). Nedd4-2$^{-/-}$ mice have enhanced ENaC expression and function; however, this genetic manipulation has

lethal consequences (24). In contrast, overexpression of the ligase causes a decrease in ENaC density at the plasma membrane (PM) and reduces Na^+ transport (25).

Previous studies have proposed the involvement of phosphorylation in the mechanisms regulating Nedd4-2 binding to ENaC (26, 27). For example, extracellular signal-regulated kinase (ERK), c-Jun N-terminal kinase (JNK), and recently also the cellular energy sensor, AMP-activated protein kinase (AMPK), have been described as potential modulators of the ENaC/Nedd4-2 interaction by phosphorylating the E3 ligase or the target (28–32). We have previously described that hypercapnia markedly impairs AFC and initiates a specific signaling pattern in the alveolar epithelium, including rapid activation of ERK, AMPK, and JNK and subsequent downregulation of the Na,K-ATPase (7, 8, 33). Considering the pivotal role of ENaC in AFR and that several kinases, which have previously been suggested to alter ENaC/Nedd4-2 interaction, are activated by elevated CO_2 levels, in the current study we sought to determine whether ENaC is effected by hypercapnia and provide evidence that excess CO_2 initiates ERK-mediated β-ENaC phosphorylation and AMPK/JNK-dependent activation of Nedd4-2 leading to an enhancement of β-ENaC polyubiquitination and, thus, to endocytosis of the ENaC complex form the cell surface. Since ENaC activity is essential for optimal lung fluid balance, the hypercapnia-induced alterations in ENaC cell surface stability may cause further aggravation of lung injury.

MATERIALS AND METHODS

Cell Culture

Human epithelial A549 cells (ATCC, CCL 185) were grown in DMEM supplemented with 10% fetal bovine serum and 100 U/ml penicillin, 100 μg/ml streptomycin as previously described (8). Experiments were performed on subconfluent monolayers of cells. Cells were incubated in a humidified atmosphere of 5% CO_2/95% air at 37°C.

CO$_2$ Exposure

A549 cells were treated with 40 or 120 mmHg CO_2 (normocapnia and hypercapnia, respectively). Before each experiment, fresh solutions were prepared with DMEM-Ham's F-12 medium and Tris base. The buffering capacity of the experimental media was modified by changing the initial pH using Tris base to obtain a pH of 7.4 at 40 and 120 mmHg CO_2 (8). The desired CO_2 concentrations and pH levels were obtained by equilibrating the experimental media overnight in a humidified chamber from BioSpherix Ltd. (NY, USA). The C-Chamber's atmosphere was controlled with a PRO-CO_2 Carbon Dioxide controller (Biospherix Ltd.). In the chamber, cells were treated with a pCO_2 of 40 or 120 mmHg while keeping 21% O_2 balanced with N_2. Before and after CO_2 exposure, pH, pCO_2, and pO_2 levels in the media were measured using a Rapidlab blood gas analyzer (Siemens, Erlangen, Germany).

Plasmids, Constructs, Site-Directed Mutagenesis, Antibodies, and Inhibitors

pEYFP-C1-expressing α-ENaC was constructed by PCR amplifying α-ENaC gene using as a template pTNT-α-ENaC and oligonucleotide primers α-ENaC forward 5'-GAATTCAATGG-AGGGGAACAAGCTGGAGG-3' and α-ENaC reverse 5'-GGATCCCTTGTCATCGTCATCCTTGTAATCGGGCCCC CCCAGAGGAC-3'. The resulting amplicon was digested with EcoRI/BamH1 and ligated to the multiple cloning site (MCS) of pEYFP-C1 plasmid. The pEYFP-C1 vector contained the epitope-tag eYFP at the N-terminus and a FLAG-tag at the C-terminus. Thus, anti-GFP or anti-FLAG antibodies recognize the α-ENaC construct at a predicted size of 118 kDa, 1,073 amino acids [α-ENaC (90 kDa) plus YFP (27 kDa) and FLAG (1 kDa)]. pcDNA3.1V5/His expressing β-ENaC was constructed by PCR amplifying β-ENaC gene using as a template cDNA transcribed from total mRNA isolated from A549 cells and oligonucleotide primers β-ENaC forward 5'-CTCGGATCCACATGCACGTGAAGAAGTACCT-3' and β-ENaC reverse 5'-GCACTCGAGGATGGCATCACCCT-CACTGT-3'. The resulting amplicon was digested with Xho1/BamH1 and ligated to MCS of pcDNA3.1V5/His plasmid. Finally, E. coli DH5α were transformed using the constructed plasmid. Anti-V5 antibodies recognize the β-ENaC construct at a predicted size of 96 kDa, 872 amino acids [β-ENaC plus V5 at the C-terminus (1 kDa)]. pCMV-HA-C-expressing γ-ENaC was constructed by PCR amplifying γ-ENaC gene using as a template pTNT-γENaC and oligonucleotide primers γ-ENaC forward 5'-AGGCCCGAATTCATGGCACCCGGAGAGAAGAT-3' and γ-ENaC reverse 5'-GTAGCCGGTACCGAGCTCATC-CAGCATCTGGG-3'. The resulting amplicon was digested and ligated to MCS of pCMV-HA-C plasmid. The pCMV-HA-C vector contained the epitope-tag myc at the N-terminus and an HA-tag at the C-terminus. Anti-HA antibodies recognize γ-ENaC at a predicted size of 97 kDa, 881 amino acids [γ-ENaC plus myc (1 kDa) and HA (1 kDa)]. pRK5-HA-ubiquitin was a gift from Ted Dawson [Addgene 17608 (34)] and the pCI HA NEDD4L plasmid was a gift from Joan Massague [Addgene 27000 (35)]. Site-directed mutagenesis was used to perform point mutation of T899A in human Nedd4-2 using Quick Change Mutagenesis Kit from Stratagene (La Jolla, CA, USA) in accordance to the manufacturer's instructions. The primer sequences were as follows: Nedd4-2 forward: 5'-ACTGCAGTTTGTCGCAGGGACATCG-CGAG-3', Nedd4-2 reverse: 5' CTCGCGATGTCCCTGCGAC-AAACTGCAGT-3'. Immunoblot analysis of epitope-tagged ENaC expressed in A549 cells were performed with a mouse anti-GFP antibody from Roche (Basel, Switzerland), a mouse anti-HA antibody (Covance, Princeton, NJ, USA), a mouse anti-V5 antibody and a mouse antibody against transferrin receptor used as loading control of biotinylated proteins from Invitrogen (Waltham, MA, USA; Figure S1 in Supplementary Material). A rabbit antibody directed against β-actin was used as loading control of cytoplasmic ENaC and was purchased from Sigma Aldrich (Saint Louis, MO, USA). The inhibitor of AMPK, Compound C, was from Merck Millipore (Darmstadt, Germany). The inhibitor of MEK, U0126 was from Promega (Fitchburg, WI, USA). siRNA against AMPK-α1 and Nedd4-2 and scrambled siRNA control were purchased from Santa Cruz Biotechnology (Dallas, TX, USA).

Transient Transfection

A549 cells were transiently transfected with eYFP-α-ENaC, β-ENaC-V5, HA-ubiquitin, HA-Nedd4-2 wild type, or mutant by using nucleofection, as previously described (36). Briefly,

cells were resuspended in 100 μl of the nucleofection solution SF (Lonza, Cologne, Germany), and 4–6 μg of DNA was added. Cells were placed in a cuvette and pulsed with the specified cell-type nucleofector program. After 10 min of incubation time, cells were cultured in DMEM supplemented with 10% FBS, 100 U/ml penicillin, and 100 μg/ml streptomycin. In some studies, 24 h before nucleofection with ENaC plasmids, cells were transfected with siRNA using Lipofectamine RNAiMAX (Invitrogen, Waltham, MA, USA) according to the instructions of the manufacturer. Experiments were performed 48 h later.

Cell Surface Biotinylation

A549 cells were labeled for 20 min using 1 mg/ml EZ-Link NHS-SS-biotin (Pierce Biotechnology, Waltham, MA, USA) and lysed in lysis buffer (50 mM HEPES, 150 mM NaCl, 1 mM EGTA, 10% glycerol, 1% TritonX100). Surface proteins were pulled down with streptavidin-agarose beads from Pierce Biotechnology (Waltham, MA, USA) and analyzed by SDS-PAGE and immuno-blot, as described previously (8).

Ubiquitination Studies

A549 cells were transfected with ENaC plasmids (2 μg of each) and HA-ubiquitin (3 μg). In some studies, cells were co-transfected with a plasmid coding HA-Nedd4-2 (wild type or mutant T899A, 2 μg) or siRNAs (against AMPK-α1, Nedd4-2, or scrambled). Cells were exposed to 40 mmHg CO_2 (Ctrl) or to 120 mmHg CO_2 (CO_2) for 15 or 30 min and lysed on ice in lysis buffer (50 mM HEPES, 150 mM NaCl, 1 mM EGTA, 10% glycerol, 1% TritonX100), containing a protease inhibitor cocktail from Roche. After lysing the samples, proteins were resolved in 8% polyacrylamide gel, transferred to nitrocellulose membrane (Optitran; Schleicher & Schuell, Dassel, Germany) using a semidry apparatus from Bio-Rad (Hercules, Berkeley, CA, USA). Membranes were blocked in 5% fat-free dried milk powder and immunoblotted with anti-GFP or anti-V5 to detect α- or β-ENaC, respectively. Films were overexposed to detect ENaC ubiquitin conjugates.

Phosphorylation Experiments

Phosphorylation studies of ERK1/2, AMPK-α1, and c-Jun were performed using antibodies from Cell Signaling (Danvers, MA, USA). The anti-phospho-β-ENaC (T615) antibody was from Abcam (Cambridge, UK). A549 cells were treated with normal or elevated CO_2 concentrations (40 or 120 mmHg, respectively) for the desired times, and then were washed with PBS twice and were lysed on ice in lysis buffer (50 mM HEPES, 150 mM NaCl, 1 mM EGTA, 10% glycerol, 1% TritonX100). Samples having the same amount of protein were resuspended in Laemmli sample buffer and boiled for 10 min at 98°C and immunoblotted with specific antibodies.

Statistics

Data are presented as mean ± SEM and were analyzed using one-way analysis of variance (ANOVA) followed by a multiple comparison with the Dunnet test. p values of less than 0.05 were considered significant. GraphPad prism 6 (GraphPad software, San Diego, CA, USA) was used for the analysis and presentation of data.

RESULTS

Acute Exposure to Elevated CO_2 Levels Leads to ENaC Endocytosis by Promoting Polyubiquitination of β-ENaC

To test whether high CO_2 levels promote endocytosis of ENaC, A549 cells were co-transfected with plasmids encoding the human α- and β-subunit of ENaC and the PM abundance of these proteins was measured after exposure of cells to physiological (pCO_2 40 mmHg; normocapnia) or elevated (pCO_2 120 mmHg; hypercapnia) CO_2 concentrations at a pH_e of 7.4 for 30 min. Exposure of cells to elevated CO_2 levels decreased α- and β-ENaC cell surface abundance by approximately 60% (**Figure 1A**), whereas the total protein level remained unaffected (**Figure 1B**). To determine whether elevated CO_2 levels lead to ubiquitination of either ENaC subunit, A549 cells were co-transfected with α- or β-ENaC and ubiquitin containing HA-tag (HA-Ub) and exposed the cells to 40 or 120 mmHg CO_2 for 15 min. Whereas no ubiquitination of α-ENaC in response to hypercapnia was

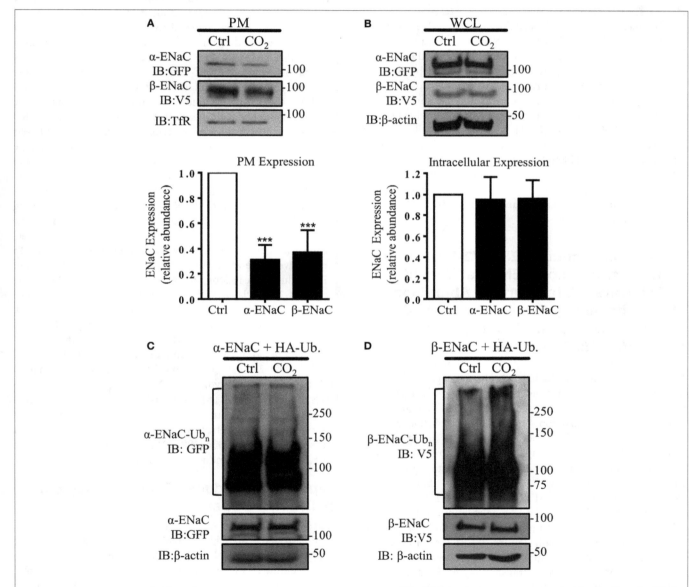

FIGURE 1 | Acute exposure to elevated CO_2 levels leads to epithelial sodium channel (ENaC) endocytosis by promoting polyubiquitination of β-ENaC.
(A) A549 cells were co-transfected with α- and β-ENaC and were exposed to 40 mmHg CO_2 (Ctrl) or 120 mmHg CO_2 (CO_2) for 30 min at a pH_e of 7.4. Plasma membrane (PM) proteins were determined by streptavidin pull-downs and immunoblotting with anti-GFP to detect α-ENaC and anti-V5 to detect β-ENaC. Representative immunoblots of α-, β-ENaC, and transferrin receptor (TfR) at the PM are shown. **(B)** A549 cells were co-transfected with α- and β-ENaC and were treated as described above. Protein abundance in whole cell lysate (WCL) was measured by immunoblotting. Representative immunoblots of α-, β-ENaC, and β-actin are shown. Bars represent mean ± SEM [n (number of independent experiments) = 3; ***$p < 0.001$]. **(C,D)**, A549 cells were co-transfected with ubiquitin containing HA-tag (HA-Ub) and α-ENaC **(C)** or β-ENaC **(D)** and were exposed to 40 or 120 mmHg CO_2 for 15 min. Total ubiquitinated α-ENaC and β-ENaC was detected by immunoblots with anti-GFP or anti-V5 antibody.

evident (**Figure 1C**), a marked increase in β-ENaC ubiquitination in total cell lysates was observed when cells were treated with elevated CO_2 and immunoblotted with an antibody against V5 (**Figure 1D**). We detected a "polyubiquitin smear" above the molecular size of ENaC suggesting the presence of β-ENaC ubiquitin conjugates. This observation suggested that β-ENaC is a substrate of CO_2-induced ubiquitination.

Nedd4-2 Mediates the Hypercapnia-Induced ENaC Polyubiquitination and Endocytosis

In subsequent studies, we silenced the endogenous Nedd4-2 with a specific siRNA to study whether Nedd4-2 mediates β-ENaC polyubiquitination during hypercapnia. Of note, the elevated CO_2-induced ENaC ubiquitination was prevented by Nedd4-2 silencing (**Figure 2A**). To further test whether Nedd4-2 silencing altered ENaC PM stability, we measured cell surface ENaC abundance in A549 cells co-transfected with a scrambled siRNA (si-Scr.) or siRNA against Nedd4-2. Importantly, cells exposed to increased CO_2 concentrations treated with siRNA targeting Nedd4-2 had increased ENaC α- and β-subunit density at the PM (**Figure 2B**). Thus, upon hypercapnia, Nedd4-2 targets β-ENaC, leading to polyubiquitination of the β-subunit of the channel, which results in decreased abundance of the α/β-ENaC complex at the cell surface.

Hypercapnia Induces ERK1/2-Dependent Phosphorylation of β-ENaC at Thr615 and Downregulates Surface Abundance of the Channel by Facilitating β-ENaC Polyubiquitination and Endocytosis of the α/β-ENaC Complex

In agreement with a previous report describing increased ERK 1/2 activity in alveolar epithelial cells (AECs) exposed to hypercapnia (33), we found a rapid and transient phosphorylation of ERK1/2 in A549 cells exposed to elevated CO_2 (**Figure 3A**). Moreover, ERK1/2 activation was paralleled by phosphorylation of β-ENaC at the Thr 615 residue (**Figure 3B**). To test whether ERK-dependent β-ENaC phosphorylation was sufficient to promote polyubiquitination of β-ENaC in response to high CO_2, we co-transfected A549 cells with β-ENaC and HA-ubiquitin. Cells were pre-treated with the MEK (upstream of ERK) inhibitor U0126 and exposed to elevated CO_2 concentrations for 30 min. Inhibition of ERK prevented phosphorylation and polyubiquitination of the ENaC β-subunit (**Figure 3C**). To further prove that the hypercapnia-induced ENaC cell surface retrieval is dependent on ERK1/2, A549 cells were co-transfected with ENaC plasmids, and exposed to normo- or hypercapnia as described above and observed that inhibition of ERK1/2 markedly increased the number of the ENaC molecules at the cell surface upon hypercapnia exposure (**Figure 3D**). Together, these data indicate that the hypercapnia-induced ERK1/2 activation promotes ENaC internalization by phosphorylation-dependent ubiquitination of the β-subunit of the channel.

JNK1/2-Dependent Nedd4-2 Phosphorylation at Thr899 Facilitates β-ENaC Polyubiquitination and Endocytosis

Because JNK activation has been implicated in the CO_2-induced signaling pattern in AEC, which led to inhibition of the Na, K-ATPase (7), we next investigated the effects of JNK phosphorylation in AEC exposed to hypercapnia on ENaC. Activity of JNK1/2 was assessed by phosphorylation of c-Jun, a downstream target of JNK1/2. In line with the previously published data, we observed a rapid and time-dependent JNK activation induced by hypercapnia, which returned to baseline within 30 min of exposure to elevated CO_2 levels (**Figure 4A**). To further investigate whether increased activity of Nedd4-2 is crucial to decrease hypercapnia-induced ENaC cell surface abundance, we next mutated a single amino acid in the catalytic domain of Nedd4-2 (T899A). The Thr899 residue within the HECT domain of the E3 ligase has previously been reported to be involved in the Nedd4-2-mediated ubiquitination of α-ENaC (37). A549 cells were co-transfected with HA-Ub and HA-Nedd4-2 wild type (WT) or HA-Nedd4-2 mutant (T899) constructs and exposed to 40 or 120 mmHg CO_2 for 30 min. Of note, we found that phosphorylation of Thr899 played a central role in the hypercapnia-induced ubiquitination of β-ENaC, as in A549 cells expressing the Nedd4-2 in which the Thr899 has been mutated to an alanine (T899A), which cannot be phosphorylated, the level of β-ENaC polyubiquitination significantly decreased (**Figure 4B**). To further investigate whether this decrease in the ubiquitination of β-ENaC due to the lack of phosphorylation at the Thr899 residue of Nedd4-2 correlated with an increase in ENaC cell surface stability, cell surface biotinylation studies were performed. Importantly, overexpression of the Nedd4-2 mutant (T899A) also prevented endocytosis of the α/β-ENaC complex during hypercapnia (**Figure 4C**). Moreover and further confirming the central role of Nedd4-2 phosphorylation at Thr899 in the ubiquitination and subsequent endocytosis of ENaC, we observed increased levels of ENaC proteins at the cell surface after overexpression of the Nedd4-2 T899A mutant. Finally and in line with the above described findings, pretreatment of A549 cells with the potent and specific JNK inhibitor, SP600125, also fully prevented the hypercapnia-induced endocytosis of ENaC (**Figure 4D**).

Hypercapnia Induces ENaC Endocytosis by ERK1/2-Dependent AMPK-α1 Activation

AMP-activated protein kinase, which has been shown to activate Nedd4-2 and inhibit ENaC (29), has also been described as one of the central mediators of the hypercapnia-induced alveolar epithelial dysfunction and a downstream target of ERK upon CO_2 exposure (8, 33). Furthermore, we have previously observed that AMPK activates JNK1/2 in AEC when exposed to elevated CO_2 levels (7). In line with these previously published observations, we measured a rapid and transient phosphorylation of AMPK-α1 in A549 cells exposed to hypercapnia (**Figure 5A**), which was dependent on activation of ERK (**Figure 5B**) and

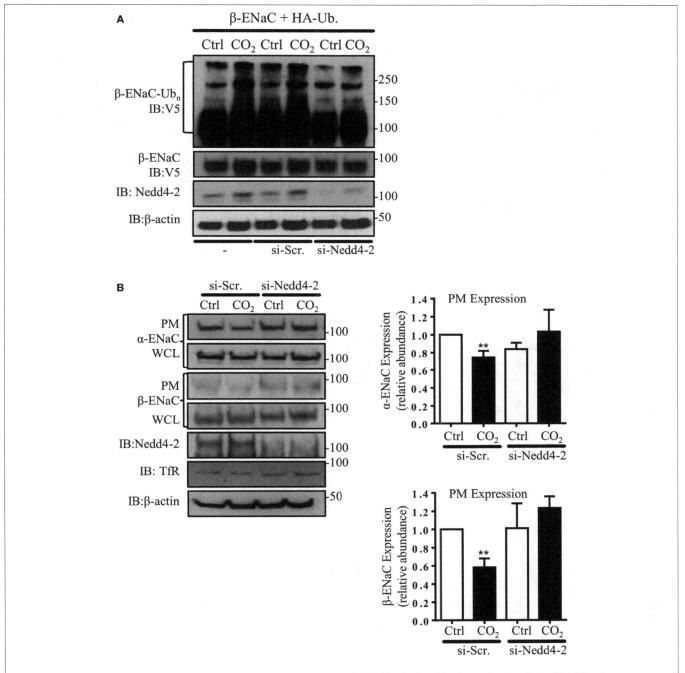

FIGURE 2 | Nedd4-2 mediates hypercapnia-induced epithelial sodium channel (ENaC) polyubiquitination and endocytosis. (A) A549 cells were co-transfected with β-ENaC, HA-ubiquitin, and siRNA against Nedd4-2 or a scrambled siRNA (si-Scr.) and were treated with 40 or 120 mmHg CO_2 for 30 min and β-ENaC polyubiquitinated isoforms were determined. (B) A549 cells were co-transfected with α-, β-ENaC, and siRNA targeting Nedd4-2 or scrambled siRNA. Biotinylated ENaC proteins were detected by immunoblotting. Representative immunoblots of α-, β-ENaC, and transferrin receptor (TfR) at the plasma membrane (PM) and total protein abundance [whole cell lysate (WCL)] of ENaC proteins, β-actin, and Nedd4-2 are shown. Bars represent mean ± SEM (n = 3; ** p < 0.01).

upstream of JNK (Figure S2 in Supplementary Material). To determine whether activation of AMPK was necessary for the hypercapnia-induced polyubiquitination of β-ENaC, A549 cells were co-transfected with β-ENaC, HA-ubiquitin, and a specific siRNA against AMPK-α1 (or a scrambled siRNA) and were exposed to normal or elevated CO_2 levels and observed a significant decrease in polyubiquitination of β-ENaC after CO_2 exposure (**Figure 5C**). As a second approach, endogenous AMPK was inhibited by compound C after co-transfection of A549 cells with β-ENaC and HA-ubiquitin. Similar to our data that we obtained with AMPK silencing, exposure of the cells to hypercapnia in the presence of the inhibitor markedly

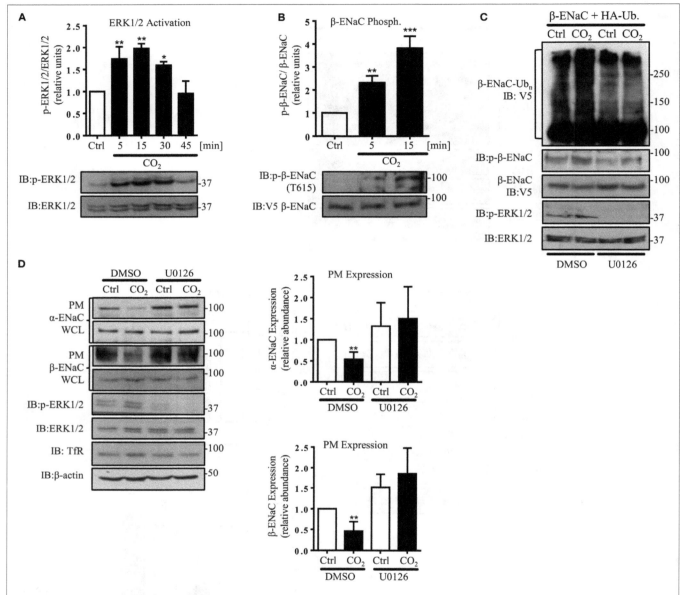

FIGURE 3 | Hypercapnia induces extracellular signal-regulated kinase (ERK)1/2-dependent phosphorylation of β-ENaC at T615 facilitating β-ENaC polyubiquitination and endocytosis of the α/β-ENaC complex. (A) A549 cells were exposed to 40 mmHg CO₂ (Ctrl) for 15 min or to 120 mmHg CO₂ (CO₂) for 5–45 min at a pH₉ of 7.4. Phosphorylation of ERK1/2 and the total amount of ERK1/2 were measured. The graph represents the p-ERK1/2/ERK1/2 ratio. Representative immunoblots of p-ERK1/2 and total ERK1/2 are shown. (B) A549 cells were co-transfected with β-ENaC and were treated with 40 mmHg CO₂ for 15 min or 120 mmHg CO₂ for 5 and 15 min at a pH₉ of 7.4. Phosphorylation of β-ENaC at T615 (p-β-ENaC) and total β-ENaC were determined by immunoblotting. Graphs represent p-β-ENaC/β-ENaC ratio. Representative immunoblots of p-β-ENaC and β-ENaC are shown. Values are expressed as mean ± SEM (n = 3; *p < 0.05; **p < 0.01). (C) A549 cells were transfected with β-ENaC, HA-ubiquitin, and were exposed to 40 mmHg CO₂ or 120 mmHg CO₂ for 30 min at a pH₉ of 7.4 in the presence or absence of U0126 (10 μM, 30 min pretreatment). Total ubiquitinated β-ENaC was detected by immunoblotting with anti-V5 antibody. (D) A549 cells were co-transfected with α- and β-ENaC and were exposed to CO₂ as described above. ENaC subunits at the plasma membrane (PM) were determined by biotin-streptavidin pull-downs and immunoblotting. Representative immunoblots of α- and β-ENaC at the PM, total protein abundance of epithelial sodium channel (ENaC) and p-ERK 1/2 are shown. Bars represent mean ± SEM (n = 3; *p < 0.05; ***p < 0.001).

decreased the hypercapnia-induced β-ENaC polyubiquitination (**Figure 5D**). To further confirm the role of AMPK-α1 in the CO₂-induced downregulation of ENaC, we transfected A549 cells with α- and β-ENaC and exposed to elevated CO₂ levels for 30 min in the presence or absence of the above mentioned siRNA against AMPK-α1 (**Figure 5E**) or compound C (Figure S3 in Supplementary Material) and observed that silencing or inhibition of AMPK stabilized ENaC proteins at the PM upon hypercapnia. Taken together, these latter studies suggest that AMPK by activation of JNK and subsequent phosphorylation of Nedd4-2 plays a central role in the hypercapnia-induced ubiquitination and endocytosis of ENaC.

DISCUSSION

In the present study, we show that elevated CO_2 levels initiate a specific signaling pattern leading to ubiquitination-mediated retrieval of ENaC from the PM, thereby reducing cell surface abundance of the channel in a human AEC line. Hypercapnia is associated with a number of acute and chronic pulmonary diseases; however, it is not evident to what extent and by which mechanisms these elevated levels of CO_2 may further impact on disease states. While hypercapnia and the associated acidosis have been shown to have anti-inflammatory effects, which might be advantageous at sites of excessive inflammation, recently, it has been clearly demonstrated that by impairing innate immunity, cellular repair, and alveolar epithelial function, elevated CO_2 may play a role in the pathogenesis of ARDS and COPD (2, 5, 9, 10, 38). Furthermore, it is increasingly evident that patients with ARDS and COPD who present with hypercapnia have worse outcomes (3, 39, 40).

A major function of the alveolar epithelium is the clearance of excess alveolar fluid, thereby promoting effective gas exchange. This clearance is mediated by the concerted action of various sodium transporters, among which the apically located ENaC

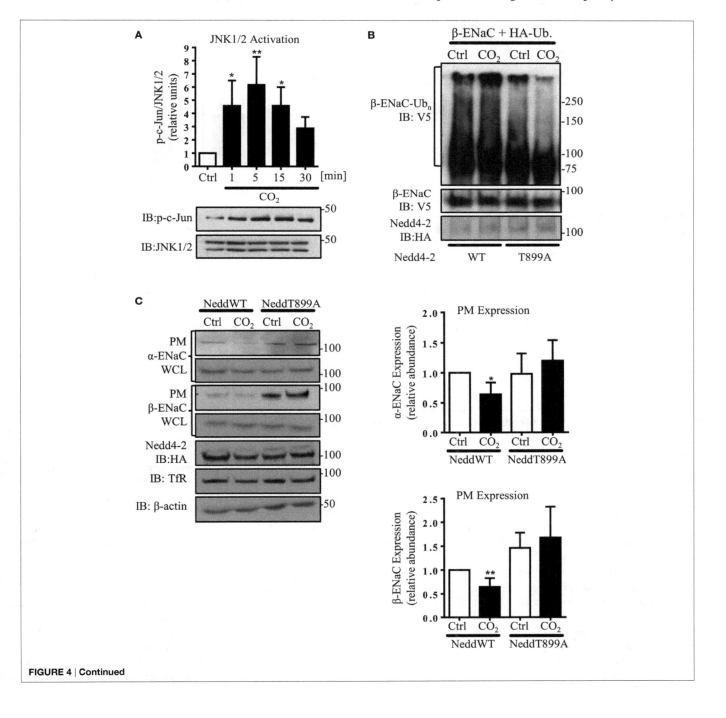

FIGURE 4 | Continued

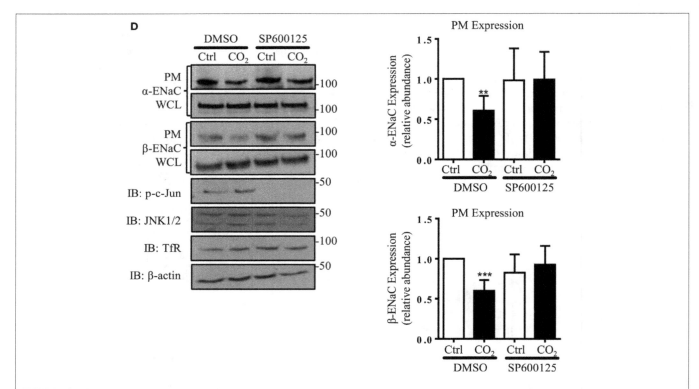

FIGURE 4 | c-Jun N-terminal kinase (JNK)1/2-dependent Nedd4-2 phosphorylation at Thr899 facilitates β-ENaC polyubiquitination and endocytosis. (A) A549 cells were exposed to 40 mmHg CO_2 (Ctrl) for 15 min or to 120 mmHg CO_2 (CO_2) for 1 to 30 min at a pH$_e$ of 7.4 and the phosphorylation of c-Jun and the total amount of JNK1/2 were measured by immunoblotting. Graph represents the p-c-Jun/JNK1/2 ratio. Representative immunoblots of p-c-Jun and total JNK1/2 levels are shown. Values are expressed as mean ± SEM (n = 3; *p < 0.05; **p < 0.01). (B) A549 cells were co-transfected with β-ENaC, HA-ubiquitin, and HA-Nedd4-2 wild type (WT) or mutant (T899A). Cells were treated with 40 mmHg CO_2 or 120 mmHg CO_2 for 30 min at a pH$_e$ of 7.4. Total ubiquitinated β-ENaC was detected by immunoblotting with anti-V5 antibody. (C) A549 cells were co-transfected with α- and β-ENaC and Nedd4-2 wild type or mutant and were exposed to CO_2 as described above. Epithelial sodium channel (ENaC) at the plasma membrane (PM) was determined by biotin-streptavidin pull-downs and immunoblotting. Representative immunoblots of α- and β-ENaC at the PM, total protein abundance of ENaC, Nedd4-2, and β-actin are shown. Mean ± SEM (n = 3; *p < 0.05). (D) A549 cells were co-transfected with α- and β-ENaC exposed to 40 mmHg CO_2 or 120 mmHg CO_2 for 30 min at a pH$_e$ of 7.4 in the presence or absence of SP600125 (25 µM, 30 min pretreatment). ENaC at the PM was determined by biotin-streptavidin pull-downs and immunoblotting. Representative immunoblots of α- and β-ENaC at the PM, total protein abundance of ENaC, p-c-Jun, JNK1/2, and β-actin are shown. Bars represent mean ± SEM (n = 5; **p < 0.01; ***p < 0.001).

and the basolateral Na,K-ATPase have been identified as key players. Indeed, we have previously shown that the Na,K-ATPase is downregulated by hypercapnia; however, a potential regulation of ENaC by carbon dioxide has not been previously investigated. Various factors have been shown to affect ENaC cell surface abundance and function, including interleukin-1β, interleukin-4, transforming growth factor-β, LPS, or hypoxia (41–45), which similar to hypercapnia are often observed in patients with respiratory failure. As reducing hypercapnia without further damaging the lung is challenging, a better understanding of the molecular patterns initiated by elevated CO_2 levels may help us to interfere with the deleterious signals, thereby rescuing or at least not further aggravating lung damage.

Ubiquitination is a posttranslational modification that regulates trafficking and stability of proteins (46). Numerous studies described that depending on the stimulus ENaC subunits may undergo multimono- or polyubiquitination leading to channel retrieval from the cell surface or degradation of ENaC (47–49). It is also well documented that the phosphorylation status of target molecules and the E3 ubiquitin ligase often play a pivotal role in the initiation of ubiquitination (50, 51). Previous findings established the significance of mitogen-activated protein kinase (MAPK) in the hypercapnia-induced impairment of AFC (7, 33). Moreover, it has also been described that ERK and JNK, two prominent members of the MAPK family, may alter the phosphorylation status of ENaC and the E3 ligase of the channel, Nedd4-2, respectively (31, 37).

Thus, we first investigated whether elevated CO_2 concentrations affect ENaC cell surface stability by a mechanism involving ubiquitination of the channel and whether the MAPK pathway is involved in the hypercapnia-induced signaling events. Of note, a remarkable and rapid increase in polyubiquitination of β-ENaC and a significant reduction of the cell surface abundance of the α/β-ENAC complex were observed in AEC exposed to hypercapnia, as early as 30 min after CO_2 exposure, suggesting that ENaC function is probably sensitive to changes in CO_2 levels. In contrast, in the first half an hour after CO_2 exposure, total intracellular levels of ENaC remained unchanged, suggesting that CO_2 influenced

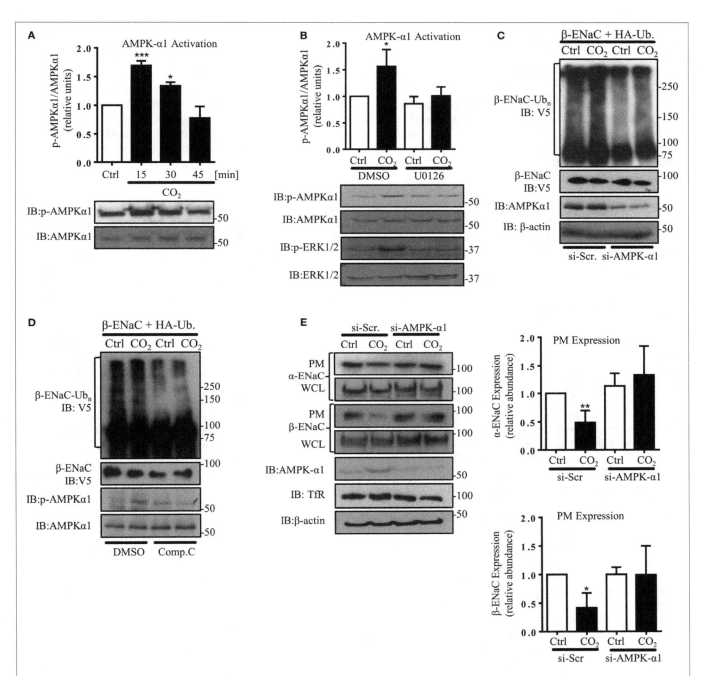

FIGURE 5 | Hypercapnia induces epithelial sodium channel (ENaC) endocytosis *via* extracellular signal-regulated kinase (ERK)1/2-dependent AMPK-α1 activation. **(A)** A549 cells were exposed to 40 mmHg CO_2 (Ctrl) for 15 min or to 120 mmHg CO_2 (CO_2) for 15–45 min at a pH$_e$ of 7.4. The phosphorylation of AMPK-α1 at Thr172 and the total amount of AMPK-α1 were measured by immunoblotting. Graph represents the p-AMPK-α1/AMPK-α1 ratio. Representative immunoblots of p-AMPK-α1 and total AMPK-α1 are shown. **(B)** A549 cells were treated with 40 mmHg CO_2 (Ctrl) or with 120 mmHg CO_2 (CO_2) for 15 min at a pH$_e$ of 7.4 in the presence or absence of 10 μM U0126 (30 min pretreatment). Phosphorylation of AMPK-α1 at Thr172, p-ERK1/2, and the total amount of both proteins were determined by immunoblotting. Graph represents the p-AMPK-α1/AMPK-α1 ratio. Representative immunoblots of p-AMPK-α1, p-ERK1/2 and total level of AMPK-α1 and ERK1/2 are shown. Values are expressed as mean ± SEM ($n = 3$; *$p < 0.05$; ***$p < 0.001$). **(C)** A549 cells were co-transfected with β-ENaC, HA-ubiquitin, and siRNA targeting AMPK-α1 or a scrambled siRNA and were treated with 40 or 120 mmHg CO_2 for 30 min. β-ENaC polyubiquitinated isoforms were determined with anti-V5 antibody. Representative immunoblots of β-ENaC, AMPK-α1, and β-actin are shown. **(D)** A549 cells were co-transfected with β-ENaC and HA-ubiquitin and were treated with 40 mmHg CO_2 or 120 mmHg CO_2 for 30 min at a pH$_e$ of 7.4 in the presence or absence of compound C (20 μM, 30 min pretreatment). Total ubiquitinated β-ENaC was detected as described above. Representative immunoblots of β-ENaC, p-AMPK-α1, and total AMPK-α1 are shown. **(E)** Cells were co-transfected with α- and β-ENaC and siRNA targeting AMPK-α1 or a scrambled siRNA and exposed to 40 mmHg CO_2 or 120 mmHg CO_2 for 30 min at a pH$_e$ of 7.4. Biotinylated ENaC proteins were detected by immunoblotting. Representative western blots of α- and β-ENaC at the plasma membrane (PM) and total protein abundance of ENaC, p-AMPK-α1, and AMPK-α1 are shown. Bars present mean ± SEM ($n = 3$; *$p < 0.05$; **$p < 0.01$).

the trafficking of the channel rather than protein degradation. Furthermore, no significant changes in the ubiquitination status of α-ENaC have been detected upon hypercapnic treatment, highlighting and further confirming the central regulatory role of β-ENaC in the trafficking of the channel (52).

Our data demonstrate that elevated CO_2 levels cause a rapid and time-dependent ERK1/2 activation followed by phosphorylation of β-ENaC at the Thr615 residue. Moreover, genetic inhibition of Nedd4-2, the E3 ubiquitin ligase that drives ubiquitination of the various ENaC subunits (49), by a specific siRNA reduced β-ENaC polyubiquitination and prevented the hypercapnia-induced redistribution of α- and β-ENaC from the PM to the intracellular store, indicating a central role for Nedd4-2 in ENaC ubiquitination and endocytosis in AEC exposed to hypercapnia. Indeed, ERK1/2 has previously been described as a negative regulator of ENaC. For example, Eaton et al. showed that protein kinase C-δ drives ERK activation leading to ENaC internalization (30). Another study established that the ERK-mediated ENaC downregulation is promoted by phosphorylation β- and γ-ENaC, resulting in enhancement of Nedd4-2/ENaC interaction and thus, decreased Na^+ transport (31). Therefore, hypercapnia by enhancing ERK activity promotes phosphorylation of the ENaC β-subunit, which may increase the affinity of the E3 ubiquitin ligase to ENaC.

We have previously shown that JNK is also implicated in CO_2 responses and that phosphorylation of the kinase is required for the CO_2-induced inhibition of the Na,K-ATPase in the alveolar epithelium (7). The significance of JNK in cellular adaptation to stress has been shown by several studies (53). Of note, the possible role of JNK in modulating Nedd4-2 activity and ENaC current has been reported in polarized kidney epithelial cells (28). Remarkably, this study also showed that the Thr899 residue in the HECT (homologous to the E6-AP carboxyl terminus) domain of Nedd4-2 may be phosphorylated by JNK1, which was required for ubiquitination of α-ENaC (28). To assess the potential involvement of JNK-mediated Nedd4-2 phosphorylation in the hypercapnia-induced downregulation of ENaC, we mutated Thr899 to Ala to prevent phosphorylation of the E3 ligase at this residue. Importantly, this point mutation largely prevented the CO_2-induced polyubiquitination of β-ENaC although activation of JNK was evident and stabilized α- and β-ENaC at the cell surface. Thus, our data together with the previously published literature suggest that phosphorylation of Nedd4-2 by JNK at the Thr899 residue is critical for the hypercapnia-induced ubiquitination of β–ENaC, which drives endocytosis of the ENaC complex from the PM in AEC.

We have previously shown that AMPK, a cellular metabolic sensor that inhibits several ion transporters including the cystic fibrosis transmembrane conductance regulator, Na,K-ATPase, and ENaC, is rapidly activated by hypercapnia (8, 29, 54). Regarding the regulation of ENaC, it has been shown that chemical stimulation of AMPK by 5-aminoimidazole-4-carboxamide-1-beta-4-ribofuranoside inhibited ENaC activity in lung epithelial cells (55). Moreover, enhanced abundance of ENaC channels at the cell surface was reported in the distal airways in AMPK-$\alpha1^{-/-}$ mice (28). Interestingly, AMPK has also been reported to regulate Nedd4-2 activity (26, 29). In the current study, treatment of AEC with a specific siRNA against AMPK-$\alpha1$

or an AMPK-α inhibitor, compound C markedly decreased CO_2-induced β-ENaC polyubiquitination and endocytosis of α-, and β-ENaC, which is consistent with previous findings showing that in human embryonic kidney cells, AMPK activation promoted Nedd4-2/ENaC association (26). Furthermore, and in line with a previously published study (7), we also show that in the context of hypercapnia, AMPK is an upstream regulator of JNK. Thus, it is probable that the AMPK-regulated effects of CO_2 on Nedd4-2 and ENaC are indirect and mediated by JNK. Moreover, although AMPK is an early element of the CO_2-induced signaling pattern, its activation appears to be downstream of ERK upon hypercapnic exposure. This is of particular importance as ERK appears two have a dual role in the hypercapnia-induced downregulation of ENaC. On the one hand, it rapidly phosphorylates the β-subunit of the channel and by activating AMPK and JNK, it indirectly promotes phosphorylation of the E3 ligase Nedd4-2 as well. Of note, both of these phosphorylation events seem to be critically required for the CO_2-induced ubiquitination and subsequent endocytosis of ENaC, probably by enhancing the association of the E3 ligase and the target molecule.

Our study has some clear limitations. Although we show a rapid activation of ERK and a subsequent phosphorylation of β-ENaC at the Thr615 residue, which is a known target of ERK, we have not investigated the potential rescue of β-ENaC ubiquitination or trafficking of the ENaC complex after preventing phosphorylation at this specific site. A mutation of this residue will be necessary to definitely prove that ERK-promoted phosphorylation of β-ENaC at this residue drives the downregulation of the channel upon hypercapnia. Moreover, the current study was performed exclusively in AECs and further *in vivo* investigations will be necessary to establish the role of the hypercapnia-induced signaling events identified in the current manuscript in ENaC-driven AFC and alveolar epithelial barrier dysfunction in an animal model of hypercapnic acute lung injury.

Taken together, our study shows for the first time that upon exposure to elevated CO_2 levels, ENaC cell surface abundance is rapidly downregulated in a human AEC line by a specific, CO_2-induced and ERK-, AMPK-, and JNK-mediated signaling pathway, which promotes phosphorylation of both β-ENaC and Nedd4-2, leading to ubiquitination of β-ENaC and subsequent internalization of the α/β-ENaC complex. This novel signaling pathway may contribute to the persistence of alveolar edema and thus, interfering with these molecular mechanisms may improve alveolar fluid balance and lead to better outcomes in patients with ARDS and hypercapnia.

AUTHOR CONTRIBUTIONS

Conception or design of the work: PG and IV; acquisition, analysis, or interpretation of data: PG, BB, KM, SH, RM, WS, and IV; drafting the work: PG and IV; revising it critically for important intellectual content: PG, BB, KM, SH, RM, WS, and IV. All the authors approved the final version of the manuscript and agreed to be accountable for all aspects of the work in ensuring that questions related to the accuracy or integrity of any part of the work are appropriately investigated and resolved.

ACKNOWLEDGMENTS

The authors thank Mrs. Miriam Wessendorf (Universities of Giessen and Marburg Lung Center) for her excellent technical assistance.

REFERENCES

1. Putnam RW, Filosa JA, Ritucci NA. Cellular mechanisms involved in CO(2) and acid signaling in chemosensitive neurons. *Am J Physiol Cell Physiol* (2004) 287(6):C1493–526. doi:10.1152/ajpcell.00282.2004
2. Vadasz I, Hubmayr RD, Nin N, Sporn PH, Sznajder JI. Hypercapnia: a nonpermissive environment for the lung. *Am J Respir Cell Mol Biol* (2012) 46(4):417–21. doi:10.1165/rcmb.2011-0395PS
3. Nin N, Muriel A, Penuelas O, Brochard L, Lorente JA, Ferguson ND, et al. Severe hypercapnia and outcome of mechanically ventilated patients with moderate or severe acute respiratory distress syndrome. *Intensive Care Med* (2017) 43(2):200–8. doi:10.1007/s00134-016-4611-1
4. Cummins EP, Selfridge AC, Sporn PH, Sznajder JI, Taylor CT. Carbon dioxide-sensing in organisms and its implications for human disease. *Cell Mol Life Sci* (2014) 71(5):831–45. doi:10.1007/s00018-013-1470-6
5. Briva A, Vadasz I, Lecuona E, Welch LC, Chen J, Dada LA, et al. High CO2 levels impair alveolar epithelial function independently of pH. *PLoS One* (2007) 2(11):e1238. doi:10.1371/journal.pone.0001238
6. Gates KL, Howell HA, Nair A, Vohwinkel CU, Welch LC, Beitel GJ, et al. Hypercapnia impairs lung neutrophil function and increases mortality in murine pseudomonas pneumonia. *Am J Respir Cell Mol Biol* (2013) 49 (5):821–8. doi:10.1165/rcmb.2012-0487OC
7. Vadasz I, Dada LA, Briva A, Helenius IT, Sharabi K, Welch LC, et al. Evolutionary conserved role of c-Jun-N-terminal kinase in CO2-induced epithelial dysfunction. *PLoS One* (2012) 7(10):e46696. doi:10.1371/journal.pone.0046696
8. Vadasz I, Dada LA, Briva A, Trejo HE, Welch LC, Chen J, et al. AMP-activated protein kinase regulates CO2-induced alveolar epithelial dysfunction in rats and human cells by promoting Na,K-ATPase endocytosis. *J Clin Invest* (2008) 118(2):752–62. doi:10.1172/JCI29723
9. Vohwinkel CU, Lecuona E, Sun H, Sommer N, Vadasz I, Chandel NS, et al. Elevated CO(2) levels cause mitochondrial dysfunction and impair cell proliferation. *J Biol Chem* (2011) 286(43):37067–76. doi:10.1074/jbc.M111.290056
10. Laffey JG, Honan D, Hopkins N, Hyvelin JM, Boylan JF, McLoughlin P. Hypercapnic acidosis attenuates endotoxin-induced acute lung injury. *Am J Respir Crit Care Med* (2004) 169(1):46–56. doi:10.1164/rccm.200205-394OC
11. Matthay MA, Folkesson HG, Clerici C. Lung epithelial fluid transport and the resolution of pulmonary edema. *Physiol Rev* (2002) 82(3):569–600. doi:10.1152/physrev.00003.2002
12. Mutlu GM, Sznajder JI. Mechanisms of pulmonary edema clearance. *Am J Physiol Lung Cell Mol Physiol* (2005) 289(5):L685–95. doi:10.1152/ajplung.00247.2005
13. Ware LB, Matthay MA. Alveolar fluid clearance is impaired in the majority of patients with acute lung injury and the acute respiratory distress syndrome. *Am J Respir Crit Care Med* (2001) 163(6):1376–83. doi:10.1164/ajrccm.163.6.2004035
14. Enuka Y, Hanukoglu I, Edelheit O, Vaknine H, Hanukoglu A. Epithelial sodium channels (ENaC) are uniformly distributed on motile cilia in the oviduct and the respiratory airways. *Histochem Cell Biol* (2012) 137(3):339–53. doi:10.1007/s00418-011-0904-1
15. Bhalla V, Hallows KR. Mechanisms of ENaC regulation and clinical implications. *J Am Soc Nephrol* (2008) 19(10):1845–54. doi:10.1681/ASN.2008020225
16. Matalon S, Bartoszewski R, Collawn JF. Role of epithelial sodium channels in the regulation of lung fluid homeostasis. *Am J Physiol Lung Cell Mol Physiol* (2015) 309(11):L1229–38. doi:10.1152/ajplung.00319.2015
17. Hanukoglu I, Hanukoglu A. Epithelial sodium channel (ENaC) family: phylogeny, structure-function, tissue distribution, and associated inherited diseases. *Gene* (2016) 579(2):95–132. doi:10.1016/j.gene.2015.12.061
18. Canessa CM, Schild L, Buell G, Thorens B, Gautschi I, Horisberger JD, et al. Amiloride-sensitive epithelial Na+ channel is made of three homologous subunits. *Nature* (1994) 367(6462):463–7. doi:10.1038/367463a0
19. Hummler E, Barker P, Gatzy J, Beermann F, Verdumo C, Schmidt A, et al. Early death due to defective neonatal lung liquid clearance in alpha-ENaC-deficient mice. *Nat Genet* (1996) 12(3):325–8. doi:10.1038/ng0396-325
20. Mall M, Grubb BR, Harkema JR, O'Neal WK, Boucher RC. Increased airway epithelial Na+ absorption produces cystic fibrosis-like lung disease in mice. *Nat Med* (2004) 10(5):487–93. doi:10.1038/nm1028
21. Abriel H, Loffing J, Rebhun JF, Pratt JH, Schild L, Horisberger JD, et al. Defective regulation of the epithelial Na+ channel by Nedd4 in Liddle's syndrome. *J Clin Invest* (1999) 103(5):667–73. doi:10.1172/JCI5713
22. Snyder PM, Olson DR, McDonald FJ, Bucher DB. Multiple WW domains, but not the C2 domain, are required for inhibition of the epithelial Na+ channel by human Nedd4. *J Biol Chem* (2001) 276(30):28321–6. doi:10.1074/jbc.M011487200
23. Rotin D, Staub O. Role of the ubiquitin system in regulating ion transport. *Pflugers Arch* (2011) 461(1):1–21. doi:10.1007/s00424-010-0893-2
24. Boase NA, Rychkov GY, Townley SL, Dinudom A, Candi E, Voss AK, et al. Respiratory distress and perinatal lethality in Nedd4-2-deficient mice. *Nat Commun* (2011) 2:287. doi:10.1038/ncomms1284
25. Knight KK, Olson DR, Zhou R, Snyder PM. Liddle's syndrome mutations increase Na+ transport through dual effects on epithelial Na+ channel surface expression and proteolytic cleavage. *Proc Natl Acad Sci U S A* (2006) 103(8):2805–8. doi:10.1073/pnas.0511184103
26. Carattino MD, Edinger RS, Grieser HJ, Wise R, Neumann D, Schlattner U, et al. Epithelial sodium channel inhibition by AMP-activated protein kinase in oocytes and polarized renal epithelial cells. *J Biol Chem* (2005) 280(18):17608–16. doi:10.1074/jbc.M501770200
27. Debonneville C, Flores SY, Kamynina E, Plant PJ, Tauxe C, Thomas MA, et al. Phosphorylation of Nedd4-2 by Sgk1 regulates epithelial Na(+) channel cell surface expression. *EMBO J* (2001) 20(24):7052–9. doi:10.1093/emboj/20.24.7052
28. Almaca J, Kongsuphol P, Hieke B, Ousingsawat J, Viollet B, Schreiber R, et al. AMPK controls epithelial Na(+) channels through Nedd4-2 and causes an epithelial phenotype when mutated. *Pflugers Arch* (2009) 458(4):713–21. doi:10.1007/s00424-009-0660-4
29. Bhalla V, Oyster NM, Fitch AC, Wijngaarden MA, Neumann D, Schlattner U, et al. AMP-activated kinase inhibits the epithelial Na+ channel through functional regulation of the ubiquitin ligase Nedd4-2. *J Biol Chem* (2006) 281(36):26159–69. doi:10.1074/jbc.M606045200
30. Eaton AF, Yue Q, Eaton DC, Bao HF. ENaC activity and expression is decreased in the lungs of protein kinase C-alpha knockout mice. *Am J Physiol Lung Cell Mol Physiol* (2014) 307(5):L374–85. doi:10.1152/ajplung.00040.2014
31. Shi H, Asher C, Chigaev A, Yung Y, Reuveny E, Seger R, et al. Interactions of beta and gamma ENaC with Nedd4 can be facilitated by an ERK-mediated phosphorylation. *J Biol Chem* (2002) 277(16):13539–47. doi:10.1074/jbc.M111717200
32. Yang LM, Rinke R, Korbmacher C. Stimulation of the epithelial sodium channel (ENaC) by cAMP involves putative ERK phosphorylation sites in the C termini of the channel's beta- and gamma-subunit. *J Biol Chem* (2006) 281(15):9859–68. doi:10.1074/jbc.M512046200
33. Welch LC, Lecuona E, Briva A, Trejo HE, Dada LA, Sznajder JI. Extracellular signal-regulated kinase (ERK) participates in the hypercapnia-induced Na, K-ATPase downregulation. *FEBS Lett* (2010) 584(18):3985–9. doi:10.1016/j.febslet.2010.08.002
34. Lim KL, Chew KC, Tan JM, Wang C, Chung KK, Zhang Y, et al. Parkin mediates nonclassical, proteasomal-independent ubiquitination of synphilin-1: implications for Lewy body formation. *J Neurosci* (2005) 25(8):2002–9. doi:10.1523/JNEUROSCI.4474-04.2005
35. Gao S, Alarcon C, Sapkota G, Rahman S, Chen PY, Goerner N, et al. Ubiquitin ligase Nedd4L targets activated Smad2/3 to limit TGF-beta signaling. *Mol Cell* (2009) 36(3):457–68. doi:10.1016/j.molcel.2009.09.043

36. Grzesik BA, Vohwinkel CU, Morty RE, Mayer K, Herold S, Seeger W, et al. Efficient gene delivery to primary alveolar epithelial cells by nucleofection. *Am J Physiol Lung Cell Mol Physiol* (2013) 305(11):L786–94. doi:10.1152/ajplung.00191.2013

37. Hallows KR, Bhalla V, Oyster NM, Wijngaarden MA, Lee JK, Li H, et al. Phosphopeptide screen uncovers novel phosphorylation sites of Nedd4-2 that potentiate its inhibition of the epithelial Na+ channel. *J Biol Chem* (2010) 285(28):21671–8. doi:10.1074/jbc.M109.084731

38. Doerr CH, Gajic O, Berrios JC, Caples S, Abdel M, Lymp JF, et al. Hypercapnic acidosis impairs plasma membrane wound resealing in ventilator-injured lungs. *Am J Respir Crit Care Med* (2005) 171(12):1371–7. doi:10.1164/rccm.200309-1223OC

39. Kohnlein T, Windisch W, Kohler D, Drabik A, Geiseler J, Hartl S, et al. Non-invasive positive pressure ventilation for the treatment of severe stable chronic obstructive pulmonary disease: a prospective, multicentre, randomised, controlled clinical trial. *Lancet Respir Med* (2014) 2(9):698–705. doi:10.1016/S2213-2600(14)70153-5

40. Bellani G, Laffey JG, Pham T, Fan E, Brochard L, Esteban A, et al. Epidemiology, patterns of care, and mortality for patients with acute respiratory distress syndrome in intensive care units in 50 countries. *JAMA* (2016) 315(8):788–800. doi:10.1001/jama.2016.0291

41. Galietta LJV, Pagesy P, Folli C, Caci E, Romio L, Costes B, et al. IL-4 is a potent modulator of ion transport in the human bronchial epithelium in vitro. *J Immunol* (2002) 168(2):839–45. doi:10.4049/jimmunol.168.2.839

42. Gille T, Randrianarison-Pellan N, Goolaerts A, Dard N, Uzunhan Y, Ferrary E, et al. Hypoxia-induced inhibition of epithelial Na(+) channels in the lung. Role of Nedd4-2 and the ubiquitin-proteasome pathway. *Am J Respir Cell Mol Biol* (2014) 50(3):526–37. doi:10.1165/rcmb.2012-0518OC

43. Migneault F, Boncoeur E, Morneau F, Pascariu M, Dagenais A, Berthiaume Y. Cycloheximide and lipopolysaccharide downregulate alphaENaC mRNA *via* different mechanisms in alveolar epithelial cells. *Am J Physiol Lung Cell Mol Physiol* (2013) 305(10):L747–55. doi:10.1152/ajplung.00023.2013

44. Roux J, Kawakatsu H, Gartland B, Pespeni M, Sheppard D, Matthay MA, et al. Interleukin-1beta decreases expression of the epithelial sodium channel alpha-subunit in alveolar epithelial cells *via* a p38 MAPK-dependent signaling pathway. *J Biol Chem* (2005) 280(19):18579–89. doi:10.1074/jbc.M410561200

45. Peters DM, Vadász I, Wujak L, Wygrecka M, Olschewski A, Becker C, et al. TGF-beta directs trafficking of the epithelial sodium channel ENaC which has implications for ion and fluid transport in acute lung injury. *Proc Natl Acad Sci U S A* (2014) 111(3):E374–83. doi:10.1073/pnas.1306798111

46. Hershko A, Ciechanover A. The ubiquitin system. *Annu Rev Biochem* (1998) 67:425–79. doi:10.1146/annurev.biochem.67.1.425

47. Butterworth MB, Edinger RS, Ovaa H, Burg D, Johnson JP, Frizzell RA. The deubiquitinating enzyme UCH-L3 regulates the apical membrane recycling of the epithelial sodium channel. *J Biol Chem* (2007) 282(52):37885–93. doi:10.1074/jbc.M707989200

48. Wiemuth D, Ke Y, Rohlfs M, McDonald FJ. Epithelial sodium channel (ENaC) is multi-ubiquitinated at the cell surface. *Biochem J* (2007) 405(1):147–55. doi:10.1042/BJ20060747

49. Zhou R, Patel SV, Snyder PM. Nedd4-2 catalyzes ubiquitination and degradation of cell surface ENaC. *J Biol Chem* (2007) 282(28):20207–12. doi:10.1074/jbc.M611329200

50. Butterworth MB, Frizzell RA, Johnson JP, Peters KW, Edinger RS. PKA-dependent ENaC trafficking requires the SNARE-binding protein complexin. *Am J Physiol Renal Physiol* (2005) 289(5):F969–77. doi:10.1152/ajprenal.00390.2003

51. Hunter T. The age of crosstalk: phosphorylation, ubiquitination, and beyond. *Mol Cell* (2007) 28(5):730–8. doi:10.1016/j.molcel.2007.11.019

52. Firsov D, Schild L, Gautschi I, Merillat AM, Schneeberger E, Rossier BC. Cell surface expression of the epithelial Na channel and a mutant causing Liddle syndrome: a quantitative approach. *Proc Natl Acad Sci U S A* (1996) 93(26):15370–5. doi:10.1073/pnas.93.26.15370

53. Weston CR, Davis RJ. The JNK signal transduction pathway. *Curr Opin Cell Biol* (2007) 19(2):142–9. doi:10.1016/j.ceb.2007.02.001

54. Hallows KR, Raghuram V, Kemp BE, Witters LA, Foskett JK. Inhibition of cystic fibrosis transmembrane conductance regulator by novel interaction with the metabolic sensor AMP-activated protein kinase. *J Clin Invest* (2000) 105(12):1711–21. doi:10.1172/JCI9622

55. Woollhead AM, Scott JW, Hardie DG, Baines DL. Phenformin and 5-aminoimidazole-4-carboxamide-1-beta-D-ribofuranoside (AICAR) activation of AMP-activated protein kinase inhibits transepithelial Na+ transport across H441 lung cells. *J Physiol* (2005) 566(Pt 3):781–92. doi:10.1113/jphysiol.2005.088674

11

Gas Exchange Disturbances Regulate Alveolar Fluid Clearance during Acute Lung Injury

István Vadász[1]* and Jacob I. Sznajder[2]

[1] Department of Internal Medicine, Justus Liebig University, Universities of Giessen and Marburg Lung Center, Giessen, Germany, [2] Division of Pulmonary and Critical Care Medicine, Feinberg School of Medicine, Northwestern University, Chicago, IL, United States

*Correspondence:
István Vadász
istvan.vadasz@innere.med.
uni-giessen.de

Disruption of the alveolar–capillary barrier and accumulation of pulmonary edema, if not resolved, result in poor alveolar gas exchange leading to hypoxia and hypercapnia, which are hallmarks of acute lung injury and the acute respiratory distress syndrome (ARDS). Alveolar fluid clearance (AFC) is a major function of the alveolar epithelium and is mediated by the concerted action of apically-located Na^+ channels [epithelial Na^+ channel (ENaC)] and the basolateral Na,K-ATPase driving vectorial Na^+ transport. Importantly, those patients with ARDS who cannot clear alveolar edema efficiently have worse outcomes. While hypoxia can be improved in most cases by O_2 supplementation and mechanical ventilation, the use of lung protective ventilation settings can lead to further CO_2 retention. Whether the increase in CO_2 concentrations has deleterious or beneficial effects have been a topic of significant controversy. Of note, both low O_2 and elevated CO_2 levels are sensed by the alveolar epithelium and by distinct and specific molecular mechanisms impair the function of the Na,K-ATPase and ENaC thereby inhibiting AFC and leading to persistence of alveolar edema. This review discusses recent discoveries on the sensing and signaling events initiated by hypoxia and hypercapnia and the relevance of these results in identification of potential novel therapeutic targets in the treatment of ARDS.

Keywords: hypoxia, hypercapnia, alveolar fluid clearance, Na,K-ATPase, epithelial Na^+ channel, acute respiratory distress syndrome, acute lung injury

A major function of the alveolar epithelium is to maintain alveolar fluid balance resulting in minimal epithelial lining fluid, thus providing optimal gas exchange (1). However, during acute lung injury (ALI) and the clinical acute respiratory distress syndrome (ARDS) the alveolar–capillary barrier fails, which leads to flooding of the alveolar space and causes a severe impairment of gas exchange (2). It is well established that clearance of alveolar edema is markedly impaired in most patients with ARDS and that this impairment is associated with worse outcomes (3). Thus, removal of the excess alveolar fluid is of significant clinical importance. The primary mechanism driving fluid reabsorption from the alveolar space is the active vectorial flux of sodium from the airspaces into the lung interstitium and the pulmonary circulation (1). Sodium, in exchange to potassium, is pumped out of the alveolar epithelial cells (AEC) basolaterally by the Na,K-ATPase, whereas Na^+ enters the cells apically through the amiloride-sensitive and -insensitive epithelial Na^+ channel (ENaC) (1, 4). This vectorial sodium transport process creates an osmotic gradient that drives clearance of fluid from the alveolar space (1). Failure of the alveolar–capillary barrier function leads to alveolar edema and thus to alveolar hypoventilation, resulting in hypoxemia and often elevated CO_2 concentrations in the blood (hypercapnia) in patients with ARDS (1, 4). This is of particular importance, as several studies have shown that these conditions are not only consequences of alveolar edema but also further exacerbate alveolar fluid dysbalance by promoting formation and inhibiting reabsorption of the edema fluid (5–7). In this review, we will focus on the mechanisms by which hypoxia and hypercapnia impair alveolar fluid clearance (AFC), concentrating on the regulation of the Na,K-ATPase and ENaC in the context of ALI.

ROLE OF HYPOXIA IN INFLAMMATION AND ALVEOLAR FLUID BALANCE IN ALI

Adaptation to hypoxia is critically important for cellular survival as oxygen is required for ATP synthesis in the mitochondria by oxidative phosphorylation (8). During hypoxia, production of ATP is reduced by inhibition of the electron transport chain. In order to reduce energy consumption, protein translation is down-regulated and various processes with high energy demand are inhibited (8). In the context of ALI/ARDS, alveolar hypoxia and systemic hypoxemia occur as the inflamed/injured alveolar–capillary barrier fails. It is generally accepted that hypoxia is intimately coupled to inflammatory states in various organs (9). For example, inflammatory hypoxia, a manifestation of locally increased metabolism and reduced oxygen supply, may drive and further exacerbate inflammatory bowel diseases, such as ulcerative colitis or Crohn's disease (10). While hypoxia *per se* can be an inflammatory stimulus, which up-regulates inflammatory cytokine levels, stabilization of hypoxia-inducible factor (HIF)-1α and activation of adenosine A_{2A} receptor-mediated mechanisms secondary to hypoxia may have significant anti-inflammatory effects in the lung (11, 12). Other than regulating inflammation, it is well established that hypoxia impairs alveolar fluid balance. The first preclinical studies over 15 years ago addressing the effects of hypoxia in intact rat lungs suggested that the impaired fluid balance upon exposing animals to low O_2 levels was due to an inhibition of transepithelial sodium transport processes (5, 13). Importantly, these negative effects of hypoxia on AFC can also be observed in humans and prophylactic administration of salmeterol, a β_2-adrenergic receptor agonist, prevents lung edema in subjects who are susceptible to high-altitude pulmonary edema, probably due to up-regulation of the Na,K-ATPase and/or ENaC (14).

EFFECTS OF SHORT-TERM HYPOXIA ON ALVEOLAR EPITHELIAL Na+ TRANSPORT

The molecular mechanisms by which hypoxia down-regulates Na+ transporters depend on the duration of exposure to low O_2 levels and have been studied in various AEC lines. Severe hypoxia leads to rapid (within minutes) endocytosis of the Na,K-ATPase molecules from the plasma membrane (PM) into intracellular pools, thereby decreasing activity of the enzyme (15). It appears that in the first hour of hypoxic exposure this trafficking event is solely responsible for the hypoxia-induced impairment of Na,K-ATPase function as the total cellular abundance of the

transporter remains unchanged, excluding the possibility of accelerated degradation of the transporter upon short-term hypoxia. In line with this notion, the endocytosis of the Na,K-ATPase upon hypoxia is promptly reversible upon reoxygenation (15). Furthermore, it has been reported that the effects of hypoxia on the Na,K-ATPase are mediated by mitochondrial reactive oxygen species as in ρ^0-A549 cells, which are incapable of mitochondrial respiration, and thus unable to generate mitochondrial ROS, hypoxia does not alter the cell surface stability of the Na,K-ATPase (15, 16). Release of mitochondrial ROS upon hypoxic exposure initiates Ca^{2+} release from the endoplasmic reticulum (ER) and redistribution of the calcium sensor STIM1 to the ER PM junctions, thereby resulting in calcium entry through Ca^{2+} release-activated Ca^{2+} channels, which in turn activates Ca^{2+}/calmodulin-dependent kinase kinase (CAMKK)-β, a well-known inducer of the metabolic sensor AMP-activated protein kinase (AMPK) (17). Of note, AMPK is a major regulator of cellular energy balance and activation of the kinase leads to inhibition of processes that require high energy (18); thus, playing a central role in the adaptation to hypoxia. As the Na,K-ATPase accounts for ~30–80% of the energy expenditure of cells (8), rapid down-regulation of the transporter driven by AMPK appears to be key in this adaptation process. Once activated, AMPK-$\alpha 1$ directly phosphorylates protein kinase C (PKC)-ζ at the Thr410 residue (19). This is of relevance as phosphorylation of PKC-ζ at Thr410 drives translocation of the protein kinase to the PM where it phosphorylates the Na,K-ATPase at Ser18. It is well documented that phosphorylation of this serine residue promotes endocytosis of the Na+ pump from the PM (15). In parallel, upon hypoxic exposure mitochondrial ROS activate RhoA, a member of the Rho GTPase family and its downstream effector, the Rho-associated serine/threonine kinase (ROCK), a central regulator of filamentous actin reorganization, which has been implicated in the control of endocytosis (20, 21). Thus, in the alveolar epithelium the mitochondria serve as hypoxia sensors and release of mitochondrial ROS initiates a rapid and highly specific signaling cascade that leads to endocytosis of the Na,K-ATPase from the PM and thereby alveolar epithelial dysfunction (**Figure 1**).

Moreover, reactive oxygen and nitrogen species (RONS) have also been implicated in the down-regulation of ENaC (22). Recently, two Tyr residues located in the extracellular loop of the α-subunit of ENaC, Tyr279 and 283, have been identified as potential targets of oxidation by RONS (23). Various additional ion channels have been shown to be modulated (mainly down-regulated) by ROS and RONS by regulation of channel transcription, direct oxidation, nitration or nitrosylation of channels, and via interference with signaling patterns regulating activity, trafficking or expression of channels (24).

EFFECTS OF SUSTAINED HYPOXIA ON THE Na,K-ATPase AND ENaC

Sustained hypoxia down-regulates sodium transporter function in the alveolar epithelium by at least two independent mechanisms. As discussed above, during cellular adaptation to hypoxia protein translation is down-regulated to reduce energy

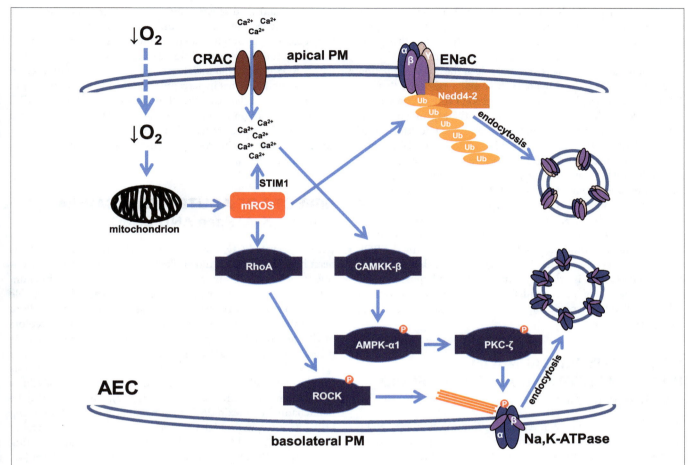

FIGURE 1 | Schematic depiction of the signaling cascades impairing cell surface expression of the Na,K-ATPase and epithelial Na+ channel (ENaC) upon acute hypoxia. In alveolar epithelial cells (AEC), hypoxia is sensed by mitochondria, which in response release mROS. Increased mROS concentrations lead to Ca^{2+} entry through Ca^{2+} release-activated Ca^{2+} (CRAC) channels by activation of STIM1. Elevated intracellular Ca^{2+} levels result in activation of Ca^{2+}/calmodulin-dependent kinase kinase (CAMKK)-β, which in turn phosphorylates and activates AMP-activated protein kinase (AMPK). Subsequently, AMPK promotes translocation of protein kinase C (PKC)-ζ to the plasma membrane (PM) where it phosphorylates the Na,K-ATPase α-subunit, thereby promoting endocytosis of the transporter. Hypoxia-induced endocytosis of the Na,K-ATPase also requires filamentous actin reorganization, which is mediated by mROS-induced activation of RhoA and ROCK. In parallel, increased mROS levels activate the E3 ubiquitin ligase Nedd4-2, which conjugates ubiquitin molecules to the ENaC β-subunit, thereby leading to endocytosis of the ENaC complex. This down-regulation of both Na,K-ATPase and ENaC cell surface expression results in impaired alveolar fluid clearance during hypoxia.

consumption (8). Indeed, several reports documented that upon long-term hypoxia both mRNA and total protein levels of the Na,K-ATPase and ENaC are decreased (25). A second, and more specific mechanism is the ubiquitination and directed degradation of the transporters. Ubiquitination is a post-translational modification during which ubiquitin molecules are conjugated (mostly but not exclusively) to specific lysine residues of target proteins, thereby controlling stability, function, and localization of the target (26, 27). Regarding the regulation of Na,K-ATPase upon prolonged hypoxic exposure, it has been documented that degradation of the enzyme occurs first (after approximately 2 h) in the PM, whereas exposing AEC to severe hypoxia for up to 24 h results in degradation of the Na,K-ATPase in intracellular pools (16). Considering that the Na,K-ATPase accounts for a significant proportion of the energy expenditure of cells, as mentioned above, it appears logical that as an adaptive mechanism to hypoxia the active Na,K-ATPase molecules (located at the PM) will be removed from the surface and degraded more rapidly than degradation of the inactive molecules (located in the intracellular pools) occurs to reduce cellular energy consumption and thus promote survival (8). A subsequent study established that four Lys residues (Lys16, 17, 19, and 20) surrounding the PKC-ζ phosphorylation site (Ser18) at the N-terminus of the Na,K-ATPase α-subunit are required for ubiquitin conjugation (28). Of note, phosphorylation of the Na+ pump by PKC-ζ at Ser18 is necessary for ubiquitination, perhaps by increasing affinity of ubiquitin to the phosphorylated target, highlighting the possibility of cross-talk between phosphorylation and ubiquitination (28). The E3 ubiquitin ligase of the Na,K-ATPase remains to be identified. Although the E3 ubiquitin ligase, von Hippel Lindau protein has been implicated in the degradation of the Na,K-ATPase upon hypoxia, it has also been shown that this E3 ligase does not directly target the Na$^+$ pump (29). Further research on the E3 ligase targeting the Na,K-ATPase will be of particular importance, as that molecule may represent a highly specific druggable target of impaired AFC upon gas exchange disturbances.

Ubiquitination also plays a central role in the down-regulation of ENaC upon sustained hypoxia. It is well established that the E3 ubiquitin ligase, Nedd4-2 plays a pivotal role in the regulation of ENaC cell surface stability by directly targeting α-, β-, or γ-ENaC depending on the stimulus leading to endocytosis and/or degradation of the channel (30). It has been reported that upon hypoxic exposure for 24 h in mice carrying a truncation of the C-terminus of β-ENaC (homozygous β-Liddle mouse strain), thus preventing interactions with Nedd4-2, amiloride-sensitive AFC remains normal, whereas in wild-type mice AFC is decreased by approximately 70%. Furthermore, a marked reduction in the amiloride-sensitive apical Na$^+$ current upon hypoxia can be fully prevented by inhibition of the proteasome and by the ROS scavenger N-acetyl-cysteine (31), suggesting that the ubiquitin–proteasome system is critically required for the hypoxia-driven down-regulation of ENaC and further confirming the central role of ROS in the hypoxic impairment of alveolar epithelial Na$^+$ transport processes.

ROLE OF HYPERCAPNIA IN INFLAMMATION AND ALVEOLAR FLUID BALANCE IN ALI

While in most patients with ARDS hypoxia can be corrected by the use of mechanical ventilation with elevated inspired fractions of oxygen, hypercapnia often persists in part due to the low tidal volume ventilation strategy, which is required to minimize further ventilator-induced lung injury (32). While "protective" mechanical ventilation with low tidal volumes is clearly beneficial (33), the effects of hypercapnia in the context of lung injury remain a topic of intense debate. Several studies suggested that hypercapnia is tolerable or even beneficial whereas others documented that various aspects of the hypercapnic effects on alveolar epithelial function are deleterious, leading to the terms of permissive, therapeutic, and non-permissive hypercapnia, respectively (6, 34). It is very well established that excessive inflammation plays a central role in the pathogenesis ARDS (35). Moreover, respiratory acidosis (a decrease in the pH of the blood secondary to hypercapnia) has several anti-inflammatory properties, such as reduction of pro-inflammatory cytokines, impairment of neutrophil function, and inhibition of generation of free radicals (36). Thus, it appears logical that hypercapnia (or the associated acidosis) may be beneficial in the context of ARDS. In contrast, a recent secondary analysis of three large prospective non-interventional clinical studies recruiting mechanically ventilated patients with moderate and severe ARDS in over 900 ICUs from 40 countries documented that hypercapnia is independently associated with a markedly higher ICU mortality (37), which is further supported by another study in which hypercapnic acidosis in the first 24 h after ICU admission was associated with higher hospital mortality (38). There are several factors that may lead to worse outcomes of hypercapnic patients with ARDS.

Although, and as discussed above, the hypercapnia-associated acidosis may exhibit early anti-inflammatory effects; recently, it has become increasingly evident that hypercapnia impairs innate immunity, thereby potentially increasing susceptibility of patients with ARDS to bacterial infections (39, 40). Furthermore, recent studies established that hypercapnia, independently of changes in pH, impairs alveolar epithelial fluid balance by inhibiting AFC, and thus resolution of pulmonary edema (41–43). As it is well documented that clearance of the excess, protein-rich alveolar edema in patients with ARDS is critical for survival, this aspect is of clinical relevance.

EFFECTS OF ACUTE HYPERCAPNIA ON THE Na,K-ATPase AND ENaC

Because elevated CO_2 levels impair AFC within minutes, it has been hypothesized that much like variations in oxygen concentration, levels of CO_2 may be sensed by the alveolar epithelium (41, 43–45). It was described several decades ago that excitable cells, such as specialized brainstem neurons or the glomus cells of the carotid body serve as central and peripheral chemoreceptors of CO_2 and depolarize upon hypercapnia (46). In contrast, only recently it became evident that elevated CO_2 levels also initiate specific signaling patterns in non-excitable cell types, such as the alveolar epithelium, independently of intra- or extracellular pH, carbonic anhydrases, or ROS (41, 42). Most recently, the hemichannel connexin 26 has been implicated in CO_2 sensing (47). Interestingly, the high CO_2-induced signaling leads to a rapid down-regulation of the Na,K-ATPase activity, thereby inhibiting AFC, one of the major functions of the alveolar epithelium (41, 42). This hypercapnia-induced signaling pattern has been dissected in the past years and we now know that elevated CO_2 levels increase intracellular Ca^{2+} concentrations within seconds leading to activation of CAMKK-β, which stimulates the metabolic sensor AMPK. Similarly to the effects of hypoxic exposure, the hypercapnia-induced activation of AMPK leads to translocation of PKC-ζ to the PM, where the kinase phosphorylates the Na,K-ATPase α-subunit, thereby promoting endocytosis of the transporter from the PM (41, 43). The endocytosis of the Na,K-ATPase also requires activation of the c-Jun N-terminal kinase (JNK), which is similarly to PKC-ζ also downstream of AMPK in the CO_2-induced signaling cascade (48). Upon hypercapnia, activated JNK phosphorylates the scaffolding protein LMO7b at the Ser1295 residue, which enables interaction of the scaffolding protein with the Na,K-ATPase at the PM of AEC, thereby promoting endocytosis and thus inhibition of the transporter (49). Of note, the requirement of JNK in the hypercapnia-induced inhibition of the Na,K-ATPase was not only shown in mice, rats, and human cells but also in *Drosophila melanogaster*, suggesting that at least some elements of the CO_2-induced signaling pattern are evolutionarily conserved (48). Interestingly, this pathway overlaps with that of initiated by acute hypoxia; however, the effects of hypercapnia are independent of mitochondrial ROS. Furthermore, unlike in hypoxia the source of Ca^{2+} upon hypercapnic exposure of the alveolar epithelium remains unknown and the regulation of the endocytic machinery appears to be different in hypoxia and hypercapnia, where activation of RhoA and ROCK as opposed to JNK and LMO7b are required, respectively (**Figure 2**). Moreover, some effects of hypercapnia and hypoxia are opposing, as elevated CO_2 levels inhibit the HIF-driven adaptation mechanisms to hypoxia (50). Recently, an alternative and AMPK-independent pathway has also been identified in the elevated CO_2-induced down-regulation of the Na,K-ATPase. It has been reported that hypercapnia also activates the recently identified metabolic sensor CO_2/HCO_3^- responsive soluble adenylyl cyclase (CO_2/HCO_3-sAC), which by producing cAMP in specific microdomains in the proximity of the PM led to activation of protein kinase A (PKA) type Iα that phosphorylated the actin cytoskeleton component α-adducin at Ser726, thereby promoting endocytosis of the Na,K-ATPase (51). This novel pathway is AMPK-independent as AMPK phosphorylation upon hypercapnia also occurs in the presence of an siRNA against CO_2/HCO_3-sAC, similarly to PKA activation in AEC after AMPK silencing, suggesting that both pathways are required for the hypercapnia-induced down-regulation of Na,K-ATPase cell surface stability.

Most recently, the molecular mechanism impairing ENaC cell surface stability in AEC upon acute hypercapnic exposure has been described (52). Upon hypercapnia, extracellular signal-regulated kinase (ERK), which has been previously identified in the CO_2-induced signaling pattern as an activator of AMPK (53), directly phosphorylates the ENaC β-subunit at Thr615. Moreover, JNK, which is activated by AMPK upon activation of the latter kinase by ERK, phosphorylates Nedd4-2 at Thr899, thereby increasing the activity of the E3 ubiquitin ligase (52). These phosphorylation events promote the interaction of β-ENaC and Nedd4-2 and lead to polyubiquitination

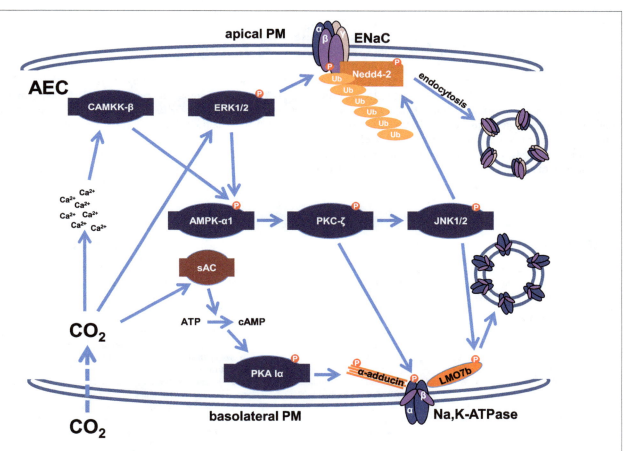

FIGURE 2 | Schematic representation of the signaling signatures down-regulating the Na,K-ATPase and epithelial Na+ channel (ENaC) upon acute hypercapnia. Hypercapnia leads to phosphorylation and subsequent endocytosis of Na,K-ATPase by an AMP-activated protein kinase (AMPK)-dependent and an AMPK-independent mechanism. An acute elevation in CO_2 levels in alveolar epithelial cells (AEC) leads to an increased intracellular Ca^{2+} concentration by a yet unidentified mechanism. A subsequent activation of the Ca^{2+}/calmodulin-dependent kinase kinase (CAMKK)-β/AMPK-α/protein kinase C (PKC)-ζ signaling cascade results in phosphorylation of the Na,K-ATPase α-subunit. PKC-ζ also activates c-Jun N-terminal kinase (JNK), which phosphorylates the scaffolding protein LMO7b, thereby promoting endocytosis of the Na,K-ATPase. Furthermore, elevated CO_2 is sensed by the sAC, which in turn activates protein kinase A (PKA) type Iα by cAMP in microdomains at close proximity of the basolateral membrane, resulting in phosphorylation of α-adducin, which is required for the rearrangement of the actin cytoskeleton necessary for endocytosis. Moreover, CO_2 activates extracellular signal-regulated kinase (ERK), which is also required for AMPK stimulation. ERK phosphorylates the ENaC β-subunit, thereby attracting the E3 ubiquitin ligase Nedd4-2, which is phosphorylated and activated by JNK upon hypercapnic exposure, leading to polyubiquitination of β-ENaC, and a reduction of ENaC abundance at the apical PM. Collectively, these mechanisms impair the function of both the Na,K-ATPase and ENaC and are responsible for the hypercapnia-induced inhibition of alveolar edema clearance.

of β-ENaC and subsequent endocytosis of the ENaC complex, thereby reducing cell surface stability of the channel.

EFFECTS OF SUSTAINED HYPERCAPNIA ON ALVEOLAR EPITHELIAL Na⁺ TRANSPORT AND REPAIR

Interestingly, the effects of long-term elevated CO_2 levels on the Na,K-ATPase are reversible. Exposing rats to elevated CO_2 concentrations for up to 1 week leads to a sustained and marked decrease in AFC (43). Similarly, exposure of AEC to elevated CO_2 levels for up to 24 h causes a sustained reduction of Na,K-ATPase abundance at the PM (43). However, when exposing rat lungs to normocapnia after a hypercapnic treatment for 1 h, levels of AFC rapidly return to normal (41). Furthermore, treatment of rat lungs with the β-adrenergic receptor agonist, isoproterenol not only prevents but also reverses the hypercapnia-induced decrease in AFC, confirming that the high CO_2-induced AFC impairment is reversible at least in the first hour of hypercapnia (43). Moreover, sustained hypercapnia induces the microRNA, miR-183, which down-regulates isocitrate dehydrogenase 2, an enzyme that catalyzes the conversion of isocitrate to α-ketoglutarate during the tricarboxylic acid cycle (54). This effect leads to mitochondrial dysfunction thus, inhibiting proliferation of AEC, which may impair repair mechanisms and resolution of lung injury.

CONCLUSION

Gas exchange disturbances are hallmarks of ALI and ARDS. Both low O_2 and elevated CO_2 levels are rapidly sensed by the alveolar epithelium, the site of oxygen uptake and CO_2 elimination, leading to adaptation but also deleterious effects on cellular function. Both hypoxia and hypercapnia are intimately coupled to inflammation and by highly specific and partially described signaling pathways, which inhibit epithelial sodium transport processes impair AFC. As alveolar hypoxia and hypercapnia cannot always be corrected at the areas of severe injury, interfering with these deleterious signals may lead to novel therapies against ARDS.

AUTHOR CONTRIBUTIONS

IV: drafting the work and preparing figures. JS and IV: revising it critically for important intellectual content. Both authors approved the final version of the manuscript.

FUNDING

This work was supported by grants from the Excellence Cluster "Cardio Pulmonary System" (ECCPS), the German Center for Lung Research (DZL), the Landes-Offensive zur Entwicklung Wissenschaftlich-ökonomischer Exzellenz (LOEWE) of the Hessen State Ministry of Higher Education, Research and the Arts and the Deutsche Forschungsgemeinschaft (Clinical Research Unit KFO309/1) (for IV), and by the National Institutes of Health (HL-71643 and HL-85534) (for JS).

REFERENCES

1. Matthay MA, Folkesson HG, Clerici C. Lung epithelial fluid transport and the resolution of pulmonary edema. *Physiol Rev* (2002) 82(3):569–600. doi:10.1152/physrev.00003.2002
2. Ware LB, Matthay MA. The acute respiratory distress syndrome. *N Engl J Med* (2000) 342(18):1334–49. doi:10.1056/NEJM200005043421806
3. Ware LB, Matthay MA. Alveolar fluid clearance is impaired in the majority of patients with acute lung injury and the acute respiratory distress syndrome. *Am J Respir Crit Care Med* (2001) 163(6):1376–83. doi:10.1164/ajrccm.163.6.2004035
4. Vadasz I, Raviv S, Sznajder JI. Alveolar epithelium and Na,K-ATPase in acute lung injury. *Intensive Care Med* (2007) 33(7):1243–51. doi:10.1007/s00134-007-0661-8
5. Suzuki S, Noda M, Sugita M, Ono S, Koike K, Fujimura S. Impairment of transalveolar fluid transport and lung Na(+)-K(+)-ATPase function by hypoxia in rats. *J Appl Physiol (1985)* (1999) 87(3):962–8.
6. Vadasz I, Hubmayr RD, Nin N, Sporn PH, Sznajder JI. Hypercapnia: a nonpermissive environment for the lung. *Am J Respir Cell Mol Biol* (2012) 46(4):417–21. doi:10.1165/rcmb.2011-0395PS
7. Zhou G, Dada LA, Sznajder JI. Regulation of alveolar epithelial function by hypoxia. *Eur Respir J* (2008) 31(5):1107–13. doi:10.1183/09031936.00155507
8. Wheaton WW, Chandel NS. Hypoxia. 2. Hypoxia regulates cellular metabolism. *Am J Physiol Cell Physiol* (2011) 300(3):C385–93. doi:10.1152/ajpcell.00485.2010
9. Eltzschig HK, Bratton DL, Colgan SP. Targeting hypoxia signalling for the treatment of ischaemic and inflammatory diseases. *Nat Rev Drug Discov* (2014) 13(11):852–69. doi:10.1038/nrd4422

10. Colgan SP, Taylor CT. Hypoxia: an alarm signal during intestinal inflammation. *Nat Rev Gastroenterol Hepatol* (2010) 7(5):281–7. doi:10.1038/nrgastro.2010.39
11. Thiel M, Chouker A, Ohta A, Jackson E, Caldwell C, Smith P, et al. Oxygenation inhibits the physiological tissue-protecting mechanism and thereby exacerbates acute inflammatory lung injury. *PLoS Biol* (2005) 3(6):e174. doi:10.1371/journal.pbio.0030174
12. Eckle T, Brodsky K, Bonney M, Packard T, Han J, Borchers CH, et al. HIF1A reduces acute lung injury by optimizing carbohydrate metabolism in the alveolar epithelium. *PLoS Biol* (2013) 11(9):e1001665. doi:10.1371/journal.pbio.1001665
13. Suzuki S, Sugita M, Noda M, Tsubochi H, Fujimura S. Effects of intraalveolar oxygen concentration on alveolar fluid absorption and metabolism in isolated rat lungs. *Respir Physiol* (1999) 115(3):325–32. doi:10.1016/S0034-5687(99)00009-2
14. Sartori C, Allemann Y, Duplain H, Lepori M, Egli M, Lipp E, et al. Salmeterol for the prevention of high-altitude pulmonary edema. *N Engl J Med* (2002) 346(21):1631–6. doi:10.1056/NEJMoa013183
15. Dada LA, Chandel NS, Ridge KM, Pedemonte C, Bertorello AM, Sznajder JI. Hypoxia-induced endocytosis of Na,K-ATPase in alveolar epithelial cells is mediated by mitochondrial reactive oxygen species and PKC-zeta. *J Clin Invest* (2003) 111(7):1057–64. doi:10.1172/JCI16826
16. Comellas AP, Dada LA, Lecuona E, Pesce LM, Chandel NS, Quesada N, et al. Hypoxia-mediated degradation of Na,K-ATPase via mitochondrial reactive oxygen species and the ubiquitin-conjugating system. *Circ Res* (2006) 98(10):1314–22. doi:10.1161/01.RES.0000222418.99976.1d
17. Gusarova GA, Trejo HE, Dada LA, Briva A, Welch LC, Hamanaka RB, et al. Hypoxia leads to Na,K-ATPase downregulation via Ca(2+) release-activated Ca(2+) channels and AMPK activation. *Mol Cell Biol* (2011) 31(17):3546–56. doi:10.1128/MCB.05114-11

18. Carling D. AMPK signalling in health and disease. *Curr Opin Cell Biol* (2017) 45:31–7. doi:10.1016/j.ceb.2017.01.005
19. Gusarova GA, Dada LA, Kelly AM, Brodie C, Witters LA, Chandel NS, et al. Alpha1-AMP-activated protein kinase regulates hypoxia-induced Na,K-ATPase endocytosis via direct phosphorylation of protein kinase C zeta. *Mol Cell Biol* (2009) 29(13):3455–64. doi:10.1128/MCB.00054-09
20. Dada LA, Novoa E, Lecuona E, Sun H, Sznajder JI. Role of the small GTPase RhoA in the hypoxia-induced decrease of plasma membrane Na,K-ATPase in A549 cells. *J Cell Sci* (2007) 120(Pt 13):2214–22. doi:10.1242/jcs.003038
21. Lamaze C, Chuang TH, Terlecky LJ, Bokoch GM, Schmid SL. Regulation of receptor-mediated endocytosis by Rho and Rac. *Nature* (1996) 382(6587):177–9. doi:10.1038/382177a0
22. Song W, Matalon S. Modulation of alveolar fluid clearance by reactive oxygen-nitrogen intermediates. *Am J Physiol Lung Cell Mol Physiol* (2007) 293(4):L855–8. doi:10.1152/ajplung.00305.2007
23. Chen L, Fuller CM, Kleyman TR, Matalon S. Mutations in the extra-cellular loop of alpha-rENaC alter sensitivity to amiloride and reactive species. *Am J Physiol Renal Physiol* (2004) 286(6):F1202–8. doi:10.1152/ajprenal.00352.2003
24. Matalon S, Hardiman KM, Jain L, Eaton DC, Kotlikoff M, Eu JP, et al. Regulation of ion channel structure and function by reactive oxygen-nitrogen species. *Am J Physiol Lung Cell Mol Physiol* (2003) 285(6):L1184–9. doi:10.1152/ajplung.00281.2003
25. Wodopia R, Ko HS, Billian J, Wiesner R, Bartsch P, Mairbaurl H. Hypoxia decreases proteins involved in epithelial electrolyte transport in A549 cells and rat lung. *Am J Physiol Lung Cell Mol Physiol* (2000) 279(6):L1110–9.
26. Vadasz I, Weiss CH, Sznajder JI. Ubiquitination and proteolysis in acute lung injury. *Chest* (2012) 141(3):763–71. doi:10.1378/chest.11-1660
27. Queisser MA, Dada LA, Deiss-Yehiely N, Angulo M, Zhou G, Kouri FM, et al. HOIL-1L functions as the PKCzeta ubiquitin ligase to promote lung tumor growth. *Am J Respir Crit Care Med* (2014) 190(6):688–98. doi:10.1164/rccm.201403-0463OC
28. Dada LA, Welch LC, Zhou G, Ben-Saadon R, Ciechanover A, Sznajder JI. Phosphorylation and ubiquitination are necessary for Na,K-ATPase endocytosis during hypoxia. *Cell Signal* (2007) 19(9):1893–8. doi:10.1016/j.cellsig.2007.04.013
29. Zhou G, Dada LA, Chandel NS, Iwai K, Lecuona E, Ciechanover A, et al. Hypoxia-mediated Na-K-ATPase degradation requires von Hippel Lindau protein. *FASEB J* (2008) 22(5):1335–42. doi:10.1096/fj.07-8369com
30. Rotin D, Staub O. Role of the ubiquitin system in regulating ion transport. *Pflugers Arch* (2011) 461(1):1–21. doi:10.1007/s00424-010-0893-2
31. Planes C, Blot-Chabaud M, Matthay MA, Couette S, Uchida T, Clerici C. Hypoxia and beta 2-agonists regulate cell surface expression of the epithelial sodium channel in native alveolar epithelial cells. *J Biol Chem* (2002) 277(49):47318–24. doi:10.1074/jbc.M209158200
32. Bellani G, Laffey JG, Pham T, Fan E, Brochard L, Esteban A, et al. Epidemiology, patterns of care, and mortality for patients with acute respiratory distress syndrome in intensive care units in 50 countries. *JAMA* (2016) 315(8):788–800. doi:10.1001/jama.2016.0291
33. Acute Respiratory Distress Syndrome Network, Brower RG, Matthay MA, Morris A, Schoenfeld D, Thompson BT, et al. Ventilation with lower tidal volumes as compared with traditional tidal volumes for acute lung injury and the acute respiratory distress syndrome. *N Engl J Med* (2000) 342(18):1301–8. doi:10.1056/NEJM200005043421801
34. Kavanagh BP, Laffey JG. Hypercapnia: permissive and therapeutic. *Minerva Anestesiol* (2006) 72(6):567–76.
35. Herold S, Gabrielli NM, Vadasz I. Novel concepts of acute lung injury and alveolar-capillary barrier dysfunction. *Am J Physiol Lung Cell Mol Physiol* (2013) 305(10):L665–81. doi:10.1152/ajplung.00232.2013
36. Curley G, Contreras MM, Nichol AD, Higgins BD, Laffey JG. Hypercapnia and acidosis in sepsis: a double-edged sword? *Anesthesiology* (2010) 112(2):462–72. doi:10.1097/ALN.0b013e3181ca361f
37. Nin N, Muriel A, Penuelas O, Brochard L, Lorente JA, Ferguson ND, et al. Severe hypercapnia and outcome of mechanically ventilated patients with moderate or severe acute respiratory distress syndrome. *Intensive Care Med* (2017) 43(2):200–8. doi:10.1007/s00134-016-4611-1
38. Tiruvoipati R, Pilcher D, Buscher H, Botha J, Bailey M. Effects of hypercapnia and hypercapnic acidosis on hospital mortality in mechanically ventilated patients. *Crit Care Med* (2017) 45(7):e649–56. doi:10.1097/CCM.0000000000002332

39. Helenius IT, Krupinski T, Turnbull DW, Gruenbaum Y, Silverman N, Johnson EA, et al. Elevated CO_2 suppresses specific *Drosophila* innate immune responses and resistance to bacterial infection. *Proc Natl Acad Sci USA* (2009) 106(44):18710–5. doi:10.1073/pnas.0905925106
40. Wang N, Gates KL, Trejo H, Favoreto S Jr, Schleimer RP, Sznajder JI, et al. Elevated CO_2 selectively inhibits interleukin-6 and tumor necrosis factor expression and decreases phagocytosis in the macrophage. *FASEB J* (2010) 24(7):2178–90. doi:10.1096/fj.09-136895
41. Briva A, Vadasz I, Lecuona E, Welch LC, Chen J, Dada LA, et al. High CO_2 levels impair alveolar epithelial function independently of pH. *PLoS One* (2007) 2(11):e1238. doi:10.1371/journal.pone.0001238
42. Chen J, Lecuona E, Briva A, Welch LC, Sznajder JI. Carbonic anhydrase II and alveolar fluid reabsorption during hypercapnia. *Am J Respir Cell Mol Biol* (2008) 38(1):32–7. doi:10.1165/rcmb.2007-0121OC
43. Vadasz I, Dada LA, Briva A, Trejo HE, Welch LC, Chen J, et al. AMP-activated protein kinase regulates CO_2-induced alveolar epithelial dysfunction in rats and human cells by promoting Na,K-ATPase endocytosis. *J Clin Invest* (2008) 118(2):752–62. doi:10.1172/JCI29723
44. Sharabi K, Lecuona E, Helenius IT, Beitel GJ, Sznajder JI, Gruenbaum Y. Sensing, physiological effects and molecular response to elevated CO_2 levels in eukaryotes. *J Cell Mol Med* (2009) 13(11–12):4304–18. doi:10.1111/j.1582-4934.2009.00952.x
45. Cummins EP, Selfridge AC, Sporn PH, Sznajder JI, Taylor CT. Carbon dioxide-sensing in organisms and its implications for human disease. *Cell Mol Life Sci* (2014) 71(5):831–45. doi:10.1007/s00018-013-1470-6
46. Putnam RW, Filosa JA, Ritucci NA. Cellular mechanisms involved in CO(2) and acid signaling in chemosensitive neurons. *Am J Physiol Cell Physiol* (2004) 287(6):C1493–526. doi:10.1152/ajpcell.00282.2004
47. de Wolf E, Cook J, Dale N. Evolutionary adaptation of the sensitivity of connexin26 hemichannels to CO_2. *Proc Biol Sci* (2017) 284(1848):20162723. doi:10.1098/rspb.2016.2723
48. Vadasz I, Dada LA, Briva A, Helenius IT, Sharabi K, Welch LC, et al. Evolutionary conserved role of c-Jun-N-terminal kinase in CO_2-induced epithelial dysfunction. *PLoS One* (2012) 7(10):e46696. doi:10.1371/journal.pone.0046696
49. Dada LA, Trejo Bittar HE, Welch LC, Vagin O, Deiss-Yehiely N, Kelly AM, et al. High CO_2 leads to Na,K-ATPase endocytosis via c-Jun amino-terminal kinase-induced LMO7b phosphorylation. *Mol Cell Biol* (2015) 35(23):3962–73. doi:10.1128/MCB.00813-15
50. Selfridge AC, Cavadas MA, Scholz CC, Campbell EL, Welch LC, Lecuona E, et al. Hypercapnia suppresses the HIF-dependent adaptive response to hypoxia. *J Biol Chem* (2016) 291(22):11800–8. doi:10.1074/jbc.M116.713941
51. Lecuona E, Sun H, Chen J, Trejo HE, Baker MA, Sznajder JI. Protein kinase A-Ialpha regulates Na,K-ATPase endocytosis in alveolar epithelial cells exposed to high CO(2) concentrations. *Am J Respir Cell Mol Biol* (2013) 48(5):626–34. doi:10.1165/rcmb.2012-0373OC
52. Gwozdzinska P, Buchbinder BA, Mayer K, Herold S, Morty RE, Seeger W, et al. Hypercapnia impairs ENaC cell surface stability by promoting phosphorylation, polyubiquitination and endocytosis of β-ENaC in a human alveolar epithelial cell line. *Front Immunol* (2017) 8:591. doi:10.3389/fimmu.2017.00591
53. Welch LC, Lecuona E, Briva A, Trejo HE, Dada LA, Sznajder JI. Extracellular signal-regulated kinase (ERK) participates in the hypercapnia-induced Na,K-ATPase downregulation. *FEBS Lett* (2010) 584(18):3985–9. doi:10.1016/j.febslet.2010.08.002
54. Vohwinkel CU, Lecuona E, Sun H, Sommer N, Vadasz I, Chandel NS, et al. Elevated CO(2) levels cause mitochondrial dysfunction and impair cell proliferation. *J Biol Chem* (2011) 286(43):37067–76. doi:10.1074/jbc.M111.290056

12

Involvement of Cytokines in the Pathogenesis of Salt and Water Imbalance in Congestive Heart Failure

Zaher S. Azzam[1,2]*, Safa Kinaneh[1], Fadel Bahouth[1], Reem Ismael-Badarneh[1], Emad Khoury[1] and Zaid Abassi[1]

[1] Department of Physiology and Biophysics, Technion, Israel Institute of Technology, Haifa, Israel, [2] Internal Medicine "B", Rambam Health Care Campus, Haifa, Israel

*Correspondence:
Zaher S. Azzam
z_azzam@rambam.health.gov.il

Congestive heart failure (CHF) has become a major medical problem in the western world with high morbidity and mortality rates. CHF adversely affects several systems, mainly the kidneys and the lungs. While the involvement of the renin–angiotensin–aldosterone system and the sympathetic nervous system in the progression of cardiovascular, pulmonary, and renal dysfunction in experimental and clinical CHF is well established, the importance of pro-inflammatory mediators in the pathogenesis of this clinical setting is still evolving. In this context, CHF is associated with overexpression of pro-inflammatory cytokines, such as tumor necrosis factor-α, interleukin (IL)-1, and IL-6, which are activated in response to environmental injury. This family of cytokines has been implicated in the deterioration of CHF, where it plays an important role in initiating and integrating homeostatic responses both at the myocardium and circulatory levels. We and others showed that angiotensin II decreased the ability of the lungs to clear edema and enhanced the fibrosis process *via* phosphorylation of the mitogen-activated protein kinases p38 and p42/44, which are generally involved in cellular responses to pro-inflammatory cytokines. Literature data also indicate the involvement of these effectors in modulating ion channel activity. It has been reported that in heart failure due to mitral stenosis; there were varying degrees of vascular and other associated parenchymal changes such as edema and fibrosis. In this review, we will discuss the effects of cytokines and other inflammatory mediators on the kidneys and the lungs in heart failure; especially their role in renal and alveolar ion channels activity and fluid balance.

Keywords: heart failure, alveolar epithelium, renal cells, inflammation, cytokines, alveolar fluid clearance

INTRODUCTION

Congestive heart failure (CHF) has recently become a major medical problem in the developed countries with increased rates of mortality and morbidity, particularly among the elderly population. CHF constitutes an enormous economic burden on health service because of the expensive costs of the various therapeutic modalities, frequent hospital admissions, and poor quality of life. In the developed countries, it is estimated that up to 2% of the adult population suffers from this syndrome; whereas, in patients $\geq$65 years of age, the prevalence surges to more than 10% (1). The pathophysiologic conditions of CHF are various and include either decreased cardiac output due to loss of cardiac muscle tissue as it is observed in myocardial infarction, myocarditis and dilated cardiomyopathy; or increased filling pressures of the heart as it is evident in hypertension, hypertrophic and restrictive cardiomyopathies, and certain valvular diseases. CHF can also develop due to a volume overload deriving from arteriovenous shunts or fistulas and administration of fluid excess.

Understanding the underlying mechanisms leading to the development of CHF and its complications is therefore essential for optimizing the treatment of CHF and exploring novel therapies that aim to improve the outcome of the disease (2). Since the early 1980s, the importance of vasoconstrictor neurohormonal systems in the pathogenesis of CHF has been increasingly recognized. Numerous studies in patients and in experimental models of CHF have established the important role of the renin–angiotensin–aldosterone system (RAAS) and the sympathetic nervous system (SNS) in the progression of cardiovascular and renal dysfunction in CHF. It is now accepted that excessive neurohormonal activation may adversely affect cardiac function and the hemodynamic condition by enhancement of systemic vasoconstriction and promoting salt and water retention by the kidney. In addition, prolonged activation of the SNS and RAAS may have direct deleterious actions on the myocardium, independent of their systemic hemodynamic effects (3–5). However, generally, inflammation plays an important role in most cardiac diseases, and receptor-mediated innate immunity is primarily investigated with respect to toll-like receptors. However, the role of the innate immune system in heart failure has been controversial (6).

Cytokines that are composed of a vast array of relatively low molecular weight, pharmacologically active proteins; have been implicated in the progression of CHF. The most important cytokines are tumor necrosis factor-α (TNF-α), interleukin (IL) 1β, and IL-6. These cytokines share some of their major characteristics (redundancy), and all act in a pro-inflammatory sense (7). Adhesion molecules, autoantibodies, nitric oxide (NO), and endothelin-1 are also thought to be relevant to the pathogenesis of CHF (8).

Recently, it was shown in patients with acute decompensated heart failure (ADHF) that following standard treatment of ADHF, the monocyte profile and circulating inflammatory markers (C-reactive protein and IL-6) shifts to more closely resemble those of healthy controls, suggesting the contribution of systemic inflammation to the pathophysiology of ADHF (9). We and others have shown the deleterious consequences of heart failure on the lungs and the kidneys; therefore, we decided in this review to focus on the effects of cytokines and other inflammatory mediators on the lungs and the kidneys in heart failure; especially their role in renal and alveolar ion channels activity and fluid balance.

THE CONTRIBUTION OF THE IMMUNE SYSTEM TO HEART FAILURE

There are several theories regarding the activation of the immune system in heart failure (10). One hypothesis is based on the consequences of heart failure, that is, systemic venous congestion including the mesenteric venous system with consequent bowel edema and increased permeability that leads to bacterial translocation, endotoxin release and resultant activation of the immune system (11). The second theory is related to the ability of the failing heart to produce cytokines; Torre-Amione et al. have shown that TNF-α mRNA and TNF-α protein were present in the explanted hearts from dilated cardiomyopathy and ischemic heart disease patients but not in non-failing hearts (12).

In the third hypothesis, the state decreased cardiac output in heart failure causes systemic tissue hypoxia with subsequent systemic inflammation, which in turn may be the primary stimulus for increased TNF-α production (13).

The heart undergoes extensive structural and functional remodeling in response to injury, central to which is the hypertrophy of cardiac myocytes, with excessive deposition of extracellular matrix (14). Myocardial fibrosis is commonly categorized as one of two types: reactive fibrosis or replacement fibrosis. Reactive fibrosis occurs in perivascular spaces and corresponds to similar fibrogenic responses in other tissues; replacement fibrosis occurs at the site of myocyte loss.

Myocardial fibrosis is attributed to cardiac fibroblasts, which resides in the myocardium and is confirmed to be abundant (15). Following myocardial injury, all types of fibroblasts proliferate and differentiate into myofibroblasts, a process that is orchestrated by classic mediators such as TGF-β1, endothelin-1, and angiotensin II (Ang II). Notably, fibrosis is accelerated as result of intercellular interaction and cross talk; in this case, between activated fibroblasts and cardiomyocytes (16).

The effects of fibrosis on the heart muscle are various and include impairment of cardiac function, both systolic and diastolic. It also caused electrical instability and the development of fatal ventricular arrhythmias. This arrhythmogenic activity occurs in areas that couple fibroblasts and cardiomyocytes due to discontinuous slowing of conduction and consequent arrhythmia (17).

The CORONA study that included 1,464 patients with chronic ischemic systolic HF demonstrated that serum levels of TNF-α, soluble TNF receptors type I and II (sTNF-RI and sTNF-RII), and the chemokines monocyte chemoattractant protein-1 and interleukin-8 (IL-8) were independent predictors of all endpoints (all-cause mortality, cardiovascular mortality, and worsening heart failure). After further adjustment for estimated glomerular filtration rate (GFR), the ApoB/ApoA-1 ratio, NT-proBNP, and high-sensitivity C-reactive protein, only IL-8 remained a significant predictor of all endpoints (except the coronary endpoint), while sTNF-RI remained independently associated with CV mortality (18). Recently, in concordance of this study, it was reported IL-8 was negatively correlated with the left ventricular end-diastolic diameter and positively with left ventricular systolic volume (19). However, it should be emphasized that the elevated levels of cytokines in general and in heart failure, in particular, may not be responsible for tissue injury, rather it may reflect a concomitant phenomenon where cytokines could be used as biomarkers for heart failure but not effectors.

Pulmonary System

The alveoli are composed of thin layer of epithelial cells; alveolar epithelial cells type I and type II (AECI and AECII, respectively) that occupy together 99% of surface area of the lungs and play a crucial role in breathing and preserving lung homeostasis. There are also alveolar residential macrophages that protect the lungs from pathogens and regulate lung immune response (20).

Alveolar macrophages—AMφ comprise 95% of bronchoalveolar lavage and are part of cellular compartment of innate immunity that has an essential role in pathogen defense. Another type of macrophages is interstitial macrophages or bone-marrow derived macrophages that are also involved in the process of lung defense (21).

Alveolar Fluid Clearance (AFC)

Active sodium (Na$^+$) transport across the alveolar-capillary barrier is important in keeping the airspaces free of fluid in healthy conditions and for the resorption of lung edema in pathologic conditions. Briefly, Na$^+$ enters the alveolar epithelial cells through apical amiloride sensitive Na$^+$ channels (ENaC), and by a process that consumes energy is pumped out of the cell by the Na,K-ATPase located in the basolateral membrane in exchange for potassium entry on a ratio of 3:2 Na$^+$–K$^+$ against their chemical gradient (20, 22–27) (**Figure 1**). ENaC constitutes the rate limiting step for sodium absorption in epithelial cells of various sites including distal renal tubule, distal colon, exocrine glands, and lungs. Concerning the latter, ENaC plays a critical role in AFC. A support for this notion was derived from Hummler et al. who demonstrated that AFC in knockout mice to ENaC was severely attenuated with resultant fatal respiratory distress (27). Notably, non-selective Na$^+$ channels (NSC) and cyclic nucleotide-gated channel have been shown to be involved in the process of AFC, however to a lesser extent than ENaC (28). In addition, K$^+$ ions are recycled by basolateral K$^+$ channels, which also participate in the control of Na$^+$ and fluid absorption (26). It has been shown that AFC is modulated by several pharmacologic modalities and interventions; such as catecholamines, angiotensin, vasopressin, endothelin, gene therapy, hypercapnia, hyperoxia, sepsis, and others (20, 29–33). Notably, Ang II decreased AFC *via* c-AMP–Na, K-ATPase pathway. Whereas, it was reported that Ang II plays a role in

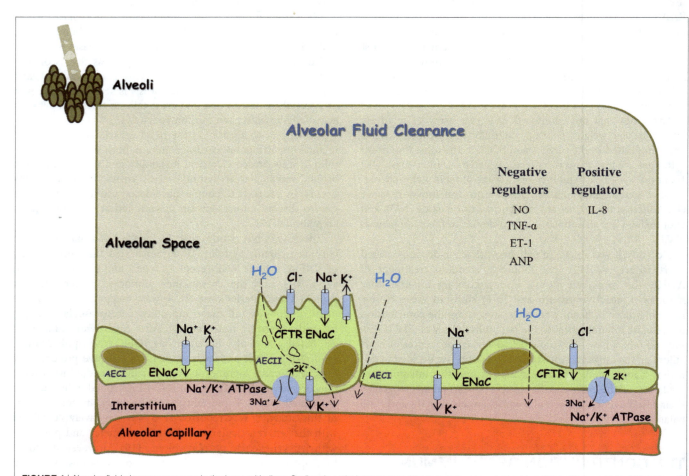

FIGURE 1 | Alveolar fluid clearance process in the lung epithelium. Sodium is actively transported from alveolar space to the lungs' interstitium and blood vessels; achieved mainly by apical ENaC and basolateral Na$^+$/K$^+$ ATPase located at AECI and AECII. This results in the formation of osmotic gradient, which drives transcellular and paracellular movements of water molecules. Some regulators, including cytokines, negatively affect this process while others appear to be with positive effects. AECI, alveolar epithelial cells type I; AECII, alveolar epithelial cells type II.

lung fibrosis by phosphorylating p38 and p42/44 kinases (also called extracellular signal-regulated protein kinases, ERK 1/2) (31). Ang II-induced mitogen-activated protein kinase (MAPK) activation has been implicated in myocardial hypertrophy, inflammation and neurotransmitter catecholamine synthesis, and release in the brain (34–36). These two kinases play a distinct role in the induction and signaling of pro-inflammatory cytokines. Specifically, fibroblasts stimulated with Ang II showed a strong time-dependent expression of COX-2 protein. The p38 MAPK inhibitor SB203580 but not the p42/44 MAPK-inhibitor PD98059 suppressed Ang II-induced COX-2 protein expression, a pro inflammatory enzyme (37). Likewise, blockade of Ang II receptors type I and II (AT1 and AT2, respectively) reduced the levels of TNF-α and its damage on renal tubular cell injury, thus exerting cytoprotective effects (38). Concerning the interaction between the RAAS and CNS systems, Wei et al. demonstrated that Ang II stimulates MAPK to upregulate brain AT1 receptors in rats with HF (39). Similarly, these authors demonstrated that Ang II-activated MAPK signaling pathways contribute to sympathetic excitation in HF (40). Specifically, intracerebroventricular administration of two selective p44/42 MAPK inhibitors, PD98059 and UO126, induced significant decreases in mean arterial pressure, heart rate, and renal sympathetic nerve activity in rats with HF but did not affect these parameters in sham controls. In addition, MAPK can be activated by other factors, such as pro-inflammatory cytokines and reactive oxygen species (41, 42), which are known to increase during inflammatory, pulmonary, and cardiac diseases. ERK1 and ERK2 play a crucial role in the pathogenesis of cardiac and vascular diseases. In this context, it was found that ERK1/2 and p38 MAPK activation occurred within 10 min of transverse aortic constriction, a model of pressure load heart failure (43). Similarly, activation of ERK, Jun kinase (JNK), and p38 MAPK has been demonstrated in other clinical and experimental heart failure (44).

The ability of the lungs to clear edema is impaired in acutely increased left atrial pressure (45–48). The underlying mechanisms are not fully understood; it has been assumed that NO synthesized in the alveolar endothelial cells attenuated the ability of the lungs to clear fluids *via* alveolar endothelial–epithelial interactions (45). The addition of Ang II to cultured vascular smooth muscle cells did not induce neither nuclear factor kappa B (NF-κB) activation nor iNOS or VCAM-1 expression. However, when added together with IL-1β, Ang II, through activation of the (AT1) receptor, inhibited iNOS expression and enhanced VCAM-1 expression induced by the cytokine. The inhibitory effect of Ang II on iNOS expression was associated with a downregulation of the sustained activation of extracellular signal-regulated kinase (ERK) and NF-κB by IL-1β, whereas the effect on VCAM-1 was independent of ERK activation. The effect of Ang II on iNOS was abolished by inhibition of p38 MAPK with SB203580. The authors concluded that Ang II, by a mechanism that involves p38 MAPK, differentially regulates the expression of NF-κB-dependent genes in response to IL-1β stimulation by controlling the duration of activation of ERK and NF-κB (49).

In chronic heart failure, however, the ability of the lungs to clear edema is increased particularly in compensated CHF

(50, 51). Verghese et al. have shown that in most of the patients with hydrostatic pulmonary edema, AFC is intact or even increased. Notably, in this population, there was a trend though insignificant toward better outcomes (52).

De Vito reported that Na$^+$/H$^+$ Exchanger isoform 1 might be a possible mediator of immunity involved in cytoplasmic pH (pH$_i$) homeostasis and expression of cytokines and chemokines (53). Our laboratory is currently investigating the expression pattern of Na$^+$/H$^+$ Exchanger (NHE) isoforms in alveolar epithelial cells and to evaluate their involvement in AFC process in both control and heart failure rats. CHF was induced by the placement of arteriovenous fistula between the abdominal aorta and vena cava (50). Notably, one should bear in mind that many of the immune cell functions are coupled with pH$_i$ modification. Specifically, an increase in pH$_i$ represents an important signal for cytokine and chemokine release, whereas a decrease in phagosomal pH can induce an efficient antigen presentation (53). Thus, our hypothesis in this regard speculates a potential role of one of the NHE isoforms in the inflammatory aspect of heart failure in general and pulmonary system in particular.

The Effects of Cytokines on AFC
The effects of cytokines on AFC were examined on a variety of acute lung injury (ALI) models and found to play a controversial role (18, 19, 54).

The role of the immune system in patients with acute respiratory distress syndrome (ARDS) and ALI is well known; briefly, soon after lung injury, endothelial cells are damaged with gap formation that allows fluid permeability, activation, and migration of neutrophils with activation of pro-inflammatory cytokines such as TNF-α, IL-1β, and the transcriptional regulatory NF-κB. Notably, in response to stimuli, such as infection, NF-κB is activated with consequent cellular responses that lead to pulmonary edema due to ALI/ARDS (55). Peteranderl et al. recently demonstrated that in mice lungs infected with influenza A (IAV), the rate of AFC was decreased *via* inhibiting the recruitment of Na,K-ATPase α subunit to the plasma membrane (54). It was demonstrated that this process was mediated by a paracrine cross talk between the infected and non-infected AEC and alveolar macrophages. The mediators that were involved in this interaction were principally interferon α and to lesser degree IFNβ and an IFN-dependent elevation of macrophage TNF-related apoptosis-inducing ligand. Interestingly, interruption of this cellular cross talk accelerates the rate edema resolution, which is of biologic and clinical importance to patients with IAV-induced lung injury (56).

TNF-α levels are known to be increased in heart failure. It was shown that LV ejection fraction was depressed in transgenic mice overexpressing TNF-α in cardiomyocytes; this effect was dependent on TNF-α gene dosage (57). However, the knowledge regarding the role of cytokines on AFC in the context of heart failure is limited. Rezaiguia et al. have shown that TNF-α instilled in normal rats increased alveolar liquid clearance by 43% over 1 h compared with control rats; conceivably, due to ENaC stimulation. TNF-α, which is secreted from alveolar macrophages binds to TNF receptors located on alveolar epithelial cells, where it induces its effects probably *via* upregulating of G proteins coupled ENaC. This effect is mediated *via* the lectin-like domain of TNF-α (58, 59). Another suggested mechanism is recruitment of ion channels to the cell membranes (60, 61). Moreover, it was demonstrated that in a model of ischemia–reperfusion in rats; AFC was upregulated, at least partly *via* TNF-α-dependent mechanism (62). On the other hand, it was reported that treating alveolar epithelial cells with TNF-α, the mRNA expression of ENaC subunits was decreased with compatible decrease in activity (63, 64). Therefore, these studies demonstrated that exposure to TNFα decreases ENaC mRNA and protein expression, as well as ENaC function both in alveolar type II cells and in injured lungs.

In models of ALI, it was demonstrated that IL-8 mediated injury to both the endothelium and epithelium, with consequent high permeability edema formation and decreased AFC (54). In addition, pretreatment with anti-IL-8 antibodies successfully restored the rate of AFC to normal probably by attenuating injury to the epithelium (18, 19).

The Effect of NO and Endothelin on AFC

Endothelin-1 (ET-1), a potent vasoactive peptide produced by endothelial cells and released during injurious stimuli such as pulmonary hypertension and heart failure. It has been shown that elevated concentrations of ET-1 predict mortality and hospitalizations in HF patients (65). It is noteworthy that ET-1 has an inhibitory effect on lung edema clearance *via* an endothelial epithelial interaction. The underlying mechanism involves activation of endothelial ETB receptors and NO generation leading to alveolar epithelial Na,K-ATPase downregulation in a cyclic guanosine monophosphate (cGMP)-independent manner (32).

Kaestle et al. have explored the role of NO in both acute and chronic heart failure. They have shown that in isolated mouse lungs, hydrostatic edema formation was attenuated by NO synthase (NOS) inhibition. Similarly, edema formation was decreased in isolated mouse lungs of endothelial NOS-deficient mice. Whereas, in chronic heart failure model; AFC was preserved as a result of endothelial dysfunction and decreased NO generation. This effect is mediated by endothelial-derived NO acting as an intercompartmental signaling molecule at the alveolo-capillary barrier (45) (**Figure 1**).

Renal System

Kidney dysfunction is common in heart failure and is associated with an increased risk of mortality. The interaction between the heart and kidney in this setting is complex, involving multiple interdependent mechanisms including hemodynamic alterations and activation of multiple neurohormonal as well as pro-inflammatory systems (**Figure 2**).

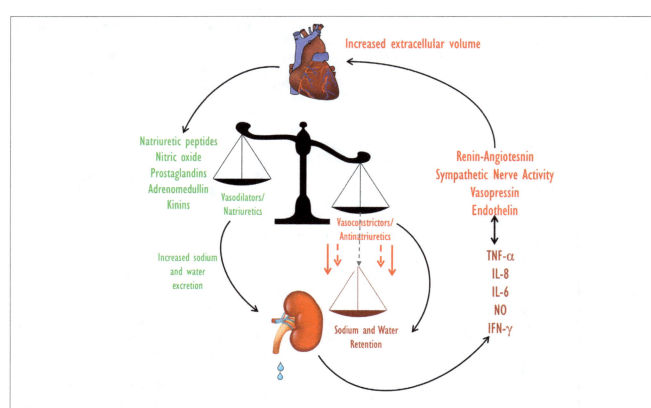

FIGURE 2 | Extracellular fluid volume control in CHF. Volume homeostasis in CHF is determined by the balance between the natriuretic and the anti-natriuretic arms. In decompensated CHF, enhanced activities of the Na⁺-retaining systems along with activation of pro inflammatory substances overcome the effects of the vasodilatory/natriuretic systems, leading to a net reduction in Na⁺ excretion and eventually to an increase in ECF volume. CHF, congestive heart failure; ECF, extracellular fluid.

Effects of Cytokines on Renal Handling of Water and Salt

The kidney is a major target organ of various hormones, and paracrine and autocrine substances. Many of the latter belong to the cytokines family, and some of the hormones that act on the kidney possess pro inflammatory properties. CHF is known to cause amplification of several pro-inflammatory mediators that can be detected at high concentrations in several vital organs and blood stream. The biologic sources of this chronic inflammatory state in CHF are not fully recognized. However, the heart and the kidneys produce a wide range of pro-inflammatory cytokines in response to activation of various neurohormonal systems and endotoxin accumulation as described below. Moreover, the hypo perfusion of the kidney during cardiorenal syndrome (CRS) results in sodium and water retention with further venous congestion. The biomechanical stretch of the vascular endothelium stimulates cytokine production (66).

The Renin–Angiotensin System

The RAAS plays a major role in the pathogenesis of heart failure and responsible for the cardiovascular and renal manifestations of this disease (67–69). At the initial phase of CHF, the RAAS exerts beneficial effects aimed at BP maintenance by direct systemic vasoconstriction, or indirectly *via* augmentation of the SNS activity and by promoting renal sodium retention. However, as CHF progress, the biological activities of the RAAS turn to be deleterious and contribute significantly to the disease aggravation (67). The main active substances of the RAAS are Ang II and aldosterone, which play a key role in the adverse cardiac and renal manifestations of severe CHF (3). Concerning the kidney, both Ang II and aldosterone act directly on the proximal tubule and collecting dust where they enhance Na⁺ reabsorption *via* NHE3 and ENaC, respectively (**Figure 3**). Specifically, two-thirds of filtered sodium is reabsorbed in the proximal tubule *via* cotransporters along amino acid, glucose, phosphor as well as NHE3. Water follows sodium *via* aquaporin 1. At the distal tubule, sodium is reabsorbed by Na, K-cotransporter sensitive to thiazide. In the collecting ducts, a minimal amount of sodium (2–3%) is reabsorbed *via* amiloride sensitive ENaC that is upregulated by aldosterone. Water is reabsorbed in the collecting ducts *via* aquaporin 2 induced by vasopressin (70, 71). Furthermore, it is conceivable to reason that the anti-natriuretic effect of the RAAS is counterbalanced by the natriuretic/vasodilatory effect of atrial natriuretic peptide (ANP) on the kidney, thereby leading to substantial urinary retention of sodium and water retention with resultant edema formation (72, 73). In addition, increased activity of the RAAS contributes to the attenuated endothelial-dependent renal vasodilatation and the development of endothelial dysfunction characterizing CHF (74). Concerning the latter, it is attributed to several factors including the immune system. In support of this notion, it has been reported that T cells and various T cell-derived cytokines play a role in the pathogenesis of fluid/salt imbalance and elevated vascular resistance. For instance, various stimuli including Ang II, aldosterone, and catecholamines, which are known to be activated in CHF and hypertension increase the count of effector like T cells, which infiltrate the renal tissue in the perivascular regions of both arteries and arterioles (66, 75). There is also accumulation of monocyte/macrophages in these vascular beds (75). Both cell types release several cytokines including IL-17, IFN-γ, tumor necrosis factor-α (TNF-α), and IL-6, which cause renal damage and vascular dysfunction, resulting in avid sodium retention and elevated vascular resistance (75). By applying MI model induced by left coronary artery ligation in rats, Cho et al. demonstrated elevated activated monocytes (CC chemokine receptor 2⁺ ED-1⁺) in peripheral blood, along with the infiltration of ED-1⁺ macrophages and the increment of nuclear p65 in the kidney of MI rats, suggesting the contribution of NF-κB-mediated inflammation in the development of type I CRS. The inflammatory cytokines, IL-6, and tumor necrosis factor-α (TNF-α) mRNA expression, as well as microvascular endothelial permeability and

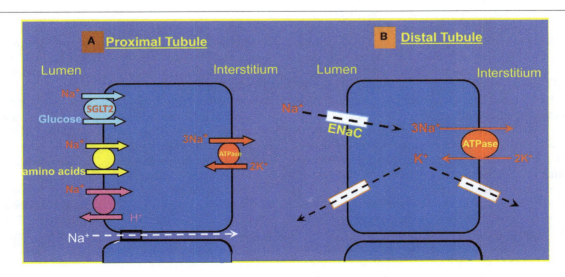

FIGURE 3 | **(A)** Sodium transport in the proximal tubule. **(B)** Reabsorption of Na⁺ and K⁺ transport in the principle cells of the collecting duct.

tubular cell apoptosis, significantly enhanced in the kidneys of MI rats. These findings support the involvement of the immune activation/inflammation in the pathophysiology of CRS besides the hemodynamic alteration, pathological compensatory neurohormonal activation and oxidative stress (76).

As mentioned above, the RAAS activates the immune system but also the immune system activates certain components of RAAS (8). In this context, TNF-α and IL-6 stimulate the generation of angiotensinogen, exaggerate sodium retention and enhance renal fibrosis (77). One of the most famous representatives of the adverse cytokines in CHF is TNF-α, whose circulatory levels increase in correlation with the severity of the disease (66). In line with the deleterious pro-inflammatory role of Ang II in CHF, pharmacological blockade of the AT1 receptors in this clinical setting decreased the levels of pro-inflammatory cytokines including TNF-α (78, 79). Similarly, *in vivo* studies demonstrated that Ang II enhanced the expression of both TNF-α and IL-6 in the cardiomyocytes and in renal cortical and tubular cells (78, 80). These findings support the notion that the RAAS, especially Ang II, triggers the production of pro-inflammatory molecules in CHF.

Finally, several studies provided a keen linkage between oxidative stress and immune activation in several cardiovascular diseases including CHF and hypertension (81, 82). Interestingly, long-term activation of the RAAS impairs mitochondrial function, and increase oxidative stress burden which in turn can lead to renal injury and sodium and water retention (81). The major prooxidative stress stimulator is Ang II, where administration of the latter enhances renal mitochondrial oxidative stress and reduces GFR in rats with heart failure.

Sympathetic Nervous System

Activation of SNS is one of the hallmarks of CHF. It is well established the SNS mediates system and renal vasoconstrictor and salt retaining biological actions (83). However, experimental studies have demonstrated the involvement of pro-inflammatory cytokines TNF-α, IL-6, and IL-1β in CHF rats that were exposed to chronic stimulation of β-adrenergic stimulation with isoproterenol for 12 weeks as manifested by increased mRNA expression of these cytokines in cardiomyocytes and cardiac blood vessels. Nevertheless, the mRNA expression of NO was not increased. Thus, it is presumed that one mechanism underlying the beneficial effects of β-adrenergic blockade in heart failure may involve attenuation of TNF-α and IL-1β expression independent of iNOS and NO. In this context, β-blockade with metoprolol causes significant decline in TNF-α and IL-1β, but not IL-6 expression in the myocardium (84). It should be emphasized that the kidneys are preferentially innervate by sympathetic nerve fibers and the activity of renal sympathetic nerve is markedly increased in CHF. Stimulation of the renal nerve augments sodium reabsorption, decreases renal blood flow (RBF) *via* renal artery constriction, and stimulates renin release through $\beta1$ receptors on the juxtaglomerular apparatus (85).

Whether enhanced circulatory levels or locally produced cytokines in response to SNS or RAAS activation in CHF mediate some of the adverse renal actions of these systems remained largely to be elucidated. However, previous studies have shown that pro-inflammatory mediators such as TNF-α, IL-6, and CRP play a role in the pathophysiology of progressive renal injury and probably in salt and water imbalance characterizing various acute and chronic kidney diseases including CRS. As mentioned above, volume expansion associated with CHF promotes secretion of cytokines by endothelial cells. In this context, it was reported that TNF-α caused renal dysfunction as was evident by intravascular volume expansion due to salt and water retention (86). Likewise, oxidative stress enhances NaCl absorption by the thick ascending limb through activation of protein kinase C (87). Additional explanation to the avid sodium retention and water imbalance in heart failure is renal epithelial and endothelial damage, which leads to a loss of endo–epithelial barrier integrity and function. In this respect, Cho et al. have shown that CRS type I and II was associated with increased tubular damage marker as was evident by elevated levels of NGAL and tubular cell apoptosis. Moreover, macrophage infiltration and inflammatory cytokine expression possibly mediated by the NF-κB pathway, and microvascular endothelial damage increased significantly in kidneys at 3 days post-induction of MI, suggesting the important contribution of inflammation in the pathogenesis of type I CRS. These changes ultimately led to renal interstitial fibrosis along with chronically decreased heart function (type II CRS) (76). Although the direct effects of cytokines on ion transports in the kidney were no studied yet, the observation that heart failure is associated with enhanced renal TNF-α and IL-6 expression along tubular cell apoptosis supports such a role. In addition, microvascular endothelial injury characterized by endothelial cell apoptosis, alteration of actin cytoskeleton, or increased expression of leukocyte adhesion molecules has mediated the early phase of renal injury following ischemia and by facilitating leukocyte transmigration; it substantially contributes to tissue inflammation. In the long run, activation of the Ang II and SNS along renal hypoperfusion causes further activation of pro-inflammatory cytokines, which in their turn enhance neurohormonal activation thus creating a vicious cycle (88).

Endothelin

ET peptides are synthesized as preproETs in endothelium, heart, and kidney, processed into a big precursor and then converted into biologically active peptides such as ET-1 by 2 ET-converting-enzyme isoforms. Active ET-1 binds to ETA and ETB receptors (ETAR/ETBR) expressed in the kidney, lung, brain and cardiovascular system. ETAR activation generally causes vasoconstriction, while ETBR produces vasodilation. The status of the major components of the ET system in the kidney during CHF has been subject to intensive investigation. As outlined above, the endothelin system is over activated in CHF as evident by elevated levels of ET-1 in the circulation, cardiac and renal tissues as well as urinary excretion of this peptide (89–92). The deleterious and beneficial renal and cardiac ET effects are usually attributed to ETAR and ETBR, respectively (93, 94). However, ETAR blockade failed to improve cardiovascular outcomes and caused edema in clinical trials (95–98).

The heart and kidney are both important sources and key targets for ET. Cardiac myocytes and the renal glomerulus, vessels, and tubular epithelium each express ETA and ETB receptors (91).

Elevated ET-1 levels correlate with CHF, hemodynamic dysfunction, and symptom severity (15, 99) and result in cardiac ETA upregulation along ETB downregulation (100–102). ET receptor antagonists attenuate experimental cardiac pathophysiology (103–107). ET-mediated renal pathology during CHF is an area of debate, but the potent reductions in RBF, GFR, natriuresis, and urine volume when ET-1 is increased to CHF levels supports a deleterious role for ET (108). ET levels also strongly correlate with renal dysfunction in patients with CRS (109, 110). However, a sustained cortical vasoconstriction and transient medullary vasodilation indicate renal responses to ET-1 are complex (108, 111). ET also produces dose-dependent changes in renal Na^+ and water excretion, with high levels causing anti-natriuretic and antidiuretic effects, due to reduced GFR and RBF. In contrast, lower doses or local tubular *in situ* epithelial delivery produced ET-1 decrease tubular salt and water reabsorption, which are blocked by ETB antagonists (112).

Collectively, these findings suggest that ET signaling contributes to cardiac and renal dysfunction. Besides its endocrine/paracrine role in the regulation of the cardio vascular and renal hemodynamic and salt balance, ET-1 possesses pro-inflammatory and pro-fibrotic properties in pulmonary, cardiac, and renal diseases. Under these disease conditions, increases in ET-1 are critically involved in initiating and maintaining inflammation and injury, thereby promoting perturbations among the rest of salt and water balance. At the renal level, ET-1 stimulates the aggregation and accumulation of neutrophils, thus propagating glomerular inflammation, a process that can be inhibited by ETA receptor blockade (113).

Natriuretic Peptides (NPs)
This family consists of three members of the NPs: ANP, brain natriuretic peptide (BNP), and C-natriuretic peptides (114, 115). ANP and BNP are secreted mainly from the atria and ventricles, respectively, upon atrial distention and volume overload (116, 117). By binding to the NPR-A receptor, ANP and BNP induce the production of cGMP, which in turn promotes vasodilation, diuresis, natriuresis, and prevent cardiac remodeling, thus playing a major role in the homeostasis of blood pressure as well as of water and salt balance.

Interestingly, clinical and experimental heart failure are associated with high levels of circulating NPs, and today these peptides serve as biomarkers for HF. However, few studies have demonstrated that *de novo* synthesis of NPs in the renal tissue constitutes an essential pathway for maintaining normal blood pressure and fluid balance besides the NPs of cardiac origin. Ritter et al. were the first to report that primary cultures of neonatal and adult rat kidney cells produce and secrete ANP-like prohormone (118). Soon after, by using immunohistochemical staining, Greenwald et al. detected proANP predominantly in the distal cortical nephron (119). It was later that Ramirez et al. reported that all forms of proANP/ANP were found in the kidney, mainly in the proximal and distal nephron (120). ANP and their receptor, NPR-A, were highly expressed as well in these parts of the tubule. The natriuretic and diuretic effects of ANP are attributed to its stimulatory effect on GFR but also to its inhibitory action on ENaC in the collecting duct (121).

Interestingly, several studies demonstrated that ANP also act as autocrine/paracrine factor where it modulates various immune functions (122). There is keen evidence that ANP is locally produced by several immune cells, which also present specific natriuretic receptors. For instance, ANP stimulates the phagocytosis of macrophage and killing activity by ROS production, thus improving the innate immunity (123). Moreover, ANP inhibits lipopolysaccharide-induced NO release by macrophage cells and promotes the inactivation of NF-κB *via* cGMP (53, 123). In a recent study by Mitaka et al. (124), ANP pretreatment prevented kidney–lung cross talk in a rat model of renal ischemic reperfusion injury. Interestingly, this group has also shown that ANP posttreatment ameliorated injuries in kidney and lung by direct tissue protective effect and anti-inflammatory effects, which potentially inhibited interorgan cross talk (125). Zhu et al. have shown that ANP reduced the levels pro-inflammatory cytokines such as IL-1β, IL-6, IL-10, and TNF-α in rats with oleic acid-induced ALI (126). In agreement with its anti-inflammatory properties, ANP interferes with the expression of adhesion molecules such as ICAM-1 and E-selectin (66, 77).

Finally, in critically ill patients, BNP and NT-proBNP levels correlated with inflammatory markers such as CRP and leukocyte count (127). Likewise, patients with septic shock had elevated BNP concentration regardless of the presence of CHF condition. Although the involvement of these anti-inflammatory effects of NPs in the pathogenesis of renal function in CHF has not been completely understood, it may represent a counterbalance compensatory response to the activation of the adverse neurohormonal systems including RAAS, SNS, and ET-1.

NO System
Renal NO is a molecule synthesized from its precursor, L-arginine by the enzyme, NOS; this process takes place in several sites, mainly in the endothelial cells of the renal blood vessels but also in the tubular epithelial and mesangial cells. Notably, three different isoforms of NOS; NOS 1 (bNOS), NOS 2 (iNOS) and NOS 3 (eNOS). NO plays an important role in the regulation of renal hemodynamics and excretory function. Specifically, locally produced NO is involved in the regulation RPF, salt excretion, and renin release. The action of NO is mediated by activation of a soluble guanylate cyclase in adjacent vascular smooth muscle cells, thereby increasing intracellular levels of its second messenger, cGMP (128, 129).

It has been shown that iNOS has been implicated in many human diseases associated with inflammation *via* the activation of the c-JNK, p42/44 MAPK, and p38 kinase pathways (130, 131). This isoform of NOS is responsible for the generation of excessive amounts of NO, which leads to tissue injury due to exaggerated generation of oxidative radicals such peroxynitrate. For instance, iNOS is overexpressed in the venous endothelial cells harvested from patients with decompensation CHF (132). Likewise, excessive NO in the heart leads to myocardial depression and reduced contractility in patients and experimental animals with CHF (133).

These findings lead to the "cytokine hypothesis," which suggests that cytokines play an important pathogenic role in development of HF. This notion is further supported by two studies demonstrating that iNOS knockout mice display less cardiac dysfunction after myocardial infarction than wild-type controls (134). Interestingly, there is negative interplay between iNOS and ANP, where the latter *via* cGMP production increases intracellular calcium levels in murine macrophages resulting in decreased iNOS expression (135).

SUMMARY AND CONCLUSION

In summary, inflammation and neurohormonal systems appear to interplay one with each other leading to worsening cardiac, pulmonary, and renal functions, which negatively affect patients' outcome. While the adverse role of the RAAS, SNS, and ET-1 in the pathogenesis of CHF is well established, the involvement of the innate and adaptive immune in the cardiac, renal, and pulmonary manifestations of CHF is still evolving. Although we have shown that the inflammatory system plays a substantial direct and indirect role in heart failure, this observation does not prove unequivocally a causal role in CHF. Therefore, another possibility should be considered, such as that these cytokines are elevated in heart failure in response to the underlying injury, and that they may serve as markers rather than drivers of the disease process. The therapeutic interventions aimed at reducing the activation of the immune cells or blockade of certain cytokines were unsatisfactory. Milestones studies that investigated the effect of TNF-α antagonists, etanercept (136), and infliximab (137) on the composite clinical outcomes of mortality and worsening heart failure in the range of several weeks, in patients with chronic systolic heart failure failed to show any benefit. Infliximab failed to show beneficial effect; this was related possibly to the short term treatment. The RENEWAL investigators suggested several possibilities for the lack of benefit of etanercept; among them, lower investigated doses of etanercept, cytokines may not play an important role in heart failure or alternatively, there is a need to simultaneously target several inflammatory mediators and the predisposition for infection due to etanercept. A recent review of these studies argued that the unfavorable outcomes might be attributed to the population cohorts that were mostly severe with

advanced heart failure, toxicity of the treatment, and genetic polymorphism (138). Recently, it was shown in a small cohort of 30 patients with systolic heart failure and acute decompensation; the administration of IL-1 blocker, anakinra reduced the inflammatory burden as shown by reduced C-reactive protein levels within 72 h. However, this study did not address clinical outcomes (139). Cavalli et al. have reported that in a patient who developed fulminant myocarditis with biventricular failure and cardiogenic shock, the administration of anakinra restored cardiac function with clinical improvement (140). Yet, we should await more well-designed studies that may prove to be beneficial in reducing target organ damage and preventing congestion characterizing heart failure.

In light of the limited therapeutic tools of congestion of pulmonary and cardiac etiologies, anti-inflammatory treatment strategies may turn to be a novel approach with promising prognostic consequences in the CRS. Yet, further research is required to understand in depth the interaction between the classic neurohormonal systems and the inflammatory ones, the sources of the latter in the CRS, and their effect on the specific mediators of salt and water transporters at the pulmonary and renal tissues.

AUTHOR CONTRIBUTIONS

ZSA and ZA conceived and designed the manuscript structure. ZSA, SK, FB, RI-B, EK, and ZA contributed to writing and reviewing the paper. SK, ZSA, and ZA contributed in preparing the figures.

FUNDING

This work was supported by Israel Foundation (ISF), Grant No. 625/08; The Office of Chief Scientist (Grant No. 6267-1); Ministry of Health, Israel; Manlam Office, Jess & Mildred Fisher Family (Fund No. 2020201), Technion, The Israel Institute of Technology, and The Rappaport Family Institute for Research in the Medical Sciences, Technion, Israel Institute of Technology, Haifa.

REFERENCES

1. Ponikowski P, Voors AA, Anker SD, Bueno H, Cleland JG, Coats AJ, et al. 2016 ESC Guidelines for the diagnosis and treatment of acute and chronic heart failure: The Task Force for the diagnosis and treatment of acute and chronic heart failure of the European Society of Cardiology (ESC). Developed with the special contribution of the Heart Failure Association (HFA) of the ESC. *Eur J Heart Fail* (2016) 18(8):891–975. doi:10.1002/ejhf.592
2. Jessup M, Brozena S. Heart failure. *N Engl J Med* (2003) 348(20):2007–18. doi:10.1056/NEJMra021498
3. Francis GS, Goldsmith SR, Levine TB, Olivari MT, Cohn JN. The neurohumoral axis in congestive heart failure. *Ann Intern Med* (1984) 101(3):370–7. doi:10.7326/0003-4819-101-3-370
4. Katz AM. Cardiomyopathy of overload. A major determinant of prognosis in congestive heart failure. *N Engl J Med* (1990) 322(2):100–10. doi:10.1056/NEJM199001113220206
5. Packer M. The neurohormonal hypothesis: a theory to explain the mechanism of disease progression in heart failure. *J Am Coll Cardiol* (1992) 20(1):248–54. doi:10.1016/0735-1097(92)90167-L
6. Wagner KB, Felix SB, Riad A. Innate immune receptors in heart failure: side effect or potential therapeutic target? *World J Cardiol* (2014) 6(8):791–801. doi:10.4330/wjc.v6.i8.791

7. Anker SD, von Haehling S. Inflammatory mediators in chronic heart failure: an overview. *Heart* (2004) 90(4):464–70. doi:10.1136/hrt.2002.007005
8. Sharma R, Coats AJ, Anker SD. The role of inflammatory mediators in chronic heart failure: cytokines, nitric oxide, and endothelin-1. *Int J Cardiol* (2000) 72(2):175–86. doi:10.1016/S0167-5273(99)00186-2
9. Goonewardena SN, Stein AB, Tsuchida RE, Rattan R, Shah D, Hummel SL. Monocyte subsets and inflammatory cytokines in acute decompensated heart failure. *J Card Fail* (2016) 22(5):358–65. doi:10.1016/j.cardfail.2015.12.014
10. Sharma R, Anker SD. Immune and neurohormonal pathways in chronic heart failure. *Congest Heart Fail* (2002) 8(1):23–8, 48. doi:10.1111/j.1527-5299.2002.00724.x
11. Anker SD, Egerer KR, Volk HD, Kox WJ, Poole-Wilson PA, Coats AJ. Elevated soluble CD14 receptors and altered cytokines in chronic heart failure. *Am J Cardiol* (1997) 79(10):1426–30. doi:10.1016/S0002-9149(97)00159-8
12. Torre-Amione G, Kapadia S, Lee J, Durand JB, Bies RD, Young JB, et al. Tumor necrosis factor-alpha and tumor necrosis factor receptors in the failing human heart. *Circulation* (1996) 93(4):704–11. doi:10.1161/01.CIR.93.4.704
13. Hasper D, Hummel M, Kleber FX, Reindl I, Volk HD. Systemic inflammation in patients with heart failure. *Eur Heart J* (1998) 19(5):761–5. doi:10.1053/euhj.1997.0858

14. Hill JA, Olson EN. Cardiac plasticity. *N Engl J Med* (2008) 358(13):1370–80. doi:10.1056/NEJMra072139
15. Moore-Morris T, Guimaraes-Camboa N, Banerjee I, Zambon AC, Kisseleva T, Velayoudon A, et al. Resident fibroblast lineages mediate pressure overload-induced cardiac fibrosis. *J Clin Invest* (2014) 124(7):2921–34. doi:10.1172/JCI74783
16. Burchfield JS, Xie M, Hill JA. Pathological ventricular remodeling: mechanisms: part 1 of 2. *Circulation* (2013) 128(4):388–400. doi:10.1161/CIRCULATIONAHA.113.001878
17. Spinale FG. Myocardial matrix remodeling and the matrix metalloproteinases: influence on cardiac form and function. *Physiol Rev* (2007) 87(4):1285–342. doi:10.1152/physrev.00012.2007
18. Laffon M, Pittet JF, Modelska K, Matthay MA, Young DM. Interleukin-8 mediates injury from smoke inhalation to both the lung endothelial and the alveolar epithelial barriers in rabbits. *Am J Respir Crit Care Med* (1999) 160 (5 Pt 1):1443–9. doi:10.1164/ajrccm.160.5.9901097
19. Modelska K, Pittet JF, Folkesson HG, Courtney Broaddus V, Matthay MA. Acid-induced lung injury. Protective effect of anti-interleukin-8 pretreatment on alveolar epithelial barrier function in rabbits. *Am J Respir Crit Care Med* (1999) 160(5 Pt 1):1450–6. doi:10.1164/ajrccm.160.5.9901096
20. Azzam ZS, Sznajder JI. Lung edema clearance: relevance to patients with lung injury. *Rambam Maimonides Med J* (2015) 6(3). doi:10.5041/RMMJ.10210
21. Divangahi M, King IL, Pernet E. Alveolar macrophages and type I IFN in airway homeostasis and immunity. *Trends Immunol* (2015) 36(5):307–14. doi:10.1016/j.it.2015.03.005
22. Basset G, Crone C, Saumon G. Significance of active ion transport in transalveolar water absorption: a study on isolated rat lung. *J Physiol* (1987) 384:311–24. doi:10.1113/jphysiol.1987.sp016456
23. Matthay MA, Folkesson HG, Clerici C. Lung epithelial fluid transport and the resolution of pulmonary edema. *Physiol Rev* (2002) 82(3):569–600. doi:10.1152/physrev.00003.2002
24. Saumon G, Basset G. Electrolyte and fluid transport across the mature alveolar epithelium. *J Appl Physiol* (1993) 74(1):1–15.
25. Sakuma T, Takahashi K, Ohya N, Nakada T, Matthay MA. Effects of ATP-sensitive potassium channel opener on potassium transport and alveolar fluid clearance in the resected human lung. *Pharmacol Toxicol* (1998) 83(1):16–22. doi:10.1111/j.1600-0773.1998.tb01436.x
26. Bardou O, Prive A, Migneault F, Roy-Camille K, Dagenais A, Berthiaume Y, et al. K+ channels regulate ENaC expression via changes in promoter activity and control fluid clearance in alveolar epithelial cells. *Biochim Biophys Acta* (2012) 1818(7):1682–90. doi:10.1016/j.bbamem.2012.02.025
27. Hummler E, Barker P, Gatzy J, Beermann F, Verdumo C, Schmidt A, et al. Early death due to defective neonatal lung liquid clearance in alpha-ENaC-deficient mice. *Nat Genet* (1996) 12(3):325–8. doi:10.1038/ng0396-325
28. O'Brodovich H, Yang P, Gandhi S, Otulakowski G. Amiloride-insensitive Na+ and fluid absorption in the mammalian distal lung. *Am J Physiol Lung Cell Mol Physiol* (2008) 294(3):L401–8. doi:10.1152/ajplung.00431.2007
29. Berger G, Guetta J, Klorin G, Badarneh R, Braun E, Brod V, et al. Sepsis impairs alveolar epithelial function by downregulating Na-K-ATPase pump. *Am J Physiol Lung Cell Mol Physiol* (2011) 301(1):L23–30. doi:10.1152/ajplung.00010.2010
30. Guidot DM, Folkesson HG, Jain L, Sznajder JI, Pittet JF, Matthay MA. Integrating acute lung injury and regulation of alveolar fluid clearance. *Am J Physiol Lung Cell Mol Physiol* (2006) 291(3):L301–6. doi:10.1152/ajplung.00153.2006
31. Konigshoff M, Wilhelm A, Jahn A, Sedding D, Amarie OV, Eul B, et al. The angiotensin II receptor 2 is expressed and mediates angiotensin II signaling in lung fibrosis. *Am J Respir Cell Mol Biol* (2007) 37(6):640–50. doi:10.1165/rcmb.2006-0379TR
32. Comellas AP, Briva A, Dada LA, Butti ML, Trejo HE, Yshii C, et al. Endothelin-1 impairs alveolar epithelial function via endothelial ETB receptor. *Am J Respir Crit Care Med* (2009) 179(2):113–22. doi:10.1164/rccm.200804-540OC
33. Ismael-Badarneh R, Guetta J, Klorin G, Berger G, Abu-Saleh N, Abassi Z, et al. The role of angiotensin II and cyclic AMP in alveolar active sodium transport. *PLoS One* (2015) 10(7):e0137118. doi:10.1371/journal.pone.0137118
34. Lu D, Yang H, Raizada MK. Angiotensin II regulation of neuromodulation: downstream signaling mechanism from activation of mitogen-activated

protein kinase. *J Cell Biol* (1996) 135(6 Pt 1):1609–17. doi:10.1083/jcb.135.6.1609
35. Vaziri ND, Xu ZG, Shahkarami A, Huang KT, Rodriguez-Iturbe B, Natarajan R. Role of AT-1 receptor in regulation of vascular MCP-1, IL-6, PAI-1, MAP kinase, and matrix expressions in obesity. *Kidney Int* (2005) 68(6):2787–93. doi:10.1111/j.1523-1755.2005.00750.x
36. Pellieux C, Sauthier T, Aubert JF, Brunner HR, Pedrazzini T. Angiotensin II-induced cardiac hypertrophy is associated with different mitogen-activated protein kinase activation in normotensive and hypertensive mice. *J Hypertens* (2000) 18(9):1307–17. doi:10.1097/00004872-200018090-00017
37. Scheuren N, Jacobs M, Ertl G, Schorb W. Cyclooxygenase-2 in myocardium stimulation by angiotensin-II in cultured cardiac fibroblasts and role at acute myocardial infarction. *J Mol Cell Cardiol* (2002) 34(1):29–37. doi:10.1006/jmcc.2001.1484
38. Kagawa T, Takao T, Horino T, Matsumoto R, Inoue K, Morita T, et al. Angiotensin II receptor blocker inhibits tumour necrosis factor-alpha-induced cell damage in human renal proximal tubular epithelial cells. *Nephrology (Carlton)* (2008) 13(4):309–15. doi:10.1111/j.1440-1797.2008.00918.x
39. Wei SG, Yu Y, Zhang ZH, Felder RB. Activated mitogen-activated protein kinase contributes to the up-regulation of angiotensin type 1 receptors in the brain of heart failure rats. *Circulation* (2006) 114(Suppl 18):310.
40. Wei SG, Yu Y, Zhang ZH, Weiss RM, Felder RB. Angiotensin II-triggered p44/42 mitogen-activated protein kinase mediates sympathetic excitation in heart failure rats. *Hypertension* (2008) 52(2):342–50. doi:10.1161/HYPERTENSIONAHA.108.110445
41. Viedt C, Soto U, Krieger-Brauer HI, Fei J, Elsing C, Kubler W, et al. Differential activation of mitogen-activated protein kinases in smooth muscle cells by angiotensin II: involvement of p22phox and reactive oxygen species. *Arterioscler Thromb Vasc Biol* (2000) 20(4):940–8. doi:10.1161/01.ATV.20.4.940
42. Boone E, Vandevoorde V, De Wilde G, Haegeman G. Activation of p42/p44 mitogen-activated protein kinases (MAPK) and p38 MAPK by tumor necrosis factor (TNF) is mediated through the death domain of the 55-kDa TNF receptor. *FEBS Lett* (1998) 441(2):275–80. doi:10.1016/S0014-5793(98)01567-1
43. Purcell NH, Wilkins BJ, York A, Saba-El-Leil MK, Meloche S, Robbins J, et al. Genetic inhibition of cardiac ERK1/2 promotes stress-induced apoptosis and heart failure but has no effect on hypertrophy in vivo. *Proc Natl Acad Sci U S A* (2007) 104(35):14074–9. doi:10.1073/pnas.0610906104
44. Haq S, Choukroun G, Lim H, Tymitz KM, del Monte F, Gwathmey J, et al. Differential activation of signal transduction pathways in human hearts with hypertrophy versus advanced heart failure. *Circulation* (2001) 103(5):670–7. doi:10.1161/01.CIR.103.5.670
45. Kaestle SM, Reich CA, Yin N, Habazettl H, Weimann J, Kuebler WM. Nitric oxide-dependent inhibition of alveolar fluid clearance in hydrostatic lung edema. *Am J Physiol Lung Cell Mol Physiol* (2007) 293(4):L859–69. doi:10.1152/ajplung.00008.2007
46. Saldias FJ, Azzam ZS, Ridge KM, Yeldandi A, Rutschman DH, Schraufnagel D, et al. Alveolar fluid reabsorption is impaired by increased left atrial pressures in rats. *Am J Physiol Lung Cell Mol Physiol* (2001) 281(3):L591–7.
47. Campbell AR, Folkesson HG, Berthiaume Y, Gutkowska J, Suzuki S, Matthay MA. Alveolar epithelial fluid clearance persists in the presence of moderate left atrial hypertension in sheep. *J Appl Physiol* (1999) 86(1):139–51.
48. Raj JU, Bland RD. Lung luminal liquid clearance in newborn lambs. Effect of pulmonary microvascular pressure elevation. *Am Rev Respir Dis* (1986) 134(2):305–10.
49. Jiang B, Xu S, Hou X, Pimentel DR, Cohen RA. Angiotensin II differentially regulates interleukin-1-beta-inducible NO synthase (iNOS) and vascular cell adhesion molecule-1 (VCAM-1) expression: role of p38 MAPK. *J Biol Chem* (2004) 279(19):20363–8. doi:10.1074/jbc.M314172200
50. Azzam ZS, Adir Y, Welch L, Chen J, Winaver J, Factor P, et al. Alveolar fluid reabsorption is increased in rats with compensated heart failure. *Am J Physiol Lung Cell Mol Physiol* (2006) 291(5):L1094–100. doi:10.1152/ajplung.00180.2005
51. Huang W, Kingsbury MP, Turner MA, Donnelly JL, Flores NA, Sheridan DJ. Capillary filtration is reduced in lungs adapted to chronic heart failure: morphological and haemodynamic correlates. *Cardiovasc Res* (2001) 49(1):207–17. doi:10.1016/S0008-6363(00)00223-6

52. Verghese GM, Ware LB, Matthay BA, Matthay MA. Alveolar epithelial fluid transport and the resolution of clinically severe hydrostatic pulmonary edema. *J Appl Physiol* (1999) 87(4):1301–12.

53. De Vito P. The sodium/hydrogen exchanger: a possible mediator of immunity. *Cell Immunol* (2006) 240(2):69–85. doi:10.1016/j.cellimm.2006.07.001

54. Zemans RL, Matthay MA. Bench-to-bedside review: the role of the alveolar epithelium in the resolution of pulmonary edema in acute lung injury. *Crit Care* (2004) 8(6):469–77. doi:10.1186/cc2906

55. Gonzales JN, Lucas R, Verin AD. The acute respiratory distress syndrome: mechanisms and perspective therapeutic approaches. *Austin J Vasc Med* (2015) 2(1):1009–22.

56. Peteranderl C, Morales-Nebreda L, Selvakumar B, Lecuona E, Vadasz I, Morty RE, et al. Macrophage-epithelial paracrine crosstalk inhibits lung edema clearance during influenza infection. *J Clin Invest* (2016) 126(4): 1566–80. doi:10.1172/JCI83931

57. Mann DL. Innate immunity and the failing heart: the cytokine hypothesis revisited. *Circ Res* (2015) 116(7):1254–68. doi:10.1161/CIRCRESAHA.116. 302317

58. Vadasz I, Schermuly RT, Ghofrani HA, Rummel S, Wehner S, Muhldorfer I, et al. The lectin-like domain of tumor necrosis factor-alpha improves alveolar fluid balance in injured isolated rabbit lungs. *Crit Care Med* (2008) 36(5):1543–50. doi:10.1097/CCM.0b013e31816f485e

59. Yang G, Hamacher J, Gorshkov B, White R, Sridhar S, Verin A, et al. The dual role of TNF in pulmonary edema. *J Cardiovasc Dis Res* (2010) 1(1):29–36. doi:10.4103/0975-3583.59983

60. Rezaiguia S, Garat C, Delclaux C, Meignan M, Fleury J, Legrand P, et al. Acute bacterial pneumonia in rats increases alveolar epithelial fluid clearance by a tumor necrosis factor-alpha-dependent mechanism. *J Clin Invest* (1997) 99(2):325–35. doi:10.1172/JCI119161

61. Fukuda N, Jayr C, Lazrak A, Wang Y, Lucas R, Matalon S, et al. Mechanisms of TNF-alpha stimulation of amiloride-sensitive sodium transport across alveolar epithelium. *Am J Physiol Lung Cell Mol Physiol* (2001) 280(6): L1258–65.

62. Borjesson A, Norlin A, Wang X, Andersson R, Folkesson HG. TNF-alpha stimulates alveolar liquid clearance during intestinal ischemia-reperfusion in rats. *Am J Physiol Lung Cell Mol Physiol* (2000) 278(1):L3–12.

63. Yamagata T, Yamagata Y, Nishimoto T, Hirano T, Nakanishi M, Minakata Y, et al. The regulation of amiloride-sensitive epithelial sodium channels by tumor necrosis factor-alpha in injured lungs and alveolar type II cells. *Respir Physiol Neurobiol* (2009) 166(1):16–23. doi:10.1016/j.resp.2008.12.008

64. Dagenais A, Frechette R, Yamagata Y, Yamagata T, Carmel JF, Clermont ME, et al. Downregulation of ENaC activity and expression by TNF-alpha in alveolar epithelial cells. *Am J Physiol Lung Cell Mol Physiol* (2004) 286(2):L301–11. doi:10.1152/ajplung.00326.2002

65. Gottlieb SS, Harris K, Todd J, Estis J, Christenson RH, Torres V, et al. Prognostic significance of active and modified forms of endothelin 1 in patients with heart failure with reduced ejection fraction. *Clin Biochem* (2015) 48(4–5):292–6. doi:10.1016/j.clinbiochem.2014.12.012

66. Colombo PC, Ganda A, Lin J, Onat D, Harxhi A, Iyasere JE, et al. Inflammatory activation: cardiac, renal, and cardio-renal interactions in patients with the cardiorenal syndrome. *Heart Fail Rev* (2012) 17(2):177–90. doi:10.1007/s10741-011-9261-3

67. Packer M. Adaptive and maladaptive actions of angiotensin II in patients with severe congestive heart failure. *Am J Kidney Dis* (1987) 10(1 Suppl 1):66–73.

68. Pieruzzi F, Abassi ZA, Keiser HR. Expression of renin-angiotensin system components in the heart, kidneys, and lungs of rats with experimental heart failure. *Circulation* (1995) 92(10):3105–12. doi:10.1161/01.CIR.92. 10.3105

69. Winaver J, Hoffman A, Burnett JC Jr, Haramati A. Hormonal determinants of sodium excretion in rats with experimental high-output heart failure. *Am J Physiol* (1988) 254(5 Pt 2):R776–84.

70. Knepper MA, Kwon TH, Nielsen S. Molecular physiology of water balance. *N Engl J Med* (2015) 372(14):1349–58. doi:10.1056/NEJMra1404726

71. Palmer LG, Schnermann J. Integrated control of Na transport along the nephron. *Clin J Am Soc Nephrol* (2015) 10(4):676–87. doi:10.2215/CJN. 12391213

72. Villarreal D, Freeman RH. ANF and the renin-angiotensin system in the regulation of sodium balance: longitudinal studies in experimental heart failure. *J Lab Clin Med* (1991) 118(6):515–22.

73. Winaver J, Hoffman A, Abassi Z, Haramati A. Does the heart's hormone, ANP, help in congestive heart failure? *News Physiol Sci* (1995) 10(6): 247–53.

74. Abassi ZA, Gurbanov K, Mulroney SE, Potlog C, Opgenorth TJ, Hoffman A, et al. Impaired nitric oxide-mediated renal vasodilation in rats with experimental heart failure: role of angiotensin II. *Circulation* (1997) 96(10):3655–64. doi:10.1161/01.CIR.96.10.3655

75. McMaster WG, Kirabo A, Madhur MS, Harrison DG. Inflammation, immunity, and hypertensive end-organ damage. *Circ Res* (2015) 116(6):1022–33. doi:10.1161/CIRCRESAHA.116.303697

76. Cho E, Kim M, Ko YS, Lee HY, Song M, Kim MG, et al. Role of inflammation in the pathogenesis of cardiorenal syndrome in a rat myocardial infarction model. *Nephrol Dial Transplant* (2013) 28(11):2766–78. doi:10.1093/ndt/gft376

77. Satou R, Miyata K, Gonzalez-Villalobos RA, Ingelfinger JR, Navar LG, Kobori H. Interferon-gamma biphasically regulates angiotensinogen expression via a JAK-STAT pathway and suppressor of cytokine signaling 1 (SOCS1) in renal proximal tubular cells. *FASEB J* (2012) 26(5):1821–30. doi:10.1096/fj.11-195198

78. Ruiz-Ortega M, Ruperez M, Lorenzo O, Esteban V, Blanco J, Mezzano S, et al. Angiotensin II regulates the synthesis of proinflammatory cytokines and chemokines in the kidney. *Kidney Int Suppl* (2002) 82:S12–22. doi:10.1046/j.1523-1755.62.s82.4.x

79. Tsutamoto T, Wada A, Maeda K, Mabuchi N, Hayashi M, Tsutsui T, et al. Angiotensin II type 1 receptor antagonist decreases plasma levels of tumor necrosis factor alpha, interleukin-6 and soluble adhesion molecules in patients with chronic heart failure. *J Am Coll Cardiol* (2000) 35(3):714–21. doi:10.1016/S0735-1097(99)00594-X

80. Moriyama T, Fujibayashi M, Fujiwara Y, Kaneko T, Xia C, Imai E, et al. Angiotensin II stimulates interleukin-6 release from cultured mouse mesangial cells. *J Am Soc Nephrol* (1995) 6(1):95–101.

81. Giam B, Kaye DM, Rajapakse NW. Role of renal oxidative stress in the pathogenesis of the cardiorenal syndrome. *Heart Lung Circ* (2016) 25(8):874–80. doi:10.1016/j.hlc.2016.02.022

82. Kaur K, Sharma AK, Dhingra S, Singal PK. Interplay of TNF-alpha and IL-10 in regulating oxidative stress in isolated adult cardiac myocytes. *J Mol Cell Cardiol* (2006) 41(6):1023–30. doi:10.1016/j.yjmcc.2006.08.005

83. Skorecki KL, Winaver J, Abassi ZA. Extracellular fluid and edema formation. 8th ed. In: Brenner BM, editor. *The Kidney*. Philadelphia: Saunders Elsevier (2008). p. 398–458.

84. Prabhu SD, Chandrasekar B, Murray DR, Freeman GL. beta-adrenergic blockade in developing heart failure: effects on myocardial inflammatory cytokines, nitric oxide, and remodeling. *Circulation* (2000) 101(17):2103–9. doi:10.1161/01.CIR.101.17.2103

85. Goldsmith SR, Sobotka PA, Bart BA. The sympathorenal axis in hypertension and heart failure. *J Card Fail* (2010) 16(5):369–73. doi:10.1016/j.cardfail.2009.12.022

86. DiPetrillo K, Coutermarsh B, Gesek FA. Urinary tumor necrosis factor contributes to sodium retention and renal hypertrophy during diabetes. *Am J Physiol Renal Physiol* (2003) 284(1):F113–21. doi:10.1152/ajprenal.00026.2002

87. Garvin JL, Ortiz PA. The role of reactive oxygen species in the regulation of tubular function. *Acta Physiol Scand* (2003) 179(3):225–32. doi:10.1046/j.0001-6772.2003.01203.x

88. Damman K, Navis G, Smilde TD, Voors AA, van der Bij W, van Veldhuisen DJ, et al. Decreased cardiac output, venous congestion and the association with renal impairment in patients with cardiac dysfunction. *Eur J Heart Fail* (2007) 9(9):872–8. doi:10.1016/j.ejheart.2007.05.010

89. Abassi Z, Gurbanov K, Rubinstein I, Better OS, Hoffman A, Winaver J. Regulation of intrarenal blood flow in experimental heart failure: role of endothelin and nitric oxide. *Am J Physiol* (1998) 274(4 Pt 2):F766–74.

90. Barton M, Yanagisawa M. Endothelin: 20 years from discovery to therapy. *Can J Physiol Pharmacol* (2008) 86(8):485–98. doi:10.1139/Y08-059

91. Kohan DE, Rossi NF, Inscho EW, Pollock DM. Regulation of blood pressure and salt homeostasis by endothelin. *Physiol Rev* (2011) 91(1):1–77. doi:10.1152/physrev.00060.2009

92. Schiffrin EL. Vascular endothelin in hypertension. *Vascul Pharmacol* (2005) 43(1):19–29. doi:10.1016/j.vph.2005.03.004

93. Abassi Z, Francis B, Wessale J, Ovcharenko E, Winaver J, Hoffman A. Effects of endothelin receptors ET(A) and ET(B) blockade on renal

94. Abassi Z, Goltsman I, Karram T, Winaver J, Hoffman A. Aortocaval fistula in rat: a unique model of volume-overload congestive heart failure and cardiac hypertrophy. *J Biomed Biotechnol* (2011) 2011:729497. doi:10.1155/2011/729497

95. Anand I, McMurray J, Cohn JN, Konstam MA, Notter T, Quitzau K, et al. Long-term effects of darusentan on left-ventricular remodelling and clinical outcomes in the EndothelinA Receptor Antagonist Trial in Heart Failure (EARTH): randomised, double-blind, placebo-controlled trial. *Lancet* (2004) 364(9431):347–54. doi:10.1016/S0140-6736(04)16723-8

96. Kelland NF, Webb DJ. Clinical trials of endothelin antagonists in heart failure: a question of dose? *Exp Biol Med (Maywood)* (2006) 231(6):696–9.

97. Shapiro S, Pollock DM, Gillies H, Henig N, Allard M, Blair C, et al. Frequency of edema in patients with pulmonary arterial hypertension receiving ambrisentan. *Am J Cardiol* (2012) 110(9):1373–7. doi:10.1016/j.amjcard.2012.06.040

98. Weber MA, Black H, Bakris G, Krum H, Linas S, Weiss R, et al. A selective endothelin-receptor antagonist to reduce blood pressure in patients with treatment-resistant hypertension: a randomised, double-blind, placebo-controlled trial. *Lancet* (2009) 374(9699):1423–31. doi:10.1016/S0140-6736(09)61500-2

99. McMurray JJ, Ray SG, Abdullah I, Dargie HJ, Morton JJ. Plasma endothelin in chronic heart failure. *Circulation* (1992) 85(4):1374–9. doi:10.1161/01.CIR.85.4.1374

100. Brown LA, Nunez DJ, Brookes CI, Wilkins MR. Selective increase in endothelin-1 and endothelin A receptor subtype in the hypertrophied myocardium of the aorto-venacaval fistula rat. *Cardiovasc Res* (1995) 29(6):768–74. doi:10.1016/0008-6363(96)88611-1

101. Lerman A, Kubo SH, Tschumperlin LK, Burnett JC Jr. Plasma endothelin concentrations in humans with end-stage heart failure and after heart transplantation. *J Am Coll Cardiol* (1992) 20(4):849–53. doi:10.1016/0735-1097(92)90183-N

102. Spieker LE, Noll G, Ruschitzka FT, Luscher TF. Endothelin receptor antagonists in congestive heart failure: a new therapeutic principle for the future? *J Am Coll Cardiol* (2001) 37(6):1493–505. doi:10.1016/S0735-1097(01)01210-4

103. Bauersachs J, Braun C, Fraccarollo D, Widder J, Ertl G, Schilling L, et al. Improvement of renal dysfunction in rats with chronic heart failure after myocardial infarction by treatment with the endothelin A receptor antagonist, LU 135252. *J Hypertens* (2000) 18(10):1507–14. doi:10.1097/00004872-200018100-00020

104. Borgeson DD, Grantham JA, Williamson EE, Luchner A, Redfield MM, Opgenorth TJ, et al. Chronic oral endothelin type A receptor antagonism in experimental heart failure. *Hypertension* (1998) 31(3):766–70. doi:10.1161/01.HYP.31.3.766

105. Ding SS, Qiu C, Hess P, Xi JF, Clozel JP, Clozel M. Chronic endothelin receptor blockade prevents renal vasoconstriction and sodium retention in rats with chronic heart failure. *Cardiovasc Res* (2002) 53(4):963–70. doi:10.1016/S0008-6363(01)00558-2

106. Gurbanov K, Rubinstein I, Hoffman A, Abassi Z, Better OS, Winaver J. Bosentan improves renal regional blood flow in rats with experimental congestive heart failure. *Eur J Pharmacol* (1996) 310(2–3):193–6. doi:10.1016/0014-2999(96)00494-3

107. Kiowski W, Sutsch G, Hunziker P, Muller P, Kim J, Oechslin E, et al. Evidence for endothelin-1-mediated vasoconstriction in severe chronic heart failure. *Lancet* (1995) 346(8977):732–6. doi:10.1016/S0140-6736(95)91504-4

108. Brodsky S, Abassi Z, Wessale J, Ramadan R, Winaver J, Hoffman A. Effects of A-192621.1, a specific endothelin-B antagonist, on intrarenal hemodynamic responses to endothelin-1. *J Cardiovasc Pharmacol* (2000) 36(5 Suppl 1):S311–3. doi:10.1097/00005344-200036001-00090

109. Dhaun N, Webb DJ, Kluth DC. Endothelin-1 and the kidney – beyond BP. *Br J Pharmacol* (2012) 167(4):720–31. doi:10.1111/j.1476-5381.2012.02070.x

110. Sorokin A, Kohan DE. Physiology and pathology of endothelin-1 in renal mesangium. *Am J Physiol Renal Physiol* (2003) 285(4):F579–89. doi:10.1152/ajprenal.00019.2003

111. Gurbanov K, Rubinstein I, Hoffman A, Abassi Z, Better OS, Winaver J. Differential regulation of renal regional blood flow by endothelin-1. *Am J Physiol* (1996) 271(6 Pt 2):F1166–72.

112. Nakano D, Pollock D. New concepts in endothelin control of sodium balance. *Clin Exp Pharmacol Physiol* (2012) 39(1):104–10. doi:10.1111/j.1440-1681.2011.05517.x

113. Barton M, Nett PC, Amann K, Teixeira MM. Anti-inflammatory effects of endothelin receptor antagonists and their importance for treating human disease. In: Chaudhary I, Ur-Rahman A, editors. *Frontiers in Cardiovascular Drug Discovery*. Oak Park, IL, USA: Bentham Science Publishers Ltd (2010). p. 236–58.

114. Dietz JR. Mechanisms of atrial natriuretic peptide secretion from the atrium. *Cardiovasc Res* (2005) 68(1):8–17. doi:10.1016/j.cardiores.2005.06.008

115. Kuhn M. Molecular physiology of natriuretic peptide signalling. *Basic Res Cardiol* (2004) 99(2):76–82. doi:10.1007/s00395-004-0460-0

116. Braunwald E. Biomarkers in heart failure. *N Engl J Med* (2008) 358(20):2148–59. doi:10.1056/NEJMra0800239

117. Potter LR, Abbey-Hosch S, Dickey DM. Natriuretic peptides, their receptors, and cyclic guanosine monophosphate-dependent signaling functions. *Endocr Rev* (2006) 27(1):47–72. doi:10.1210/er.2005-0014

118. Ritter D, Chao J, Needleman P, Tetens E, Greenwald JE. Localization, synthetic regulation, and biology of renal atriopeptin-like prohormone. *Am J Physiol* (1992) 263(3 Pt 2):F503–9.

119. Greenwald JE, Needleman P, Wilkins MR, Schreiner GF. Renal synthesis of atriopeptin-like protein in physiology and pathophysiology. *Am J Physiol* (1991) 260(4 Pt 2):F602–7.

120. Ramirez G, Saba SR, Dietz JR, Vesely DL. Immunocytochemical localization of proANF 1-30, proANF 31-67 and atrial natriuretic factor in the kidney. *Kidney Int* (1992) 41(2):334–41. doi:10.1038/ki.1992.46

121. Zeidel ML. Hormonal regulation of inner medullary collecting duct sodium transport. *Am J Physiol* (1993) 265(2 Pt 2):F159–73.

122. De Vito P. Atrial natriuretic peptide: an old hormone or a new cytokine? *Peptides* (2014) 58:108–16. doi:10.1016/j.peptides.2014.06.011

123. Vollmar AM. The role of atrial natriuretic peptide in the immune system. *Peptides* (2005) 26(6):1086–94. doi:10.1016/j.peptides.2004.08.034

124. Mitaka C, Si MK, Tulafu M, Yu Q, Uchida T, Abe S, et al. Effects of atrial natriuretic peptide on inter-organ crosstalk among the kidney, lung, and heart in a rat model of renal ischemia-reperfusion injury. *Intensive Care Med Exp* (2014) 2(1):28. doi:10.1186/s40635-014-0028-8

125. Tulafu M, Mitaka C, Hnin Si MK, Abe S, Kitagawa M, Ikeda S, et al. Atrial natriuretic peptide attenuates kidney-lung crosstalk in kidney injury. *J Surg Res* (2014) 186(1):217–25. doi:10.1016/j.jss.2013.07.033

126. Zhu YB, Zhang YB, Liu DH, Li XF, Liu AJ, Fan XM, et al. Atrial natriuretic peptide attenuates inflammatory responses on oleic acid-induced acute lung injury model in rats. *Chin Med J (Engl)* (2013) 126(4):747–50.

127. Rudiger A, Fischler M, Harpes P, Gasser S, Hornemann T, von Eckardstein A, et al. In critically ill patients, B-type natriuretic peptide (BNP) and N-terminal pro-BNP levels correlate with C-reactive protein values and leukocyte counts. *Int J Cardiol* (2008) 126(1):28–31. doi:10.1016/j.ijcard.2007.03.108

128. Kone BC, Baylis C. Biosynthesis and homeostatic roles of nitric oxide in the normal kidney. *Am J Physiol* (1997) 272(5 Pt 2):F561–78.

129. Herrera M, Garvin JL. Recent advances in the regulation of nitric oxide in the kidney. *Hypertension* (2005) 45(6):1062–7. doi:10.1161/01.HYP.0000159760.88697.1e

130. LaPointe MC, Isenovic E. Interleukin-1beta regulation of inducible nitric oxide synthase and cyclooxygenase-2 involves the p42/44 and p38 MAPK signaling pathways in cardiac myocytes. *Hypertension* (1999) 33(1 Pt 2):276–82. doi:10.1161/01.HYP.33.1.276

131. Fujimoto M, Shimizu N, Kunii K, Martyn JA, Ueki K, Kaneki M. A role for iNOS in fasting hyperglycemia and impaired insulin signaling in the liver of obese diabetic mice. *Diabetes* (2005) 54(5):1340–8. doi:10.2337/diabetes.54.5.1340

132. Onat D, Jelic S, Schmidt AM, Pile-Spellman J, Homma S, Padeletti M, et al. Vascular endothelial sampling and analysis of gene transcripts: a new quantitative approach to monitor vascular inflammation. *J Appl Physiol (1985)* (2007) 103(5):1873–8. doi:10.1152/japplphysiol.00367.2007

133. Gealekman O, Abassi Z, Rubinstein I, Winaver J, Binah O. Role of myocardial inducible nitric oxide synthase in contractile dysfunction and beta-adrenergic hyporesponsiveness in rats with experimental volume-overload

heart failure. *Circulation* (2002) 105(2):236–43. doi:10.1161/hc0202. 102015

134. Feng Q, Lu X, Jones DL, Shen J, Arnold JM. Increased inducible nitric oxide synthase expression contributes to myocardial dysfunction and higher mortality after myocardial infarction in mice. *Circulation* (2001) 104(6): 700–4. doi:10.1161/hc3201.092284

135. Kiemer AK, Vollmar AM. Elevation of intracellular calcium levels contributes to the inhibition of nitric oxide production by atrial natriuretic peptide. *Immunol Cell Biol* (2001) 79(1):11–7. doi:10.1046/j.1440-1711.2001. 00969.x

136. Mann DL, McMurray JJ, Packer M, Swedberg K, Borer JS, Colucci WS, et al. Targeted anticytokine therapy in patients with chronic heart failure: results of the Randomized Etanercept Worldwide Evaluation (RENEWAL). *Circulation* (2004) 109(13):1594–602. doi:10.1161/01.CIR.0000124490. 27666.B2

137. Chung ES, Packer M, Lo KH, Fasanmade AA, Willerson JT; Anti-TNF Therapy Against Congestive Heart Failure Investigators. Randomized, double-blind, placebo-controlled, pilot trial of infliximab, a chimeric monoclonal antibody to tumor necrosis factor-alpha, in patients with moderate-to-severe heart failure: results of the anti-TNF Therapy Against Congestive Heart Failure (ATTACH) trial. *Circulation* (2003) 107(25):3133–40.

138. Javed Q, Murtaza I. Therapeutic potential of tumour necrosis factor-alpha antagonists in patients with chronic heart failure. *Heart Lung Circ* (2013) 22(5):323–7. doi:10.1016/j.hlc.2012.12.002

139. Van Tassell BW, Abouzaki NA, Oddi Erdle C, Carbone S, Trankle CR, Melchior RD, et al. Interleukin-1 blockade in acute decompensated heart failure: a randomized, double-blinded, placebo-controlled pilot study. *J Cardiovasc Pharmacol* (2016) 67(6):544–51. doi:10.1097/FJC.0000000000000378

140. Cavalli G, Foppoli M, Cabrini L, Dinarello CA, Tresoldi M, Dagna L. Interleukin-1 receptor blockade rescues myocarditis-associated end-stage heart failure. *Front Immunol* (2017) 8:131. doi:10.3389/fimmu.2017.00131

13

Inhibition of TNF Receptor p55 by a Domain Antibody Attenuates the Initial Phase of Acid-Induced Lung Injury in Mice

Michael R. Wilson[1†], Kenji Wakabayashi[1,2†], Szabolcs Bertok[1], Charlotte M. Oakley[1], Brijesh V. Patel[1], Kieran P. O'Dea[1], Joanna C. Cordy[3], Peter J. Morley[3], Andrew I. Bayliffe[3] and Masao Takata[1*]

[1]Section of Anaesthetics, Pain Medicine and Intensive Care, Faculty of Medicine, Imperial College London, Chelsea and Westminster Hospital, London, UK, [2]Department of Intensive Care Medicine, Tokyo Medical and Dental University, Tokyo, Japan, [3]Biopharm Molecular Discovery, GlaxoSmithKline R&D, Stevenage, UK

*Correspondence:
Masao Takata
m.takata@imperial.ac.uk

[†]These authors have contributed equally to this work.

Background: Tumor necrosis factor-α (TNF) is strongly implicated in the development of acute respiratory distress syndrome (ARDS), but its potential as a therapeutic target has been hampered by its complex biology. TNF signals through two receptors, p55 and p75, which play differential roles in pulmonary edema formation during ARDS. We have recently shown that inhibition of p55 by a novel domain antibody (dAb™) attenuated ventilator-induced lung injury. In the current study, we explored the efficacy of this antibody in mouse models of acid-induced lung injury to investigate the longer consequences of treatment.

Methods: We employed two acid-induced injury models, an acute ventilated model and a resolving spontaneously breathing model. C57BL/6 mice were pretreated intratracheally or intranasally with p55-targeting dAb or non-targeting "dummy" dAb, 1 or 4 h before acid instillation.

Results: Acid instillation in the dummy dAb group caused hypoxemia, increased respiratory system elastance, pulmonary inflammation, and edema in both the ventilated and resolving models. Pretreatment with p55-targeting dAb significantly attenuated physiological markers of ARDS in both models. p55-targeting dAb also attenuated pulmonary inflammation in the ventilated model, with signs that altered cytokine production and leukocyte recruitment persisted beyond the very acute phase.

Conclusion: These results demonstrate that the p55-targeting dAb attenuates lung injury and edema formation in models of ARDS induced by acid aspiration, with protection from a single dose lasting up to 24 h. Together with our previous data, the current study lends support toward the clinical targeting of p55 for patients with, or at risk of ARDS.

Keywords: CD120a, TNFRSF1a, acid aspiration, inflammation, respiratory mechanics

INTRODUCTION

Acute respiratory distress syndrome (ARDS) is a major cause of patient morbidity and mortality within the ICU, constituting ~10% of ICU admissions worldwide with an associated mortality of 30–50% (1). ARDS can result from various insults, of which aspiration of acidic gastric contents is a major contributor both within the community and in the operating theater during anesthesia

(2). Inflammation has been considered to be key in developing ARDS, but attempts to minimize "global" inflammation, e.g., by use of corticosteroids have delivered limited mortality benefits (3–7), suggesting the need for a more targeted approach. Among all potential targets, tumor necrosis factor-α (TNF) is one of the strongest candidates for such interventions—it is one of the earliest expressed "gate-keeper" cytokines in response to almost any potentially damaging situation, modulating subsequent inflammatory responses, and has been repeatedly implicated in the development and progression of ARDS (8), including direct effects on pulmonary edema formation and clearance. Despite this, previous clinical trials of anti-TNF therapy have shown little beneficial impact within the ICU setting (9). This may be partly attributed to the biophysical properties of the inhibitors used (e.g., affinity and tissue penetration), and also likely related to the complex nature of TNF signaling.

Tumor necrosis factor signals through two cell surface receptors, TNF receptor (TNFR) type I (p55) and TNFR type II (p75). Historically, p75 signaling was considered to be adjunct to the p55 pathway (10, 11), but it is now becoming clear that each TNFR subtype has signaling capabilities of its own, which in particular circumstances may lead to directly opposing consequences (12–16). In line with this, we have previously shown using genetically modified mice that specific absence of p55 is protective in the very acute phase of ARDS induced by mechanical ventilation (17), while absence of p75 seems to be detrimental. We have also found that p55 signaling triggers alveolar epithelial cell dysfunction in the early phase of ARDS, promoting lung permeability as well as impairing alveolar fluid reabsorption (18). These findings suggest that while total TNF signaling blockade would likely be counterproductive, specific therapeutic strategies targeting the individual TNFRs could be effective in ARDS.

We have recently demonstrated efficacy of selective pharmacological blockade of p55 signaling in an acute model of mouse ventilator-induced lung injury (VILI), using a novel IgG fragment known as a domain antibody (Biopharmaceuticals R&D, GlaxoSmithKline, Stevenage, UK) (19). Domain antibodies (dAb™) offer multiple advantages over conventional antibody technology (20)—for example, they have fewer off-target effects and can be delivered at much higher concentrations per unit mass compared to conventional antibodies due to the lack of an Fc region and can be manufactured to be suitable for local delivery such as inhalation. In the current study, we tested the efficacy of a dAb antagonist of murine p55, in mouse models of acute and resolving acid aspiration-induced lung injury (21). This enabled us to both evaluate the acute benefits of pharmacological p55 blockade in a highly clinically relevant model and explore whether any beneficial effects persisted beyond the acute stage. A similar dAb antagonist of human p55 has recently entered early clinical development for lung injury (22).

MATERIALS AND METHODS

All protocols were approved by the Ethical Review Board of Imperial College London and carried out under the authority of the UK Home Office in accordance with the Animals (Scientific Procedures) Act 1986, UK. Male C57BL/6 mice (Charles River, Margate, UK) aged 9–12 weeks old, weighing 25–30 g were used throughout.

The p55-targeting dAb sequence was identified from a phage display library. To determine binding kinetics, murine p55 or p75 was immobilized on an IgG surface, varying concentrations of dAb (from 0.25 to 16 nM) were passed over the surface, and interactions were evaluated via surface plasmon resonance using a Biacore T200 system. Association constant (ka) of the dAb for p55 was determined as 3.455×10^7 (1/Ms) and dissociation constant (kd) was 0.0014 (1/s), indicating high affinity of binding (KD) of 4.05×10^{-11}M, assuming a 1:1 binding stoichiometry. In contrast, no specific binding was observed to p75.

Ventilated Acid Aspiration Model

We have previously shown that genetic absence of TNFR p55 signaling attenuates pulmonary edema formation during the first 2–3 h after acid instillation in mice (18). Therefore, initial experiments were carried out to determine whether p55 dAb administration would have a similar influence during the acute phase of acid aspiration-induced lung injury.

Mice were anesthetized (intraperitoneal ketamine 80 mg/kg and xylazine 8 mg/kg), tracheostomized, and connected to a custom-made ventilator/pulmonary function testing system as described previously (23). Animals had a cannula placed in the carotid artery for monitoring of blood pressure, blood gas analysis, and fluid replacement. All animals were ventilated using 7 ml/kg tidal volume, 2.5 cmH₂O positive end-expiratory pressure (PEEP), and respiratory rate of 120/min, with 100% O₂. Following instrumentation, either specific murine TNFR p55 blocking dAb (Dom-1m-15-12, GSK) or non-targeting control dAb ("dummy") was intratracheally delivered in bolus form (25 μg of antibody in a volume of 50 μl) via a fine cannula passed through the endotracheal tube. The lungs were then immediately recruited with four sustained inflation maneuvers (35 cmH₂O, 5 s) to maximize distribution of the antibody into the lungs. Mice were ventilated for 1 h to allow respiratory mechanics to return toward normal, and then 65 μl of 0.075M hydrochloric acid (HCl) was instilled into the trachea through the endotracheal tube. Lungs were again recruited by sustained inflations, and mice were ventilated for a further 3 h. Anesthesia was maintained by bolus administrations of intraperitoneal ketamine (40 mg/kg) and xylazine (4 mg/kg) every 20–25 min.

Airway pressure and arterial blood pressure were monitored continuously. Plateau pressure, and respiratory system elastance and resistance were determined every 20 min by the end-inflation occlusion technique, followed each time by sustained inflation (35 cmH₂O for 5 s) to avoid the development of atelectasis (23). Arterial blood gases were assessed at predetermined points throughout the protocol (immediately before, 60, 120, and 180 min after acid instillation). At the end of the experiments, animals were exsanguinated, lung lavage was performed using 750 μl of saline, and lung tissue samples were taken for further analysis. Each animal was experimented on a separate day, so each observation reflects an independent experiment.

Spontaneously Breathing Model of Acid Aspiration

While the use of mechanical ventilation provides many advantages, including real-time cardiorespiratory monitoring and an ability to directly compare findings with those of our previous studies in genetically modified animals (18), by definition the model is limited to investigation within the acute phase. We have recently developed a spontaneously resolving model of acid aspiration-induced lung injury (21), which, unlike a number of other models, mimics most of the features of clinical ARDS over up to 5–10 days (24–26). We therefore employed this resolving model to investigate the impact of intranasally delivered p55-targeting dAb on the later phases of injury/start of the repair process.

All animals were anesthetized briefly with inhalational isoflurane (2%) and intranasally dosed with 100 μg (50 μl total volume, divided into two nostrils) of either p55-targeting dAb or dummy dAb. Four hours after dosing (a period designed to allow distribution of the antibody and full recovery of respiratory mechanics from the nasal dosing procedure under non-ventilated conditions), animals were reanesthetized either for physiological analysis (see below—0 h mice) or for acid instillation according to our previously published protocols (21). In brief, mice were suspended vertically for orotracheal instillation, and a fine catheter passed through the vocal cords. A total of 75 μl of an isoosmolar solution of 0.1M hydrochloric acid (pH 1.0) was instilled, and mice received an intraperitoneal bolus of 0.9% saline for fluid resuscitation. Mice were maintained in a humidified chamber containing supplemental oxygen (decreasing from FiO_2 1.0–0.4) over the next 4 h and were then returned to individually ventilated cages. Due to the nature of the dosing technique and postdosing care requirements, a maximum of three animals were dosed with acid/antibody on a single day. Each set of data shown in the Section "Results," of any given combination of treatment (dummy versus p55-targeting dAb) and time point (0, 24, 48, and 72 h), therefore represents observations from 5 to 8 mice, obtained from 3 to 4 independent experiments.

Physiological analysis was carried out at predetermined end points, i.e., 0, 24, 48, or 72 h post acid. Mice were anesthetized (ketamine 80 mg/kg, xylazine 8 mg/kg) and instrumented as described for the acute ventilated model. Immediately after completing surgical preparation, lungs were recruited by sustained inflation (35 cmH_2O for 5 s). Mice were then ventilated with 7 ml/kg tidal volume, 2.5 cmH_2O PEEP, and respiratory rate of 120/min using 100% O_2 for 30 min, in order to standardize the volume history of the lung and determine the PaO_2/FiO_2 ratio from carotid blood samples (21). At the end of 30 min ventilation, respiratory mechanics and blood gases were evaluated, and animals were terminated by exsanguination. The right lung was tied off at the hilum, weighed, and placed in an oven at 60°C for determination of wet:dry weight ratio. The left lung was lavaged using 400 μl saline and dissected out for further analysis.

Evaluation of Injury and Inflammation in Lavage Samples

Total protein concentration in lung lavage fluid was measured as an indicator of alveolar-capillary permeability (Bio-Rad, Hertfordshire, UK). Concentrations of interleukin 6 (IL-6), the neutrophil chemoattractants CXCL1 and CXCL2, and the monocyte chemoattractant CCL2 were measured by ELISA (R&D Systems, Abingdon, UK). The number of neutrophils in lavage fluid was determined by microscopic cytology using hemocytometer and Cytospin-prepared slides.

Lung Tissue Flow Cytometry

The identification and quantification of leukocytes within lung tissue was performed by flow cytometry using methods described and validated previously. For the acute ventilated model, lung samples were removed, minced, and passed through a 40 μm filter (19, 27). Samples were resuspended in a washing buffer (PBS with 2% FCS, 0.1% sodium azide, and 5 mM EDTA) and stained for 30 min in the dark at 4°C with fluorophore-conjugated anti-mouse antibodies for CD11b (clone M1/70), Gr-1 (RB6-8C5) (both BD BioSciences), and F4/80 (CI:A3-1) (Biolegend). For the spontaneously breathing resolution model, the potential for influx of other cell types over time led us to modify this approach for further identification of leukocyte subpopulations (18). Lung tissues were excised and fixed with Cytofix/Cytoperm (BD Biosciences, Oxford, UK), mechanically disrupted by gentleMACS Dissociator (Miltenyi Biotech, Surrey, UK) and passed through a 40 μm filter to prepare single-cell suspensions. Samples were then stained for 30 min in the dark at 4°C with fluorophore-conjugated anti-mouse antibodies for CD11b, Gr-1, Ly6C (AL-21), and NK1.1 (PK136) (BD BioSciences). Importantly, we showed previously (28) that although the Gr-1 antibody used (clone RB6-8C5) binds both Ly6G and Ly6C epitopes under non-fixed conditions (i.e., for the acute ventilated model), the use of Cytofix/Cytoperm results in loss of Ly6C recognition by the antibody. Therefore, in the context of the resolution model, Gr-1 staining is representative solely of cell Ly6G expression. Cell samples were analyzed by a CyAn flow cytometer with Summit software (Beckman Coulter, High Wycombe, UK), and further data analysis was performed by FlowJo software (Tree Star, Ashland, OR). Absolute leukocyte counts were determined using microsphere beads (Invitrogen, Paisley, UK).

Statistical Analysis

Statistical analyses were performed using SPSS version 22 (IBM, Portsmouth, UK). The normality of model residuals was assessed by QQ plot and Shapiro–Wilk test. Data that were not normally distributed were transformed (see legends for details), and subsequent parametric distribution confirmed before analyses were carried out. Data that could not be normalized by transformation were analyzed using non-parametric tests. Time-course data in the acute ventilated model were analyzed by repeated measures analysis of variance (ANOVA) followed by pairwise analysis of individual time points, while end-point analyses were carried out by Student's t-test. In the resolving injury model, differences between treatment groups were evaluated on each day, using either Student's t-test or Mann–Whitney U-test. A value of $p < 0.05$ was considered significant.

RESULTS

Acute Model

We first carried out experiments to determine the influence of p55-targeting dAb administration on the acute phase of acid aspiration-induced lung injury. As part of the model development, experiments were performed comparing the physiological consequences of acid instillation versus those of saline instillation. Initial administration of dummy dAb led to a transient increase in peak inspiratory pressure (**Figure 1A**), which returned toward normal as fluid was distributed and absorbed within the lungs (the same pattern was apparent following administration of p55-targeting dAb; data not shown). Instillation of either saline or acid 60 min later caused similar increases in airway pressure. In animals receiving saline, peak inspiratory pressure decreased and plateaued. In contrast, animals that received acid instillation showed an initial improvement in airway pressure, which then deteriorated over the final 60 min. Intratracheal administrations also caused small, transient decreases in blood pressure, most likely secondary to the sustained inflation maneuvers carried out to distribute instilled fluids (**Figure 1B**). Blood pressure was otherwise well maintained throughout the experiments until the final 60 min during which it deteriorated somewhat, particularly in acid-treated animals.

The physiological consequences of acid instillation were then compared between animals pretreated with either the dummy non-targeting dAb or the p55-targeting dAb ($N = 6$ independent experiments/group). The initial mechanics response to acid was similar between the two groups (**Figure 2A**), consisting of a transient spike in elastance followed by a return toward pre-instillation levels. In the dummy dAb group, elastance then increased from ~100 min until the end, whereas in contrast, the p55-targeting dAb-treated mice showed little increase, resulting in a significantly attenuated elastance change (p value for interaction <0.01, although pairwise analysis did not detect significant differences at individual time points). Respiratory system resistance showed similar patterns in both groups, consisting of a decrease following acid instillation that remained relatively stable thereafter (**Figure 2B**). There was also a decrease in arterial pO_2 and an increase in pCO_2 during the final hour of ventilation in dummy-treated animals (**Figures 2C,D**). These impairments in gas exchange were significantly attenuated by treatment with the p55-targeting dAb (p-value for interaction <0.05, with pairwise analysis showing significant difference at the 180 min time point).

Lung lavage fluid in the dummy-treated group contained a substantial amount of protein, indicating an increase in epithelial/endothelial barrier permeability (**Figure 3A**, dotted line represents data from saline-treated animals for visual comparison). This was somewhat, though not significantly, reduced by p55-targeting dAb. Evaluation of pro-inflammatory cytokines in lung lavage fluid showed that IL-6 and CXCL1 showed a tendency to be reduced, while CXCL2 and CCL2 were significantly attenuated in p55-targeting dAb-treated mice (**Figures 3B–E**).

Finally, lung leukocyte recruitment was determined in each group of mice. Neutrophil infiltration into the alveolar space (evaluated by microscopic cytology of lung lavage fluid) was significantly attenuated by p55-targeting dAb (**Figures 4A,B**). Total lung tissue neutrophil and monocyte recruitment were evaluated by flow cytometry (**Figure 4C**). Neutrophil recruitment was somewhat (though not significantly) reduced following p55-targeting dAb, while inflammatory Ly6C^{hi} monocyte numbers were significantly attenuated (**Figures 4D,E**).

Resolving Model

While the data from the acute model indicate that intratracheal inhibition of p55 using the dAb attenuates both pulmonary edema and inflammation during the early phase of ALI/VILI, it does not necessarily follow that this would translate to a prolonged benefit. We therefore carried out experiments to investigate the consequences of p55-targeting dAb on the later phase of ALI using the resolving model.

Acid instillation caused a clear physiological lung injury in dummy dAb-treated animals, consistent with previous reports using this model (21, 29). Respiratory system elastance (determined after 30 min of ventilation) was increased at 24 h after acid, and subsequently returned toward baseline although did not reach normal values by day 3 (**Figure 5A**). Similarly, arterial pO_2 was substantially decreased (**Figure 5B**) and pCO_2 increased

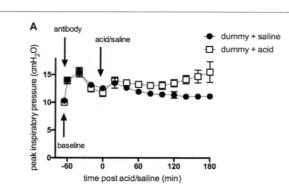
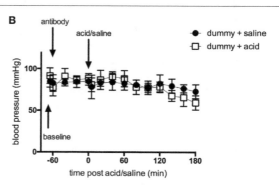

FIGURE 1 | Peak inspiratory pressure (A) and arterial blood pressure (B) in ventilated animals following intratracheal treatment with dummy dAb, followed by challenge with either intratracheal saline or hydrochloric acid. $N = 4$ (dummy + saline), or 6 (dummy + acid) at each time point. Data are expressed as mean ± SD.

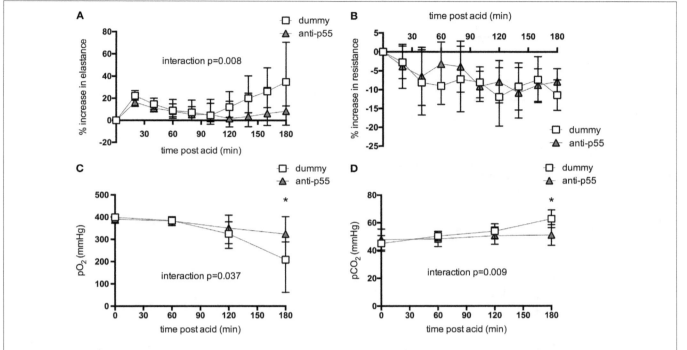

FIGURE 2 | Respiratory system elastance (A) and resistance (B), and arterial pO₂ (C) and pCO₂ (D) following acid instillation in animals treated with dummy or p55-targeting dAb. Mechanics data are expressed as % increase following acid. Elastance data (A) were log-transformed to achieve normal distribution, while pO₂ (C) was normalized by raising to the power of 2. These data are displayed as back-transformed mean with error bars representing 90% confidence intervals. Resistance data and pCO₂ were normally distributed and thus displayed as mean ± SD. Repeated measures analysis of variance revealed significant interactions between treatment and time for elastance change ($p < 0.01$), pO₂ ($p < 0.05$), and pCO₂ ($p < 0.01$). *$p < 0.05$ between dummy and dAb-treated animals at 180 min after acid. N = 5–6 observations from independent experiments at each time point.

(**Figure 5C**) 1 day after acid. pO₂ remained low at day 2 and then started to recover at day 3, while pCO₂ showed some signs of return toward normal at day 2. The single pretreatment with p55-targeting dAb led to a significant attenuation in each of these parameters at 24 h. It was clear however that by 48 h most of the protection afforded by the dAb was lost, with animals appearing as injured as dummy dAb-treated mice. Acid instillation also caused increases in pulmonary edema/permeability, assessed by lavage fluid protein (**Figure 5D**) and lung wet:dry weight ratio (**Figure 5E**). Both of these markers peaked around days 1–2 before returning toward (but not achieving) baseline levels by day 3. Pretreatment with the p55-targeting dAb reduced lavage fluid protein levels (again, only at day 1) and lung wet:dry ratio (at days 1 and 2).

Finally, the effect of p55-targeting dAb on inflammation within the lungs was evaluated after acid instillation. Lavage fluid CXCL1 (**Figure 6A**) was increased to a variable degree in dummy dAb-treated animals, but still significantly attenuated at days 1 and 2 following p55-targeting dAb. In contrast, levels of CCL2 (**Figure 6B**) were similar between the treatment groups on all days, and unlike CXCL1, did not return to baseline by day 3. Neutrophil infiltration into the alveolar space (by differential cytology) was highly variable and showed little difference between treatment groups (**Figures 6C,D**), apart from a small reduction in neutrophil percentage at day 2 following p55-targeting dAb. Lung tissue recruitment of neutrophils and Ly6C^{hi} monocytes, evaluated by flow cytometry (**Figure 6E**), showed large increases between 24 and 48 h after acid in dummy dAb-treated animals (**Figures 6F,G**), consistent with previously published kinetics in this model of injury (30). However, there was no significant difference in cell recruitment with p55-targeting dAb, apart from a reduction in Ly6C^{hi} monocytes at day 3.

DISCUSSION

Despite much research, and major advances in our understanding of the pathophysiology, effective pharmacological therapies for ARDS patients remain elusive. It is generally accepted that inflammation plays an important role in ARDS, and numerous drug targets have been identified within preclinical settings, but none of these have translated into clinical treatment. The reasons for this have been widely discussed, including the recent debate regarding the similarity of inflammatory responses between rodents and humans (31, 32), and the possible different responses of ARDS subphenotypes (33). Perhaps more to the point is that animal models of ARDS generally replicate a limited number of the features seen in patients (24, 25). Many models are either too severe/invasive to explore longer consequences (i.e., animals cannot be studied beyond the acute phase) or too mild to replicate the complex pathology. Thus, these models often have very limited predictive power, particularly when they are considered in isolation, in terms of the consequences of inhibiting pathways.

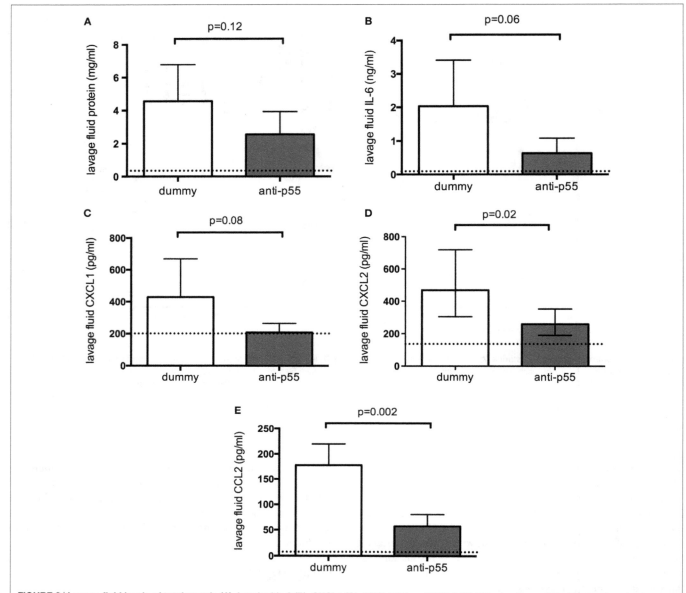

FIGURE 3 | Lavage fluid levels of total protein (A), interleukin 6 (B), CXCL1 (C), CXCL2 (D), and CCL2 (E) 180 min after acid instillation in animals treated with dummy or p55-targeting domain antibody. Dotted lines represent data from saline-treated animals for visual comparison. Lavage fluid CXCL2 (D) required log-transformation to normal distribution and is therefore displayed as geometric mean with error bars representing 90% confidence intervals. All other data were normally distributed and thus are displayed as arithmetic mean ± SD. T-tests were used to evaluate differences between treatments. N = 5 observations from independent experiments for each group (corresponding to the total number of mice assessed for these parameters).

For this reason, in the current study, we explored the impact of a domain antibody (dAb™) targeting the p55 TNFR, which we previously showed to be efficacious in attenuating VILI in mice (19), in more clinically relevant acute and resolving models of acid aspiration-induced lung injury.

In the acute ventilated model, the data demonstrate a very clear attenuation of injury in the animals receiving p55-targeting dAb. Specifically, respiratory mechanics and blood gases were significantly preserved. While pairwise analysis of individual time points indicated that only pO_2 and pCO_2 showed significant differences, and then only at the final time point, repeated measures ANOVA demonstrated clear interaction effects for elastance, pO_2 and pCO_2. Given that the repeated measures ANOVA both maximizes the data being utilized within any given analysis and decreases the chance of type II error by reducing within group variability, these data show that the development of "physiological injury" over time was attenuated by the administration of p55-targeting dAb. We did not evaluate lung histology in these animals, although respiratory system mechanics and blood gasses are clinically important parameters crucial for the diagnosis of ARDS, which are not always evaluated within animal models. We have previously evaluated histological changes

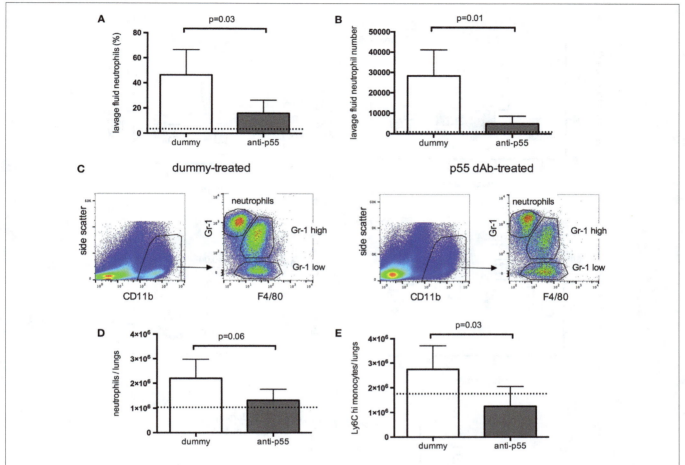

FIGURE 4 | Recruitment of leukocytes into the alveolar space (A,B), and lung tissue (C–E), 180 min after acid instillation in animals treated with dummy or p55-targeting domain antibody. For the acute ventilated model, tissue neutrophils were identified as CD11b^{high}, Gr-1^{high}, F4/80 negative events, while monocytes were identified as CD11b^{high}, F4/80 positive events, and differentiated by their expression of Gr-1. Under the non-fixed conditions used for these experiments, the Gr-1 antibody used (clone RB6-8C5) binds both Ly6G and Ly6C epitopes. Panel **(C)** shows side-by-side representative flow cytometric plots for lungs from dummy dAb and p55-targeting dAb-treated animals. Cell numbers were determined by use of fluorescent counting beads and expressed as total cell counts in both lungs **(D,E)**. Data are displayed as mean ± SD, with t-tests used to evaluate differences. N = 4–5 observations from independent experiments for each group (corresponding to the total number of mice assessed for these parameters).

within the acute and resolving acid-induced injury models (18, 21) and showed that it correlates well with these other markers. In addition to the changes observed, lung permeability showed a tendency toward protection. Overall, these data are consistent with our previous investigations into acid-induced lung injury in genetically modified animals (18), confirming the importance of the p55 TNFR pathway in this model of pulmonary injury and edema formation. Interestingly, in that previous study, we found that "classic" inflammatory mediators (IL-6, CXCL1, CCL2) and leukocyte recruitment were unaffected by the absence of p55 signaling (18), while here we found quite clearly that the acute intratracheal inhibition of p55 using the dAb led to significant attenuation of alveolar cytokine/chemokine levels, and reduced recruitment of neutrophils and inflammatory Ly6C^{hi} monocytes. The reasons for this apparent difference may relate to consequences of compartmentalized inhibition of p55 signaling versus whole body absence of p55, or the effects of chronic compensation of signaling pathways in genetically modified animals. A similar phenomenon is apparent when comparing genetic modification versus acute inhibition of p55 in models of VILI (17, 19) so although the underlying reasons are unclear, they are not model specific. An alternative explanation could be that the dAb has some additional "off-target" effects. We believe this is unlikely, as binding data demonstrated that dAb has high affinity binding to the p55 TNFR and no specific binding to the closely related p75 receptor. This could be clarified in future experiments by exploring the consequences of p55 dAb administration into p55 knockout mice.

A major aspect of the current study was to explore the influence of p55 inhibition beyond the very acute (3–4 h) phase; it may be dangerous to assume that any early consequences of p55 inhibition will continue to be beneficial into the later stages of disease progression, without understanding the knock-on effects of interfering with this pathway. For this reason, we

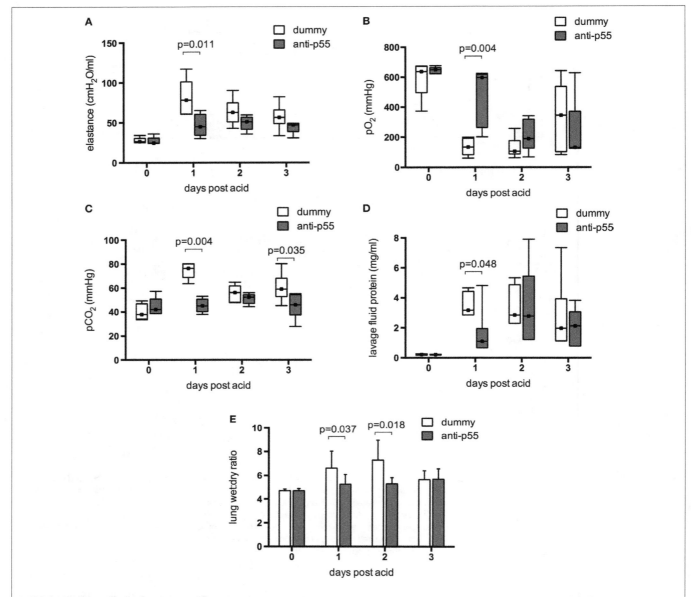

FIGURE 5 | **Physiological indications of injury in the resolution model were determined in terms of elastance (A), arterial pO$_2$ (B), and pCO$_2$ (C) measured after 30 min ventilation with 100% O$_2$**. Data were evaluated for differences due to treatment on each day. Data did not achieve normal distribution even with transformation, and thus are displayed as box-whisker plots and analyzed using Mann–Whitney U-test. Error bars extend to maximum and minimum values, while markers within boxes show the median. Physiological parameters of injury were significantly attenuated by p55-targeting dAb treatment at day 1, but this was mostly lost by day 2. N = 5–8 for elastance and 5–7 for blood gases at each time point. Permeability/edema was evaluated by lavage fluid protein **(D)** and wet:dry weight ratio **(E)**. Lavage fluid protein is displayed as box-whisker plots and was analyzed using Mann–Whitney U-test, while wet:dry weight is displayed as mean ± SD and was analyzed using Student's t-test. N = 5–7 for lavage protein and 5–8 for wet:dry ratio at each time point.

utilized a more chronic model of acid aspiration-induced injury developed within our research group (21). For the purposes of this study, we investigated the first 72 h after injury, a time frame that from our previous work encompasses the peak of injury and beginnings of a return toward homeostasis. In order to avoid frequent airway manipulation, we chose to use the intranasal route for delivery of domain antibody, followed by intratracheal acid instillation. Studies have estimated that the intranasal administration technique achieves approximately 50% delivery into the airspaces (34). This, combined with the fact that we were looking for consequences of domain antibody administration over a much longer time period, led us to increase the antibody dose from 25 µg in the acute model to 100 µg. Within these experiments, we found that markers of respiratory system mechanics, blood gases, and edema/permeability were significantly improved by the single pretreatment with p55-targeting dAb. However, for a number of these markers, most notably arterial pO$_2$ and lavage fluid protein, the injury induced by acid

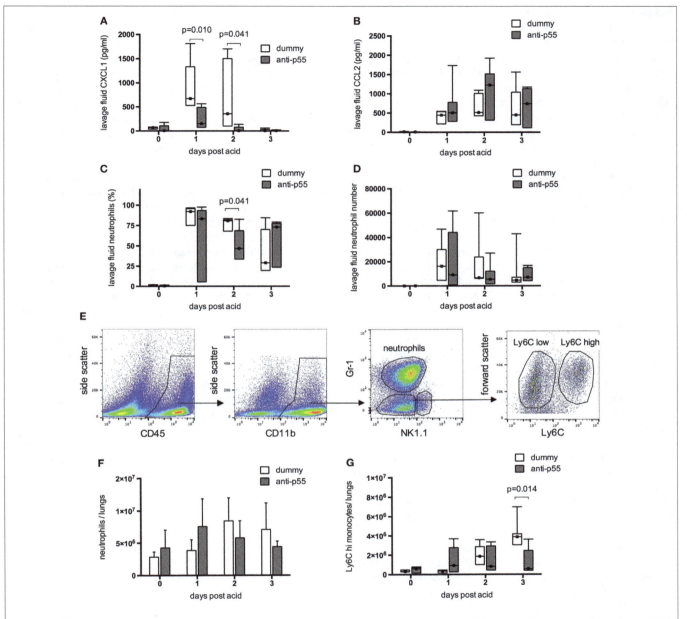

FIGURE 6 | **Inflammation within the resolution model was evaluated in terms of lavage fluid cytokines and leukocyte recruitment**. Data were evaluated for differences due to treatment on each day. Lavage fluid CXCL1 **(A)** and CCL2 **(B)** could not be normalized and are displayed as box-whisker plots with analysis by Mann–Whitney U-test (N = 4–7 at each time point). CXCL1 levels were significantly attenuated following pretreatment with p55-targeting dAb, while CCL2 was unaffected. Neutrophil infiltration into the alveolar space **(C,D)** was highly variable. Neutrophil percentage was reduced at day 2 by dAb treatment, although numbers recruited were not significantly attenuated. For the resolution model neutrophils, monocytes, and NK cells within lung tissue were identified as CD45 positive, CD11b^{high} events using flow cytometry, and differentiated by their expression of Gr-1 and NK1.1 [representative plots from dummy-treated mouse at 24 h after acid shown in panel **(E)**]. NK cells were identified as NK1.1 positive events. We showed previously (28) that although the Gr-1 antibody used (clone RB6-8C5) binds both Ly6G and Ly6C epitopes under non-fixed conditions, the use of Cytofix/Cytoperm results in loss of Ly6C recognition by the antibody. Therefore, in the current context, Gr-1 staining is representative of cell Ly6G expression. Within the NK1.1 negative events, neutrophils were thus identified as Gr-1 (Ly6G) high events, while Gr-1 (Ly6G) low events were designated as monocytes. These were further subcategorized based on expression of Ly6C. Total lung tissue recruitment of neutrophils **(F)** and Ly6C^{hi} monocytes **(G)** were not different following dummy or p55-targeting dAb treatment, apart from a reduction in Ly6C^{hi} monocytes at day 3. Neutrophil numbers in lung tissue **(F)** are displayed as mean ± SD, while Ly6C^{hi} monocyte numbers **(G)** and neutrophils in lavage fluid **(C,D)** could not be normalized and are displayed as box-whisker plots (evaluated using Mann–Whitney U-test). N = 5–7 for each time point.

was delayed rather than prevented. Thus, in general, most of the protective effects of a single dose of p55-targeting dAb treatment in terms of physiology were lost after 24 h.

p55-targeting dAb treatment also influenced inflammatory markers within the chronic model, although these were less pronounced than the physiological findings. Levels of CXCL1 and lavage fluid neutrophils (percentage of alveolar cells) were attenuated at days 1–2, but CCL2 levels were not. Interestingly, there was no clear difference in numbers of lung tissue leukocytes on day 1 (or 2) after acid, at which point physiological injury was clearly attenuated following p55-targeting dAb. Ly6C^{hi} monocyte recruitment was attenuated at day 3, and while these cells have been reported as being injurious in the acute phase of injury (27, 35, 36), the physiological relevance of the current finding is unclear. It is possible that this later phase of monocyte recruitment represents transmigration of a reparative subset (37), although this remains speculation.

Tumor necrosis factor-α, as a highly pleiotropic cytokine, plays a multitude of roles during the pathogenesis of ARDS, and these roles may themselves change during the progression of the syndrome from acute exudative to chronic resolution phases. The data from this study and our previous investigations (17–19) indicate that while TNF p55 signaling is involved in both physiological injury/pulmonary edema formation and lung leukocyte recruitment, there is a clear lack of correlation between these two processes. Other pathophysiological mechanisms mediated by TNF may be more important in determining alveolar epithelial barrier function and fluid balance during ARDS than its role in recruiting leukocytes, which may involve more redundant pathways. Specifically, TNF has a complicated involvement in clearance of pulmonary edema fluid (38). We have previously shown that inhibition of p55 signaling was able to prevent caspase-8 activation within epithelial cells and thus allow maintenance of barrier function and alveolar fluid clearance (18). Inhibition of TNF may also aid fluid clearance by reduction of downstream CXCL1 expression (seen in the current study), the human homolog of which (CXCL8) depresses fluid transport (39). However, TNF has also been shown in opposition to this, to promote clearance of water from the lung via direct activation of epithelial sodium channels (40), prevention of which could be highly damaging. We did not evaluate alveolar fluid clearance in this study, but there was no clear evidence that our treatment regime had adverse effects on physiological parameters, possibly because the fluid clearance promoting activity of TNF seemingly occurs mainly through a receptor-independent pathway (41). Within our acute experiments, the earliest detectable consequence of p55 inhibition occurred around 120 min after acid injury, at which point elastance started to diverge from dummy dAb-treated animals. Future study of such early time points may therefore yield important information regarding the links between TNF, leukocytes, and physiological injury.

In the current study, we chose to use a prophylactic strategy of dosing animals before induction of injury to identify the true potential of p55 inhibition using the dAb. Once their lungs are significantly injured by acid to the level comparable to clinical ARDS, mice do not tolerate anesthesia and intra-airway drug delivery (either intratracheal or intranasal) very well. For this reason, it was not possible to give repeated dosings of antibody, which may have enhanced or prolonged the protective effects observed. The domain antibody used within this study has been formulated specifically for airway administration and has a very short half-life in the circulation, so unfortunately systemic dosing to explore later consequences was also not possible here. Future work may include testing of a recently characterized p55-targeting dAb (DMS5540, GSK), which has been modified to provide an extended circulating half-life (42), although it remains unclear whether this would be able to penetrate into the alveolar space (or indeed whether this would be necessary). While it could be argued that prophylactic dosing in preclinical models of disease may not represent the most clinically relevant scenario, it is perhaps not so unreasonable in the case of ARDS. Recent studies report that up to 75% of patients suffering from ARDS acquired or developed it after entering hospital or during their ICU stay (43, 44). Identification of treatments that work safely when delivered prophylactically to "at risk" patients, or very early during the onset of disease, may therefore be a useful strategy to prevent progression to ARDS, although the same interventions should not be expected to be therapeutically efficacious in patients with established disease.

In conclusion, our data show clearly that targeting of the p55 TNFR with use of an intrapulmonary domain antibody attenuates many physiological indications of acid aspiration-induced lung injury, including respiratory mechanics, blood gases, and markers of edema/permeability. These data show the persistent importance of p55 TNF signaling in both the very acute and later phases of lung injury, and thus strongly support a role for p55 inhibition in patients with or at risk of lung injury, an approach that is currently being developed clinically. Although in the current study the beneficial effects were mainly lost after 24 h of injury, the protection up to this point was achieved with just a single intranasal dosing. Subsequent experiments will be necessary to determine the potential for modified dosing regimes to prolong the attenuation in injury observed.

AUTHOR CONTRIBUTIONS

MW, MT, PM, and AB were involved in the initial design of the study. MW, KW, SB, CO, BP, KO, and JC were involved in the acquisition and analysis of data. MW, KW, and MT prepared the manuscript. MW, KW, SB, CO, BP, KO, JC, PM, AB, and MT were involved in revising the manuscript and approving it for publication.

ACKNOWLEDGMENTS

The authors thank Elliot Thompson and Emilie Madura (GSK) for generation of the dAb-binding affinity data.

REFERENCES

1. Bellani G, Laffey JG, Pham T, Fan E, Brochard L, Esteban A, et al. Epidemiology, patterns of care, and mortality for patients with acute respiratory distress syndrome in intensive care units in 50 countries. *JAMA* (2016) 315:788–800. doi:10.1001/jama.2016.0291

2. Raghavendran K, Nemzek J, Napolitano LM, Knight PR. Aspiration-induced lung injury. *Crit Care Med* (2011) 39:818–26. doi:10.1097/CCM.0b013e31820a856b

3. Steinberg KP, Hudson LD, Goodman RB, Hough CL, Lanken PN, Hyzy R, et al. Efficacy and safety of corticosteroids for persistent acute respira

tory distress syndrome. *N Engl J Med* (2006) 354:1671–84. doi:10.1056/NEJMoa051693

4. Spieth PM, Zhang H. Pharmacological therapies for acute respiratory distress syndrome. *Curr Opin Crit Care* (2014) 20:113–21. doi:10.1097/MCC.0000000000000056

5. Adhikari N, Burns KE, Meade MO. Pharmacologic therapies for adults with acute lung injury and acute respiratory distress syndrome. *Cochrane Database Syst Rev* (2004) CD004477. doi:10.1002/14651858.CD004477.pub2

6. Adhikari NK, Dellinger RP, Lundin S, Payen D, Vallet B, Gerlach H, et al. Inhaled nitric oxide does not reduce mortality in patients with acute respiratory distress syndrome regardless of severity: systematic review and meta-analysis. *Crit Care Med* (2014) 42:404–12. doi:10.1097/CCM.0b013e3182a27909

7. Tang BM, Craig JC, Eslick GD, Seppelt I, McLean AS. Use of corticosteroids in acute lung injury and acute respiratory distress syndrome: a systematic review and meta-analysis. *Crit Care Med* (2009) 37:1594–603. doi:10.1097/CCM.0b013e31819fb507

8. Mukhopadhyay S, Hoidal JR, Mukherjee TK. Role of TNFalpha in pulmonary pathophysiology. *Respir Res* (2006) 7:125. doi:10.1186/1465-9921-7-125

9. Qiu P, Cui X, Sun J, Welsh J, Natanson C, Eichacker PQ. Antitumor necrosis factor therapy is associated with improved survival in clinical sepsis trials: a meta-analysis. *Crit Care Med* (2013) 41:2419–29. doi:10.1097/CCM.0b013e3182982add

10. Fang L, Fang J, Chen CQ. TNF receptor-associated factor-2 binding site is involved in TNFR75-dependent enhancement of TNFR55-induced cell death. *Cell Res* (2001) 11:217–22. doi:10.1038/sj.cr.7290089

11. Wajant H, Pfizenmaier K, Scheurich P. Tumor necrosis factor signaling. *Cell Death Differ* (2003) 10:45–65. doi:10.1038/sj.cdd.4401189

12. Fontaine V, Mohand-Said S, Hanoteau N, Fuchs C, Pfizenmaier K, Eisel U. Neurodegenerative and neuroprotective effects of tumor necrosis factor (TNF) in retinal ischemia: opposite roles of TNF receptor 1 and TNF receptor 2. *J Neurosci* (2002) 22:RC216.

13. Ebach DR, Riehl TE, Stenson WF. Opposing effects of tumor necrosis factor receptor 1 and 2 in sepsis due to cecal ligation and puncture. *Shock* (2005) 23:311–8. doi:10.1097/01.shk.0000157301.87051.77

14. Monden Y, Kubota T, Inoue T, Tsutsumi T, Kawano S, Ide T, et al. Tumor necrosis factor-alpha is toxic via receptor 1 and protective via receptor 2 in a murine model of myocardial infarction. *Am J Physiol Heart Circ Physiol* (2007) 293:H743–53. doi:10.1152/ajpheart.00166.2007

15. Kawano S, Kubota T, Monden Y, Tsutsumi T, Inoue T, Kawamura N, et al. Blockade of NF-kappaB improves cardiac function and survival after myocardial infarction. *Am J Physiol Heart Circ Physiol* (2006) 291:H1337–44. doi:10.1152/ajpheart.01175.2005

16. Al-Lamki RS, Brookes AP, Wang J, Reid MJ, Parameshwar J, Goddard MJ, et al. TNF receptors differentially signal and are differentially expressed and regulated in the human heart. *Am J Transplant* (2009) 9:2679–96. doi:10.1111/j.1600-6143.2009.02831.x

17. Wilson MR, Goddard ME, O'Dea KP, Choudhury S, Takata M. Differential roles of p55 and p75 tumor necrosis factor receptors on stretch-induced pulmonary edema in mice. *Am J Physiol Lung Cell Mol Physiol* (2007) 293:L60–8. doi:10.1152/ajplung.00284.2006

18. Patel BV, Wilson MR, O'Dea KP, Takata M. TNF-induced death signaling triggers alveolar epithelial dysfunction in acute lung injury. *J Immunol* (2013) 190:4274–82. doi:10.4049/jimmunol.1202437

19. Bertok S, Wilson MR, Morley PJ, de Wildt R, Bayliffe A, Takata M. Selective inhibition of intra-alveolar p55 TNF receptor attenuates ventilator-induced lung injury. *Thorax* (2012) 67:244–51. doi:10.1136/thoraxjnl-2011-200590

20. Holt LJ, Herring C, Jespers LS, Woolven BP, Tomlinson IM. Domain antibodies: proteins for therapy. *Trends Biotechnol* (2003) 21:484–90. doi:10.1016/j.tibtech.2003.08.007

21. Patel BV, Wilson MR, Takata M. Resolution of acute lung injury and inflammation: a translational mouse model. *Eur Respir J* (2012) 39:1162–70. doi:10.1183/09031936.00093911

22. Cordy JC, Morley PJ, Wright TJ, Birchler MA, Lewis AP, Emmins R, et al. Specificity of human anti-variable heavy (VH) chain autoantibodies and impact on the design and clinical testing of a VH domain antibody antagonist of tumour necrosis factor-alpha receptor 1. *Clin Exp Immunol* (2015) 182:139–48. doi:10.1111/cei.12680

23. Wilson MR, Patel BV, Takata M. Ventilation with "clinically relevant" high tidal volumes does not promote stretch-induced injury in the lungs of healthy mice. *Crit Care Med* (2012) 40:2850–7. doi:10.1097/CCM.0b013e318 25b91ef

24. Matute-Bello G, Frevert CW, Martin TR. Animal models of acute lung injury. *Am J Physiol Lung Cell Mol Physiol* (2008) 295:L379–99. doi:10.1152/ajplung.00010.2008

25. Matute-Bello G, Downey G, Moore BB, Groshong SD, Matthay MA, Slutsky AS, et al. An official American Thoracic Society workshop report: features and measurements of experimental acute lung injury in animals. *Am J Respir Cell Mol Biol* (2011) 44:725–38. doi:10.1165/rcmb.2009-0210ST

26. Matthay MA, Howard JP. Progress in modelling acute lung injury in a pre-clinical mouse model. *Eur Respir J* (2012) 39:1062–3. doi:10.1183/09031936.00204211

27. O'Dea KP, Wilson MR, Dokpesi JO, Wakabayashi K, Tatton L, van Rooijen N, et al. Mobilization and margination of bone marrow Gr-1high monocytes during subclinical endotoxemia predisposes the lungs toward acute injury. *J Immunol* (2009) 182:1155–66. doi:10.4049/jimmunol.182.2.1155

28. O'Dea KP, Dokpesi JO, Tatham KC, Wilson MR, Takata M. Regulation of monocyte subset proinflammatory responses within the lung microvasculature by the p38 MAPK/MK2 pathway. *Am J Physiol Lung Cell Mol Physiol* (2011) 301:L812–21. doi:10.1152/ajplung.00092.2011

29. Jabaudon M, Blondonnet R, Roszyk L, Bouvier D, Audard J, Clairefond G, et al. Soluble receptor for advanced glycation end-products predicts impaired alveolar fluid clearance in acute respiratory distress syndrome. *Am J Respir Crit Care Med* (2015) 192:191–9. doi:10.1164/rccm.201501-0020OC

30. Patel BV, Tatham KC, Wilson MR, O'Dea KP, Takata M. In vivo compartmental analysis of leukocytes in mouse lungs. *Am J Physiol Lung Cell Mol Physiol* (2015) 309:L639–52. doi:10.1152/ajplung.00140.2015

31. Seok J, Warren HS, Cuenca AG, Mindrinos MN, Baker HV, Xu W, et al. Genomic responses in mouse models poorly mimic human inflammatory diseases. *Proc Natl Acad Sci U S A* (2013) 110:3507–12. doi:10.1073/pnas.1222878110

32. Takao K, Miyakawa T. Genomic responses in mouse models greatly mimic human inflammatory diseases. *Proc Natl Acad Sci U S A* (2015) 112:1167–72. doi:10.1073/pnas.1401965111

33. Calfee CS, Delucchi K, Parsons PE, Thompson BT, Ware LB, Matthay MA, et al. Subphenotypes in acute respiratory distress syndrome: latent class analysis of data from two randomised controlled trials. *Lancet Respir Med* (2014) 2:611–20. doi:10.1016/S2213-2600(14)70097-9

34. Southam DS, Dolovich M, O'Byrne PM, Inman MD. Distribution of intranasal instillations in mice: effects of volume, time, body position, and anesthesia. *Am J Physiol Lung Cell Mol Physiol* (2002) 282:L833–9. doi:10.1152/ajplung.00173.2001

35. Wilson MR, O'Dea KP, Zhang D, Shearman AD, van Rooijen N, Takata M. Role of lung-marginated monocytes in an in vivo mouse model of ventilator-induced lung injury. *Am J Respir Crit Care Med* (2009) 179:914–22. doi:10.1164/rccm.200806-877OC

36. Dhaliwal K, Scholefield E, Ferenbach D, Gibbons M, Duffin R, Dorward DA, et al. Monocytes control second-phase neutrophil emigration in established lipopolysaccharide-induced murine lung injury. *Am J Respir Crit Care Med* (2012) 186:514–24. doi:10.1164/rccm.201112-2132OC

37. Herold S, Tabar TS, Janssen H, Hoegner K, Cabanski M, Lewe-Schlosser P, et al. Exudate macrophages attenuate lung injury by the release of IL-1 receptor antagonist in gram-negative pneumonia. *Am J Respir Crit Care Med* (2011) 183:1380–90. doi:10.1164/rccm.201009-1431OC

38. Braun C, Hamacher J, Morel DR, Wendel A, Lucas R. Dichotomal role of TNF in experimental pulmonary edema reabsorption. *J Immunol* (2005) 175:3402–8. doi:10.4049/jimmunol.175.5.3402

39. Wagener BM, Roux J, Carles M, Pittet JF. Synergistic inhibition of beta2-adrenergic receptor-mediated alveolar epithelial fluid transport by interleukin-8 and transforming growth factor-beta. *Anesthesiology* (2015) 122:1084–92. doi:10.1097/ALN.0000000000000595

40. Czikora I, Alli A, Bao HF, Kaftan D, Sridhar S, Apell HJ, et al. A novel tumor necrosis factor-mediated mechanism of direct epithelial sodium channel activation. *Am J Respir Crit Care Med* (2014) 190:522–32. doi:10.1164/rccm.201405-0833OC

41. Elia N, Tapponnier M, Matthay MA, Hamacher J, Pache JC, Brundler MA, et al. Functional identification of the alveolar edema reabsorption activity of murine tumor necrosis factor-alpha. *Am J Respir Crit Care Med* (2003) 168:1043–50. doi:10.1164/rccm.200206-618OC

42. Goodall LJ, Ovecka M, Rycroft D, Friel SL, Sanderson A, Mistry P, et al. Pharmacokinetic and pharmacodynamic characterisation of an anti-mouse TNF receptor 1 domain antibody formatted for in vivo half-life extension. *PLoS One* (2015) 10:e0137065. doi:10.1371/journal.pone.0137065

43. Li G, Malinchoc M, Cartin-Ceba R, Venkata CV, Kor DJ, Peters SG, et al. Eight-year trend of acute respiratory distress syndrome: a population-based study in Olmsted County, Minnesota. *Am J Respir Crit Care Med* (2011) 183:59–66. doi:10.1164/rccm.201003-0436OC

44. Kao KC, Hu HC, Hsieh MJ, Tsai YH, Huang CC. Comparison of community-acquired, hospital-acquired, and intensive care unit-acquired acute respiratory distress syndrome: a prospective observational cohort study. *Crit Care* (2015) 19:384. doi:10.1186/s13054-015-1096-1

14

Regulation of Lung Epithelial Sodium Channels by Cytokines and Chemokines

Brandi M. Wynne [1,2,3]*, Li Zou [2], Valerie Linck [2], Robert S. Hoover [1,2,4], He-Ping Ma [2,3] and Douglas C. Eaton [2,3]

[1] Department of Medicine, Nephrology, Emory University, Atlanta, GA, United States, [2] Department of Physiology, Emory University, Atlanta, GA, United States, [3] The Center for Cell and Molecular Signaling, Emory University, Atlanta, GA, United States, [4] Research Service, Atlanta Veteran's Administration Medical Center, Decatur, GA, United States

*Correspondence:
Brandi M. Wynne
bwynne@emory.edu

Acute lung injury leading to acute respiratory distress (ARDS) is a global health concern. ARDS patients have significant pulmonary inflammation leading to flooding of the pulmonary alveoli. This prevents normal gas exchange with consequent hypoxemia and causes mortality. A thin fluid layer in the alveoli is normal. The maintenance of this thin layer results from fluid movement out of the pulmonary capillaries into the alveolar interstitium driven by vascular hydrostatic pressure and then through alveolar tight junctions. This is then balanced by fluid reabsorption from the alveolar space mediated by transepithelial salt and water transport through alveolar cells. Reabsorption is a two-step process: first, sodium enters *via* sodium-permeable channels in the apical membranes of alveolar type 1 and 2 cells followed by active extrusion of sodium into the interstitium by the basolateral Na^+, K^+-ATPase. Anions follow the cationic charge gradient and water follows the salt-induced osmotic gradient. The proximate cause of alveolar flooding is the result of a failure to reabsorb sufficient salt and water or a failure of the tight junctions to prevent excessive movement of fluid from the interstitium to alveolar lumen. Cytokine- and chemokine-induced inflammation can have a particularly profound effect on lung sodium transport since they can alter both ion channel and barrier function. Cytokines and chemokines affect alveolar amiloride-sensitive epithelial sodium channels (ENaCs), which play a crucial role in sodium transport and fluid reabsorption in the lung. This review discusses the regulation of ENaC *via* local and systemic cytokines during inflammatory disease and the effect on lung fluid balance.

Keywords: lung, sodium channels, epithelial sodium channel, cytokines, physiology, inflammation, acute lung injury, acute respiratory distress syndrome

INTRODUCTION

The maintenance of a thin fluid layer on the surface of the alveolar epithelium is critical for respiration. Two primary mechanisms regulate this fluid layer: Starling's forces and active sodium (Na^+) transport. Starling's forces determine the movement of water from intravascular to extravascular or interstitial spaces caused by hydrostatic and oncotic pressures. An increase in pulmonary vascular pressure accounts for the increased alveolar flooding seen in cardiogenic pulmonary edema. However, the other regulator of the thickness of the alveolar fluid layer is the active transport of Na^+, followed by potential-driven anion movement through cystic fibrosis transmembrane conductance regulator, and the aquaporin-mediated transport of water. The epithelial sodium channel (ENaC) is critical in the maintenance of the epithelial fluid layer. This review focuses on the primary physiological mechanisms required to maintain and regulate this layer and is an overview of the pathophysiological mechanisms of cytokine-mediated ENaC regulation in the lung (**Figure 1**).

PULMONARY PHYSIOLOGY

The primary function of the airways is exchange of gases; thus, both the anatomy and physiology of the lung have evolved to distribute gases efficiently. The diffusion of gases is facilitated in the alveoli by the large total surface area, coupled with thin, yet strong and elastic membranes (1). Human lungs are composed of a series of branched tubes, where conducting airways lead to the terminal respiratory units that are in close proximity to the vasculature (2–4).

The primary respiratory units, or alveoli, are composed of a single, polarized, epithelial cell layer that separates a gas-filled compartment and the pulmonary circulation (5). The two predominant cell types in this cell barrier are the squamous type 1 (AT1) and cuboidal type 2 (AT2) cells. The majority of the alveolar surface area consists of AT1 cells: the remainder of the area (≈2–5%) is AT2 cells. Both cell types contribute to alveolar fluid transport (6–10). These cells are responsible for Na^+ transport from the apical to basolateral surface and maintenance of a thin layer of isotonic fluid on the alveolar surface. The AT2 cells have an additional function: they are also responsible for the secretion of surfactant, which is necessary to lower the surface tension at the interface of air and water and increase lung compliance. Overall, this anatomical structure and physiology ensures that the alveolar spaces remain open for gas exchange.

Paradigm for Fluid Transport: Role of the ENaC

Regulation of the fluid interface occurs primarily through regulating Na^+ uptake *via* ENaC in both AT1 and AT2 cells. After ENaC-mediated entry of Na^+ across the apical membrane, Na^+ leaves the cell across the basolateral membrane *via* the Na^+–K^+ ATPase and enters the interstitium where it is in equilibrium with vascular Na^+. Some investigators have suggested that regulation of the ATPase also plays a role in controlling trans-epithelial Na^+ transport (11–15); however, we will not consider ATPase regulation in this review. The paradigm in which vectorial Na^+ transport is considered a primary drive for fluid transport from the alveolar surface has been established by numerous studies where pharmacological inhibitors of apical Na^+ channels have been shown to reduce the rate at which fluid is cleared (16–21).

Regulation of ENaC in the Airway

Epithelial sodium channel is composed of three homologous subunits, such as α, β, and γ. Together, these subunits assemble in the endoplasmic reticulum and traffic to the apical membrane and are highly selective for Na^+ (22). Using ENaCα-subunit knock-out mice, investigators first showed the importance of

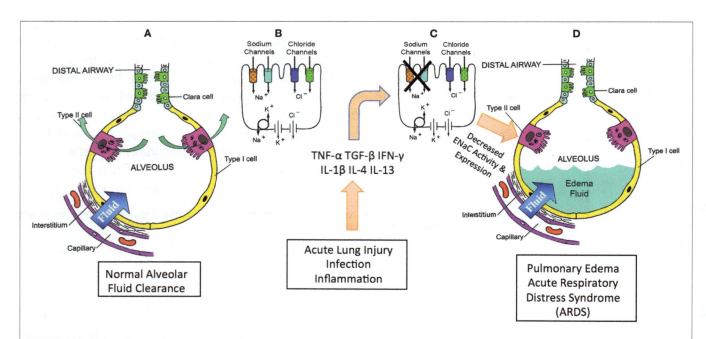

FIGURE 1 | Summary schematic for role of cytokines in mediating pulmonary edema and acute respiratory distress syndrome (ARDS). Acute lung injury (ALI), ARDS, and pneumonia are all pathologies characterized by lung edema and alveolar flooding. Pneumonia mortality is typically caused by flooding of the pulmonary alveoli, preventing normal gas exchange and consequent hypoxemia. Airways normally have a critically regulated fluid layer essential for normal gas exchange and removal of foreign particulates from the airway **(A)**. Maintaining this fluid layer in the alveoli depends critically on sodium reabsorption mediated by epithelial sodium channels (ENaCs) and CFTR chloride channels **(B)**. During ALI, sepsis, inflammation or infection, inflammatory cytokines are produced that inhibit ENaC **(C)**. A decrease in ENaC reabsorption allows fluid to accumulate in the alveoli causing alveolar flood in loss of normal gas exchange and consequent hypoxemia **(D)**.

ENaCα for proper lung function: neonates lacking ENaCα died within 40 h of birth (23). The α subunit is the ionophoric component of the heteromultimer and is required for the expression and assembly of functional ENaCs at the apical membrane. The importance of ENaC to normal lung function is underscored by the phenotype of several monogenetic disorders that affect ENaC. Patients with pseudohypoaldosteronism (PHA), a condition resulting from ENaC partial loss-of-function, were found to have twice the volume of airway surface liquid compared normal levels (24). Mice lacking the ubiquitin ligase, NEDD4-2, had increased levels of ENaC expression and increased ENaC-mediated current in AT2 cells (25). Additionally, overexpression of ENaCβ in an ENaCβ transgenic mouse model leads to airway dehydration and mucous obstruction, comparable to many features observed in cystic fibrosis (CF) (26). Together, these studies highlight the importance of proper ENaC expression and regulation for the airways.

Understanding the regulation of ENaC is significant for understanding lung fluid balance, as ENaC dysregulation is the source of pathological lung edema. In recent years, probably because monogenetic disorders often alter ENaC trafficking, much of the focus has examined how regulation of the number of channels at the apical membrane of alveolar epithelial cells can alter Na^+ transport. However, since ENaC is an ion channel, regulating how much of the time the channel spends open (the open probability, P_o) is also important. Both Liddle's syndrome and PHA type 1 (PHA 1) are conventionally described as changes in channel density (an increase and decrease, respectively); however, examination of single ENaCs in these two syndromes shows that ENaC P_o also changes. There are an observed increase in channel activity in Liddle's (27) and a decrease in activity in PHA I (28). Steroid hormones increase Na^+ transport and are often thought to do so by increasing subunit transcription and translation. Although Frindt and Palmer (29) have shown in Na^+-transporting epithelial tissue that this is indeed true, the increase in subunit density accounts for less than 25% of the increase in trans-epithelial Na^+ current implying that the remaining 75% is due to an increase in single channel P_o. Single channel recordings show that acute application of steroids dramatically increases single channel P_o (30–32).

Kleyman, Hughey, and their co-workers have shown that the α and γ subunits of ENaC must be proteolytically cleaved to be active loops (33–37). Some investigators have suggested that such cleavage might be a mechanism by which ENaC in the apical membrane could be regulated. In fact, proteolysis does appear to be required for ENaC to have any appreciable activity, and may be required for it to reach the membrane. As such, proteolysis appears to be, more or less, an all-or-none phenomenon: channels that are uncleaved are capable of little if any activity. However, under conditions of normal Na^+ transport most channels are cleaved. Under these conditions, cleaved channels are capable of a wide range of activity by changing their P_o.

Changes in membrane ENaC can occur by changing the rate of insertion into the membrane after transcription and translation (38). However, in any time frame less than 24 h, ENaC in the membrane is altered by recycling from intracellular pools into the membrane (22) or internalization of ENaC into recycling or degradative pools. Removal of ENaC occurs primarily *via* the ubiquitin ligase, NEDD 4-2, which targets ENaC for removal and proteosomal degradation (39, 40).

Therefore, in this review, we address both the regulation of P_o in cleaved channels and change in membrane channel protein density.

The regulation of ENaC occurs *via* multiple, redundant systems to ensure that Na^+ transport is not limited. ENaC is regulated by a many agents including transmitters interacting with G-protein-coupled receptors (GPCRs), circulating hormones, cytokines and chemokines, and reactive oxygen and nitrogen species. The regulation of ENaC *via* hormones and GPCRs is not a primary focus of this review, but we briefly review ENaC activation and regulation *via* steroids since their actions often interact with the activities of cytokines and chemokines.

In the lung, the glucocorticoid receptor (GR) is the primary receptor for corticosteroids (41–43). Once activated, the GR activates response elements inducing the transcription of signaling kinases, such as the serum- and glucocorticoid-regulated kinase 1 (30, 44, 45). Ligand-mediated activation of the GR *via* corticosteroids is used clinically as an anti-inflammatory treatment. The positive effects of corticosteroid therapy lie in the ability of the GR to bind to and inhibit nuclear factor kappa-light-chain-enhancer of activated B cells (Nf-κB) (46–48). Nf-κB is an important mediator of cytokine signaling. This transcription factor increases cyclooxygenase 2-induced prostaglandin production, as well as increases other proinflammatory factors (49). Corticosteroids reduce inflammation propagated *via* Nf-κB-mediated mechanisms but may not affect inflammation mediated by other signaling pathways. Indeed, GR activation may actually augment some downstream signaling pathways, such as those mediated through Smad proteins (50). This distinction is important because of the many heterogeneous pathways activated by each cytokine (51–54).

PULMONARY PATHOPHYSIOLOGY

Regulation of the air/water interface is crucial for gas exchange, as the amount of the alveolar fluid layer must be precise. With injury, the inability of the lungs to clear this fluid can lead to pulmonary edema. Increased fluid accumulation can result from compromised ENaC function or when there is an asymmetrical hydrostatic force from the vasculature, pushing fluid from capillaries into the alveolar space (e.g., pulmonary hypertension) (5). In addition, tight junctions that maintain structural integrity and a tight epithelial layer can be disrupted, resulting in increased permeability. In fact, high levels of pulmonary inflammation causing airway tight junction damage that compromise alveolar barrier function is a primary cause of epithelial injury (55). And lastly, many proinflammatory and noxious factors cause changes in Na^+ transport. Dysfunction in any single factor can lead to a dysregulation of the alveolar fluid (5). Because of the increased morbidity and mortality associated with alveolar fluid accumulation, understanding the mechanisms that regulate these factors are vital.

Immune Responses in the Airway

During inflammation most cells are capable of secreting a variety of small molecular weight proteins, called cytokines and chemokines, which communicate the inflammatory signals. In the airway, resident immune cells are mostly the alveolar macrophages; however, during infection or inflammation, other mononuclear and granular immune cells infiltrate (56). Several studies have proposed a role for the airway epithelium in propagating the immune response, especially as a "first responder" since the airway is the first to sense viral and bacterial pathogens as they enter the body. This layer can be an active participant in the immune response, producing a variety of cytokines and chemokines, as well as exclusive epithelial-derived cytokines (55, 57, 58).

Direct interaction with pathogens, such as influenza, reduces ENaC activity (59). However, other evidence suggests that some of the more chronic effects of pathogens may be *via* noxae-stimulated chronic cytokine production (60–62). Additionally, inflammatory activation of the airway epithelium can result in local nitric oxide (NO) production, most likely *via* increased cytokine production, further reducing ENaC activity and fluid transport (59, 63–67). Cytokines frequently increase local levels of reactive oxygen species (ROS) as well. Interestingly, ROS has been shown to activate ENaC at relatively low concentrations but to inhibit ENaC at higher concentrations often associated with massive pathogen-induced cytokine production (40, 68, 69). The overall redox environment of the alveoli is crucial and can rapidly change, often driven by high levels of Rac1-NADPH oxidase activity in AT1 cells (67, 70).

CYTOKINE-MEDIATED REGULATION OF ENaC

Some of the earliest studies revealed a correlation between large and sustained proinflammatory cytokine increases in bronchio-alveolar lavage (BAL) fluid and an unfavorable outcome in acute respiratory distress syndrome (ARDS) (71). Overall, increased cytokine levels from lung injury can quickly lead to the accumulation of alveolar fluid, edema, and then acute respiratory distress. Thus, proinflammatory cytokines and chemokines produce a feed forward cycle decreasing lung Na^+ transporter expression, as well as activity.

Regulation of ENaC *via* Tumor Necrosis Factor (TNF)-α

The TNF super family comprises 19 members and was originally named for its role in apoptosis (53). The best-studied member of this family is TNF-α, which plays a role in propagating the immune response and secretion of other cytokines. TNF-α was implicated in the pathogenesis of pulmonary edema, and increased levels were observed in patients with ARDS (72, 73). Monocytes and macrophages produce significant TNF-α, but it is also produced by alveolar epithelial cells following lipopolysaccharide stimulation (74).

Although TNF-α can bind to two different receptors that are linked to separate signaling pathways, much of the work in the airway has focused on TNF receptor 1. The effect that TNF-α elicits on ENaC function, and alveolar liquid clearance, seems to be critically dependent upon receptor activation or receptor-independent mechanisms and has been shown using both *in vitro* and *in vivo* models (75–78).

Tumor necrosis factor receptor 1-mediated activation of NF-κB increases cytokine (IL-1, IL-8, IL-6) and chemokine production. It also increases the expression of adhesion molecules including selectins, vascular cell adhesion molecules, and intercellular adhesion molecule (ICAM)-1 (53, 79, 80). In freshly isolated AT2 cells, TNF-α decreased α- and γ-ENaC mRNA and protein levels and reduced amiloride-sensitive trans-epithelial current (75, 78).

Tumor necrosis factor-α also plays an especially important role in endothelial activation, as well as disturbing the epithelial tight junction barrier. Disruption of the tight junctions not only leads to respiratory distress and increased exudate but also may reduce alveolar fluid clearance as well (81). TNF-α reduces the expression of tight junction proteins, including the claudins and zonula occludens protein 1, thus increasing alveolar permeability (55, 82). Consequently, TNF-α has a critical and multi-faceted role in the development of ARDS. TNF-α not only regulates Na^+ and water clearance but also disrupts tight junction barriers and endothelial integrity and contributes to a pro-inflammatory environment.

Interestingly, TNF-α contains not only a receptor-binding domain but also a lectin-like domain (referred to as a TIP domain) that is spatially distinct from the receptor-binding site (83, 84). TNF-α produces an opposite response when there is binding of the lectin-like domain, or TIP, to certain oligosaccharides at high concentrations of TNF-α. This process increases Na^+ uptake in AT2 cells and may account for the differential responses to TNF-α (85–87). *In vivo*, a peptide analog of TIP increased clearance in a murine flooded-lung model (85). Czikora and colleagues also demonstrated that this TIP domain directly binds to and, then, activates ENaC (83). This implies an endogenous mechanism to limit the effects of high TNF-α concentrations. Use of this may become a novel method in counteracting reduced alveolar clearance.

Regulation of ENaC *via* Transforming Growth Factor (TGF)-β1

Transforming growth factor-β1 is a pathogenic cytokine, which has been implicated in the early phase of acute lung injury (ALI) prior to ARDS (72, 88). TGF-β1 levels were increased in ARDS patients compared to healthy controls (89). Furthermore, active TGF-β1 levels were more than doubled in the epithelial lining fluid from ARDS patients (90). As mentioned earlier, corticosteroids are a common tool to reduce inflammation and aid in lung clearance. Interestingly, TGF-β actually reduces the ability to produce multiple steroids, possibly leading to the inability for self-healing and furthering inflammatory damage, in addition to the activation of multiple Smad pathways (50, 52). Some of these pathways may be insensitive to corticosteroid treatment. However, there is still much to learn regarding which Smad-mediated pathways are downstream of TGF-β signaling during ALI and ARDS.

Other studies have specifically have explored the role of TGF-β in alveolar flooding. Using a bleomycin-induced lung injury model, TGF-β1-inducible genes were dramatically increased as early as 2 days, suggesting that TGF-β1 may precede alveolar flooding (91). Of interest, TGF-β may actually remain latent locally, covalently attached to a latency-associated peptide (LAP); pulmonary epithelial cells can activate and cause dissociation of TGF-β from LAP (92–94). One member of the integrin family, αvβ6, was recently shown to be a ligand for LAP (93). αvβ6 is expressed normally at lower levels, yet increased significantly with injury revealing a novel mechanism for rapid and local TGF-β activation (95). TGF-β is also redox sensitive, and *in vitro* models of increased ROS *via* ionizing radiation revealed another mechanism for TGF-β activation (96). Together, these studies show multiple, redundant possibilities for systemic and paracrine TGF-β activation during lung injury.

One of the first studies to directly implicate TGF-β1 in regulating ENaC was by Frank and colleagues. They showed that TGF-β1 reduced amiloride-sensitive Na$^+$ transport in lung epithelial cells. Additionally, TGF-β1 reduced αENaC mRNA and protein expression *via* an ERK1/2 pathway in a model of ALI, thus promoting alveolar edema (97). *In vivo* studies then showed that TGF-β1 reduces vectorial Na$^+$ and water transport and that this process occurs independently from increases in epithelial permeability (97, 98). Interestingly, TGF-β was also found to have an integral role in ENaC trafficking. Peters and colleagues were the first to demonstrate this acute regulation of ENaC in the lung; they found that TGF-β induces ENaC internalization *via* interaction with ENaCβ (99). In summary, TGF-β has been implicated in multiple mechanisms reducing ENaC expression and apical localization, thus contributing to the pathophysiology of ARDS and pulmonary edema (100).

Regulation of ENaC by Interferon-γ

The interferons (IFN) are a family of proteins originally classified by their ability to reduce viral replication. This family consists of both Type I and Type II IFNs; INF-γ is the only member of the Type II IFN family and is structurally unrelated to the other IFNs. During inflammation, INF-γ is secreted by multiple immune cells, but mostly by T lymphocytes. INF-γ increases ICAM-1 levels and increases NO production *via* inducible nitric oxide synthase. Little is known about the role of INF-γ in ENaC regulation; however, studies using human bronchial epithelial cells (BECs) showed that INF-γ treatment significantly reduced trans-epithelial Na$^+$ transport in normal human BECs (101).

Regulation of ENaC by the Interleukins: IL-1β, IL-4, and IL-13

ENaC Regulation by IL-1β

Several interleukins are correlated with the early stages of ALI; however, the best studied is IL-1β. This cytokine plays a diverse role in the pathogenesis of ALI and ARDS. IL-1β levels are increased in the BAL fluid, as well as the pulmonary edema fluid, of patients with ALI (102–106). IL-1β levels are higher in the pulmonary lavage fluids compared to serum suggesting that there is a local, pulmonary source for IL-1β similar to that of TGF-β (71, 104). An earlier study by Pugin and colleagues suggested

that of the cytokines present in the BAL fluid, IL-1β is the most biologically active, and others have suggested that the source may be from early-infiltrating neutrophils (103, 107). BAL fluids from ARDS patients applied to AT2 cells increased ICAM-1 expression, while IL-1 inhibition reduced the increase in ICAM-1 (103).

IL-1β also seems to have significant effects on endothelial leakage and permeability. *In vitro*, IL-1β treatment significantly increased microvascular permeability (108). Several studies have also demonstrated that when given intratracheally, IL-1β increased endothelial permeability and lung leak (108–111). More recently, IL-1β has been shown to directly affect ENaC expression. Incubation with IL-1β reduced ENaC mRNA protein expression, possibly through promoter inhibition and a p38 MAPK-dependent mechanism. Additionally, IL-1β application reduced apical ENaC protein and amiloride-sensitive trans-epithelial current and Na$^+$ flux (112).

Other studies have tried to reverse IL-1β effects. *In vitro* modeling suggests that the reduction of IL-1β, *via* suppressor of cytokine signaling-1, can rescue the IL-1β-mediated suppression of ENaCs (113). When investigating patients with ALI, those who had an increased activation of the stress protein response (SPR) positively correlated with preserved alveolar clearance rates (114). Thus, activation of this SPR during immune-related injury may ameliorate effects of IL-1β, if used as a "preconditioning" agent (115).

ENaC Regulation by IL-4 and IL-13

Classically, increases in IL-4 and IL-13 are associated with an increased goblet-cell hyperplasia and mucous secretion. These cytokines are implicated in allergic airway diseases and CF and contribute to reduced ciliary movement reducing the ability to clear the airways. These related cytokines frequently share signaling cascades and receptor subunits, such as the IL-4 receptor (116). However, studies in airway epithelial cells from human bronchi suggest that these cytokines may also alter ion transport. IL-4 significantly reduced ENaC subunits γ and β; interestingly, αENaC levels were not altered. IL-4 and IL-13 treatments reduced amiloride-sensitive short circuit current (using an Ussing chamber), which was reversed with an IL-4 receptor antagonist (116). Although these studies were investigating allergic diseases, one could infer a similar involvement in a variety of other inflammatory conditions where there are increased IL-4/IL-13 levels and reduced ENaC function.

CONCLUSION: BALANCING THE INFLAMMATORY MILIEU

Delineating the role of pro-inflammatory cytokines is important for the understanding of alveolar flooding and ALI; however, the lack of anti-inflammatory cytokines also plays a crucial role in mediating the "balance" necessary for regulating the epithelial fluid lining. Studies have shown that there is an increased mortality when there are reduced levels of "anti-inflammatory" cytokines, such as IL-10 and the IL-1 receptor antagonists (117). Much work is needed to understand the diverse and redundant roles of cytokines in disease progression. Nonetheless, pro-inflammatory cytokines seem to reduce the total expression, apical localization, and activity of ENaC in the lungs *via* multiple mechanisms (**Figure 1**). Given the prominent role for ENaC in maintaining alveolar fluid levels, understanding how inflammatory cytokines regulate ENaC will allow for the development of therapies to treat these complex diseases.

AUTHOR CONTRIBUTIONS

BW and DE conceived and wrote the manuscript. LZ, VL, H-PM, and RH edited and approved the manuscript.

REFERENCES

1. West JB. Comparative physiology of the pulmonary circulation. *Compr Physiol* (2011) 1:1525–39. doi:10.1002/cphy.c090001
2. KH SNaA. *The Structure of the Lungs Relative to Their Principle Function.* Philadelphia, PA: Saunders (1988).
3. Matthay MA, Folkesson HG, Clerici C. Lung epithelial fluid transport and the resolution of pulmonary edema. *Physiol Rev* (2002) 82:569–600. doi:10.1152/physrev.00003.2002
4. Phalen RF, Oldham MJ. Tracheobronchial airway structure as revealed by casting techniques. *Am Rev Respir Dis* (1983) 128:S1–4.
5. Eaton DC, Helms MN, Koval M, Bao HF, Jain L. The contribution of epithelial sodium channels to alveolar function in health and disease. *Annu Rev Physiol* (2009) 71:403–23. doi:10.1146/annurev.physiol.010908.163250
6. Borok Z, Liebler JM, Lubman RL, Foster MJ, Zhou B, Li X, et al. Na transport proteins are expressed by rat alveolar epithelial type I cells. *Am J Physiol Lung Cell Mol Physiol* (2002) 282:L599–608. doi:10.1152/ajplung.00130.2000
7. Flodby P, Kim YH, Beard LL, Gao D, Ji Y, Kage H, et al. Knockout mice reveal a major role for alveolar epithelial type I cells in alveolar fluid clearance. *Am J Respir Cell Mol Biol* (2016) 55:395–406. doi:10.1165/rcmb.2016-0005OC
8. Helms MN, Chen XJ, Ramosevac S, Eaton DC, Jain L. Dopamine regulation of amiloride-sensitive sodium channels in lung cells. *Am J Physiol Lung Cell Mol Physiol* (2006) 290:L710–22. doi:10.1152/ajplung.00486.2004
9. Helms MN, Self J, Bao HF, Job LC, Jain L, Eaton DC. Dopamine activates amiloride-sensitive sodium channels in alveolar type I cells in lung slice preparations. *Am J Physiol Lung Cell Mol Physiol* (2006) 291:L610–8. doi:10.1152/ajplung.00426.2005
10. Johnson MD, Bao HF, Helms MN, Chen XJ, Tigue Z, Jain L, et al. Functional ion channels in pulmonary alveolar type I cells support a role for type I cells in lung ion transport. *Proc Natl Acad Sci U S A* (2006) 103:4964–9. doi:10.1073/pnas.0600855103
11. Adir Y, Welch LC, Dumasius V, Factor P, Sznajder JI, Ridge KM. Overexpression of the Na-K-ATPase alpha2-subunit improves lung liquid clearance during ventilation-induced lung injury. *Am J Physiol Lung Cell Mol Physiol* (2008) 294:L1233–7. doi:10.1152/ajplung.00076.2007
12. Comellas AP, Kelly AM, Trejo HE, Briva A, Lee J, Sznajder JI, et al. Insulin regulates alveolar epithelial function by inducing Na+/K+-ATPase translocation to the plasma membrane in a process mediated by the action of Akt. *J Cell Sci* (2010) 123:1343–51. doi:10.1242/jcs.066464
13. Gusarova GA, Trejo HE, Dada LA, Briva A, Welch LC, Hamanaka RB, et al. Hypoxia leads to Na,K-ATPase downregulation via Ca(2+) release-activated Ca(2+) channels and AMPK activation. *Mol Cell Biol* (2011) 31:3546–56. doi:10.1128/MCB.05114-11
14. Lecuona E, Sun H, Chen J, Trejo HE, Baker MA, Sznajder JI. Protein kinase A-Ialpha regulates Na,K-ATPase endocytosis in alveolar epithelial cells exposed to high CO(2) concentrations. *Am J Respir Cell Mol Biol* (2013) 48:626–34. doi:10.1165/rcmb.2012-0373OC
15. Lecuona E, Trejo HE, Sznajder JI. Regulation of Na,K-ATPase during acute lung injury. *J Bioenerg Biomembr* (2007) 39:391–5. doi:10.1007/s10863-007-9102-1
16. Berthiaume Y, Staub NC, Matthay MA. Beta-adrenergic agonists increase lung liquid clearance in anesthetized sheep. *J Clin Invest* (1987) 79:335–43. doi:10.1172/JCI112817

17. Finley N, Norlin A, Baines DL, Folkesson HG. Alveolar epithelial fluid clearance is mediated by endogenous catecholamines at birth in guinea pigs. *J Clin Invest* (1998) 101:972–81. doi:10.1172/JCI1478
18. Jain L, Chen XJ, Malik B, Al-Khalili O, Eaton DC. Antisense oligonucleotides against the alpha-subunit of ENaC decrease lung epithelial cation-channel activity. *Am J Physiol* (1999) 276:L1046–51.
19. Jayr C, Garat C, Meignan M, Pittet JF, Zelter M, Matthay MA. Alveolar liquid and protein clearance in anesthetized ventilated rats. *J Appl Physiol (1985)* (1994) 76:2636–42.
20. Matalon S. Mechanisms and regulation of ion transport in adult mammalian alveolar type II pneumocytes. *Am J Physiol* (1991) 261:C727–38.
21. Matalon S, Bridges RJ, Benos DJ. Amiloride-inhibitable Na+ conductive pathways in alveolar type II pneumocytes. *Am J Physiol* (1991) 260:L90–6.
22. Butterworth MB. Regulation of the epithelial sodium channel (ENaC) by membrane trafficking. *Biochim Biophys Acta* (2010) 1802:1166–77. doi:10.1016/j.bbadis.2010.03.010
23. Hummler E, Barker P, Gatzy J, Beermann F, Verdumo C, Schmidt A, et al. Early death due to defective neonatal lung liquid clearance in alpha-ENaC-deficient mice. *Nat Genet* (1996) 12:325–8. doi:10.1038/ng0396-325
24. Kerem E, Bistritzer T, Hanukoglu A, Hofmann T, Zhou Z, Bennett W, et al. Pulmonary epithelial sodium-channel dysfunction and excess airway liquid in pseudohypoaldosteronism. *N Engl J Med* (1999) 341:156–62. doi:10.1056/NEJM199907153410304
25. Boase NA, Rychkov GY, Townley SL, Dinudom A, Candi E, Voss AK, et al. Respiratory distress and perinatal lethality in Nedd4-2-deficient mice. *Nat Commun* (2011) 2:287. doi:10.1038/ncomms1284
26. Mall M, Grubb BR, Harkema JR, O'Neal WK, Boucher RC. Increased airway epithelial Na+ absorption produces cystic fibrosis-like lung disease in mice. *Nat Med* (2004) 10:487–93. doi:10.1038/nm1028
27. Auberson M, Hoffmann-Pochon N, Vandewalle A, Kellenberger S, Schild L. Epithelial Na+ channel mutants causing Liddle's syndrome retain ability to respond to aldosterone and vasopressin. *Am J Physiol Renal Physiol* (2003) 285:F459–71. doi:10.1152/ajprenal.00071.2003
28. Kucher V, Boiko N, Pochynyuk O, Stockand JD. Voltage-dependent gating underlies loss of ENaC function in pseudohypoaldosteronism type 1. *Biophys J* (2011) 100:1930–9. doi:10.1016/j.bpj.2011.02.046
29. Frindt G, Palmer LG. Acute effects of aldosterone on the epithelial Na channel in rat kidney. *Am J Physiol Renal Physiol* (2015) 308:F572–8. doi:10.1152/ajprenal.00585.2014
30. Itani OA, Auerbach SD, Husted RF, Volk KA, Ageloff S, Knepper MA, et al. Glucocorticoid-stimulated lung epithelial Na(+) transport is associated with regulated ENaC and sgk1 expression. *Am J Physiol Lung Cell Mol Physiol* (2002) 282:L631–41. doi:10.1152/ajplung.00085.2001
31. Jain L, Chen XJ, Ramosevac S, Brown LA, Eaton DC. Expression of highly selective sodium channels in alveolar type II cells is determined by culture conditions. *Am J Physiol Lung Cell Mol Physiol* (2001) 280:L646–58.
32. Kemendy AE, Kleyman TR, Eaton DC. Aldosterone alters the open probability of amiloride-blockable sodium channels in A6 epithelia. *Am J Physiol* (1992) 263:C825–37.
33. Bruns JB, Carattino MD, Sheng S, Maarouf AB, Weisz OA, Pilewski JM, et al. Epithelial Na+ channels are fully activated by furin- and prostasin-dependent release of an inhibitory peptide from the gamma-subunit. *J Biol Chem* (2007) 282:6153–60. doi:10.1074/jbc.M610636200

ACKNOWLEDGMENTS

We would like to thank Dr. Rudolph Lucas for extensive discussions and suggestions.

34. Caldwell RA, Boucher RC, Stutts MJ. Serine protease activation of near-silent epithelial Na+ channels. *Am J Physiol Cell Physiol* (2004) 286:C190–4. doi:10.1152/ajpcell.00342.2003

35. Caldwell RA, Boucher RC, Stutts MJ. Neutrophil elastase activates near-silent epithelial Na+ channels and increases airway epithelial Na+ transport. *Am J Physiol Lung Cell Mol Physiol* (2005) 288:L813–9. doi:10.1152/ajplung.00435.2004

36. Hughey RP, Carattino MD, Kleyman TR. Role of proteolysis in the activation of epithelial sodium channels. *Curr Opin Nephrol Hypertens* (2007) 16:444–50. doi:10.1097/MNH.0b013e32821f6072

37. Sheng S, Maarouf AB, Bruns JB, Hughey RP, Kleyman TR. Functional role of extracellular loop cysteine residues of the epithelial Na+ channel in Na+ self-inhibition. *J Biol Chem* (2007) 282:20180–90. doi:10.1074/jbc.M611761200

38. Rossier BC, Baker ME, Studer RA. Epithelial sodium transport and its control by aldosterone: the story of our internal environment revisited. *Physiol Rev* (2015) 95:297–340. doi:10.1152/physrev.00011.2014

39. Loffing-Cueni D, Flores SY, Sauter D, Daidie D, Siegrist N, Meneton P, et al. Dietary sodium intake regulates the ubiquitin-protein ligase nedd4-2 in the renal collecting system. *J Am Soc Nephrol* (2006) 17:1264–74. doi:10.1681/ASN.2005060659

40. Snyder PM. Intoxicated Na(+) channels. Focus on "ethanol stimulates epithelial sodium channels by elevating reactive oxygen species". *Am J Physiol Cell Physiol* (2012) 303:C1125–6. doi:10.1152/ajpcell.00301.2012

41. Folkesson HG, Norlin A, Wang Y, Abedinpour P, Matthay MA. Dexamethasone and thyroid hormone pretreatment upregulate alveolar epithelial fluid clearance in adult rats. *J Appl Physiol (1985)* (2000) 88:416–24.

42. McTavish N, Getty J, Burchell A, Wilson SM. Glucocorticoids can activate the alpha-ENaC gene promoter independently of SGK1. *Biochem J* (2009) 423:189–97. doi:10.1042/BJ20090366

43. Nakamura K, Stokes JB, McCray PB Jr. Endogenous and exogenous glucocorticoid regulation of ENaC mRNA expression in developing kidney and lung. *Am J Physiol Cell Physiol* (2002) 283:C762–72. doi:10.1152/ajpcell.00029.2002

44. Brennan FE, Fuller PJ. Rapid upregulation of serum and glucocorticoid-regulated kinase (sgk) gene expression by corticosteroids in vivo. *Mol Cell Endocrinol* (2000) 166:129–36. doi:10.1016/S0303-7207(00)00274-4

45. Chen SY, Bhargava A, Mastroberardino L, Meijer OC, Wang J, Buse P, et al. Epithelial sodium channel regulated by aldosterone-induced protein sgk. *Proc Natl Acad Sci U S A* (1999) 96:2514–9. doi:10.1073/pnas.96.5.2514

46. De Bosscher K, Vanden Berghe W, Haegeman G. The interplay between the glucocorticoid receptor and nuclear factor-kappaB or activator protein-1: molecular mechanisms for gene repression. *Endocr Rev* (2003) 24:488–522. doi:10.1210/er.2002-0006

47. McKay LI, Cidlowski JA. Molecular control of immune/inflammatory responses: interactions between nuclear factor-kappa B and steroid receptor-signaling pathways. *Endocr Rev* (1999) 20:435–59. doi:10.1210/er.20.4.435

48. Rhen T, Cidlowski JA. Antiinflammatory action of glucocorticoids – new mechanisms for old drugs. *N Engl J Med* (2005) 353:1711–23. doi:10.1056/NEJMra050541

49. Tanabe T, Tohnai N. Cyclooxygenase isozymes and their gene structures and expression. *Prostaglandins Other Lipid Mediat* (2002) 68-69:95–114. doi:10.1016/S0090-6980(02)00024-2

50. Schwartze JT, Becker S, Sakkas E, Wujak LA, Niess G, Usemann J, et al. Glucocorticoids recruit Tgfbr3 and Smad1 to shift transforming growth factor-beta signaling from the Tgfbr1/Smad2/3 axis to the Acvrl1/Smad1 axis in lung fibroblasts. *J Biol Chem* (2014) 289:3262–75. doi:10.1074/jbc.M113.541052

51. Halwani R, Al-Muhsen S, Al-Jahdali H, Hamid Q. Role of transforming growth factor-beta in airway remodeling in asthma. *Am J Respir Cell Mol Biol* (2011) 44:127–33. doi:10.1165/rcmb.2010-0027TR

52. Matsuki K, Hathaway CK, Lawrence MG, Smithies O, Kakoki M. The role of transforming growth factor beta1 in the regulation of blood pressure. *Curr Hypertens Rev* (2014) 10:223–38. doi:10.2174/1573402110041503191233313

53. Thomas PS. Tumour necrosis factor-alpha: the role of this multi-functional cytokine in asthma. *Immunol Cell Biol* (2001) 79:132–40. doi:10.1046/j.1440-1711.2001.00980.x

54. Yanagisawa J, Yanagi Y, Masuhiro Y, Suzawa M, Watanabe M, Kashiwagi K, et al. Convergence of transforming growth factor-beta and vitamin D signaling pathways on SMAD transcriptional coactivators. *Science* (1999) 283:1317–21. doi:10.1126/science.283.5406.1317

55. Wittekindt OH. Tight junctions in pulmonary epithelia during lung inflammation. *Pflugers Arch* (2017) 469:135–47. doi:10.1007/s00424-016-1917-3

56. Martin TR, Frevert CW. Innate immunity in the lungs. *Proc Am Thorac Soc* (2005) 2:403–11. doi:10.1513/pats.200508-090JS

57. Cromwell O, Hamid Q, Corrigan CJ, Barkans J, Meng Q, Collins PD, et al. Expression and generation of interleukin-8, IL-6 and granulocyte-macrophage colony-stimulating factor by bronchial epithelial cells and enhancement by IL-1 beta and tumour necrosis factor-alpha. *Immunology* (1992) 77:330–7.

58. Kato A, Schleimer RP. Beyond inflammation: airway epithelial cells are at the interface of innate and adaptive immunity. *Curr Opin Immunol* (2007) 19:711–20. doi:10.1016/j.coi.2007.08.004

59. Chen XJ, Seth S, Yue G, Kamat P, Compans RW, Guidot D, et al. Influenza virus inhibits ENaC and lung fluid clearance. *Am J Physiol Lung Cell Mol Physiol* (2004) 287:L366–73. doi:10.1152/ajplung.00011.2004

60. Eisenhut M, Sidaras D, Barton P, Newland P, Southern KW. Elevated sweat sodium associated with pulmonary oedema in meningococcal sepsis. *Eur J Clin Invest* (2004) 34:576–9. doi:10.1111/j.1365-2362.2004.01386.x

61. Eisenhut M, Southern KW. Positive sweat test following meningococcal septicaemia. *Acta Paediatr* (2002) 91:361–2. doi:10.1111/j.1651-2227.2002.tb01731.x

62. Eisenhut M, Wallace H, Barton P, Gaillard E, Newland P, Diver M, et al. Pulmonary edema in meningococcal septicemia associated with reduced epithelial chloride transport. *Pediatr Crit Care Med* (2006) 7:119–24. doi:10.1097/01.PCC.0000200944.98424.E0

63. Belshe RB. Influenza prevention and treatment: current practices and new horizons. *Ann Intern Med* (1999) 131:621–4. doi:10.7326/0003-4819-131-8-199910190-00013

64. Doyle WJ, Skoner DP, Hayden F, Buchman CA, Seroky JT, Fireman P. Nasal and otologic effects of experimental influenza A virus infection. *Ann Otol Rhinol Laryngol* (1994) 103:59–69. doi:10.1177/000348949410300111

65. Greenberg SB. Respiratory viral infections in adults. *Curr Opin Pulm Med* (2002) 8:201–8. doi:10.1097/00063198-200205000-00009

66. Helms MN, Yu L, Malik B, Kleinhenz DJ, Hart CM, Eaton DC. Role of SGK1 in nitric oxide inhibition of ENaC in Na+-transporting epithelia. *Am J Physiol Cell Physiol* (2005) 289:C717–26. doi:10.1152/ajpcell.00006.2005

67. Matalon S, Hardiman KM, Jain L, Eaton DC, Kotlikoff M, Eu JP, et al. Regulation of ion channel structure and function by reactive oxygen-nitrogen species. *Am J Physiol Lung Cell Mol Physiol* (2003) 285:L1184–9. doi:10.1152/ajplung.00281.2003

68. Helms MN, Jain L, Self JL, Eaton DC. Redox regulation of epithelial sodium channels examined in alveolar type 1 and 2 cells patch-clamped in lung slice tissue. *J Biol Chem* (2008) 283:22875–83. doi:10.1074/jbc.M801363200

69. Yu L, Bao HF, Self JL, Eaton DC, Helms MN. Aldosterone-induced increases in superoxide production counters nitric oxide inhibition of epithelial Na channel activity in A6 distal nephron cells. *Am J Physiol Renal Physiol* (2007) 293:F1666–77. doi:10.1152/ajprenal.00444.2006

70. Takemura Y, Goodson P, Bao HF, Jain L, Helms MN. Rac1-mediated NADPH oxidase release of O2- regulates epithelial sodium channel activity in the alveolar epithelium. *Am J Physiol Lung Cell Mol Physiol* (2010) 298:L509–20. doi:10.1152/ajplung.00230.2009

71. Meduri GU, Kohler G, Headley S, Tolley E, Stentz F, Postlethwaite A. Inflammatory cytokines in the BAL of patients with ARDS. Persistent elevation over time predicts poor outcome. *Chest* (1995) 108:1303–14. doi:10.1378/chest.108.5.1303

72. Hamacher J, Lucas R, Lijnen HR, Buschke S, Dunant Y, Wendel A, et al. Tumor necrosis factor-alpha and angiostatin are mediators of endothelial cytotoxicity in bronchoalveolar lavages of patients with acute respiratory distress syndrome. *Am J Respir Crit Care Med* (2002) 166:651–6. doi:10.1164/rccm.2109004

73. Horgan MJ, Palace GP, Everitt JE, Malik AB. TNF-alpha release in endotoxemia contributes to neutrophil-dependent pulmonary edema. *Am J Physiol* (1993) 264:H1161–5.

74. McRitchie DI, Isowa N, Edelson JD, Xavier AM, Cai L, Man HY, et al. Production of tumour necrosis factor alpha by primary cultured rat alveolar epithelial cells. *Cytokine* (2000) 12:644–54. doi:10.1006/cyto.1999.0656

75. Dagenais A, Frechette R, Yamagata Y, Yamagata T, Carmel JF, Clermont ME, et al. Downregulation of ENaC activity and expression by TNF-alpha in alveolar epithelial cells. *Am J Physiol Lung Cell Mol Physiol* (2004) 286:L301–11. doi:10.1152/ajplung.00326.2002

76. Elia N, Tapponnier M, Matthay MA, Hamacher J, Pache JC, Brundler MA, et al. Functional identification of the alveolar edema reabsorption activity of murine tumor necrosis factor-alpha. *Am J Respir Crit Care Med* (2003) 168:1043–50. doi:10.1164/rccm.200206-618OC

77. Fukuda N, Jayr C, Lazrak A, Wang Y, Lucas R, Matalon S, et al. Mechanisms of TNF-alpha stimulation of amiloride-sensitive sodium transport across alveolar epithelium. *Am J Physiol Lung Cell Mol Physiol* (2001) 280:L1258–65.

78. Yamagata T, Yamagata Y, Nishimoto T, Hirano T, Nakanishi M, Minakata Y, et al. The regulation of amiloride-sensitive epithelial sodium channels by tumor necrosis factor-alpha in injured lungs and alveolar type II cells. *Respir Physiol Neurobiol* (2009) 166:16–23. doi:10.1016/j.resp.2008.12.008

79. Lassalle P, Gosset P, Delneste Y, Tsicopoulos A, Capron A, Joseph M, et al. Modulation of adhesion molecule expression on endothelial cells during the late asthmatic reaction: role of macrophage-derived tumour necrosis factor-alpha. *Clin Exp Immunol* (1993) 94:105–10. doi:10.1111/j.1365-2249.1993.tb05985.x

80. Pober JS, Gimbrone MA Jr, Lapierre LA, Mendrick DL, Fiers W, Rothlein R, et al. Overlapping patterns of activation of human endothelial cells by interleukin 1, tumor necrosis factor, and immune interferon. *J Immunol* (1986) 137:1893–6.

81. Rokkam D, Lafemina MJ, Lee JW, Matthay MA, Frank JA. Claudin-4 levels are associated with intact alveolar fluid clearance in human lungs. *Am J Pathol* (2011) 179:1081–7. doi:10.1016/j.ajpath.2011.05.017

82. Mazzon E, Cuzzocrea S. Role of TNF-alpha in lung tight junction alteration in mouse model of acute lung inflammation. *Respir Res* (2007) 8:75. doi:10.1186/1465-9921-8-75

83. Czikora I, Alli A, Bao HF, Kaftan D, Sridhar S, Apell HJ, et al. A novel tumor necrosis factor-mediated mechanism of direct epithelial sodium channel activation. *Am J Respir Crit Care Med* (2014) 190:522–32. doi:10.1164/rccm.201405-0833OC

84. Yang G, Hamacher J, Gorshkov B, White R, Sridhar S, Verin A, et al. The dual role of TNF in pulmonary edema. *J Cardiovasc Dis Res* (2010) 1:29–36. doi:10.4103/0975-3583.59983

85. Braun C, Hamacher J, Morel DR, Wendel A, Lucas R. Dichotomal role of TNF in experimental pulmonary edema reabsorption. *J Immunol* (2005) 175:3402–8. doi:10.4049/jimmunol.175.5.3402

86. Rezaiguia S, Garat C, Delclaux C, Meignan M, Fleury J, Legrand P, et al. Acute bacterial pneumonia in rats increases alveolar epithelial fluid clearance by a tumor necrosis factor-alpha-dependent mechanism. *J Clin Invest* (1997) 99:325–35. doi:10.1172/JCI119161

87. Tillie-Leblond I, Guery BP, Janin A, Leberre R, Just N, Pittet JF, et al. Chronic bronchial allergic inflammation increases alveolar liquid clearance by TNF-alpha-dependent mechanism. *Am J Physiol Lung Cell Mol Physiol* (2002) 283:L1303–9. doi:10.1152/ajplung.00147.2002

88. Wagener BM, Roux J, Carles M, Pittet JF. Synergistic inhibition of beta2-adrenergic receptor-mediated alveolar epithelial fluid transport by interleukin-8 and transforming growth factor-beta. *Anesthesiology* (2015) 122:1084–92. doi:10.1097/ALN.0000000000000595

89. Fahy RJ, Lichtenberger F, McKeegan CB, Nuovo GJ, Marsh CB, Wewers MD. The acute respiratory distress syndrome: a role for transforming growth factor-beta 1. *Am J Respir Cell Mol Biol* (2003) 28:499–503. doi:10.1165/rcmb.2002-0092OC

90. Wakefield LM, Letterio JJ, Chen T, Danielpour D, Allison RS, Pai LH, et al. Transforming growth factor-beta1 circulates in normal human plasma and is unchanged in advanced metastatic breast cancer. *Clin Cancer Res* (1995) 1:129–36.

91. Kaminski N, Allard JD, Pittet JF, Zuo F, Griffiths MJ, Morris D, et al. Global analysis of gene expression in pulmonary fibrosis reveals distinct programs regulating lung inflammation and fibrosis. *Proc Natl Acad Sci U S A* (2000) 97:1778–83. doi:10.1073/pnas.97.4.1778

92. Annes JP, Chen Y, Munger JS, Rifkin DB. Integrin alphaVbeta6-mediated activation of latent TGF-beta requires the latent TGF-beta binding protein-1. *J Cell Biol* (2004) 165:723–34. doi:10.1083/jcb.200312172

93. Annes JP, Rifkin DB, Munger JS. The integrin alphaVbeta6 binds and activates latent TGFbeta3. *FEBS Lett* (2002) 511:65–8. doi:10.1016/S0014-5793(01)03280-X

94. Munger JS, Huang X, Kawakatsu H, Griffiths MJ, Dalton SL, Wu J, et al. The integrin alpha v beta 6 binds and activates latent TGF beta 1: a mechanism for regulating pulmonary inflammation and fibrosis. *Cell* (1999) 96:319–28. doi:10.1016/S0092-8674(00)80545-0

95. Breuss JM, Gallo J, DeLisser HM, Klimanskaya IV, Folkesson HG, Pittet JF, et al. Expression of the beta 6 integrin subunit in development, neoplasia and tissue repair suggests a role in epithelial remodeling. *J Cell Sci* (1995) 108(Pt 6):2241–51.

96. Barcellos-Hoff MH, Dix TA. Redox-mediated activation of latent transforming growth factor-beta 1. *Mol Endocrinol* (1996) 10:1077–83. doi:10.1210/me.10.9.1077

97. Frank J, Roux J, Kawakatsu H, Su G, Dagenais A, Berthiaume Y, et al. Transforming growth factor-beta1 decreases expression of the epithelial sodium channel alphaENaC and alveolar epithelial vectorial sodium and fluid transport via an ERK1/2-dependent mechanism. *J Biol Chem* (2003) 278:43939–50. doi:10.1074/jbc.M304882200

98. Pittet JF, Griffiths MJ, Geiser T, Kaminski N, Dalton SL, Huang X, et al. TGF-beta is a critical mediator of acute lung injury. *J Clin Invest* (2001) 107:1537–44. doi:10.1172/JCI11963

99. Peters DM, Vadasz I, Wujak L, Wygrecka M, Olschewski A, Becker C, et al. TGF-beta directs trafficking of the epithelial sodium channel ENaC which has implications for ion and fluid transport in acute lung injury. *Proc Natl Acad Sci U S A* (2014) 111:E374–83. doi:10.1073/pnas.1306798111

100. Frank JA, Matthay MA. TGF-beta and lung fluid balance in ARDS. *Proc Natl Acad Sci U S A* (2014) 111:885–6. doi:10.1073/pnas.1322478111

101. Galietta LJ, Folli C, Marchetti C, Romano L, Carpani D, Conese M, et al. Modification of transepithelial ion transport in human cultured bronchial epithelial cells by interferon-gamma. *Am J Physiol Lung Cell Mol Physiol* (2000) 278:L1186–94.

102. Olman MA, White KE, Ware LB, Cross MT, Zhu S, Matthay MA. Microarray analysis indicates that pulmonary edema fluid from patients with acute lung injury mediates inflammation, mitogen gene expression, and fibroblast proliferation through bioactive interleukin-1. *Chest* (2002) 121:69S–70S. doi:10.1378/chest.121.3_suppl.69S

103. Pugin J, Ricou B, Steinberg KP, Suter PM, Martin TR. Proinflammatory activity in bronchoalveolar lavage fluids from patients with ARDS, a prominent role for interleukin-1. *Am J Respir Crit Care Med* (1996) 153:1850–6. doi:10.1164/ajrccm.153.6.8665045

104. Pugin J, Verghese G, Widmer MC, Matthay MA. The alveolar space is the site of intense inflammatory and profibrotic reactions in the early phase of acute respiratory distress syndrome. *Crit Care Med* (1999) 27:304–12. doi:10.1097/00003246-199902000-00036

105. Siler TM, Swierkosz JE, Hyers TM, Fowler AA, Webster RO. Immunoreactive interleukin-1 in bronchoalveolar lavage fluid of high-risk patients and patients with the adult respiratory distress syndrome. *Exp Lung Res* (1989) 15:881–94. doi:10.3109/01902148909069633

106. Suter PM, Suter S, Girardin E, Roux-Lombard P, Grau GE, Dayer JM. High bronchoalveolar levels of tumor necrosis factor and its inhibitors, interleukin-1, interferon, and elastase, in patients with adult respiratory distress syndrome after trauma, shock, or sepsis. *Am Rev Respir Dis* (1992) 145:1016–22. doi:10.1164/ajrccm/145.5.1016

107. Gonzales JN, Lucas R, Verin AD. The acute respiratory distress syndrome: mechanisms and perspective therapeutic approaches. *Austin J Vasc Med* (2015) 2:1009.

108. Lee YM, Hybertson BM, Cho HG, Terada LS, Cho O, Repine AJ, et al. Platelet-activating factor contributes to acute lung leak in rats given interleukin-1 intratracheally. *Am J Physiol Lung Cell Mol Physiol* (2000) 279:L75–80.

109. Hybertson BM, Lee YM, Cho HG, Cho OJ, Repine JE. Alveolar type II cell abnormalities and peroxide formation in lungs of rats given IL-1 intratracheally. *Inflammation* (2000) 24:289–303. doi:10.1023/A:1007092529261

110. Leff JA, Bodman ME, Cho OJ, Rohrbach S, Reiss OK, Vannice JL, et al. Post-insult treatment with interleukin-1 receptor antagonist decreases oxidative lung injury in rats given intratracheal interleukin-1. *Am J Respir Crit Care Med* (1994) 150:109–12. doi:10.1164/ajrccm.150.1.8025734

111. Repine JE. Interleukin-1-mediated acute lung injury and tolerance to oxidative injury. *Environ Health Perspect* (1994) 102(Suppl 10):75–8. doi:10.1289/ehp.94102s1075

112. Roux J, Kawakatsu H, Gartland B, Pespeni M, Sheppard D, Matthay MA, et al. Interleukin-1beta decreases expression of the epithelial sodium channel alpha-subunit in alveolar epithelial cells via a p38 MAPK-dependent signaling pathway. *J Biol Chem* (2005) 280:18579–89. doi:10.1074/jbc.M410561200

113. Galam L, Soundararajan R, Breitzig M, Rajan A, Yeruva RR, Czachor A, et al. SOCS-1 rescues IL-1beta-mediated suppression of epithelial sodium channel in mouse lung epithelial cells via ASK-1. *Oncotarget* (2016) 7:29081–91. doi:10.18632/oncotarget.8543

114. Ganter MT, Ware LB, Howard M, Roux J, Gartland B, Matthay MA, et al. Extracellular heat shock protein 72 is a marker of the stress protein response in acute lung injury. *Am J Physiol Lung Cell Mol Physiol* (2006) 291:L354–61. doi:10.1152/ajplung.00405.2005

115. Howard M, Roux J, Iles KE, Miyazawa B, Christiaans S, Anjum N, et al. Activation of the heat shock response attenuates the interleukin 1β-mediated inhibition of the amiloride-sensitive alveolar epithelial ion transport. *Shock* (2013) 39:189–96. doi:10.1097/SHK.0b013e31827e8ea3

116. Galietta LJ, Pagesy P, Folli C, Caci E, Romio L, Costes B, et al. IL-4 is a potent modulator of ion transport in the human bronchial epithelium in vitro. *J Immunol* (2002) 168:839–45. doi:10.4049/jimmunol.168.2.839

117. Donnelly SC, Strieter RM, Reid PT, Kunkel SL, Burdick MD, Armstrong I, et al. The association between mortality rates and decreased concentrations of interleukin-10 and interleukin-1 receptor antagonist in the lung fluids of patients with the adult respiratory distress syndrome. *Ann Intern Med* (1996) 125:191–6. doi:10.7326/0003-4819-125-3-199608010-00005

15

The Role of Transient Receptor Potential Vanilloid 4 in Pulmonary Inflammatory Diseases

Rachel G. Scheraga, Brian D. Southern, Lisa M. Grove and Mitchell A. Olman*

Cleveland Clinic, Department of Pathobiology, Lerner Research Institute, Cleveland, OH, USA

*Correspondence:
Mitchell A. Olman
olmanm@ccf.org

Ion channels/pumps are essential regulators of organ homeostasis and disease. In the present review, we discuss the role of the mechanosensitive cation channel, transient receptor potential vanilloid 4 (TRPV4), in cytokine secretion and pulmonary inflammatory diseases such as asthma, cystic fibrosis (CF), and acute lung injury/acute respiratory distress syndrome (ARDS). TRPV4 has been shown to play a role in lung diseases associated with lung parenchymal stretch or stiffness. TRPV4 indirectly mediates hypotonicity-induced smooth muscle contraction and airway remodeling in asthma. Further, the literature suggests that in CF TRPV4 may improve ciliary beat frequency enhancing mucociliary clearance, while at the same time increasing pro-inflammatory cytokine secretion/lung tissue injury. Currently it is understood that the role of TRPV4 in immune cell function and associated lung tissue injury/ARDS may depend on the injury stimulus. Uncovering the downstream mechanisms of TRPV4 action in pulmonary inflammatory diseases is likely important to understanding disease pathogenesis and may lead to novel therapeutics.

Keywords: transient receptor potential vanilloid 4, ion channels, asthma, pulmonary vascular disease, acute respiratory distress syndrome

INTRODUCTION

Ion channels and pumps play multiple important roles in cell homeostasis (1). They function to allow passive, agonist-induced, or voltage-dependent flux of specific ions in and out of the cell (1, 2). Dysregulation of channel function and/or expression can lead to organ dysfunction and disease (1–3). Recent studies have shown that a transient receptor potential (TRP) channel family member, transient receptor potential vanilloid 4 (TRPV4), is implicated in inflammatory lung diseases such as asthma, cystic fibrosis (CF), acute lung injury/acute respiratory distress syndrome (ARDS), and pulmonary fibrosis (4–10). In fact, these studies show that TRPV4 can regulate inflammatory cytokines that play key roles in orchestrating lung tissue homeostasis and inflammatory lung disease (4, 7, 10–14). Dysregulation of cytokines leads to alterations in cell–cell interactions, lung tissue remodeling, and repair (15). Regulating cytokine secretion through the modulation of ion channels such as TRPV4 may mediate inflammatory lung diseases. Therefore, TRPV4 may be a potential target for lung disease pathogenesis (16). This review summarizes and integrates the data from our laboratory and others to further the understanding of the TRPV4–cytokine interaction in pulmonary inflammation.

THE TRPV4 CHANNEL

Intracellular calcium is tightly regulated in a spatiotemporal manner through a system of ion channels and membrane pumps (17). One such channel is TRPV4, a transmembrane (TM) cation channel of the TRP superfamily (18). TRPV4 is an 871 amino acid protein that has 6 TM domains, an ion pore located between TM5 and 6, an NH_2 terminal intracellular sequence with several ankyrin-type repeats, and a COOH-terminal intracellular tail (19, 20). Both the NH_2 and COOH termini interact with signal kinases, other molecules [e.g., nitric oxide (NO)], and scaffolding proteins (21). The intracellular tails contain several activity-modifying phosphorylation sites. TRPV4 is sensitized and activated by both chemical [5,6-epoxyeicosatrienoic acid (EET) and 4 alpha-phorbol 12,13-didecanoate (4-αPDD)] and physical stimuli (temperature 27–35°C, membrane stretch, and hypotonicity) (22–25). TRPV4 is ubiquitously expressed in many cell types in the respiratory system. In the setting of pulmonary inflammation, TRPV4 has been found to be highly expressed and upregulated in airway smooth muscle, vascular endothelial cells, alveolar epithelial cells, and immune cells such as macrophages and neutrophils (12, 16, 21, 26–28). TRPV4 has been implicated in the pathogenesis of asthma, CF, and sterile and infection-associated ARDS (4–10, 29).

THE ROLE OF TRPV4 IN INFLAMMATORY LUNG DISEASES

Asthma

Asthma is a chronic lung disease characterized by airway inflammation and remodeling, excess bronchial secretions, and smooth muscle hypertrophy and contraction leading to airway narrowing (bronchoconstriction). Recent work shows that TRPV4 mediates airway wall thickness, goblet cell recruitment, collagen expression, fibrotic airway remodeling, and increased expression of transforming growth factor-β (TGF-β) in a house dust mite (*Dermatophagoides farinae*) mouse model of asthma (30). The authors also show that TRPV4 mediates TGF-β-dependent myofibroblast differentiation *in vitro* through the ras homolog gene family member A (RhoA), p38, and PI3Kα (30). *In vitro* exposure of airway smooth muscle or tracheal rings to hypotonic solutions causes smooth muscle cell contraction, and some asthmatic patients are hypersensitive to this stimulus. To that end, it has been found that small nucleotide polymorphisms in the G allele in the coding region and 3′ flanking region of the TRPV4 gene, as first identified in COPD, are associated with a greater reduction in pulmonary function after hypotonic saline administration (8, 31). Interestingly, the calcium and contractile response of smooth muscle cells to hypotonic saline involves interactions between the cysteinyl leukotriene pathway and TRPV4 (12, 32). These findings suggest that downregulation of TRPV4 may be a therapeutic target in some etiologies and genetic variants of asthma. Of note, different TRPV4 activation stimuli beyond hypotonicity utilize different pathways for TRPV4 activation. For example, hypotonicity induces TRPV4 activation through phospholipase A2 (PLA2)/P450

epoxygenase-dependent generation of EETs, while heat and 4αPDD are PLA2/P450-independent (25). Further study of the mode of TRPV4 activation in individual diseases would support disease-specific, pathway-targeted therapy. While asthma is an inflammatory disease, there is no current evidence linking Th2-type cytokines and TRPV4 in the pathogenesis of asthma. Hence, this is an avenue for future studies.

Cystic Fibrosis

Cystic fibrosis is characterized by a mutation in the cystic fibrosis transmembrane conductance regulator (CFTR), a membrane-based chloride channel, which initially causes dehydration of the airway surface liquid thereby increasing susceptibility to bacterial and fungal infections (e.g., *Pseudomonas*, *Staphylococcus*, *Burkholderia*, atypical mycobacterium) (33). TRPV4 interacts with CFTR on several levels. TRPV4-dependent calcium influx in response to hypotonicity is reduced in human CF epithelial cells (34). Furthermore, other hypotonicity-induced TRPV4 chemical activators (5,6-, 8,9-, 11,12-, and 14,15-EET) and their metabolites (5,6 DHET) have been measured in the sputum of CF patients (10). Although the current consensus suggests that dehydration of airway mucous is the predominant cause of impaired mucociliary clearance in CF, recent considerations have been put forth to increase ciliary function or ciliary beat frequency (CBF) as a means to improve mucociliary clearance (35, 36). Concordantly, TRPV4-deleted tracheal epithelial cells have decreased CBF in response to ATP, 4αPDD, and temperature, whereas CBF in response to hyperviscosity was similar in wild-type (WT) and TRPV4 deleted cells. These data suggest that TRPV4 agonism might increase CBF; however, the effects on CF prognosis remain to be determined (37).

The pathogenesis of CF is also characterized by cytokine-mediated airway inflammation. Recently, both cytokines/chemokines and lipid mediators secreted from epithelial cells have been identified as key components in the inflammatory process. In this regard, TRPV4 activation induces epithelial cell secretion of pro-inflammatory cytokines/chemokines and active lipid mediators (e.g., IL-8, cytosolic PLA2, prostaglandin E2, NF-κB, AA, etc.) in response to lipopolysaccharide (LPS) (10). Secretion of IL-8/KC, in both bronchial epithelial cells and in intact mice lungs in response to TPRV4 activation, was increased upon inhibition of CFTR (10). These data demonstrate that TRPV4 has pleotropic effects on CF pathogenesis. Further study of the individual molecular pathways downstream of TRPV4 in CF may identify selectivity in the TRPV4 responses that can then be marshaled for therapeutic intent.

ACUTE LUNG INJURY/ARDS

Acute respiratory distress syndrome is a syndrome characterized by patchy lung inflammation along with cytokine release leading to alveolar space edema, exudate, and collapse. The pathogenesis of ARDS is complex; it is characterized by endothelial and alveolar epithelial injury followed by recruitment and accumulation of inflammatory cells in the injured alveolus (38). ARDS is a consequence of non-infectious (trauma, hemorrhage, lung ventilator stretch) or infectious (sepsis, pneumonia) causes (39).

As the biological processes that underlie the lung injury and their molecular drivers are not fully understood, medical therapy directed at the lung inflammatory response has yet to successfully modify the course of ARDS. Experimental animal and patient studies demonstrate the lung injury and resolution phases of ARDS are mediated through a complex orchestration of cytokines/chemokines (e.g., IL-1β, TNFα, IL-8, IL-6, and IL-10) (40–44). Studies show that both sterile (e.g., ventilator-induced stretch) and infectious [e.g., intra-tracheal (IT) LPS] triggers of ARDS result in stiffening (reduced compliance) of the lung tissue (45, 46).

The role of TRPV4 in ARDS is context/etiology-dependent. It has been shown that TRPV4 mediates the lung injury response to a sterile stimulus *in vivo* [i.e., hydrochloric acid (HCl)], as assessed by inflammatory cell influx, lung vascular permeability (wet/dry ratio, Evans blue dye extravasation, and total protein), lung histopathology and physiology, and pro-inflammatory cytokine levels (IL-1β, VEGF, KC, G-CSF, MCP-1, RANTES, MIP-2, and IL-6) (7, 14). Protection from the acute lung injury response to IT HCl was noted in mice that lack TRPV4 (TRPV4 KO), or in mice that were treated with three different small molecule inhibitors of TRPV4 (7, 14). Importantly, two of these inhibitors (GSK2220691 and GSK2337429A) show efficacy when administered 30 min after IT HCl (7). Thus, these inhibitors show promise as a novel and exciting therapeutic/preventative approach for acute lung injury (7). *In vitro* stimulation of human and murine neutrophils (with platelet-activating factor or LPS) induced TRPV4-dependent calcium influx, reactive oxygen species (ROS) production, adhesion chemotaxis, and Rac activation (14). Taken together, these data suggest that neutrophils possess the capacity to mediate acute lung injury in a TRPV4-dependent manner. Whether the *in vivo* lung injury response to HCl is solely dependent on neutrophil TRPV4, as opposed to TRPV4 in other cell types, remains to be determined. In addition to TRPV4's effect on the cytokine/inflammatory changes in ARDS, TRPV4 actions can induce lung endothelial barrier dysfunction *in vitro* and *in vivo*, as well as cause disruption of alveolar type I epithelial cells leading to lung vascular leak and alveolar edema (9, 29). These findings are the rationale for a clinical trial of TRPV4 antagonists in high venous pressure-induced pulmonary edema.

TRPV4 AND MACROPHAGE FUNCTION IN LUNG INJURY

A similar TRPV4-dependent lung injury response has been demonstrated in macrophages in high volume ventilator-induced lung injury (6, 47). Mice lacking TRPV4 (TRPV4 KO) had less vascular leak, pulmonary edema (wet/dry ratio, filtration coefficient), and NO production in response to high volumes (peak inflation pressure 35 cm H_2O) when compared to WT controls. TRPV4 also seemed to partially mediate the increase in injury due to the combined effects of high volume ventilation and induced hyperthermia (40°C). Analysis of alveolar macrophages after high volume ventilation revealed that TRPV4 KO macrophages had less production of NO and ROS than those from WT mice. As in the HCl model, pretreatment with a non-selective TRP inhibitor

(ruthenium red) prevented the increase in vascular permeability from combined high volume ventilation/hyperthermia in WT mice (48). Adoptive transfer of WT macrophages to TRPV4 KO mice reestablished the lung injury seen in WT mice. These data suggest that macrophage-specific TRPV4 acts as a mechanical and temperature sensor to initiate/mediate the acute lung injury induced by high volume ventilation (47).

Our laboratory is studying the role of TRPV4 in macrophage function during infection-associated lung injury. Alveolar macrophages are known to be effector cells in bacterial and particle clearance, and in the injury/repair process (49). We chose to explore the role of the calcium ion channel, TRPV4, in macrophage phagocytosis, as intracellular calcium is known to be required for the phagocytic process, and because TRPV4 plays a role in force-dependent cytoskeletal changes in other systems/cell types (7–9, 29, 47, 50, 51). Studies show that the process of phagocytosis in macrophages requires integration of the signals from macrophage surface receptors, pathogens, and the extracellular matrix (52–54). However, the effects of matrix stiffness on the macrophage phenotypic response or its signal transduction pathways have yet to be fully elucidated.

We recently published the novel observation that TRPV4 integrates the LPS and matrix stiffness signals to control macrophage function, which promotes host defense and resolution from lung injury (4). After demonstrating that TRPV4 is expressed and functionally active in murine bone marrow-derived macrophages, we studied the macrophage response to LPS on matrices of varying physiological-range stiffnesses. We demonstrated that TRPV4 mediates LPS-stimulated macrophage phagocytosis of both opsonized particles (IgG-coated latex beads) and non-opsonized particles (*Escherichia coli*) *in vitro*. Matrix stiffness in the range seen in inflamed or fibrotic lung (>25 kPa) augmented the LPS phagocytic response by 151 ± 3% (4). Inhibition of TRPV4 by siRNA or pharmacologic inhibitors completely abrogated both the LPS effect, as well as the matrix stiffness effect, on phagocytosis. These data indicate that both the LPS and stiffness effect on macrophage phagocytosis are TRPV4 dependent (4).

As TRPV4 is required for macrophage phagocytosis *in vitro* in a stiffness-dependent manner, we next sought to examine the role of TRPV4 on macrophage phagocytosis after intratracheally (IT) administered LPS *in vivo*. Despite the influx of neutrophils, alveolar macrophages were the predominant cell type that phagocytosed IT administered IgG-coated beads following IT LPS (24 h) in WT mice (4). As seen *in vitro*, the *in vivo* enhancement effect of IT LPS on alveolar macrophage phagocytosis was lost upon deletion of TRPV4 (TRPV4 KO mice) (**Figure 1**) (4). This effect is not explained by a difference in macrophage recruitment. Concordant with the *in vitro* data, our *in vivo* data demonstrate that LPS-induced alveolar macrophage phagocytosis is TRPV4 dependent.

Studies suggest that macrophage-released cytokines modulate bacterial clearance and the lung injury/repair process, in the context of injury-related stiffened matrix (52–55). Recognizing the complexity of tissue responses to individual cytokines/chemokines, we chose to focus initially on IL-1β and IL-10, as they are well-known key mediators of lung injury/resolution (56–58). TRPV4 also modulates the LPS signal for cytokine production. Specifically, IL-1β secretion was decreased by half,

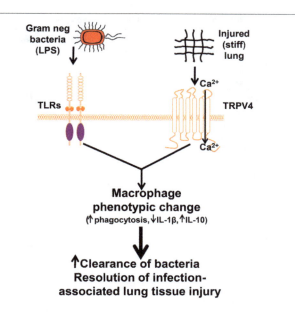

FIGURE 1 | **Working model illustrating that lipopolysaccharide (LPS) and transient receptor potential vanilloid 4 (TRPV4) signal cooperate to alter macrophage phenotypic change leading to enhanced clearance of bacteria and resolution of lung injury**. Our data suggest that TRPV4 is sensitized by extracellular matrix stiffness in the range of inflamed/fibrotic lung. Interaction between the LPS signal and the matrix stiffness signal through TRPV4 promote increased TRPV4 channel activity and macrophage phenotypic change leading to increased clearance of bacteria and resolution of infection-associated lung injury (4).

and IL-10 secretion increased approximately twofold in WT alveolar macrophages compared with TRPV4 KO macrophages in response to LPS. Such a profile would predict that TRPV4 mediates a net inflammation-suppressive response to LPS. Interestingly, this TRPV4 modulation of the LPS signal required a matrix stiffness in the range of injured or fibrotic lung (≥ 25 kPa). As illustrated in the schematic model, macrophage TRPV4 is sensitized by a stiff matrix (as seen in ARDS) to modulate the infectious (LPS—experimental surrogate for Gram-negative bacterial lung infection) signal toward an anti-inflammatory macrophage phenotype (**Figure 1**).

Collectively, our data demonstrate that TRPV4 responds to extracellular matrix stiffness, thereby altering the LPS signal to mediate macrophage phagocytosis and cytokine production (4). Despite the limitations in extrapolating our simplified experimental system to *in vivo* lung injury, the data point to TRPV4 as an important mechanosensor that mediates macrophage function differently in lung homeostasis, and in the context of pulmonary infection-induced inflammation. We speculate that under basal conditions, the resident lung macrophage response to LPS is modified (less phagocytic, more IL-1β) as a consequence of low lung tissue stiffness (i.e., 1–3 kPa) thereby enhancing recruitment of professional bactericidal cells (neutrophils) (55). After an acute inflammatory or infectious insult, a separate population of monocytes is recruited from the bone marrow to populate both interstitial and injured alveolar compartment in the context of denuded, exposed interstitial matrix (40). There are two overlapping phases of ARDS. During the initial injury phase (days 1–10), lung tissue is predominantly edematous and exudative, while during the fibroproliferative phase (days 7–28), there is increased deposition of interstitial and alveolar type I and III collagen (40). Both phases of ARDS (fibroproliferative > acute) exhibit clear evidence of increased stiffness at the whole organ level (40, 46, 59), but, limited mechanical data are available at the cellular level of resolution. A recent study shows that lung alveolar vessel wall stiffness is increased >10-fold (3 versus 43 kPa) after IT LPS (48 h) in mice compared to controls, as measured by atomic force microscopy, well within the range examined in our study (>8–25 kPa) (45, 46). We further speculate that, after injury, the macrophage phagocytic response to LPS is upregulated along with a cytokine profile that promotes resolution in a TRPV4-dependent manner as a consequence of tissue stiffening. Such a scenario would support tissue stiffness, TRPV4-dependent shift in the macrophage phenotype that is commensurate with the appropriate phase of the injury/repair process.

Thus, our findings suggest that TRPV4 regulates a feed-forward mechanism of phagocytosis in activated lung tissue macrophages when they interact with stiffened infection/injury-associated lung matrix. This concept is further supported by the observation that surfactant protein B-deficient mice have altered alveolar macrophage shape and function in association with increased alveolar surface tension (60). The macrophage activation phenotypes (M1/M2 classification) are well established *in vitro*. The classically activated M1 macrophage phenotype, induced by INFγ, TNFα, and LPS, exhibits inflammatory/bactericidal properties. In contrast, the alternatively activated M2 macrophage phenotype, induced by IL-4 and IL-13, exhibits tissue repair/fibrotic properties (49, 55). Data are emerging that the *in vivo* macrophage phenotypes are more heterogeneous and plastic than the *in vitro* derived M1/M2 classification. Our published cytokine data (↑IL-1β, ↓IL-10) with inhibition of TRPV4 indeed suggests that TRPV4 mediates polarization toward M1-like phenotype (4, 61, 62). However, a complex array of cytokines contributes to the pathogenesis of ARDS, and targeting individual cytokines has not been shown to alter the disease process, indicating the net inflammatory balance is important (41–44, 63).

Our findings regarding the role of TRPV4 in downregulating the pro-inflammatory, bacterial clearance-inducing LPS signal are opposite to those in neutrophils in response to sterile inflammation, or in macrophages upon stretch-induced tissue injury. Lung injury is dependent on cytokine production and inflammatory cell influx in response to activation of pattern recognition receptors by damage-associated molecular patterns (DAMPs) and pathogen-associated molecular patterns (PAMPs). There are multiple known ligand–receptor interactions and intracellular signaling pathways that are both DAMP/PAMP-receptor specific and overlapping. We speculate that differences in the interaction of TRPV4 signals with infectious PAMP signals versus sterile tissue injury DAMP signals might explain the differences between our infectious model and the sterile lung injury model. Defining the specific molecular pathways and interactions in individual injury models is a fruitful avenue of research that may lead to novel therapeutic targets.

TABLE 1 | *In vitro* and *in vivo* studies of the role of transient receptor potential vanilloid 4 (TRPV4) in inflammatory pulmonary diseases.

Disease	Cell type	Key findings	Reference
Asthma	Fibroblasts	Transforming growth factor-β-dependent airway remodeling	(30)
	Smooth muscle cells	Hypotonicity-induced calcium and contractile response	(12, 32)
Cystic fibrosis (CF)	Epithelial cells (tracheal and airway)	Regulates ciliary beat frequency	(10, 33–37)
		Decreased ATP-induced calcium influx	
		Pro-inflammatory cytokine production (e.g., IL-8, cytosolic PLA2, prostaglandin E2, NF-κB, arachidonic acid, etc.)	
Acute lung injury/acute respiratory distress syndrome (ARDS)	Epithelial cells	Maintains epithelial barrier function	(9, 29)
	Endothelial cells	Maintains endothelial septal barrier	(11)
	Neutrophils	Calcium influx	(7, 14)
		Reactive oxygen species production	
		Adhesion chemotaxis	
		Rac activation	
	Macrophages	Lipopolysaccharide-induced macrophage phagocytosis *in vitro* and *in vivo*	(4, 6, 47, 48)
		Anti-inflammatory cytokine production (IL-1β, IL-10)	
Pulmonary fibrosis	Fibroblasts	Myofibroblast differentiation	(5)
		Experimental pulmonary fibrosis in mice	

This table is only a partial representation of the literature, given the focused nature of the mini review. We apologize for any work omitted from this review. We summarize the cited literature on the role of TRPV4 in asthma, CF, acute lung injury/ARDS, and pulmonary fibrosis.

SUMMARY

In summary, ion channels are important in the pathogenesis of inflammatory lung diseases, and the ion channel TRPV4 plays a specific role in mediating lung diseases associated with parenchymal stretch and inflammation or infection. The data reviewed in this work on the role of TRPV4 in pulmonary inflammatory diseases are summarized in **Table 1**. TRPV4 activation and its downstream signaling pathways differ in response to varying stimuli, cell types, and contexts. In asthma, TRPV4 mediates hypotonicity-induced airway hyperresponsiveness, but not release of Th2 cytokines (12, 32). In CF, TRPV4 appears to play important, yet paradoxical, roles in CBF/mucociliary clearance and epithelial cell pro-inflammatory cytokine (IL-8/KC) secretion (35, 36). TRPV4 may also play different roles in ARDS depending on the underlying etiology (4, 7, 14, 48). We, and others, have shown that macrophage and neutrophil TRPV4 regulate

pro-inflammatory cytokine secretion. Lastly, in pulmonary fibrosis, TRPV4 has been shown to mediate the mechanosensing that drives myofibroblast differentiation and experimental lung fibrosis in mice (5). Collectively, TRPV4 is shown to play a novel role in modulating cytokine secretion and pulmonary inflammation and therefore may be involved in the pathogenesis of many respiratory diseases.

AUTHOR CONTRIBUTIONS

RS, BS, LG, and MO reviewed the literature and wrote the paper.

REFERENCES

1. Jentsch TJ, Hubner CA, Fuhrmann JC. Ion channels: function unravelled by dysfunction. *Nat Cell Biol* (2004) 6(11):1039–47. doi:10.1038/ncb1104-1039
2. Hubner CA, Jentsch TJ. Ion channel diseases. *Hum Mol Genet* (2002) 11(20):2435–45. doi:10.1093/hmg/11.20.2435
3. Eisenhut M, Wallace H. Ion channels in inflammation. *Pflugers Arch* (2011) 461(4):401–21. doi:10.1007/s00424-010-0917-y
4. Scheraga RG, Abraham S, Niese KA, Southern BD, Grove LM, Hite RD, et al. TRPV4 mechanosensitive ion channel regulates lipopolysaccharide-stimulated macrophage phagocytosis. *J Immunol* (2016) 196(1):428–36. doi:10.4049/jimmunol.1501688
5. Rahaman SO, Grove LM, Paruchuri S, Southern BD, Abraham S, Niese KA, et al. TRPV4 mediates myofibroblast differentiation and pulmonary fibrosis in mice. *J Clin Invest* (2014) 124(12):5225–38. doi:10.1172/JCI75331
6. Hamanaka K, Jian MY, Weber DS, Alvarez DF, Townsley MI, Al-Mehdi AB, et al. TRPV4 initiates the acute calcium-dependent permeability increase

during ventilator-induced lung injury in isolated mouse lungs. *Am J Physiol Lung Cell Mol Physiol* (2007) 293:L923–32. doi:10.1152/ajplung.00221.2007
7. Balakrishna S, Song W, Achanta S, Doran SF, Liu B, Kaelberer MM, et al. TRPV4 inhibition counteracts edema and inflammation and improves pulmonary function and oxygen saturation in chemically induced acute lung injury. *Am J Physiol Lung Cell Mol Physiol* (2014) 307(2):L158–72. doi:10.1152/ajplung.00065.2014
8. Zhu G; ICGN Investigators, Gulsvik A, Bakke P, Ghatta S, Anderson W, et al. Association of TRPV4 gene polymorphisms with chronic obstructive pulmonary disease. *Hum Mol Genet* (2009) 18(11):2053–62. doi:10.1093/hmg/ddp111
9. Thorneloe KS, Cheung M, Bao W, Alsaid H, Lenhard S, Jian MY, et al. An orally active TRPV4 channel blocker prevents and resolves pulmonary edema induced by heart failure. *Sci Transl Med* (2012) 4(159):ra48–48. doi:10.1126/scitranslmed.3004276
10. Henry CO, Dalloneau E, Perez-Berezo MT, Plata C, Wu Y, Guillon A, et al. In vitro and in vivo evidence for an inflammatory role of the calcium channel

TRPV4 in lung epithelium: potential involvement in cystic fibrosis. *Am J Physiol Lung Cell Mol Physiol* (2016) 311(3):L664. doi:10.1152/ajplung.00442.2015

11. Dalsgaard T, Sonkusare SK, Teuscher C, Poynter ME, Nelson MT. Pharmacological inhibitors of TRPV4 channels reduce cytokine production, restore endothelial function and increase survival in septic mice. *Sci Rep* (2016) 6:33841. doi:10.1038/srep33841

12. Jia Y, Wang X, Varty L, Rizzo CA, Yang R, Correll CC, et al. Functional TRPV4 channels are expressed in human airway smooth muscle cells. *Am J Physiol Lung Cell Mol Physiol* (2004) 287(2):L272. doi:10.1152/ajplung.00393.2003

13. Yang XR, Lin AHY, Hughes JM, Flavahan NA, Cao YN, Liedtke W, et al. Upregulation of osmo-mechanosensitive TRPV4 channel facilitates chronic hypoxia-induced myogenic tone and pulmonary hypertension. *Am J Physiol Lung Cell Mol Physiol* (2012) 302(6):L555–68. doi:10.1152/ajplung.00005.2011

14. Yin J, Michalick L, Tang C, Tabuchi A, Goldenberg N, Dan Q, et al. Role of transient receptor potential vanilloid 4 in neutrophil activation and acute lung injury. *Am J Respir Cell Mol Biol* (2015) 54(3):370–83. doi:10.1165/rcmb.2014-0225OC

15. Kelley J. Cytokines of the lung. *Am Rev Respir Dis* (1990) 141:765–88. doi:10.1164/ajrccm/141.3.765

16. Moran MM, McAlexander MA, Biro T, Szallasi A. Transient receptor potential channels as therapeutic targets. *Nat Rev Drug Discov* (2011) 10:601–20. doi:10.1038/nrd3456

17. Berridge MJ, Bootman MD, Roderick HL. Calcium signalling: dynamics, homeostasis and remodelling. *Nat Rev Mol Cell Biol* (2003) 4(7):517–29. doi:10.1038/nrm1155

18. Liedtke W. Molecular mechanisms of TRPV4-mediated neural signaling. *Ann N Y Acad Sci* (2008) 1144:42–52. doi:10.1196/annals.1418.012

19. Zhu MX. Multiple roles of calmodulin and other Ca^{2+}-binding proteins in the functional regulation of TRP channels. *Pflugers Arch* (2005) 451:105–15. doi:10.1007/s00424-005-1427-1

20. Strotmann R, Schulz G, Plant TD. Ca2+dependent potentiation of the nonselective cation channel TRPV4 is mediated by a C-terminal calmodulin binding site. *J Biol Chem* (2003) 278:26541. doi:10.1074/jbc.M302590200

21. White JPM, Cibelli M, Urban L, Nilius B, McGeown JG, Nagy I. TRPV4: molecular conductor of a diverse orchestra. *Physiol Rev* (2016) 96(3):911. doi:10.1152/physrev.00016.2015

22. Montell C, Birnbaumer L, Flockerzi V. The TRP channels, a remarkably functional family. *Cell* (2002) 108(5):595–8. doi:10.1016/S0092-8674(02)00670-0

23. Everaerts W, Nilius B, Owsianik G. The vanilloid transient receptor potential channel TRPV4: from structure to disease. *Prog Biophys Mol Biol* (2010) 103:2–17. doi:10.1016/j.pbiomolbio.2009.10.002

24. Gao X, Wu L, O'Neil RG. Temperature-modulated diversity of TRPV4 channel gating: activation by physical stresses and phorbol ester derivatives through protein kinase C-dependent and -independent pathways. *J Biol Chem* (2003) 278(29):27129–37. doi:10.1074/jbc.M302517200

25. Vriens J, Watanabe H, Janssens A, Droogmans G, Voets T, Nilius B. Cell swelling, heat, and chemical agonists use distinct pathways for the activation of the cation channel TRPV4. *Proc Natl Acad Sci U S A* (2004) 101(1):396–401. doi:10.1073/pnas.0303329101

26. Suresh K, Servinsky L, Reyes J, Baksh S, Undem C, Caterina M, et al. Hydrogen peroxide-induced calcium influx in lung microvascular endothelial cells involves TRPV4. *Am J Physiol Lung Cell Mol Physiol* (2015) 309(12):L1467. doi:10.1152/ajplung.00275.2015

27. Parpaite T, Cardouat G, Mauroux M, Gillibert-Duplantier J, Robillard P, Quignard JF, et al. Effect of hypoxia on TRPV1 and TRPV4 channels in rat pulmonary arterial smooth muscle cells. *Pflugers Arch* (2016) 468(1):111–30. doi:10.1007/s00424-015-1704-6

28. Yang XR, Lin MJ, McIntosh LS, Sham JSK. Functional expression of transient receptor potential melastatin- and vanilloid-related channels in pulmonary arterial and aortic smooth muscle. *Am J Physiol Lung Cell Mol Physiol* (2006) 290(6):L1267. doi:10.1152/ajplung.00515.2005

29. Alvarez DF, King JA, Weber D, Addison E, Liedtke W, Townsley MI. Transient receptor potential vanilloid 4-mediated disruption of the alveolar septal barrier: a novel mechanism of acute lung injury. *Circ Res* (2006) 99:988–95. doi:10.1161/01.RES.0000247065.11756.19

30. Gombedza F, Kondeti V, Al-Azzam N, Koppes S, Duah E, Patil P, et al. Mechanosensitive transient receptor potential vanilloid 4 regulates

Dermatophagoides farinae-induced airway remodeling via 2 distinct pathways modulating matrix synthesis and degradation. *FASEB J* (2017) 31(4):1556–70. doi:10.1096/fj.201601045R

31. Naumov DE, Kolosov VP, Perelman JM, Prikhodko AG. Influence of TRPV4 gene polymorphisms on the development of osmotic airway hyperresponsiveness in patients with bronchial asthma. *Dokl Biochem Biophys* (2016) 469(1):260–3. doi:10.1134/S1607672916040074

32. McAlexander MA, Luttmann MA, Hunsberger GE, Undem BJ. Transient receptor potential vanilloid 4 activation constricts the human bronchus via the release of cysteinyl leukotrienes. *J Pharmacol Exp Ther* (2014) 349(1):118. doi:10.1124/jpet.113.210203

33. Gibson RL, Burns JL, Ramsey BW. Pathophysiology and management of pulmonary infections in cystic fibrosis. *Am J Respir Crit Care Med* (2003) 168(8):918–51. doi:10.1164/rccm.200304-505SO

34. Arniges M, Vazquez E, Fernandez-Fernandez JM, Valverde MA. Swelling-activated Ca2+ entry via TRPV4 channel is defective in cystic fibrosis airway epithelia. *J Biol Chem* (2004) 279(52):54062–8. doi:10.1074/jbc.M409708200

35. Salathe M. Regulation of mammalian ciliary beating. *Annu Rev Physiol* (2007) 69:401–22. doi:10.1146/annurev.physiol.69.040705.141253

36. Satir P, Sleigh M. The physiology of cilia and mucociliary interactions. *Annu Rev Physiol* (1990) 52:137–55. doi:10.1146/annurev.physiol.52.1.137

37. Lorenzo I, Liedtke W, Sanderson M, Valverde MA. TRPV4 channel participates in receptor-operated calcium entry and ciliary beat frequency regulation in mouse airway epithelial cells. *Proc Natl Acad Sci U S A* (2008) 105(34):12611–6. doi:10.1073/pnas.0803970105

38. Han S, Mallampalli RK. The acute respiratory distress syndrome: from mechanism to translation. *J Immunol* (2015) 194(3):855–60. doi:10.4049/jimmunol.1402513

39. Hudson LD, Steinberg KP. Epidemiology of acute lung injury and ARDS. *Chest* (1999) 116:74S–82S. doi:10.1378/chest.116.suppl_1.74S-a

40. Ware LB, Matthay MA. The acute respiratory distress syndrome. *N Engl J Med* (2000) 342(18):1334–49. doi:10.1056/NEJM200005043421806

41. Martin TR, Ruzinski JT, Steinberg KP. Cytokine balance in the lungs of patients with acute respiratory distress syndrome (ARDS). *Am J Respir Crit Care Med* (1998) 157:A679.

42. Martin TR. Lung cytokines and ARDS: Roger S. Mitchell lecture. *Chest* (1999) 116:2S–8S. doi:10.1378/chest.116.suppl_1.2S

43. Meduri GU, Kohler G, Headley S, Tolley EA, Stentz F, Postlethwaite A. Inflammatory cytokines in the BAL of patients with ARDS. *Chest* (1995) 108(5):1303–14. doi:10.1378/chest.108.5.1303

44. Parsons PE, Moss M, Vannice JL, Moore EE, Moore FA, Repine JE. Circulating IL-1ra and IL-10 levels are increased but do not predict the development of acute respiratory distress syndrome in at-risk patients. *Am J Respir Crit Care Med* (1997) 155(4):1469–73. doi:10.1164/ajrccm.155.4.9105096

45. Meng F, Mambetsariev I, Tian Y, Beckham Y, Meliton A, Leff A, et al. Attenuation of LPS-induced lung vascular stiffening by lipoxin reduces lung inflammation. *Am J Respir Cell Mol Biol* (2015) 52(2):152–61. doi:10.1165/rcmb.2013-0468OC

46. Perlman CE, Lederer DJ, Bhattacharya J. Micromechanics of alveolar edema. *Am J Respir Cell Mol Biol* (2011) 44(1):34–9. doi:10.1165/rcmb.2009-0005OC

47. Hamanaka K, Jian MY, Townsley MI, King JA, Liedtke W, Weber DS, et al. TRPV4 channels augment macrophage activation and ventilator-induced lung injury. *Am J Physiol Lung Cell Mol Physiol* (2010) 299(3):L353–62. doi:10.1152/ajplung.00315.2009

48. Jurek SC, Hirano-Kobayashi M, Chiang H, Kohane DS, Matthews BD. Prevention of ventilator-induced lung edema by inhalation of nanoparticles releasing ruthenium red. *Am J Respir Cell Mol Biol* (2014) 50(6):1107–17. doi:10.1165/rcmb.2013-0163OC

49. Wynn TA, Chawla A, Pollard JW. Macrophage biology in development, homeostasis and disease. *Nature* (2013) 496(7446):445–55. doi:10.1038/nature12034

50. Wu S, Jian M, Xu Y, Zhou C, Al-Mehdi AB, Liedtke W, et al. Ca2+ entry via a1G and TRPV4 channels differentially regulated surface expression of P-selectin and barrier integrity in pulmonary capillary endothelium. *Am J Physiol Lung Cell Mol Physiol* (2009) 297(4):L650–7. doi:10.1152/ajplung.00015.2009

51. Jian MY, King JA, Al-Mehdi AB, Liedtke W, Townsley MI. High vascular pressure induced lung injury requires P450 epoxygenase dependent activation

of TRPV4. *Am J Respir Cell Mol Biol* (2008) 38(4):386–92. doi:10.1165/rcmb.2007-0192OC

52. Blakney AK, Swartzlander MD, Bryant SJ. The effects of substrate stiffness on the in vitro activation of macrophages and in vivo host response to poly(ethylene glycol)-based hydrogels. *J Biomed Mater Res A* (2012) 100A(6):1375–86. doi:10.1002/jbm.a.34104

53. Van Goethem E, Poincloux R, Gauffre F, Maridonneau-Parini I, Le Cabec V. Matrix architecture dictates three-dimensional migration modes of human macrophages: differential involvement of proteases and podosome-like structures. *J Immunol* (2010) 184(2):1049–61. doi:10.4049/jimmunol.0902223

54. Fereol S, Fodil R, Labat B, Galiacy S, Laurent VM, Louis B, et al. Sensitivity of alveolar macrophages to substrate mechanical and adhesive properties. *Cell Motil Cytoskeleton* (2006) 63(6):321–40. doi:10.1002/cm.20130

55. Murray PJ, Wynn TA. Protective and pathogenic functions of macrophage subsets. *Nat Rev Immunol* (2011) 11(11):723–37. doi:10.1038/nri3073

56. Greenberger MJ, Strieter RM, Kunkel SL, Danforth JM, Goodman RE, Standiford TJ. Neutralization of IL-10 increases survival in a murine model of *Klebsiella pneumonia*. *J Immunol* (1995) 155(2):722–9.

57. Arai T, Abe K, Matsuoka H, Yoshida M, Mori M, Goya S, et al. Introduction of the interleukin-10 gene into mice inhibited bleomycin-induced lung injury in vivo. *Am J Physiol Lung Cell Mol Physiol* (2000) 278(5):L914–22.

58. Togbe D, Schnyder-Candrian S, Schnyder B, Doz E, Noulin N, Janot L, et al. Toll-like receptor and tumour necrosis factor dependent endotoxin-induced acute lung injury. *Int J Exp Pathol* (2007) 88(6):387–91. doi:10.1111/j.1365-2613.2007.00566.x

59. Olman MA. In: Matthay MA, Lenfant C, editors. *Acute Respiratory Distress Syndrome*. New York, NY: Marcel Dekker, Inc (2003). p. 313–54.

60. Akei H, Whitsett JA, Buroker M, Ninomiya T, Tatsumi H, Weaver TE, et al. Surface tension influences cell shape and phagocytosis in alveolar macrophages. *Am J Physiol Lung Cell Mol Physiol* (2006) 291(4):L572–9. doi:10.1152/ajplung.00060.2006

61. Misharin AV, Morales-Nebreda L, Mutlu GM, Budinger GRS, Perlman H. Flow cytometric analysis of macrophages and dendritic cell subsets in the mouse lung. *Am J Respir Cell Mol Biol* (2013) 49(4):503–10. doi:10.1165/rcmb.2013-0086MA

62. Morales-Nebreda L, Misharin AV, Perlman H, Budinger GRS. The heterogeneity of lung macrophages in the susceptibility to disease. *Eur Respir Rev* (2015) 24(137):505–9. doi:10.1183/16000617.0031-2015

63. Park WY, Goodman RB, Steinberg KP, Ruzinski JT, Radella F, Park DR, et al. Cytokine balance in the lungs of patients with acute respiratory distress syndrome. *Am J Respir Crit Care Med* (2001) 164:1896–903. doi:10.1164/ajrccm.164.10.2104013

16

Role of Autophagy in Lung Inflammation

Jacob D. Painter, Lauriane Galle-Treger and Omid Akbari*

Department of Molecular Microbiology and Immunology, Keck School of Medicine, University of Southern California, Los Angeles, CA, United States

*Correspondence:
Omid Akbari
akbari@usc.edu

Autophagy is a cellular recycling system found in almost all types of eukaryotic organisms. The system is made up of a variety of proteins which function to deliver intracellular cargo to lysosomes for formation of autophagosomes in which the contents are degraded. The maintenance of cellular homeostasis is key in the survival and function of a variety of human cell populations. The interconnection between metabolism and autophagy is extensive, therefore it has a role in a variety of different cell functions. The disruption or dysfunction of autophagy in these cell types have been implicated in the development of a variety of inflammatory diseases including asthma. The role of autophagy in non-immune and immune cells both lead to the pathogenesis of lung inflammation. Autophagy in pulmonary non-immune cells leads to tissue remodeling which can develop into chronic asthma cases with long term effects. The role autophagy in the lymphoid and myeloid lineages in the pathology of asthma differ in their functions. Impaired autophagy in lymphoid populations have been shown, in general, to decrease inflammation in both asthma and inflammatory disease models. Many lymphoid cells rely on autophagy for effector function and maintained inflammation. In stark contrast, autophagy deficient antigen presenting cells have been shown to have an activated inflammasome. This is largely characterized by a T_H17 response that is accompanied with a much worse prognosis including granulocyte mediated inflammation and steroid resistance. The cell specificity associated with changes in autophagic flux complicates its targeting for amelioration of asthmatic symptoms. Differing asthmatic phenotypes between T_H2 and T_H17 mediated disease may require different autophagic modulations. Therefore, treatments call for a more cell specific and personalized approach when looking at chronic asthma cases. Viral-induced lung inflammation, such as that caused by SARS-CoV-2, also may involve autophagic modulation leading to inflammation mediated by lung resident cells. In this review, we will be discussing the role of autophagy in non-immune cells, myeloid cells, and lymphoid cells for their implications into lung inflammation and asthma. Finally, we will discuss autophagy's role viral pathogenesis, immunometabolism, and asthma with insights into autophagic modulators for amelioration of lung inflammation.

Keywords: autophagy, asthma, lung inflammation, immunometabolism, COVID-19, SARS-CoV-2

INTRODUCTION

Eukaryotic organisms need to break down intracellular constituents for a variety of reasons. These constituents can range from microbial invaders to their own cellular components, such as organelles and proteins. In the case of microbial invaders, these cells want to seek and specifically kill these smaller cells to protect themselves from infection (1, 2). However, destruction of their own cellular components is a highly regulated cellular process triggered by a variety of stimuli (1, 3, 4). This process of cellular recycling and degradation was coined autophagy in 1963 (5, 6). The name which directly translates from Greek meaning "self-eating." Common induction pathways of autophagy include stress and starvation signals. Dysregulation and malfunction of this crucial cellular component has more recently gained attention in the pathogenesis of many types of disease (1).

There are several types of autophagy in which cytosolic components are sent to the lysosome for degradation. Macroautophagy is the most prevalent form of autophagy in the cell and is responsible for much of the organelle and microbial degradation; this is through formation of a double membrane vesicle which surrounds the component and fuses to the lysosome (7, 8). This vesicle is called an autophagosome and when fused with the lysosome it becomes an autolysosome containing all the hydrolytic enzymes needed to break down its contents (4). Besides cellular components, autophagosomes can include macromolecules, such as lipids, sugars, nucleic acids, and proteins. The role of macroautophagy has been also shown to play a central role in immune function as knockout of autophagy genes in *Drosophila* make them more susceptible to both viral (vesicular stomatitis virus) and bacterial (*L. monocytogenes*) infection (9, 10). The second type of autophagy, microautophagy, deals with the degradation of cellular components largely without formation of an autophagosome. It is largely defined by the engulfment of cytoplasm and budding into the lumen of the lysosome (11, 12). The third type of autophagy is called chaperone-mediated autophagy (CMA). This type of autophagy relies on chaperones to mediate the transport of components to the lysosome for degradation; a large part of this system is reliant on lysosome-associated membrane proteins (LAMPS) for proper component processing (13, 14). These three distinct systems make up one of the most important survival systems in eukaryotic organisms and even without stimulus are still present at basal levels. Due to most studies focusing on macroautophagy, it will now be referred to as autophagy unless otherwise specified.

Regulation of autophagy is a complex cellular process involving a variety of different proteins. In this review, the models used utilize a variety of methods of autophagy-deficiency through depletion or deletion of these important proteins or genes. The general mechanism of autophagy and autophagosome formation involves three steps: initiation, nucleation, and elongation (15). The involvement of sixteen or more autophagy-related genes (Atg) products have been characterized in these three processes (15). Although there are many proteins involved in autophagy, the majority of studies covered in this review, involving genetic knockouts or otherwise, utilize autophagy-related gene 3 (Atg3), autophagy-related gene 5 (Atg5), and

autophagy-related gene 7 (Atg7). These protein products are involved in the elongation step of autophagosome formation and differ in their roles (15). In the elongation step, Atg5 and autophagy-related gene 12 (Atg12) are conjugated and associated with autophagy-related gene 16 like 1 (Atg16L1) and microtubule-associated protein 1A/1B-light chain 3 (LC3) to promote autophagosome formation (15, 16). Atg7 is involved in catalyzing the process of Atg12-Atg5 conjugation (17). Atg3 and Atg7 are involved in the lipidation process of LC3 with phospholipid phosphatidylethanolamine (PE) and are necessary for LC3 function and therefore autophagosome elongation (17). Atg3 can also indirectly affect formation of Atg12-Atg5 conjugation as mature LC3 seems to be needed for Atg12-Atg5-Atg16 complex formation (17), and Atg3-deficient mice show dramatically reduced Atg12-Atg5 conjugation (18). Therefore, in studies involving genetic modulation of Atg3, Atg5, and Atg7, it can be noted that loss of function in these proteins halt the elongation step of autophagosome formation and can be known as autophagy-deficient at some level. However, there is controversy onto what level autophagy is affected depending on what gene is being studied. In the case of Atg3, Atg5, and Atg7 mouse models, the functionality of the protein products must be maintained through birth as deletion of these genes results in neonatal lethality which points to their essential role in autophagy function *in vivo* (19). The deletion of many Atg protein products result in autophagy-deficiency which can be studied for various applications including lung inflammation (19).

Autophagy plays a key role in cellular function of a variety of different immune cell types. For example, in myeloid cells, due to the processing of antigen it is logical that autophagy would be involved heavily in these pathways. Autophagy has been since been described to play pivotal roles in a variety of different myeloid cell types. Many neutrophil functions have been linked to autophagy including differentiation (20), extracellular trap formation (21, 22), and cytokine secretion and interaction (23, 24). Eosinophils, important in allergic disease, have also been demonstrated to have diminished eosinophil extracellular trap formation (EET) when autophagy is inhibited (25). Extensive use of autophagy has also been observed in antigen presenting cells (APCs). Dendritic cells use autophagy extensively for a variety of functions including but not limited to: MHC class II antigen presentation, cytokine secretion, and activation of lymphoid cells (26). In particular, autophagy deficient macrophages have been shown to exacerbate eosinophilic inflammation through PGD_2 dysregulation (25). It is possible that this dysregulation may also lead to the recruitment of lymphoid cells, such as T cells and type two innate lymphoid cells (ILC2). Recently our lab has demonstrated that autophagy plays a critical role in the effector function of ILC2s (27). Autophagy has been shown to play a key role in a variety of T cell functions including differentiation, metabolism, survival, and activation (28). The role of autophagy within the network of these immune cells and their functions display potential for therapeutic approaches to target them for amelioration of inflammatory disease symptoms.

Due to its wide scope, autophagy has become a subject of interest in the pathology of many diseases and disorders.

Disruption of these normal pathways is currently being investigated as a causative factor variety of inflammatory and allergic diseases, such as asthma and airway hyperresponsiveness (AHR). The most common treatment option for asthma is the use of short-term inhaled corticosteroids and long-term β_2-agonists for relaxing airway smooth muscle (ASM), however these are not recommended for all chronic cases and have been found to be ineffective on 10–15% of patients (29–31). This is a significant number of the asthmatic population that is unaffected by these common treatments. Although it is a small percentage overall, these patients make up ~50% or more of asthmatic related health costs (32). Treatments seeking to target the immune cells rather than ASM itself may provide a long-term and more effective therapeutic target. Allergic asthma is largely mediated by T_H2 cells and type two innate lymphoid cells (ILC2) for production of inflammatory cytokines IL-5 and IL-13 (33–35). Chronic cases are largely due to secondary factors associated with T_H17 cell mediated neutrophilic inflammation (34, 36). Autophagy has been shown to play key roles in neutrophil mediated inflammation (21, 37). It is estimated that later stage chronic asthma has little to no T_H2 cell mediated inflammation (38). This is hypothesized to be the cause of ineffective β_2-agonist treatment on chronic asthma cases which should be effective on T_H2 asthma phenotypes. There is also a major role that airway remodeling plays in the ineffectiveness of these treatments as well (39, 40). Understanding the multiple aspects of the pathogenesis of pulmonary inflammation in these patients is key to finding clinical treatments.

Elevated levels of autophagosome formation have been reported in peripheral blood cells as well as airways in chronic asthma patients (41, 42). Recently autophagy has been shown to play a key role in T_H17 mediated asthma in APCs (43). This mechanism hints to possible causes of chronic asthma through the dysregulation and disruption of these important homeostatic pathways. Autophagy has also been observed to play a vital role in eosinophil mediated asthma as well (41, 44). Interestingly, correlations have also been drawn between high genetic polymorphisms of Atg5 in both adult and childhood asthma patients (45, 46). Emphasizing autophagy's role in a variety of inflammatory diseases, associations between Atg16L1 polymorphisms and irritable bowel disease have also been observed (47). Dysfunctional autophagy pathways also lead to metabolic remodeling that leads to airway inflammation (28, 30). Epithelial cells are also involved in exacerbating pulmonary inflammation and are available therapeutic targets (48, 49). Autophagy plays a key role in the regulation of cytokine signaling in a variety of cell types, likely leading to the pathogenesis of pulmonary diseases.

Autophagy involvement in the pathogenesis of many diseases makes it an important field of interest for clinical treatments for chronic patients. Making connections between its dysfunction in different cell types is crucial to understanding its role in these diseases. Because the overexpression or under expression of autophagic pathways has different effects on each cell type, understanding the role of autophagy in each individual cell type is needed to understand the network as a whole. The role of autophagy is different in each cell type which makes systemic treatments through autophagy for lung inflammation challenging. Contributions of autophagy in cellular metabolism also need to be discussed as it is important in the understanding of lung homeostasis. External factors, such as viruses are also relevant due to their regulation of autophagy contributing to lung remodeling and inflammation. Characterization of autophagy and its effects on myeloid, lymphoid, and epithelial cells in pulmonary systems will be explored in this review for its insights into clinical treatments of lung inflammation and asthma.

ROLE OF AUTOPHAGY IN NON-IMMUNE CELLS

Previously thought to be innocent bystanders in disease pathogenesis, cells lining the pulmonary airways, such as epithelial and mesenchymal cells have also been described to be involved in inflammatory response. Autophagy has been identified in many different cases to be a major player in the effector function of these cells. In response to cytokines, such as IL-13, it has been demonstrated that autophagy is induced in epithelial cells resulting in mucus secretion (50). Interestingly, IL-13 stimulation of pulmonary epithelial cells also showed the dependence of superoxides on autophagy levels; correlations were also found with IL-4 (51). Formation of superoxides in pulmonary airways can further lead to oxidative stress in tissues and autophagy itself. In the context of lymphoid cells, typically T_H2 cytokines inhibited autophagy while T_H1 cytokines were activating, further suggesting that autophagy needs to be studied on a cell-to-cell basis. Further adding to cell-context dependence, it has been established that IL-17A, a T_H17 cytokine, inhibits autophagy in lung epithelial cells through BCL2 degradation (52). In the stimulation of lung epithelial cells with interferon-γ (IFN-γ), autophagy was induced and was shown to control annexin A2 exomal release (exophagy) (53). These findings also suggest that there is not only cell-context dependence but also a possible cytokine dependence as well. Other sources have observed increase in autophagy in response to IFN-γ with different epithelial cell populations (54, 55). These observations could be related to the antiviral function of IFN-γ where it would induce cells to clear viral load. It has also been reported that annexin A2 could stimulate plasminogen mediated inflammatory cytokine production, mainly IL-6, by airway smooth muscle cells (56). This is an interesting situation where autophagy would impact T_H2 mediated inflammation through indirect pathways. Often it is these indirect pathways in which autophagy can have a significant effect on immune response. On the contrary, it is these same indirect pathways that make targeting of autophagy for clinical applications challenging.

Autophagy contribution in the pathogenesis of a variety of inflammatory diseases through epithelial cells is implicated in the literature. It has been described by multiple sources that attenuated or impaired autophagy leads to epithelial cell dysfunction and lung fibrosis (57). This is likely due to loss in their role of secreting both anti-fibrotic and profibrotic mediators. TGF-β, a key fibrotic modulator secreted by epithelial cells, has also been demonstrated to control autophagic activity in myofibroblasts depending on the tissue and inflammatory context (58, 59). This is due to the gene transcription in response to TGF-β being cell type, cellular condition, and microenvironment dependent. Epithelial cells in pulmonary airways are key in regulation of lung homeostasis, and maintaining healthy populations of these cells are critical for avoiding lung inflammation. Autophagy has been determined to be essential in the maintenance of epithelial cell counts in pulmonary airways (60). Loss of epithelial cells can happen through a variety of different pathways, but the most common is particulate inhalation. In protection against these particles, human bronchial epithelial cells have been found to increase mucus secretion through autophagy pathways (61). Cell death due particulates can also release inflammatory factors related to pulmonary disease. Autophagy therefore can have a direct protective role on epithelial cell populations.

Interestingly, autophagy also has been shown to play a role in airway remodeling as well. Remodeling of pulmonary airways has long lasting and irreversible effects on asthmatic patients. In remodeled asthmatic patients, epithelial thickening, reticular basement membrane, and increased airway smooth muscle bundles all important airway remodeling markers, have been observed; these patients have been described to have decreased tissue inflammation with intranasal administration of chloroquine, a known autophagy inhibitor (62). In house dust mite (HDM) induced murine allergic asthma models, autophagy inhibition with chloroquine also reduced concentration of TGF-β1 in bronchoalveolar lavage (BAL) and prevented bronchoconstriction (62). This inhibition provides a type of early treatment option for patients who may have not experienced full lung remodeling. However, regulation of autophagy by TGF-β comes on a cell to cell basis (63). Smooth muscle is also involved in the remodeling of pulmonary airways (64). Extracellular matrix depositions, such as collagen formation between muscle cells can increase bundle mass and fibrosis (65). TGF-β, and its downstream mediators, are major contributors to the maintenance and promotion of fibrosis and collagen production in these tissues (66). Interestingly there are two general hypotheses and support for both autophagy increasing and decreasing fibrosis and inflammation (67). However, the basis of these hypotheses could be based in two different contexts; these include genetic background, environment, and stage of conditioning. For example, the conditioning of one patient may result in autophagy mediated tissue fibrosis in their pulmonary airways while another patient conditioned another way may result in autophagy inhibiting fibrosis. The stage of disease is critical in understanding the role autophagy plays in pulmonary tissues and further explorations into these interactions are required.

ROLE OF AUTOPHAGY IN MYELOID CELLS

Granulocytes

The role of autophagy in myeloid cells is crucial for multiple functions in those cells. The overexpression or underexpression of this mechanism can have various effects depending on cell types (**Table 1**). In the case of granulocytes, such as neutrophils,

TABLE 1 | Summary table of autophagy in myelocytes.

Autophagy-related gene	Cell type	Function of autophagy	References
Atg5	Neutrophils	IL-1β secretion	(23)
	Dendritic cells	Inflammatory homeostasis	(30, 68, 69)
		MHC class II antigen presentation	(70–73)
		MHC class I internalization	(72, 74)
		pDC cytokine production	(75)
	Macrophage	Inflammatory homeostasis	(68, 69, 76–78)
		Monocyte differentiation	(71)
Atg7	Neutrophils	Extracellular trap formation	(37)
	Dendritic cells	Inflammatory homeostasis	(25)
	Macrophages	Inflammatory homeostasis	(25, 79)

they extensively use autophagy for a variety of essential functions, several which are implicated for inflammatory responses. Autophagy has a predominant role in degranulation which is one of the main functions of neutrophils (37). It is the process where neutrophils secrete cytoplasmic granules containing preformed antimicrobial and inflammatory proteins. Dysregulation of this process can lead to chronic disease due to constant tissue damage due to inflammatory proteins. Interestingly, knockout of Atg5 in neutrophils provided no evidence of abnormalities, such as granule proteins, apoptosis markers, migration, or effector functions (20). However, when myeloid-specific Atg5 and Atg7 autophagy-deficient murine models were tested, the results showed an actual decrease in neutrophil-mediated inflammatory and autoimmune disease models (37). These observations demonstrated that specific neutrophil knockout of Atg5 is not able to consistently reduce inflammation. Extracellular trap formation by neutrophils is also a major function in response to microbial invaders but also plays a key role in inflammatory response. Abnormal extracellular trap formation has been reported to have implications in a variety of autoimmune and autoinflammatory diseases reviewed by Delgado-Rizo et al. (80). It has been shown that lungs of asthmatic patients have increased migration of neutrophils and eosinophils to the lungs, which then exhibit extracellular trap formation (81). These neutrophil extracellular traps could cause a large amount of damage to airway epithelium as well as trigger responses by both airway epithelial cells and peripheral blood eosinophils (21). These interactions are what exacerbate the cycle of airway hyperreactivity and bronchial constriction associated with the pathology of asthma. Even though it has been established that Atg5 is not necessary for extracellular trap formation (82), multiple studies have noted abnormal extracellular trap formation in autophagy-deficient models (21, 22). Autophagy also does play a role in the priming of neutrophils for NET formation (83) and Atg7 knockouts have been determined to significantly affect NET formation (37). In the literature there is a current debate on how much involvement there is between autophagy in NET formation as there is evidence for both hypotheses (84). Neutrophils have been observed to conduct a caspase-independent form of cell death through an autophagy dependent pathway; this observation suggests a possible protective role in inflammatory contexts where it would encourage apoptosis of activated neutrophils. This mechanism is largely cytokine dependent, neutrophils exposed to GM-CSF and inflammatory cytokines went through an autophagy-dependent caspase-independent cell death associated with autophagosome formation (85). Moreover, Atg5 knockdown in neutrophils showed decreases in proinflammatory cytokines, such as IL-1β (23). Targeting neutrophil autophagy in certain phenotypes of asthma may provide a clinical avenue for treatment, however knockdown may decrease inflammation mediated through NET formation while also promoting neutrophil survival. Therefore, modulation of autophagy function in asthmatic patients does provide a treatment option in neutrophil mediated inflammation in severe asthma and other inflammatory diseases.

Autophagy has a significant role in eosinophil activation and effector function, however there are still many questions to be investigated. Eosinophils are critically involved in most asthma cases as they are recruited by the T_H2 mediated response. It has been demonstrated that eosinophils are activated by the presence of IL-5. Eosinophil activation induces autophagy and the production of eosinophil cationic protein (ECP) further leading to inflammation (41). Autophagy also likely contributes in increasing survivability of eosinophils. ECP secretion has a variety of different effects on surrounding cells, such as inflammation and mucus hypersecretion which leads to airway constriction. Interestingly it was found that knockout of autophagy, $Atg7^{-/-}$, in myeloid cell lineages showed an overall increase in eosinophils, epithelial hyperplasia, and mucosal thickening in eosinophilic chronic rhinosinusitis (25). This was largely characterized by the large increase in PGD_2 which is responsible for the inflammatory recruitment of many types of immune cells myeloid and lymphoid alike. This suggests that specific targeting of cell types is needed rather than just lineage specific or systemic knockdown. The seeming contrast between these two findings is possibly explained through the differences in disease, however IL-5 exposure may play a more predominant role than just increased autophagy in severe asthma patients. Eosinophil extracellular trap formation has also been found to be correlated with autophagy levels (21, 22), but interestingly Atg5 knockout was not necessary for their formation (82). Autophagy may have a role in the differentiation of eosinophils, however the only study of it has been through regulators, such as mTOR which regulates it indirectly (86, 87). Like neutrophils, eosinophils have also been observed to go through an autophagy-mediated caspase-independent cell death in inflammatory conditions (88). Eosinophils also are major producers of TGF-β which is heavily involved in airway remodeling and early stages of chronic asthma development (63, 89). Most findings demonstrate that there are correlations in levels of eosinophil-mediated inflammation and autophagy, however, further explorations are required to draw connections for clinical applications. Due to being one of the main cell types associated with asthma and allergic diseases, characterizing the role of autophagy in eosinophils will open avenues for clinical targets. With more study and understanding, targeting of autophagy in eosinophils in T_H2 phenotypes of asthma may ameliorate lung inflammation.

Antigen Presenting Cells

Autophagy is extensively utilized in dendritic cells (DCs) and solving its mechanism of action has possible implications for understanding lung inflammation and asthma. Autophagy and its interactions with cytokine production in dendritic cells has largely been reviewed by Harris in bacterial and viral infection (90), however its role in inflammatory disease has largely remained unexplored. In DCs derived from peripheral blood mononuclear cells (PBMCs), the inhibition of autophagy showed reduced levels of IL-10 production leading to the proliferation of T-cells (91). Regulatory T cells have also been demonstrated to downregulate autophagy in DCs which helps mediate inflammatory responses (92). Implication of these findings could be related to allergic disease; however, it has not been fully characterized. The mechanism of autophagy has also been described to regulate plasmacytoid dendritic cells (pDCs) activation. Cytokine production, mainly interferon-α (IFN-α), secreted by plasmacytoid dendritic cells is affected by Atg5 knockout (75). Functional processing of TLR7 viral antigens also requires autophagy and without Atg5, cytosolic viral replication intermediates fail to be transported into the lysosome. Therefore, autophagy has a key role in mediating antiviral response through viral ssRNA detection and subsequent cytokine response (75). Cell-specific Atg5-deletion in $CD11c^+$ cells, was found to augment lung inflammation with increased IL-17A levels in pulmonary airways leading to severe neutrophilic asthma in mice with and without HDM-challenged (30). The role of autophagy in antigen processing in DCs is the most prevalent in the literature, and improper allergen presentation leads to inflammation in multiple tissue types. Presentation to $CD8^+$ T and $CD4^+$ T cells through class-I and class-II MHC formation, respectively involves autophagy. The process in which autophagy proteins are involved in antigen presentation has been previously reviewed in the physiological context (93) so its relation to allergic disease will be described here. Atg5 has been shown to be required for MHC II antigen presentation as it is required for optimal phagosome-to-lysosome fusion. However, the same knockout did not affect MHC I presentation negatively (70). In inflammatory murine models of encephalomyelitis, Atg5 expression is required for MHC II myelin antigen presentation leading to disease pathogenesis (71). This suggests possible implications into other inflammatory diseases, such as asthma. However, knockout of autophagy, Atg5 and Atg7, has also been shown to increase MHC I antigen presentation enhancing the $CD8^+$ T cell responses to infection *in vitro* and *in vivo* (74). This induction was due to disrupted internalization of MHC I molecules which is regulated by normal autophagy pathways. Increased MHC class I presentation would be able to further polarize T cell effector response in allergic contexts, such as increased T_H17 polarization found in Suzuki et al. (30). It seems that autophagy machinery has more direct regulatory control over MHC II-restricted antigen presentation and indirectly controls MHC class I expression. Parallels can also be drawn where this antigen presentation could also increase the severity of inflammatory diseases through this increased T cell response. CMA has also been implicated to promote antigen presentation on APCs' surfaces and generate hyperactive $CD4^+$ T cells in systemic lupus erythematosus (SLE) models (94). CMA involvement in immunity has largely been unexplored as well as autophagy's role in antigen presentation in the context of asthma.

In CD11c-specific $Atg5^{-/-}$ murine models, $CD11c^+$ DCs were determined to be the cause of unprovoked neutrophilic asthma without need for HDM challenge (30). This demonstrates the importance of autophagy in the role of APCs in inflammatory contexts. These results also were found to be DC specific as $Atg5^{-/-}$ in pulmonary epithelial cells showed similarities to wild type (WT). Sublethally irradiated WT mice were inoculated with bone marrow (BM) cells isolated from $Atg5^{-/-}$ mice and developed significantly high AHR (30). These results indicated that BM-derived Atg5-deficient immune cells were the cause of severe AHR rather than other non-hematopoietic cells. Chimeric experiments inoculating irradiated $Atg5^{-/-}$ mice with WT or $Atg5^{-/-}$ bone marrow confirmed the same results with the role of autophagy in DCs (30). Further analysis with confocal microscopy revealed asthma reduced number of LC3 foci in pulmonary dendritic cells. Bone marrow derived dendritic cells were described to increase concentrations of IL-1 and IL-23 in $Atg5^{-/-}$ mice further contributing to T_H17 neutrophilic polarity (30). In response to steroid treatment, $Atg5^{-/-}$ mice were found to have no decrease in AHR showing a steroid resistant phenotype (30). As previously stated, neutrophilic asthma may account for steroid resistance in some asthma phenotypes. Challenge with HDM also demonstrated the same neutrophilic asthma phenotype as the WT suggesting that the initiation of asthma in $Atg5^{-/-}$ mice does not need to be provoked with allergen (30). This study establishes the significant impact that genetics can have in the unprovoked asthma response in patients. The role of autophagy in the pathogenesis of neutrophilic asthma is prevalent and needs more study to fully understand different phenotypes (30). In conformation of these findings, metabolic shift of APCs has been described to promote neutrophilic inflammation in the lungs through mTOR ablation, a key regulator of autophagy (43). The role of autophagy in the reprogramming of APCs into a more inflammatory phenotype can be a pivotal point of clinical interest.

Like DCs, macrophages have also been implicated with autophagy in the literature as they are also APCs. Metabolic disturbances, mTOR ablation, in macrophages have been described to directly initiate neutrophilic asthma (43). As previously mentioned, the connections between autophagy and mTOR are extensive. Autophagy also plays important roles in the differentiation of monocytes into macrophages through colony stimulating factor-1 (CSF-1) (95); further support showed that GM-CSF administration blocked cleavage of Atg5 and promoted autophagy, and without it differentiation of macrophages was attenuated along with cytokine secretions (96). Previous studies reported that hampered autophagy, through blocking of Atg5/7, LC3, and Beclin-1, led to increases in IL-1β and IL-18, suggesting a possible protective role of autophagy in inflammatory contexts

(25, 79, 96). Autophagy-deficient mice with myeloid-specific deletion of Atg5 and Atg7 with sterile lung inflammation were also shown to have increased goblet metaplasia and collagen concentrations driven by IL-18 secretion (97). In macrophages, the clearance of damaged mitochondria through autophagy is very important for these reasons. Interestingly, knockout of autophagy increased antiviral resistance but also increased inflammation and cytokine secretion (76). In obese mice models, the attenuation of autophagy in macrophages was associated with increased inflammation and acute liver injury (98, 99). Atg5 has also been reported to explicitly suppress production of IL-1β (77). In models for Crohn's disease, a prevalent autoimmune disease, a mechanistic link between macrophage autophagy and the systematic disease has been identified (100). It has also been shown that dysfunctional lysosomal and autophagic mechanisms leading to inflammasome activation in macrophages (101). In inflammatory contexts, it is important to maintain autophagy to protect against inflammasome mediated IL-1β secretion and subsequent inflammation mediated by macrophages. Effect of Atg5 knockout in APCs is summarized in **Figure 1**. Possible connections between these inflammatory disease phenotypes may be applicable for investigation into asthma phenotypes. The production of IL-1 has been proven to exacerbate neutrophilic asthma (30). Although T_H1 cytokines secreted by macrophages have been characterized, the subsequent production of T_H2 cytokines by activated T cells has been unexplored with its connection to APC autophagy. In allergic contexts, the production of colony stimulating factors increases secretion of cytokines by macrophages, however the following stimulation of T_H17 cells has yet to be explored. GM-CSF has found shown to be necessary for the maintenance of allergic asthma (102) showing that macrophage targeting with GM-CSF to induce autophagy is not a viable clinical treatment. Past studies have established that levels of GM-CSF are highly elevated in the BAL of asthmatic patients compared to healthy controls (103). These observations clearly demonstrate that other effects of GM-CSF on other cell types overpowers the macrophage inflammasome suppression effect. Therefore, preservation of the autophagic flux in macrophages must be done through other means to avoid inflammasome activation. Antigen presentation by macrophages after increased monocyte differentiation by GM-CSF could impact pulmonary inflammation through subsequent activation of T cells. Overall preservation of autophagy in macrophages is essential for suppression of the inflammasome. However, there are still open questions requiring further exploration regarding the role of autophagy in macrophages, specifically involving antigen presentation and cytokine production.

ROLE OF AUTOPHAGY IN LYMPHOID CELLS

Lymphocytes

The role of autophagy in $CD8^+$ T cells show the wide scope of its contribution in multiple cell types (**Table 2**). It has been demonstrated that autophagy plays a key role in various functions of $CD8^+$ T cells, but more specifically the proliferation, metabolism, survival, and memory function

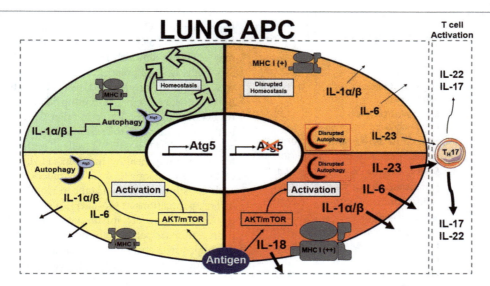

FIGURE 1 | Summary of stead state and active Atg5/Atg5$^{-/-}$ antigen presenting cells. Autophagy presence is represented by a half formed autophagosome highlighted in blue for functional and red to dysfunctional autophagy. Atg5 is a requirement for functional autophagy. Each quadrant denotes activation state of a lung APC: green represents homeostasis, yellow represents moderate activation, orange represents moderate to high activation, and red represents high activation. AKT, protein kinase B; APC, antigen presenting cell; Atg5, autophagy related 5; MHC I, major histocompatibility complex class I; mTOR, mechanistic target of rapamycin (25, 30, 74, 77, 79, 96).

(109, 110). CMA has been implicated into the function of T cells as it specifically degrades negative regulators of T cell activation (127). Multiple early studies have observed lower CD8$^+$ T cell counts in spleen and lymph nodes with increased apoptosis in Atg3, Atg5, and Atg7 deficient murine models (104, 107, 128). As these cells replicate in an inflammatory context it makes sense that autophagy is upregulated to remove unwanted reactive oxygen species (ROS) and to clear defective mitochondria through mitophagy. In these highly replicative states, involvement of mTOR is extensive as the need for protein synthesis is high (129). The interplay between mTOR and autophagy in CD8$^+$ T cells is crucial to understanding their function. The canonical model of their interaction is that mTOR is a negative regulator of autophagy (130); this is largely based on their differing roles in protein synthesis and protein recycling, respectively. However, some studies have found that this is not always the case in all CD8$^+$ T cell subsets (131). Further adding to the complexity of CD8$^+$ T cells is the metabolic reprogramming that they undergo when activated which is mediated by these autophagy and glycolytic mTOR pathways (132). AMPK is an important regulator of metabolic pathways and is able to positively regulate autophagy (133). This is through ULK phosphorylation, an important early step autophagosome protein, and also downregulation of mTOR through phosphorylation of either Raptor (134) or TSC2 (135). Regulation of AMPK can also be controlled by mTOR as it is able to inhibit ULK-AMPK interactions (133). The interaction between all these metabolic pathways provide a complex issue that needs to be addressed. Especially in the case of CD8$^+$ T cell activation where metabolism regulation is important to rapid proliferation in both bacterial and allergic inflammatory contexts.

Further understanding of this dynamic could open avenues for targeting T cell mediated asthma phenotypes. Activation of T cell receptors also has been demonstrated to co-activate both mTOR and autophagy pathways; however, it was also shown that autophagy was able to operate independently from mTOR (131). It has also been described that in CD8$^+$ CD28$^-$ T cells that TCR engagement had a decreased ability to induce autophagy, in comparison to CD28$^+$ T cells, therefore making them more likely to fail their metabolic demands and senesce when activated (131). In senescent CD8$^+$ human cells, p38 induced increased autophagy with no metabolic remodeling, with mTOR-independence, suggesting the possibility of a therapeutic knockdown in mediation of these rapidly proliferating cell populations in inflammatory contexts (136). Strikingly, Atg5 knockout in T cells displayed a more effector memory phenotype with more IFN and TNF production (137). In certain stages of asthma pathogenesis, the generation of memory T cells may exacerbate symptoms through an overreaction to antigen and lead to more chronic cases. Due to the interconnection of metabolic pathways and the role of autophagy in the cellular energetics of T cells, studies to identify novel therapeutic targets should be done. Targeting of autophagy through other metabolic systems, such as mTOR, may provide innovative approaches, but adverse effects caused by non-autophagy specific mechanisms could be induced.

In inflammatory contexts, such as asthma, CD4$^+$ T cells can play into both T$_H$17 and T$_H$2 type mediated inflammation (138) and have also been shown to utilize autophagy (139). Like their CD8$^+$ counterparts, CD4$^+$ T cells have also been found to have extensive autophagy involved in a variety of cellular functions, such as metabolism and memory (112). During

TABLE 2 | Summary table of autophagy in lymphocytes.

Autophagy-related gene	Cell type	Function of autophagy	References
Atg3	CD8+ T cells	Survival and mitochondrial maintenance	(104, 105)
	iNKT	Memory formation and mitochondrial maintenance	(106)
Atg5	CD8+T cells	Homeostasis and survival	(107, 108)
		Activation and proliferation	(107)
		Memory maintenance	(109, 110)
	CD4+ T cell	Homeostasis and survival	(107)
		Activation and proliferation	(107, 111)
		Memory maintenance	(112)
		FoxP3 expression	(113)
	B cells	Plasma cell survival and Ig production	(114, 115)
		Mature B cell homeostasis and survival	(116)
		Peripheral B cell homeostasis and survival	(117)
		Internalization of BCR to MHC-II vesicles	(118)
	ILC2	Homeostasis and survival	(27, 119)
		Effector function	(27)
		Metabolic homeostasis	(27)
	iNKT	Homeostasis and survival	(120)
		Effector function	(121)
Atg7	CD8+T cells	Homeostasis and survival	(105, 107)
		Memory maintenance	(109, 110)
	CD4+ T cell	Activation and proliferation	(122)
		Effector function	(122)
		FoxP3 expression	(113)
	B cells	Memory maintenance	(123, 124)
		B1a B cell homeostasis and survival	(125)
		Plasmablast differentiation	(126)
	iNKT	Homeostasis and survival	(120)

activation, autophagy is massively upregulated in CD4+ T cells (122, 140). Multiple proteins have been described to regulate autophagy in CD4+ T cells, such as TNFAIP3 (141) and Vps34 (142, 143), and both play roles in their cellular metabolism. In general, most literature focuses on the increase in autophagy in CD4+ T cells as the need for energy is high when in activated states. Metabolic proteins and autophagy are essential to the understanding of both T cell types in inflammatory diseases; they also provide possible therapeutic targets as well. Cell specific knockout of mTOR has been demonstrated to increase autophagy and promote CD4+ T cell survival in highly inflamed states such sepsis (144, 145). IL-21 has also been observed to engage mTOR, therefore suppressing autophagy, in CD4+ T cells leading to their dysfunction in the differentiation and effector functions in systemic lupus erythematosus (146). This shows that metabolism still plays an important role in inflammatory states of infection

or disease, and the massive role that autophagy plays in the maintenance of CD4+ T cell counts and healthy function. In the case of allergic asthma, clinical treatments targeting autophagy may be able to diminish T_H2 polarized CD4+ T cell populations. Strikingly, in T_H2 polarized CD4+ T cells, selective autophagy was found to prevent sustained TCR activation by targeting Bcl10 for degradation and limiting NF-κB activation (147). These results have not been tested in other CD4+ populations, leading to the possibility that the result is only in T_H2 polarized cells. In regulatory CD4+ FoxP3+ T cells (Treg), autophagy is essential for maintaining healthy function (113), including suppression of these pro-allergic T_H2 cell populations. In allergic diseases, such as asthma, it is important to realize the dual functionality of Treg populations as pro-allergic environments can skew Tregs to become more pro-inflammatory (148). Depending if Tregs from asthmatic patients are polarized to this pro-inflammatory or suppressive phenotype, targeting of autophagy in these cell populations would have to be case dependent. Targeting of autophagy in T_H2 polarized CD4+ cells may be helpful if the patient has a pro-inflammatory Treg phenotype. Otherwise targeting of autophagy in CD4+ populations could possibly deplete suppressive Treg populations which would exacerbate inflammation and symptoms. These changes and differences between patients make determining a route of treatment difficult. In relation, there has been an association between age and overactive autophagy causing persistence of dysfunctional mitochondria in CD4+ T cells leading to chronic inflammation and immune system impairment (149). This suggests that even over time autophagic flux can change leading to chronic disease and inflammation as well. Due to energy metabolism varying between CD4+ T cells subsets and patients targeting of these cells would be complicated due to differential impact on autophagy depletion (139).

Autophagy plays a significant role in a variety of important functions of B cells and plasma cells. It is involved in B cell memory maintenance (123, 124), homeostasis, survival, and effector function (116). More specifically autophagy, Atg7, has been described to be critical in tissue resident, B1a, B cells which play a key role in antigen presentation in pulmonary disease (125). Due to plasma cell function as immunoglobulin-secreting cells, ER stress generated by this process makes them extremely reliant on autophagy for survival (114, 115). Autophagy also plays a role in B cell differentiation to plasma cells and a larger role in subsequent immunoglobulin production in autoimmune diseases, such as lupus, which could provide a possible therapeutic target the treatment of these pathologies (117, 126). Interestingly, B cell responses to different stimuli produce different cellular responses fluctuating between canonical to non-canonical autophagy (116, 150). Recently, autophagy inducers were able to restore survival of B cells in aging patients with impaired autophagy (151). Changes in autophagic flux and mechanisms make the characterization of B cell autophagy complicated. However, their involvement in a variety of different immune branches allow them to be targeted for a large impact in therapy for lung inflammatory phenotypes. The role of B cells in asthma has been demonstrated to be detrimental as they respond to T_H2 cytokine secretion, IL-4, by upregulating autophagy, survival, IgE secretion, and enhancing antigen presentation leading to exacerbation of inflammation (152). Autophagy has also been shown to be critical for sustained inflammatory and autoimmune diseases (153) even if it is not essential for normal development of B cells (117). Secretion of IgE is primarily by plasma cells and is a major mediator in allergic response as it binds to mast cell receptors for an inflammatory response (154). Due to the critical role of autophagy in these cells, it may provide a therapeutic target. For example, specific phenotypes of disease, such as B cell activating factor from the TNF family (BAFF) induced inflammatory diseases could be targeted through regulation of intracellular Ca^{2+} level or CaMKII, AKT, or mTOR ultimately regulating autophagy and attenuating disease (155). Increased levels of BAFF have been observed in child asthma patients compared to healthy children (156). A variety of cytokines have been found to effect autophagy in B cells including IFN-α (153) and IL-4 (152). Determining which cytokines are interacting with the B cells at a patient to patient basis is essential to characterizing individual disease phenotypes. Interestingly, LAMP-2C plays a natural inhibitory role in MHC II presentation in B cells through downregulating CMA which skews presentation in response to external queues (157). Atg5 has also been established to play a role in the relocalization of internalized BCR to MHC-II containing vesicles (118). Autophagy provides a viable target for B cell mediated inflammatory disease as it plays a key role in their immunoglobulin secretion and antigen presentation. Due to their sustained inflammatory potential, they provide a great clinical avenue for treatment.

Innate-Like Lymphocytes

Autophagy also plays a crucial role in group 2 innate lymphoid cells (ILC2) (27) which are critical players in a variety of inflammatory diseases including asthma (158, 159). ILC2s are some of the first cells to receive signals through alarmin release from pulmonary epithelial cells. With these signals, ILC2s are the first producers of T_H2 cytokines which produce an allergic response and contribute to asthma pathogenesis (159). Specific targeting of ILC2s may be a therapeutic avenue to approach for these initial activating steps, possibly decreasing the downward cascade as well as asthma symptoms. Autophagy-deficiency, $Atg5^{-/-}$, in ILC2s has been shown to directly affect the homeostasis and effector function of those cells. Interestingly, the lack of critical autophagic machinery impaired ILC2 ability to produce T_H2 cytokines and lead to increases in apoptosis (27). Lower NF-κB activity also indicated less activation and cytokine secretion in Atg5 defective mice. Further analysis through Ki-67 showed that proliferation was also decreased in ILC2s in both IL-33 challenged and wild type mice. On the other hand, the induction of autophagy through the overexpression of master regulator TFEB in the Tfeb transgene ($Tfeb^{TG}$) mice was associated with higher levels of proliferation, cytokine secretion, and activated ILC2s. Autophagy overexpression and Atg5 deletion were shown to have mirrored effects on ILC2 functions (27). Other studies have also found that Atg5 has a prevalent role in the regulation of the effector function and survival of innate lymphoid cells (119), while suppression of

mTOR with inhibitors led to increase in effector function and population of innate lymphoid cells (160). These conclusions are consistent with the observations in other lymphoid cell types in which the relationship between mTOR and autophagy is dichotomous. Due to ILC2s' role as the major cytokine producers in asthma (159, 161, 162), they provide a promising target for amelioration of allergic asthma due to their tight dependence on autophagy pathways (27, 107). The multiple effects of autophagy on lymphoid cells is summarized in **Figure 2**. Further explorations are required to characterize the effect of autophagy inhibition during asthma pathogenesis in order to formulate a specific clinical approach.

Invariant natural killer T cells (iNKT) have also been shown to be affected by autophagic flux (120, 121) and have been described to play a key role in asthma pathogenesis (163, 164). With autophagy-deficiency, $Atg5^{-/-}$, T_H1 iNKTs were found to have decreased effector functions with less IL-17 and IFN-γ production when challenged with α-GalCer, an iNKT activator, *in vitro;* this finding was further supported after *in vivo* challenge with α-GalCer (121). $Atg5^{-/-}$ has also been demonstrated to induce iNKT cell death and to disrupt cell cycle progression associated with increased mitochondrial stress in multiple iNKT subsets (120). More specifically, autophagy has been reported in later stages of iNKT development to be essential in the development to mature cells (120, 121). Other autophagy proteins, such as Atg3 has been shown to be critical for iNKT memory formation. Like other autophagy-deficient models, there was increased levels of defective mitochondria and ROS when challenged, in this case with viral infection. They further described that mitochondrial proteins BNIP3 and BNIP3L were important for memory formation and autophagy knockout led to mitochondrial disruption and loss of these essential proteins (106). Important autophagy interacting proteins like Vps34 have been found to be crucial for iNKT development past early stages, however whether this is due to its interaction between autophagy or its other interactors has yet to be investigated (165). Regardless, targeting of direct and indirect proteins in the autophagy pathway may provide a clear target for treatment to ameliorate asthma symptoms. Type 2 cytokine production by T_H2 polarized iNKTs and other $CD4^+$ T cells make them significant players in asthma pathogenesis. They have also been shown to be a significant amount of the total $CD4^+$ T cell population in human asthmatic lungs, but not healthy controls (163). These iNKTs provide a very clear and present target for autophagy targeting for the amelioration of asthma.

ROLE OF AUTOPHAGY IN VIRAL-INDUCED LUNG INFLAMMATION

Viral lung infections complicate treatments in asthma patients and can lead to treatment resistance (166). Due to the role of autophagy in clearing of intracellular components, there is a lot of interaction between autophagic and viral proteins. Often bacteria and viruses find ways to attack autophagy to avoid autophagosome formation and subsequent destruction (167); in some cases they are even able to hijack and increase autophagy

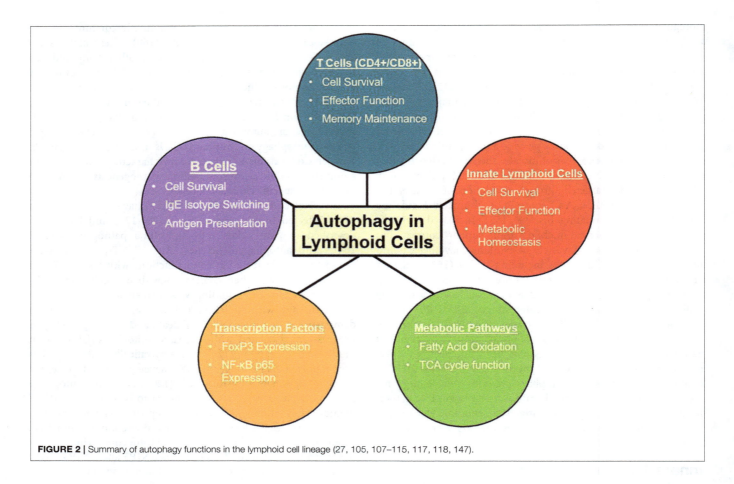

FIGURE 2 | Summary of autophagy functions in the lymphoid cell lineage (27, 105, 107–115, 117, 118, 147).

at some point in infection for increased replicative potential or aid in escape (168). Ultimate suppression of autophagy occurs after chronic viral infection. Infection of APCs and subsequent suppression of autophagy in the long term can lead to activation of the inflammasome (25, 30, 79, 96), and ultimately lead to lung remodeling. Inflammatory cytokines, such as IFN-γ and IL-22 produced by innate lymphocytes stimulated by IL-1 and IL-23 (169) may condition the pulmonary airways and contribute to airway remodeling through interactions with resident cell types. Inconsistencies in autophagic flux due to viral infection in lung resident cells may contribute to asthma pathogenesis directly with these inflammatory reactions. Older studies have noted that previous viral infection predisposes patients for late asthmatic reactions (170). In support, a high percentage of patients coming into the modern clinic have previously experienced a recent respiratory viral infection (171). Viral infection of the lungs also can contribute to airway remodeling which can have lifelong effects (172, 173). Infection of epithelial and immune cells could potentially affect the autophagic flux to exacerbate airway remodeling. Production of IL-1 and IL-23 by myeloid cells with decreased autophagy (43), due to viral infection, may contribute to enhanced asthma phenotypes. It also may contribute to steroid resistant lung inflammation as observed in murine CD11c$^+$ specific autophagy-deficient, Atg5$^{-/-}$, models (30). Disruption of autophagy by upper respiratory viruses contribute to both initiation and exacerbation of asthma. However, determination of specific effects of autophagy may prove challenging as the effect on epithelial and immune cells may be different. Tissue specific ablation of autophagy due to viral infection, especially in the lung, contributes to unwanted outcomes. Prevention of viral mediated autophagy disruption is key in avoiding future asthma onset.

Autophagy modulation is present in the pathogenesis of a variety of different viruses including influenza virus and coronaviruses (CoV), each which cause significant lung inflammation (174, 175). The involvement of autophagy in the process of CoV replication seems to be controversial with multiple papers citing different results (176). These different results likely stem from differences in viruses and autophagy proteins being tested. Overall, more investigation is needed to find the specific effect of CoVs on autophagic pathways. In human CoVs infections, such as SARS-CoV, MERS-CoV, and SARS-CoV-2, the cytokine storm following infection is largely mediated by production of IL-18, IL-1, and IL-6 (177, 178). Inflammasome activation in pulmonary resident APCs leads to the production of these proinflammatory cytokines, and this may be due to the lack of autophagy induced by viral infection. MERS-CoV infection of Vero B4 cells has been shown to decrease autophagy through Belcin1-ubiquitination (179) which, in the case of in APC infection, may lead to inflammasome activation due to the impairment of autophagy pathways (25, 30, 79, 96). It is very likely that lack of autophagy, induced by viral infection, will be responsible for activation of the inflammasome in lung resident APCs and therefore, lack of autophagy would cause production of IL-18, IL-1, and IL-6 in patients with COVID-19. This observation may be supported by the fact that air pollution, particularly PM2.5, has been reported to increase mTOR, a known inhibitory pathway of autophagy, impairing M2 macrophage polarization, and is associated with high secretion of IL-6 and IL-1β (180); however, its direct involvement in decreasing macrophage autophagy has yet to be determined. Interestingly, many recent studies support the notion that mortality rate and cytokine storm in patients exposed to air pollution was significantly higher. For example, a recent study, collected air pollution data and COVID-19 mortality rate from more than 3,000 counties in the United States, found that an increase of only 1 $\mu g/m^3$ in PM2.5 is associated with an average 8% increase in the COVID-19 death rate (181).

Production of IFN plays a crucial role in protection against viral infection, such as SARS-CoV and MERS-CoV; new studies clearly suggest that delayed induction of IFN responses from APCs contributes to the pathogenesis of disease (182). Besides epithelial cells, the only candidate that shown to be effective in IFN-α production in viral infection with SARS-CoV is pDCs (183); SARS-CoV-2 like SARS-CoV has been shown to have sensitivity to IFN (184). As pDCs are crucial in the protection against CoVs and the induction of lung inflammation leading to viral clearance, their role and function needs to be investigated in patients with COVID-19. Autophagy-deficiency, Atg5$^{-/-}$, in pDCs has been shown to halt the production of IFN-α *in vitro* and *in vivo* (75). Therefore, assessment of autophagy among various subsets of APCs, such as pDCs, after infection needs to be investigated. Based on these observations, we anticipate that autophagy inducers, particularly at early stages of infection with SARS-CoV-2, may be able to restore functional IFN-α production by pDCs and significantly reduce viral titers (75, 184). Finally, another fact that supports the notion for role of autophagy in pathogenesis of SARS-CoV-2 is the observation that patients with worse prognosis may have pre-existing conditions in regard to autophagy. Pre-existing conditions, such as obesity, hypertension, diabetes, and coronary heart disease are often associated with lack of autophagy (185, 186); therefore, it is plausible to believe that autophagy may be responsible for higher mortality rate and outcome reported after SARS-CoV-2 infection (187).

ROLE OF AUTOPHAGY IN MAINTAINING CELLULAR METABOLISM

Due to the key role of autophagy in metabolic pathways, understanding the immunometabolism mechanisms are essential. The predominant metabolic pathways, such as AMPK, mTOR, and AKT all have downstream effects regulating autophagy and ultimately affecting the inflammatory outcome. There is evidence supporting the connection between autophagy regulation and immunometabolism in a variety of different contexts. Functions regulated by autophagy can affect multiple mechanisms, such as apoptosis, mitochondrial maintenance, switches in energy-metabolism, and proteostasis. In a variety of immune cells, dysregulation of autophagy is also associated with altered cell differentiation. In the case of macrophages, the role of autophagy due to mTOR and AMPK regulation plays a role in the metabolic balance between M1 and M2 macrophages (188). Neutrophils have also been shown to have increased glycolytic activity in autophagy-deficient, Atg7$^{-/-}$, murine models. This enhanced glycolytic activity was coupled with disrupted differentiation; inhibition of autophagy-mediated lipid metabolism also resulted in halted neutrophil differentiation (189). B1 B cells, which are very active, have higher rates of energy consumption reliant on autophagy; Atg7 deletion leads to the selective loss of B1a B cells due to down-regulation of metabolic genes and dysfunctional mitochondria (125). This further supports the necessity for autophagy in immune cells to have maintained proteostasis and removal of bulk proteins for new protein translation for differentiation and survival (188). In inflammatory contexts, like asthma, the need for energy and efficient use of that energy is crucial for highly replicative and productive immune cell types. Dysregulation of delicate metabolism through autophagy deregulation or loss leads to loss in these cell populations. Metabolic reprogramming of ILC2s, major inflammatory cells in asthma pathogenesis, has been described to be extensively linked with autophagy. Deletion of Atg5 was shown to completely change the layout of ILC2 metabolism (27). Overall decrease in energy levels led to suppressed effector function of ILC2s as well as changes in glycolysis and fatty acid metabolism. Through metabolic and transcriptomic analysis, it was demonstrated that glycolysis was upregulated while fatty acid oxidation was inhibited in ILC2s (27). These metabolic changes led to a decrease in T_H2 cytokine production as well as decreased asthma and AHR. Further disruption of ILC2 metabolism was found through increases in ROS and disrupted mitochondria (27). The new and immerging field of immunometabolism is going to be key in the understanding a more in depth look at disease for the future. The connections between autophagy and immune cell metabolism are extensive and will likely play a pivotal role in this understanding.

ROLE OF AUTOPHAGY IN ASTHMA

Due to asthma and other inflammatory diseases being heterogeneous, targeting of autophagy must be assessed on a patient to patient basis. One of the largest problems faced in the asthmatic population is preconditioning of patients before getting treatment. This preconditioning results in a heterogeneity between patients, the most significant being remodeled lungs (40) and pulmonary viral infection (166). Both of which lead to either resistance to classical treatments or exacerbation of symptoms and further disease pathogenesis. Autophagy plays a prevalent role in a variety of airway remodeling processes (62). These processes can range from regulation of fibroblast populations and fibrosis (59) to increased levels of inflammatory cytokine secretion due to autophagy overactivation in key cell populations, such as ILC2s (27). Interactions between cells in a remodeled lung is completely different in comparison to healthy lung. There is definitely a link between deficits in autophagy due and asthma in the population (45, 46), still its ability to precondition patients before reaching clinical treatment and contribute to asthma pathogenesis has yet to be fully tested. The challenge faced is determining the level and start of lung remodeling in a patient as well as its cause. Autophagy does play a critical role in this development, however there are other factors. As such a large player in inflammatory diseases and general function of eukaryotic cells, autophagy does provide a large therapeutic target. However, determining the role it plays in different cell types is key to understanding how to specifically target it. Targeting of autophagy in the wrong cell type can lead to unwanted inflammation, such as suppression of healthy Treg populations (113) or healthy pulmonary epithelial cells (57). Specific targeting agents must be explored for targeting of certain disease phenotypes where a certain type of inflammation is present. Moreover, in order to reach the best clinical outcome, it is also crucial to consider the stage of development of the disease. Indeed, depending if asthmatic patients are in the initiation or exacerbation phases of the pathogenesis, the specific cell type to be targeted should be considered. The kinetics of disease development should then be a determining factor in identifying the therapeutic target. Interestingly, systemic targeting of autophagy may be able to overcome some of the detrimental effects it may have on a small subset of helpful cells, but the hypothesis is yet to be tested.

AUTOPHAGY MODULATORS AND POTENTIAL TREATMENTS FOR LUNG INFLAMMATION

Autophagy dysfunction has been involved in the pathogenesis of diverse human diseases and in particular in allergic asthma and airway inflammation, and therefore, the regulation of the autophagy mechanisms has emerged as a potential approach recently. Autophagy is a process precisely regulated by a network of proteins. Among the various autophagy modulators, there are several compounds that are FDA approved. Among them, Rapamycin is an antibiotic capable of inducing of autophagy via inhibition of mTOR activity. Rapamycin binds to the cytosolic protein FKBP-12, leading the destabilization of the mTOR complex (190). This drug is used as an immunosuppressant to prevent organ transplant rejection and could represent a potent inducer of autophagy, however its clinical application as an autophagy activator requires further investigation.

Trehalose is a natural disaccharide found in organisms, such as bacteria, fungi, and plants. It has been reported to induce autophagy via mTOR-independent pathway (191). It has been previously established that trehalose can inhibit human cytomegalovirus infection in multiple cell types (192). This result suggests that autophagy inducers could also be considered as a therapeutic option against viral-induced lung inflammation in a selective manner. As increasing autophagy in the early stages of SARS-CoV-2 infection could be beneficiary, trehalose therapeutic application in this context should be explored.

Tamoxifen is a non-steroidal estrogen receptor (ER) antagonist used widely a chemotherapeutic agent against breast cancer (193). Tamoxifen treatment is known to induce

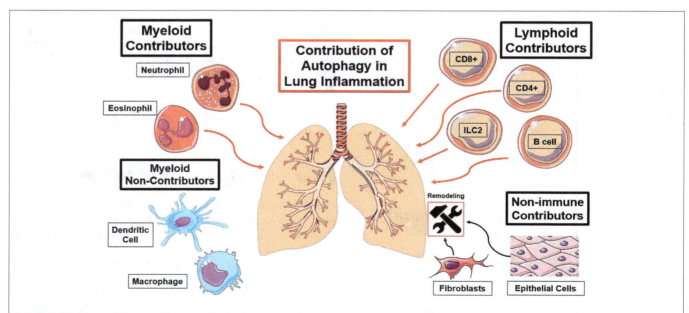

FIGURE 3 | Summary of immune cell types and the functions of autophagy contributing to lung inflammation. Red lines indicate an autophagy-mediated increase in inflammation and black lines indicate an autophagy-mediated contribution to lung remodeling [(23, 25, 27, 30, 37, 41, 57–59, 63, 66, 74, 79, 89, 96, 97, 110, 127), (116, 122, 123, 137, 140, 154)].

autophagy (194) and many recent studies suggest that tamoxifen has antiviral function and should be use in resistant virus infections (195). Interestingly, a randomized clinical trial demonstrated that Carbamazepine, an anticonvulsant drug and autophagy inducer had high efficacy in therapy of moderate or severe bronchial asthma (196). Carbamazepine decreases inositol levels (197) and it has been shown that carbamazepine induces antimicrobial autophagy through mTOR-independent pathway (198), suggesting that autophagy induction by repurposed drug could provide an easily implementable potential therapy for some asthma phenotypes. Also, FDA-approved clonidine prescribed to treat high blood pressure, binds and activates the imidazoline receptor, leading to the decrease of the level of cAMP in cells, thus triggering autophagy (199). Recently, a robust autophagy inducer was described and reported (200); α4-viral Fas-associated death domain-like interleukin-1b-converting enzyme-inhibitory protein (α4vFLIP), is conjugated to trans-activator of transcription (TAT) for cell entry, and has been shown to significantly increase autophagy *in vitro* and *in vivo*. When compared to autophagy inducers, α4-vFLIP seems to be more specific, durable, and robust particularly when utilized *in vivo* as an antiviral agent to ameliorate viral-induced lung inflammation (201).

On the other hand, some chemical compounds can also inhibit autophagic flux, such as clomipramine, which is an FDA-approved drug used for the treatment of psychiatric disorder. Clomipramine and its active metabolite desmethylclomipramine (DCMI) induced an accumulation in autophagosomal markers and a blockage of the degradation of autophagic cargo leading to an inhibition of the autophagy process (202). DCMI is also characterized by its high cytotoxicity increasing the cytotoxic effect of conventional chemotherapeutic drugs (203).

Chloroquine, a medication primarily used to prevent and treat malaria has side effects including neurotoxicity and a change in patients' QT intervals in electrocardiograms which is associated with cardiac arrhythmias. Chloroquine is also an inhibitor viral replication and autophagic flux through inhibiting PPT1 (204) and by preventing endosomal acidification; its accumulation in the endosomes and lysosomes leads to inhibition of lysosomal enzymes that require an acidic pH and prevents fusion of autophagosomes (205). However, chloroquine treatment results in multiple cellular alterations, including the disorganization of the Golgi and endo-lysosomal networks. This large range of action of chloroquine treatments makes the exploration of its autophagy inhibitor properties difficult (205). Therefore, despite anti-viral activity, probably due to inhibition of autophagy, chloroquine treatment for COVID-19 patients reported to have little or no beneficial impact (206).

Various other compounds established regulate autophagy, and many of these molecules have demonstrated to exert beneficial effects. Even though there are many studies with encouraging

results, treatments with cell type specificity are not yet available. By further characterizing the role of autophagy in specific cell populations, it could be possible to design more specific approaches aiming to modulate autophagy.

CONCLUSIONS

Autophagy is a major pathway much like many other metabolic pathways, such as mTOR, and plays a massive role in cellular function. Its role in both the initiation and subsequent allergen challenge in lung inflammatory contexts needs to be explored fully. It is important clinically to understand the effect of changes in autophagic flux in specific cell types in these stages (**Figure 3**). Due to the heterogeneous effect of autophagy on different cell types, cell-specific targeting of autophagy must be the goal for proper clinical outcomes. Systemic targeting of autophagy provides a treatment for certain asthma phenotypes but is not ideal for all patients. Different clinical profiles would require different treatment options and a need for customized medicinal approaches. Understanding the patient's inflammatory context and environment also key in this therapeutic approach. Much like any other asthma treatment, clustering of patients based on their similarities is essential. These factors need to include stage of disease as well as the autophagy requirements. Therefore, determining these different disease phenotypes before treating a chronic patient must be done. The role of autophagy in the pathogenesis of viruses, such as SARS-CoV-2, must further be explored for insight into treatment options. The ideal customized treatment targeting autophagy modulation would consider both the cell specificity and the kinetics of the pathogenesis. The acquisition of promising cell specific agents must be investigated for their modulation autophagic flux. Systemic autophagic modulation may be helpful, however ideally control of certain problematic immune cell types may avoid unwanted side effects. Clustering of patients with lung inflammation may be able to direct treatment options. Lung inflammation and asthma are heterogeneous, so personalized, and clustered approaches may be a solution for designing appropriate autophagy modulators.

AUTHOR CONTRIBUTIONS

JP wrote the manuscript and prepared illustrations. LG-T assisted in edits of the manuscript and illustrations. OA supervised and edited the manuscript. All authors contributed to the article and approved the submitted version.

REFERENCES

1. Rabinowitz J, White E. Autophagy and metabolism. *Science.* (2010) 330:1344–8. doi: 10.1126/science.1 193497

2. Deretic V. Autophagy in immunity and cell-autonomous defense against intracellular microbes. *Immunol Rev.* (2011) 240:92–104. doi: 10.1111/j.1600-065X.2010.00995.x

3. Mizushima N. Autophagy: process and function. *Genes Dev.* (2007) 21:2861–73. doi: 10.1101/gad.1599207

4. Kuma A, Mizushima N. Physiological role of autophagy as an intracellular recycling system: with an emphasis on nutrient metabolism. *Semin Cell Dev Biol.* (2010) 21:683–90. doi: 10.1016/j.semcdb.2010.03.002

5. de Duve C. The Lysosome. *Sci Am.* (1963) 208:64–73. doi: 10.1038/scientificamerican0563-64

6. Duve C, Robert W. Functions of lysosomes. *Annu Rev Physiol.* (1966) 28:435–92. doi: 10.1146/annurev.ph.28.030166.002251

7. Klionsky DJ. The molecular machinery of autophagy: unanswered questions. *J Cell Sci.* (2005) 118:7–18. doi: 10.1242/jcs.01620

8. Feng Y, He D, Yao Z, Klionsky DJ. The machinery of macroautophagy. *Cell Res.* (2014) 24:24–41. doi: 10.1038/cr.2013.168

9. Yano T, Mita S, Ohmori H, Oshima Y, Fujimoto Y, Ueda R, et al. Autophagic control of listeria through intracellular innate immune recognition in drosophila. *Nat Immunol.* (2008) 9:908–16. doi: 10.1038/ni.1634

10. Shelly S, Lukinova N, Bambina S, Berman A, Cherry S. Autophagy is an essential component of Drosophila immunity against vesicular stomatitis virus. *Immunity.* (2009) 30:588–98. doi: 10.1016/j.immuni.2009.02.009

11. Li WW, Li J, Bao JK. Microautophagy: lesser-known self-eating. *Cell Mol Life Sci.* (2012) 69:1125–36. doi: 10.1007/s00018-011-0865-5

12. Oku M, Sakai Y. Three distinct types of microautophagy based on membrane dynamics and molecular machineries. *BioEssays.* (2018) 40:1800008. doi: 10.1002/bies.201800008

13. Dice JF. Chaperone-mediated autophagy. *Autophagy.* (2007) 3:295–9. doi: 10.4161/auto.4144

14. Kaushik S, Bandyopadhyay U, Sridhar S, Kiffin R, Martinez-Vicente M, Kon M, et al. Chaperone-mediated autophagy at a glance. *J Cell Sci.* (2011) 124:495–9. doi: 10.1242/jcs.073874

15. Pyo JO, Nah J, Jung YK. Molecules and their functions in autophagy. *Exp Mol Med.* (2012) 44:73–80. doi: 10.3858/emm.2012.44.2.029

16. Fujita N, Itoh T, Omori H, Fukuda M, Noda T, Yoshimori T. The Atg16L complex specifies the site of LC3 lipidation for membrane biogenesis in autophagy. *Mol Biol Cell.* (2008) 19:2092–100. doi: 10.1091/mbc.e07-12-1257

17. Burman C, Ktistakis NT. Autophagosome formation in mammalian cells. *Semin Immunopathol.* (2010) 32:397–413. doi: 10.1007/s00281-010-0222-z

18. Sou Y, Waguri S, Iwata J, Ueno T, Fujimura T, Hara T, et al. The Atg8 conjugation system is indispensable for proper development of autophagic isolation membranes in mice. *Mol Biol Cell.* (2008) 19:4762–75. doi: 10.1091/mbc.e08-03-0309

19. Kuma A, Komatsu M, Mizushima N. Autophagy-monitoring and autophagy-deficient mice. *Autophagy.* (2017) 13:1619–28. doi: 10.1080/15548627.2017.1343770

20. Rozman S, Yousefi S, Oberson K, Kaufmann T, Benarafa C, Simon HU. The generation of neutrophils in the bone marrow is controlled by autophagy. *Cell Death Differ.* (2015) 22:445–56. doi: 10.1038/cdd.2014.169

21. Pham DL, Ban GY, Kim SH, Shin YS, Ye YM, Chwae YJ, et al. Neutrophil autophagy and extracellular DNA traps contribute to airway inflammation in severe asthma. *Clin Exp Allergy.* (2017) 47:57–70. doi: 10.1111/cea.12859

22. Skendros P, Mitroulis I, Ritis K. Autophagy in neutrophils: from granulopoiesis to neutrophil extracellular traps. *Front Cell Dev Biol.* (2018) 6:109. doi: 10.3389/fcell.2018.00109

23. Iula L, Keitelman IA, Sabbione F, Fuentes F, Guzman M, Galletti JG, et al. Autophagy mediates interleukin-1β secretion in human neutrophils. *Front Immunol.* (2018) 9:269. doi: 10.3389/fimmu.2018.00269

24. Orvedahl A, McAllaster MR, Sansone A, Dunlap BF, Desai C, Wang YT, et al. Autophagy genes in myeloid cells counteract IFNgamma-induced TNF-mediated cell death and fatal TNF-induced shock. *Proc Natl Acad Sci USA.* (2019) 116:16497–506. doi: 10.1073/pnas.1822157116

25. Choi GE, Yoon SY, Kim JY, Kang DY, Jang YJ, Kim HS. Autophagy deficiency in myeloid cells exacerbates eosinophilic inflammation in chronic rhinosinusitis. *J Allergy Clin Immunol.* (2018) 141:938–50 e912. doi: 10.1016/j.jaci.2017.10.038

26. Ghislat G, Lawrence T. Autophagy in dendritic cells. *Cell Mol Immunol.* (2018) 15:944–52. doi: 10.1038/cmi.2018.2

27. Galle-Treger L, Hurrell BP, Lewis G, Howard E, Jahani PS, Banie H, et al. Autophagy is critical for group 2 innate lymphoid cell metabolic homeostasis and effector function. *J Allergy Clin Immunol.* (2019) 145:502–17.e5. doi: 10.1016/j.jaci.2019.10.035

28. He W, Xiong W, Xia X. Autophagy regulation of mammalian immune cells. *Adv Exp Med Biol.* (2019) 1209:7–22. doi: 10.1007/978-981-15-0606-2_2

29. Choy DF, Hart KM, Borthwick LA, Shikotra A, Nagarkar DR, Siddiqui S, et al. Th2 and Th17 inflammatory pathways are reciprocally regulated in asthma. *Sci Transl Med.* (2015) 7:301ra129. doi: 10.1126/scitranslmed.aab3142

30. Suzuki Y, Maazi H, Sankaranarayanan I, Lam J, Khoo B, Soroosh P, et al. Lack of autophagy induces steroid-resistant airway inflammation. *J Allergy Clin Immunol.* (2016) 137:1382–9 e1389. doi: 10.1016/j.jaci.2015.09.033

31. Kirkland SW, Vandenberghe C, Voaklander B, Nikel T, Campbell S, Rowe BH. Combined inhaled beta-agonist and anticholinergic agents for emergency management in adults with asthma. *Cochrane Database Syst Rev.* (2017) 1:CD001284. doi: 10.1002/14651858.CD001284.pub2

32. Barnes PJ. Severe asthma: advances in current management and future therapy. *J Allergy Clin Immunol.* (2012) 129:48–59. doi: 10.1016/j.jaci.2011.11.006

33. Bartemes KR, Kephart GM, Fox SJ, Kita H. Enhanced innate type 2 immune response in peripheral blood from patients with asthma. *J Allergy Clin Immunol.* (2014) 134:671–8.e674. doi: 10.1016/j.jaci.2014.06.024

34. Vroman H, van den Blink B, Kool M. Mode of dendritic cell activation: the decisive hand in Th2/Th17 cell differentiation. Implications in asthma severity? *Immunobiology.* (2015) 220:254–61. doi: 10.1016/j.imbio.2014.09.016

35. Lewis G, Wang B, Shafiei Jahani P, Hurrell BP, Banie H, Aleman Muench GR, et al. Dietary fiber-induced microbial short chain fatty acids suppress ILC2-dependent airway inflammation. *Front Immunol.* (2019) 10:2051. doi: 10.3389/fimmu.2019.02051

36. Cosmi L, Liotta F, Maggi E, Romagnani S, Annunziato F. Th17 and non-classic Th1 cells in chronic inflammatory disorders: two sides of the same coin. *Int Arch Allergy Immunol.* (2014) 164:171–7. doi: 10.1159/000363502

37. Bhattacharya A, Wei Q, Shin JN, Abdel Fattah E, Bonilla DL, Xiang Q, et al. Autophagy is required for neutrophil-mediated inflammation. *Cell Rep.* (2015) 12:1731–9. doi: 10.1016/j.celrep.2015.08.019

38. Wenzel SE. Asthma phenotypes: the evolution from clinical to molecular approaches. *Nat Med.* (2012) 18:716–25. doi: 10.1038/nm.2678

39. Belvisi MG, Hele DJ, Birrell MA. New advances and potential therapies for the treatment of asthma. *BioDrugs.* (2004) 18:211–23. doi: 10.2165/00063030-200418040-00001

40. Yamauchi K. Airway remodeling in asthma and its influence on clinical pathophysiology. *Tohoku J Exp Med.* (2006) 209:75–87. doi: 10.1620/tjem.209.75

41. Ban GY, Pham DL, Trinh TH, Lee SI, Suh DH, Yang EM, et al. Autophagy mechanisms in sputum and peripheral blood cells of patients with severe asthma: a new therapeutic target. *Clin Exp Allergy.* (2016) 46:48–59. doi: 10.1111/cea.12585

42. Jiang X, Fang L, Wu H, Mei X, He F, Ding P, et al. TLR2 regulates allergic airway inflammation and autophagy through PI3K/Akt signaling pathway. *Inflammation.* (2017) 40:1382–92. doi: 10.1007/s10753-017-0581-x

43. Sinclair C, Bommakanti G, Gardinassi L, Loebbermann J, Johnson MJ, Hakimpour P, et al. mTOR regulates metabolic adaptation of APCs in the lung and controls the outcome of allergic inflammation. *Science.* (2017) 357:1014. doi: 10.1126/science.aaj2155

44. Silveira JS, Antunes GL, Kaiber DB, da Costa MS, Ferreira FS, Marques EP, et al. Autophagy induces eosinophil extracellular traps formation and allergic airway inflammation in a murine asthma model. *J Cell Physiol.* (2020) 235:267–80. doi: 10.1002/jcp.28966

45. Martin LJ, Gupta J, Jyothula SS, Butsch Kovacic M, Biagini Myers JM, Patterson TL, et al. Functional variant in the autophagy-related 5 gene promotor is associated with childhood asthma. *PLoS ONE.* (2012) 7:e33454. doi: 10.1371/journal.pone.0033454

46. Poon A, Eidelman D, Laprise C, Hamid Q. ATG5, autophagy and lung function in asthma. *Autophagy.* (2012) 8:694–5. doi: 10.4161/auto.19315

47. Palomino-Morales RJ, Oliver J, Gómez-García M, López-Nevot MA, Rodrigo L, Nieto A, et al. Association of ATG16L1 and IRGM genes polymorphisms with inflammatory bowel disease: a meta-analysis approach. *Genes Immun.* (2009) 10:356–64. doi: 10.1038/gene.2009.25

48. Liu T, Liu Y, Miller M, Cao L, Zhao J, Wu J, et al. Autophagy plays a role in FSTL1-induced epithelial mesenchymal transition and airway

remodeling in asthma. *Am J Physiol Lung Cell Mol Physiol.* (2017) 313:L27–40. doi: 10.1152/ajplung.00510.2016

49. Poon AH, Choy DF, Chouiali F, Ramakrishnan RK, Mahboub B, Audusseau S, et al. Increased autophagy-related 5 gene expression is associated with collagen expression in the airways of refractory asthmatics. *Front Immunol.* (2017) 8:355. doi: 10.3389/fimmu.2017.00355

50. Dickinson JD, Alevy Y, Malvin NP, Patel KK, Gunsten SP, Holtzman MJ, et al. IL13 activates autophagy to regulate secretion in airway epithelial cells. *Autophagy.* (2016) 12:397–409. doi: 10.1080/15548627.2015.1056967

51. Dickinson JD, Sweeter JM, Warren KJ, Ahmad IM, De Deken X, Zimmerman MC, et al. Autophagy regulates DUOX1 localization and superoxide production in airway epithelial cells during chronic IL-13 stimulation. *Redox Biol.* (2018) 14:272–84. doi: 10.1016/j.redox.2017.09.013

52. Liu H, Mi S, Li Z, Hua F, Hu ZW. Interleukin 17A inhibits autophagy through activation of PIK3CA to interrupt the GSK3B-mediated degradation of BCL2 in lung epithelial cells. *Autophagy.* (2013) 9:730–42. doi: 10.4161/auto.24039

53. Chen YD, Fang YT, Cheng YL, Lin CF, Hsu LJ, Wang SY, et al. Exophagy of annexin A2 via RAB11, RAB8A and RAB27A in IFN-gamma-stimulated lung epithelial cells. *Sci Rep.* (2017) 7:5676. doi: 10.1038/s41598-017-06076-4

54. Fougeray S, Mami I, Bertho G, Beaune P, Thervet E, Pallet N. Tryptophan depletion and the kinase GCN2 mediate IFN-γ-induced autophagy. *J Immunol.* (2012) 189:2954. doi: 10.4049/jimmunol.1201214

55. Wang BF, Cao PP, Wang ZC, Li ZY, Wang ZZ, Ma J, et al. Interferon-γ-induced insufficient autophagy contributes to p62-dependent apoptosis of epithelial cells in chronic rhinosinusitis with nasal polyps. *Allergy.* (2017) 72:1384–97. doi: 10.1111/all.13153

56. Schuliga M, Langenbach S, Xia YC, Qin C, Mok JS, Harris T, et al. Plasminogen-stimulated inflammatory cytokine production by airway smooth muscle cells is regulated by annexin A2. *Am J Respir Cell Mol Biol.* (2013) 49:751–8. doi: 10.1165/rcmb.2012-0404OC

57. O'Dwyer DN, Ashley SL, Moore BB. Influences of innate immunity, autophagy, and fibroblast activation in the pathogenesis of lung fibrosis. *Am J Physiol Lung Cell Mol Physiol.* (2016) 311:L590–601. doi: 10.1152/ajplung.00221.2016

58. Ghavami S, Cunnington RH, Gupta S, Yeganeh B, Filomeno KL, Freed DH, et al. Autophagy is a regulator of TGF-β1-induced fibrogenesis in primary human atrial myofibroblasts. *Cell Death Dis.* (2015) 6:e1696. doi: 10.1038/cddis.2015.36

59. Sosulski ML, Gongora R, Danchuk S, Dong C, Luo F, Sanchez CG. Deregulation of selective autophagy during aging and pulmonary fibrosis: the role of TGFbeta1. *Aging Cell.* (2015) 14:774–83. doi: 10.1111/acel.12357

60. Li K, Li M, Li W, Yu H, Sun X, Zhang Q, et al. Airway epithelial regeneration requires autophagy and glucose metabolism. *Cell Death Dis.* (2019) 10:875. doi: 10.1038/s41419-019-2111-2

61. Chen ZH, Wu YF, Wang PL, Wu YP, Li ZY, Zhao Y, et al. Autophagy is essential for ultrafine particle-induced inflammation and mucus hyperproduction in airway epithelium. *Autophagy.* (2016) 12:297–311. doi: 10.1080/15548627.2015.1124224

62. McAlinden KD, Deshpande DA, Ghavami S, Xenaki D, Sohal SS, Oliver BG, et al. Autophagy activation in asthma airways remodeling. *Am J Respir Cell Mol Biol.* (2019) 60:541–53. doi: 10.1165/rcmb.2018-0169OC

63. Makinde T, Murphy RF, Agrawal DK. The regulatory role of TGF-β in airway remodeling in asthma. *Immunol Cell Biol.* (2007) 85:348–56. doi: 10.1038/sj.icb.7100044

64. Gerthoffer WT, Schaafsma D, Sharma P, Ghavami S, Halayko AJ. Motility, survival, and proliferation. *Compr Physiol.* 2:255–281. doi: 10.1002/cphy.c110018

65. Schaafsma D, Dueck G, Ghavami S, Kroeker A, Mutawe MM, Hauff K, et al. The mevalonate cascade as a target to suppress extracellular matrix synthesis by human airway smooth muscle. *Am J Respir Cell Mol Biol.* (2011) 44:394–403. doi: 10.1165/rcmb.2010-0052OC

66. Yeganeh B, Mukherjee S, Moir LM, Kumawat K, Kashani HH, Bagchi RA, et al. Novel non-canonical TGF-β signaling networks: emerging roles in airway smooth muscle phenotype and function. *Pulmon Pharmacol Ther.* (2013) 26:50–63. doi: 10.1016/j.pupt.2012.07.006

67. Zeki AA, Yeganeh B, Kenyon NJ, Post M, Ghavami S. Autophagy in airway diseases: a new frontier in human asthma? *Allergy.* (2016) 71:5–14. doi: 10.1111/all.12761

68. Martinez J, Cunha LD, Park S, Yang M, Lu Q, Orchard R, et al. Noncanonical autophagy inhibits the autoinflammatory, lupus-like response to dying cells. *Nature.* (2016) 533:115–9. doi: 10.1038/nature17950

69. Ravindran R, Loebbermann J, Nakaya HI, Khan N, Ma H, Gama L, et al. The amino acid sensor GCN2 controls gut inflammation by inhibiting inflammasome activation. *Nature.* (2016) 531:523–7. doi: 10.1038/nature17186

70. Lee HK, Mattei LM, Steinberg BE, Alberts P, Lee YH, Chervonsky A, et al. *In vivo* requirement for Atg5 in antigen presentation by dendritic cells. *Immunity.* (2010) 32:227–39. doi: 10.1016/j.immuni.2009.12.006

71. Keller CW, Sina C, Kotur MB, Ramelli G, Mundt S, Quast I, et al. ATG-dependent phagocytosis in dendritic cells drives myelin-specific CD4+ T cell pathogenicity during CNS inflammation. *Proc Natl Acad Sci USA.* (2017) 114:E11228. doi: 10.1073/pnas.1713664114

72. Loi M, Gannagé M, Münz C. ATGs help MHC class II, but inhibit MHC class I antigen presentation. *Autophagy.* (2016) 12:1681–2. doi: 10.1080/15548627.2016.1203488

73. Oh DS, Lee HK. Autophagy protein ATG5 regulates CD36 expression and anti-tumor MHC class II antigen presentation in dendritic cells. *Autophagy.* (2019) 15:2091–106. doi: 10.1080/15548627.2019.1596493

74. Loi M, Müller A, Steinbach K, Niven J, Barreira da Silva R, Paul P, et al. Macroautophagy proteins control MHC class I levels on dendritic cells and shape anti-viral CD8+ T cell responses. *Cell Rep.* (2016) 15:1076–87. doi: 10.1016/j.celrep.2016.04.002

75. Lee HK, Lund JM, Ramanathan B, Mizushima N, Iwasaki A. Autophagy-dependent viral recognition by plasmacytoid dendritic cells. *Science.* (2007) 315:1398. doi: 10.1126/science.1136880

76. Khoury-Hanold W, Iwasaki A. Autophagy snuffs a macrophage's inner fire. *Cell Host Microbe.* (2016) 19:9–11. doi: 10.1016/j.chom.2015.12.015

77. Bechelli J, Vergara L, Smalley C, Buzhdygan TP, Bender S, Zhang W, et al. Atg5 supports *Rickettsia australis* infection in macrophages *in vitro* and *in vivo*. *Infect Immun.* (2018) 87:e00651-18. doi: 10.1128/IAI.00651-18

78. Lodder J, Denaës T, Chobert M-N, Wan J, El-Benna J, Pawlotsky J-M, et al. Macrophage autophagy protects against liver fibrosis in mice. *Autophagy.* (2015) 11:1280–92. doi: 10.1080/15548627.2015.1058473

79. Pu Q, Gan C, Li R, Li Y, Tan S, Li X, et al. Atg7 deficiency intensifies inflammasome activation and pyroptosis in *Pseudomonas sepsis*. *J Immunol.* (2017) 198:3205. doi: 10.4049/jimmunol.1601196

80. Delgado-Rizo V, Martinez-Guzman MA, Iniguez-Gutierrez L, Garcia-Orozco A, Alvarado-Navarro A, Fafutis-Morris M. Neutrophil extracellular traps and its implications in inflammation: an overview. *Front Immunol.* (2017) 8:81. doi: 10.3389/fimmu.2017.00081

81. Dworski R, Simon HU, Hoskins A, Yousefi S. Eosinophil and neutrophil extracellular DNA traps in human allergic asthmatic airways. *J Allergy Clin Immunol.* (2011) 127:1260–6. doi: 10.1016/j.jaci.2010.12.1103

82. Germic N, Stojkov D, Oberson K, Yousefi S, Simon HU. Neither eosinophils nor neutrophils require ATG5-dependent autophagy for extracellular DNA trap formation. *Immunology.* (2017) 152:517–25. doi: 10.1111/imm.12790

83. Park SY, Shrestha S, Youn Y-J, Kim J-K, Kim S-Y, Kim HJ, et al. Autophagy primes neutrophils for neutrophil extracellular trap formation during sepsis. *Am J Respir Crit Care Med.* (2017) 196:577–89. doi: 10.1164/rccm.201603-0596OC

84. Germic N, Frangez Z, Yousefi S, Simon HU. Regulation of the innate immune system by autophagy: neutrophils, eosinophils, mast cells, NK cells. *Cell Death Differ.* (2019) 26:703–14. doi: 10.1038/s41418-019-0295-8

85. Mihalache CC, Yousefi S, Conus S, Villiger PM, Schneider EM, Simon HU. Inflammation-associated autophagy-related programmed necrotic death of human neutrophils characterized by organelle fusion events. *J Immunol.* (2011) 186:6532–42. doi: 10.4049/jimmunol.1004055

86. Hua W, Liu H, Xia L-X, Tian B-P, Huang H-Q, Chen Z-Y, et al. Rapamycin inhibition of eosinophil differentiation attenuates allergic airway inflammation in mice. *Respirology.* (2015) 20:1055–65. doi: 10.1111/resp.12554

87. Zhu C, Xia L, Li F, Zhou L, Weng Q, Li Z, et al. mTOR complexes differentially orchestrates eosinophil development in allergy. *Sci Rep.* (2018) 8:6883. doi: 10.1038/s41598-018-25358-z

88. Radonjic-Hoesli S, Wang X, de Graauw E, Stoeckle C, Styp-Rekowska B, Hlushchuk R, et al. Adhesion-induced eosinophil cytolysis requires the

receptor-interacting protein kinase 3 (RIPK3)-mixed lineage kinase-like (MLKL) signaling pathway, which is counterregulated by autophagy. *J Allergy Clin Immunol.* (2017) 140:1632–42. doi: 10.1016/j.jaci.2017.01.044

89. Xu YD, Hua J, Mui A, O'Connor R, Grotendorst G, Khalil N. Release of biologically active TGF-β1 by alveolar epithelial cells results in pulmonary fibrosis. *Am J Physiol Lung Cell Mol Physiol.* (2003) 285:L527–39. doi: 10.1152/ajplung.00298.2002

90. Harris J. Autophagy and cytokines. *Cytokine.* (2011) 56:140–4. doi: 10.1016/j.cyto.2011.08.022

91. Strisciuglio C, Duijvestein M, Verhaar AP, Vos AC, van den Brink GR, Hommes DW, et al. Impaired autophagy leads to abnormal dendritic cell-epithelial cell interactions. *J Crohns Colitis.* (2013) 7:534–41. doi: 10.1016/j.crohns.2012.08.009

92. Alissafi T, Banos A, Boon L, Sparwasser T, Ghigo A, Wing K, et al. Tregs restrain dendritic cell autophagy to ameliorate autoimmunity. *J Clin Invest.* (2017) 127:2789–804. doi: 10.1172/JCI92079

93. Münz C. Autophagy proteins in antigen processing for presentation on MHC molecules. *Immunol Rev.* (2016) 272:17–27. doi: 10.1111/imr.12422

94. Wang F, Muller S. Manipulating autophagic processes in autoimmune diseases: a special focus on modulating chaperone-mediated autophagy, an emerging therapeutic target. *Front Immunol.* (2015) 6:252. doi: 10.3389/fimmu.2015.00252

95. Jacquel A, Obba S, Boyer L, Dufies M, Robert G, Gounon P, et al. Autophagy is required for CSF-1–induced macrophagic differentiation and acquisition of phagocytic functions. *Blood.* (2012) 119:4527–31. doi: 10.1182/blood-2011-11-392651

96. Zhang Y, Morgan MJ, Chen K, Choksi S, Liu ZG. Induction of autophagy is essential for monocyte-macrophage differentiation. *Blood.* (2012) 119:2895–905. doi: 10.1182/blood-2011-08-372383

97. Abdel Fattah E, Bhattacharya A, Herron A, Safdar Z, Eissa NT. Critical role for IL-18 in spontaneous lung inflammation caused by autophagy deficiency. *J Immunol.* (2015) 194:5407–16. doi: 10.4049/jimmunol.1402277

98. Liu K, Zhao E, Ilyas G, Lalazar G, Lin Y, Haseeb M, et al. Impaired macrophage autophagy increases the immune response in obese mice by promoting proinflammatory macrophage polarization. *Autophagy.* (2015) 11:271–84. doi: 10.1080/15548627.2015.1009787

99. Ilyas G, Zhao E, Liu K, Lin Y, Tesfa L, Tanaka KE, et al. Macrophage autophagy limits acute toxic liver injury in mice through down regulation of interleukin-1β. *J Hepatol.* (2016) 64:118–27. doi: 10.1016/j.jhep.2015.08.019

100. Santeford A, Wiley LA, Park S, Bamba S, Nakamura R, Gdoura A, et al. Impaired autophagy in macrophages promotes inflammatory eye disease. *Autophagy.* (2016) 12:1876–85. doi: 10.1080/15548627.2016.1207857

101. Aflaki E, Moaven N, Borger DK, Lopez G, Westbroek W, Chae JJ, et al. Lysosomal storage and impaired autophagy lead to inflammasome activation in Gaucher macrophages. *Aging Cell.* (2016) 15:77–88. doi: 10.1111/acel.12409

102. Su Y-C, Rolph MS, Hansbro NG, Mackay CR, Sewell WA. Granulocyte-macrophage colony-stimulating factor is required for bronchial eosinophilia in a murine model of allergic airway inflammation. *J Immunol.* (2008) 180:2600. doi: 10.4049/jimmunol.180.4.2600

103. Robinson DS, Hamid Q, Ying S, Tsicopoulos A, Barkans J, Bentley AM, et al. Predominant TH2-like bronchoalveolar T-lymphocyte population in atopic asthma. *N Engl J Med.* (1992) 326:298–304. doi: 10.1056/NEJM199201303260504

104. Jia W, He Y-W. Temporal regulation of intracellular organelle homeostasis in T lymphocytes by autophagy. *J Immunol.* (2011) 186:5313. doi: 10.4049/jimmunol.1002404

105. Jia W, He M-X, McLeod IX, Guo J, Ji D, He Y-W. Autophagy regulates T lymphocyte proliferation through selective degradation of the cell-cycle inhibitor CDKN1B/p27Kip1. *Autophagy.* (2015) 11:2335–45. doi: 10.1080/15548627.2015.1110666

106. O'Sullivan TE, Johnson LR, Kang HH, Sun JC. BNIP3- and BNIP3L-mediated mitophagy promotes the generation of natural killer cell memory. *Immunity.* (2015) 43:331–42. doi: 10.1016/j.immuni.2015.07.012

107. Pua HH, Dzhagalov I, Chuck M, Mizushima N, He Y-W. A critical role for the autophagy gene Atg5 in T cell survival and proliferation. *J Exp Med.* (2006) 204:25–31. doi: 10.1084/jem.20061303

108. Schlie K, Westerback A, DeVorkin L, Hughson LR, Brandon JM, MacPherson S, et al. Survival of effector CD8+T cells during influenza infection is dependent on autophagy. *J Immunol.* (2015) 194:4277. doi: 10.4049/jimmunol.1402571

109. Puleston DJ, Zhang H, Powell TJ, Lipina E, Sims S, Panse I, et al. Autophagy is a critical regulator of memory CD8(+) T cell formation. *eLife.* (2014) 3:e03706. doi: 10.7554/eLife.03706.017

110. Xu X, Araki K, Li S, Han JH, Ye L, Tan WG, et al. Autophagy is essential for effector CD8(+) T cell survival and memory formation. *Nat Immunol.* (2014) 15:1152–61. doi: 10.1038/ni.3025

111. van Loosdregt J, Rossetti M, Spreafico R, Moshref M, Olmer M, Williams GW, et al. Increased autophagy in CD4+ T cells of rheumatoid arthritis patients results in T-cell hyperactivation and apoptosis resistance. *Eur J Immunol.* (2016) 46:2862–70. doi: 10.1002/eji.201646375

112. Murera D, Arbogast F, Arnold J, Bouis D, Muller S, Gros F. CD4 T cell autophagy is integral to memory maintenance. *Sci Rep.* (2018) 8:5951. doi: 10.1038/s41598-018-23993-0

113. Wei J, Long L, Yang K, Guy C, Shrestha S, Chen Z, et al. Autophagy enforces functional integrity of regulatory T cells by coupling environmental cues and metabolic homeostasis. *Nat Immunol.* (2016) 17:277–85. doi: 10.1038/ni.3365

114. Pengo N, Scolari M, Oliva L, Milan E, Mainoldi F, Raimondi A, et al. Plasma cells require autophagy for sustainable immunoglobulin production. *Nat Immunol.* (2013) 14:298–305. doi: 10.1038/ni.2524

115. Oliva L, Cenci S. Autophagy in plasma cell pathophysiology. *Front Immunol.* (2014) 5:103. doi: 10.3389/fimmu.2014.00103

116. Sandoval H, Kodali S, Wang J. Regulation of B cell fate, survival, and function by mitochondria and autophagy. *Mitochondrion.* (2018) 41:58–65. doi: 10.1016/j.mito.2017.11.005

117. Arnold J, Murera D, Arbogast F, Fauny JD, Muller S, Gros F. Autophagy is dispensable for B-cell development but essential for humoral autoimmune responses. *Cell Death Differ.* (2016) 23:853–64. doi: 10.1038/cdd.2015.149

118. Arbogast F, Arnold J, Hammann P, Kuhn L, Chicher J, Murera D, et al. ATG5 is required for B cell polarization and presentation of particulate antigens. *Autophagy.* (2019) 15:280–94. doi: 10.1080/15548627.2018.1516327

119. O'Sullivan TE, Geary CD, Weizman OE, Geiger TL, Rapp M, Dorn GW, et al. Atg5 is essential for the development and survival of innate lymphocytes. *Cell Rep.* (2016) 15:1910–9. doi: 10.1016/j.celrep.2016.04.082

120. Pei B, Zhao M, Miller BC, Véla JL, Bruinsma MW, Virgin HW, et al. Invariant NKT cells require autophagy to coordinate proliferation and survival signals during differentiation. *J Immunol.* (2015) 194:5872–84. doi: 10.4049/jimmunol.1402154

121. Salio M, Puleston DJ, Mathan TSM, Shepherd D, Stranks AJ, Adamopoulou E, et al. Essential role for autophagy during invariant NKT cell development. *Proc Natl Acad Sci USA.* (2014) 111:E5678–87. doi: 10.1073/pnas.1413935112

122. Hubbard VM, Valdor R, Patel B, Singh R, Cuervo AM, Macian F. Macroautophagy regulates energy metabolism during effector T cell activation. *J Immunol.* (2010) 185:7349. doi: 10.4049/jimmunol.1000576

123. Chen M, Hong MJ, Sun H, Wang L, Shi X, Gilbert BE, et al. Essential role for autophagy in the maintenance of immunological memory against influenza infection. *Nat Med.* (2014) 20:503–10. doi: 10.1038/nm.3521

124. Chen M, Kodali S, Jang A, Kuai L, Wang J. Requirement for autophagy in the long-term persistence but not initial formation of memory B cells. *J Immunol.* (2015) 194:2607–15. doi: 10.4049/jimmunol.1403001

125. Clarke AJ, Riffelmacher T, Braas D, Cornall RJ, Simon AK. B1a B cells require autophagy for metabolic homeostasis and self-renewal. *J Exp Med.* (2018) 215:399–413. doi: 10.1084/jem.20170771

126. Clarke AJ, Ellinghaus U, Cortini A, Stranks A, Simon AK, Botto M, et al. Autophagy is activated in systemic lupus erythematosus and required for plasmablast development. *Ann Rheum Dis.* (2015) 74:912. doi: 10.1136/annrheumdis-2013-204343

127. Valdor R, Mocholi E, Botbol Y, Guerrero-Ros I, Chandra D, Koga H, et al. Chaperone-mediated autophagy regulates T cell responses through targeted degradation of negative regulators of T cell activation. *Nat Immunol.* (2014) 15:1046–54. doi: 10.1038/ni.3003

128. Pua HH, Guo J, Komatsu M, He Y-W. Autophagy is essential for mitochondrial clearance in mature T lymphocytes.

J Immunol. (2009) 182:4046. doi: 10.4049/jimmunol.08 01143

129. Zeng H, Chi H. mTOR signaling in the differentiation and function of regulatory and effector T cells. *Curr Opin Immunol.* (2017) 46:103–11. doi: 10.1016/j.coi.2017.04.005

130. Mizushima N. The role of the Atg1/ULK1 complex in autophagy regulation. *Curr Opin Cell Biol.* (2010) 22:132–9. doi: 10.1016/j.ceb.2009.12.004

131. Arnold CR, Pritz T, Brunner S, Knabb C, Salvenmoser W, Holzwarth B, et al. T cell receptor-mediated activation is a potent inducer of macroautophagy in human CD8(+)CD28(+) T cells but not in CD8(+)CD28(-) T cells. *Exp Gerontol.* (2014) 54:75–83. doi: 10.1016/j.exger.2014.01.018

132. Nicoli F, Papagno L, Frere JJ, Cabral-Piccin MP, Clave E, Gostick E, et al. Naive CD8(+) T-cells engage a versatile metabolic program upon activation in humans and differ energetically from memory CD8(+) T-cells. *Front Immunol.* (2018) 9:2736. doi: 10.3389/fimmu.2018.02736

133. Kim J, Kundu M, Viollet B, Guan K-L. AMPK and mTOR regulate autophagy through direct phosphorylation of Ulk1. *Nat Cell Biol.* (2011) 13:132–41. doi: 10.1038/ncb2152

134. Gwinn DM, Shackelford DB, Egan DF, Mihaylova MM, Mery A, Vasquez DS, et al. AMPK phosphorylation of raptor mediates a metabolic checkpoint. *Mol Cell.* (2008) 30:214–26. doi: 10.1016/j.molcel.2008.03.003

135. Inoki K, Zhu T, Guan K-L. TSC2 mediates cellular energy response to control cell growth and survival. *Cell.* (2003) 115:577–90. doi: 10.1016/S0092-8674(03)00929-2

136. Henson SM, Lanna A, Riddell NE, Franzese O, Macaulay R, Griffiths SJ, et al. p38 signaling inhibits mTORC1-independent autophagy in senescent human CD8(+) T cells. *J Clin Invest.* (2014) 124:4004–16. doi: 10.1172/JCI75051

137. DeVorkin L, Pavey N, Carleton G, Comber A, Ho C, Lim J, et al. Autophagy regulation of metabolism is required for CD8$^+$ T cell anti-tumor immunity. *Cell Rep.* (2019) 27:502–13.e505. doi: 10.1016/j.celrep.2019.03.037

138. Ling MF, Luster AD. Allergen-specific CD4(+) T cells in human asthma. *Ann Am Thorac Soc.* (2016) 13:S25–30. doi: 10.1513/AnnalsATS.201507-431MG

139. Jacquin E, Apetoh L. Cell-intrinsic roles for autophagy in modulating CD4 T cell functions. *Front Immunol.* (2018) 9:1023. doi: 10.3389/fimmu.2018.01023

140. Botbol Y, Patel B, Macian F. Common γ-chain cytokine signaling is required for macroautophagy induction during CD4$^+$ T-cell activation. *Autophagy.* (2015) 11:1864–77. doi: 10.1080/15548627.2015.1089374

141. Matsuzawa Y, Oshima S, Takahara M, Maeyashiki C, Nemoto Y, Kobayashi M, et al. TNFAIP3 promotes survival of CD4 T cells by restricting MTOR and promoting autophagy. *Autophagy.* (2015) 11:1052–62. doi: 10.1080/15548627.2015.1055439

142. Willinger T, Flavell RA. Canonical autophagy dependent on the class III phosphoinositide-3 kinase Vps34 is required for naive T-cell homeostasis. *Proc Natl Acad Sci USA.* (2012) 109:8670–5. doi: 10.1073/pnas.120530 5109

143. Parekh VV, Wu L, Boyd KL, Williams JA, Gaddy JA, Olivares-Villagómez D, et al. Impaired autophagy, defective T cell homeostasis, and a Wasting syndrome in mice with a T cell–specific deletion of Vps34. *J Immunol.* (2013) 190:5086. doi: 10.4049/jimmunol.1202071

144. Ying L, Zhao G-J, Wu Y, Ke H-L, Hong G-L, Zhang H, et al. Mitofusin 2 promotes apoptosis of CD4(+) T cells by inhibiting autophagy in sepsis. *Mediat Inflamm.* (2017) 2017:4926205. doi: 10.1155/2017/4926205

145. Wang H, Bai G, Cui N, Han W, Long Y. T-cell-specific mTOR deletion in mice ameliorated CD4(+) T-cell survival in lethal sepsis induced by severe invasive candidiasis. *Virulence.* (2019) 10:892–901. doi: 10.1080/21505594.2019.1685151

146. Kato H, Perl A. Blockade of Treg cell differentiation and function by the interleukin-21-mechanistic target of rapamycin axis via suppression of autophagy in patients with systemic lupus erythematosus. *Arthritis Rheumatol.* (2018) 70:427–38. doi: 10.1002/art.40380

147. Paul S, Kashyap AK, Jia W, He Y-W, Schaefer BC. Selective autophagy of the adaptor protein Bcl10 modulates T cell receptor activation of NF-κB. *Immunity.* (2012) 36:947–58. doi: 10.1016/j.immuni.2012.04.008

148. Noval Rivas M, Chatila TA. Regulatory T cells in allergic diseases. *J Allergy Clin Immunol.* (2016) 138:639–52. doi: 10.1016/j.jaci.2016.06.003

149. Bektas A, Schurman SH, Gonzalez-Freire M, Dunn CA, Singh AK, Macian F, et al. Age-associated changes in human CD4(+) T cells point to mitochondrial dysfunction consequent to impaired autophagy. *Aging.* (2019) 11:9234–63. doi: 10.18632/aging.102438

150. Martinez-Martin N, Maldonado P, Gasparrini F, Frederico B, Aggarwal S, Gaya M, et al. A switch from canonical to noncanonical autophagy shapes B cell responses. *Science.* (2017) 355:641. doi: 10.1126/science.aal3908

151. Zhang H, Simon AK. Polyamines reverse immune senescence via the translational control of autophagy. *Autophagy.* (2020) 16:181–2. doi: 10.1080/15548627.2019.1687967

152. Xia F, Deng C, Jiang Y, Qu Y, Deng J, Cai Z, et al. IL4 (interleukin 4) induces autophagy in B cells leading to exacerbated asthma. *Autophagy.* (2018) 14:450–64. doi: 10.1080/15548627.2017.1421884

153. Dong G, You M, Fan H, Ding L, Sun L, Hou Y. STS-1 promotes IFN-α induced autophagy by activating the JAK1-STAT1 signaling pathway in B cells. *Eur J Immunol.* (2015) 45:2377–88. doi: 10.1002/eji.201445349

154. Saunders SP, Ma EGM, Aranda CJ, Curotto de Lafaille MA. Non-classical B cell memory of allergic IgE responses. *Front Immunol.* (2019) 10:715. doi: 10.3389/fimmu.2019.00715

155. Dong X, Qin J, Ma J, Zeng Q, Zhang H, Zhang R, et al. BAFF inhibits autophagy promoting cell proliferation and survival by activating Ca(2+)-CaMKII-dependent Akt/mTOR signaling pathway in normal and neoplastic B-lymphoid cells. *Cell Signal.* (2019) 53:68–79. doi: 10.1016/j.cellsig.2018.09.012

156. Jee HM, Choi BS, Kim KW, Sohn MH, Han MY, Kim K-E. Increased B cell-activating factor (BAFF) level in the sputum of children with asthma. *Korean J Pediatr.* (2010) 53:795–800. doi: 10.3345/kjp.2010.53.8.795

157. Pérez L, McLetchie S, Gardiner GJ, Deffit SN, Zhou D, Blum JS. LAMP-2C inhibits MHC class II presentation of cytoplasmic antigens by disrupting chaperone-mediated autophagy. *J Immunol.* (2016) 196:2457. doi: 10.4049/jimmunol.1501476

158. Maazi H, Akbari O. ICOS regulates ILC2s in asthma. *Oncotarget.* (2015) 6:24584–5. doi: 10.18632/oncotarget.5245

159. Hurrell BP, Shafiei Jahani P, Akbari O. Social networking of group two innate lymphoid cells in allergy and asthma. *Front Immunol.* (2018) 9:2694. doi: 10.3389/fimmu.2018.02694

160. Hurez V, Dao V, Liu A, Pandeswara S, Gelfond J, Sun L, et al. Chronic mTOR inhibition in mice with rapamycin alters T, B, myeloid, and innate lymphoid cells and gut flora and prolongs life of immune-deficient mice. *Aging Cell.* (2015) 14:945–56. doi: 10.1111/acel.12380

161. Aron JL, Akbari O. Regulatory T cells and type 2 innate lymphoid cell-dependent asthma. *Allergy.* (2017) 72:1148–55. doi: 10.1111/all.13139

162. Rigas D, Lewis G, Aron JL, Wang B, Banie H, Sankaranarayanan I, et al. Type 2 innate lymphoid cell suppression by regulatory T cells attenuates airway hyperreactivity and requires inducible T-cell costimulator–inducible T-cell costimulator ligand interaction. *J Allergy Clin Immunol.* (2017) 139:1468–77.e1462. doi: 10.1016/j.jaci.2016.08.034

163. Akbari O, Faul JL, Hoyte EG, Berry GJ, Wahlström J, Kronenberg M, et al. CD4$^+$ invariant T-cell–receptor$^+$ natural killer T cells in bronchial asthma. *N Engl J Med.* (2006) 354:1117–29. doi: 10.1056/NEJMoa053614

164. Matangkasombut P, Marigowda G, Ervine A, Idris L, Pichavant M, Kim HY, et al. Natural killer T cells in the lungs of patients with asthma. *J Allergy Clin Immunol.* (2009) 123:1181–5.e1181. doi: 10.1016/j.jaci.2009.02.013

165. Yang G, Driver JP, Van Kaer L. The role of autophagy in iNKT cell development. *Front Immunol.* (2018) 9:2653. doi: 10.3389/fimmu.2018.02653

166. Oliver BGG, Robinson P, Peters M, Black J. Viral infections and asthma: an inflammatory interface? *Eur Respir J.* (2014) 44:1666. doi: 10.1183/09031936.00047714

167. Jackson WT. Viruses and the autophagy pathway. *Virology.* (2015) 479–480:450–6. doi: 10.1016/j.virol.2015.03.042

168. Pleet ML, Branscome H, DeMarino C, Pinto DO, Zadeh MA, Rodriguez M, et al. Autophagy, EVs, and infections: a perfect question for a perfect time. *Front Cell Infect Microbiol.* (2018) 8:362. doi: 10.3389/fcimb.2018.00362

169. Peral de Castro C, Jones SA, Ní Cheallaigh C, Hearnden CA, Williams L, Winter J, et al. Autophagy regulates IL-23 secretion and innate T cell responses through effects on IL-1 secretion. *J Immunol.* (2012) 189:4144. doi: 10.4049/jimmunol.1201946

170. Lemanske RF Jr, Dick EC, Swenson CA, Vrtis RF, Busse WW. Rhinovirus upper respiratory infection increases airway hyperreactivity and late

asthmatic reactions. *J Clin Invest.* (1989) 83:1–10. doi: 10.1172/JCI11 3843

171. Busse WW, Lemanske RF Jr, Gern JE. Role of viral respiratory infections in asthma and asthma exacerbations. *Lancet.* (2010) 376:826–34. doi: 10.1016/S0140-6736(10)61380-3

172. Jackson DJ, Johnston SL. The role of viruses in acute exacerbations of asthma. *J Allergy Clin Immunol.* (2010) 125:1178–87. doi: 10.1016/j.jaci.2010.04.021

173. Sly PD, Kusel M, Holt PG. Do early-life viral infections cause asthma? *J Allergy Clin Immunol.* (2010) 125:1202–5. doi: 10.1016/j.jaci.2010.01.024

174. Choi Y, Bowman JW, Jung JU. Autophagy during viral infection—a double-edged sword. *Nat Rev Microbiol.* (2018) 16:341–54. doi: 10.1038/s41579-018-0003-6

175. Gassen NC, Papies J, Bajaj T, Dethloff F, Emanuel J, Weckmann K, et al. Analysis of SARS-CoV-2-controlled autophagy reveals spermidine, MK-2206, and niclosamide as putative antiviral therapeutics. *bioRxiv.* (2020) 2020.2004.2015.997254. doi: 10.1101/2020.04.15.997254

176. Yang N, Shen H-M. Targeting the endocytic pathway and autophagy process as a novel therapeutic strategy in COVID-19. *Int J Biol Sci.* (2020) 16:1724–31. doi: 10.7150/ijbs.45498

177. Cameron MJ, Ran L, Xu L, Danesh A, Bermejo-Martin JF, Cameron CM, et al. Interferon-mediated immunopathological events are associated with atypical innate and adaptive immune responses in patients with severe acute respiratory syndrome. *J Virol.* (2007) 81:8692–706. doi: 10.1128/JVI.00527-07

178. Mehta P, McAuley DF, Brown M, Sanchez E, Tattersall RS, Manson JJ. COVID-19: consider cytokine storm syndromes and immunosuppression. *Lancet.* (2020) 395:1033–4. doi: 10.1016/S0140-6736(20)30628-0

179. Gassen NC, Niemeyer D, Muth D, Corman VM, Martinelli S, Gassen A, et al. SKP2 attenuates autophagy through Beclin1-ubiquitination and its inhibition reduces MERS-Coronavirus infection. *Nat Commun.* (2019) 10:5770. doi: 10.1038/s41467-019-13659-4

180. Zhao Q, Chen H, Yang T, Rui W, Liu F, Zhang F, et al. Direct effects of airborne PM2.5 exposure on macrophage polarizations. *Biochim Biophys Acta.* (2016) 1860:2835–43. doi: 10.1016/j.bbagen.2016.03.033

181. Wu X, Nethery RC, Sabath BM, Braun D, Dominici F. Exposure to air pollution and COVID-19 mortality in the United States: a nationwide cross-sectional study. *medRxiv.* (2020) 2020.2004.2005.20054502.

182. Channappanavar R, Fehr AR, Vijay R, Mack M, Zhao J, Meyerholz DK, et al. Dysregulated type I interferon and inflammatory monocyte-macrophage responses cause lethal pneumonia in SARS-CoV-infected mice. *Cell Host Microbe.* (2016) 19:181–93. doi: 10.1016/j.chom.2016.01.007

183. Totura AL, Whitmore A, Agnihothram S, Schäfer A, Katze MG, Heise MT, et al. Toll-like receptor 3 signaling via TRIF contributes to a protective innate immune response to severe acute respiratory syndrome coronavirus infection. *mBio.* (2015) 6:e00638. doi: 10.1128/mBio.00638-15

184. Mantlo E, Bukreyeva N, Maruyama J, Paessler S, Huang C. Antiviral activities of type I interferons to SARS-CoV-2 infection. *Antiviral Res.* (2020) 179:104811. doi: 10.1016/j.antiviral.2020.104811

185. Ren SY, Xu X. Role of autophagy in metabolic syndrome-associated heart disease. *Biochim Biophys Acta.* (2015) 1852:225–31. doi: 10.1016/j.bbadis.2014.04.029

186. Sciarretta S, Boppana VS, Umapathi M, Frati G, Sadoshima J. Boosting autophagy in the diabetic heart: a translational perspective. *Cardiovasc Diagn Ther.* (2015) 5:394–402. doi: 10.3978/j.issn.2223-3652.2015.07.02

187. Mao R, Liang J, Shen J, Ghosh S, Zhu L-R, Yang H, et al. Implications of COVID-19 for patients with pre-existing digestive diseases. *Lancet Gastroenterol Hepatol.* (2020) 5:425–7. doi: 10.1016/S2468-1253(20)30076-5

188. Riffelmacher T, Richter FC, Simon AK. Autophagy dictates metabolism and differentiation of inflammatory immune cells. *Autophagy.* (2018) 14:199–206. doi: 10.1080/15548627.2017.1362525

189. Riffelmacher T, Clarke A, Richter FC, Stranks A, Pandey S, Danielli S, et al. Autophagy-dependent generation of free fatty acids is critical for normal neutrophil differentiation. *Immunity.* (2017) 47:466–80.e465. doi: 10.1016/j.immuni.2017.08.005

190. Jacinto E, Loewith R, Schmidt A, Lin S, Rüegg MA, Hall A, et al. Mammalian TOR complex 2 controls the actin cytoskeleton and is rapamycin insensitive. *Nat Cell Biol.* (2004) 6:1122–8. doi: 10.1038/ncb1183

191. Sarkar S, Davies JE, Huang Z, Tunnacliffe A, Rubinsztein DC. Trehalose, a novel mTOR-independent autophagy enhancer, accelerates the clearance

192. Belzile J-P, Sabalza M, Craig M, Clark E, Morello CS, Spector DH. Trehalose, an mTOR-independent inducer of autophagy, inhibits human cytomegalovirus infection in multiple cell types. *J Virol.* (2016) 90:1259. doi: 10.1128/JVI.02651-15

193. Jensen EV, Jordan VC. The estrogen receptor. *Clin Cancer Res.* (2003) 9:1980.

194. Bursch W, Ellinger A, Kienzl H, Török L, Pandey S, Sikorska M, et al. Active cell death induced by the anti-estrogens tamoxifen and ICI 164 384 in human mammary carcinoma cells (MCF-7) in culture: the role of autophagy. *Carcinogenesis.* (1996) 17:1595–607. doi: 10.1093/carcin/17.8.1595

195. Cham LB, Friedrich S-K, Adomati T, Bhat H, Schiller M, Bergerhausen M, et al. Tamoxifen protects from vesicular stomatitis virus infection. *Pharmaceuticals.* (2019) 12:142. doi: 10.3390/ph12040142

196. Lomia M, Tchelidze T, Pruidze M. Bronchial asthma as neurogenic paroxysmal inflammatory disease: a randomized trial with carbamazepine. *Respir Med.* (2006) 100:1988–96. doi: 10.1016/j.rmed.2006.02.018

197. Williams RSB, Cheng L, Mudge AW, Harwood AJ. A common mechanism of action for three mood-stabilizing drugs. *Nature.* (2002) 417:292–5. doi: 10.1038/417292a

198. Schiebler M, Brown K, Hegyi K, Newton SM, Renna M, Hepburn L, et al. Functional drug screening reveals anticonvulsants as enhancers of mTOR-independent autophagic killing of *Mycobacterium tuberculosis* through inositol depletion. *EMBO Mol Med.* (2015) 7:127–39. doi: 10.15252/emmm.201404137

199. Williams A, Sarkar S, Cuddon P, Ttofi EK, Saiki S, Siddiqi FH, et al. Novel targets for Huntington's disease in an mTOR-independent autophagy pathway. *Nat Chem Biol.* (2008) 4:295–305. doi: 10.1038/nchembio.79

200. Lee J-S, Li Q, Lee J-Y, Lee S-H, Jeong JH, Lee H-R, et al. FLIP-mediated autophagy regulation in cell death control. *Nat Cell Biol.* (2009) 11:1355–62. doi: 10.1038/ncb1980

201. Moon H-J, Nikapitiya C, Lee H-C, Park M-E, Kim J-H, Kim T-H, et al. Inhibition of highly pathogenic avian influenza (HPAI) virus by a peptide derived from vFLIP through its direct destabilization of viruses. *Sci Rep.* (2017) 7:4875. doi: 10.1038/s41598-017-04777-4

202. Rossi M, Munarriz ER, Bartesaghi S, Milanese M, Dinsdale D, Guerra-Martin MA, et al. Desmethylclomipramine induces the accumulation of autophagy markers by blocking autophagic flux. *J Cell Sci.* (2009) 122:3330. doi: 10.1242/jcs.048181

203. Bongiorno-Borbone L, Giacobbe A, Compagnone M, Eramo A, De Maria R, Peschiaroli A, et al. Anti-tumoral effect of desmethylclomipramine in lung cancer stem cells. *Oncotarget.* (2015) 6:16926–38. doi: 10.18632/oncotarget.4700

204. Rebecca VW, Nicastri MC, Fennelly C, Chude CI, Barber-Rotenberg JS, Ronghe A, et al. PPT1 promotes tumor growth and is the molecular target of chloroquine derivatives in cancer. *Cancer Discov.* (2019) 9:220. doi: 10.1158/2159-8290.CD-18-0706

205. Mauthe M, Orhon I, Rocchi C, Zhou X, Luhr M, Hijlkema K-J, et al. Chloroquine inhibits autophagic flux by decreasing autophagosome-lysosome fusion. *Autophagy.* (2018) 14:1435–55. doi: 10.1080/15548627.2018.1474314

206. Meyerowitz EA, Vannier AGL, Friesen MGN, Schoenfeld S, Gelfand JA, Callahan MV, et al. Rethinking the role of hydroxychloroquine in the treatment of COVID-19. *FASEB J.* (2020) 34:6027–37. doi: 10.1096/fj.202000919

207. Turner DL, Verter J, Turner R, Cao M. Tissue. resident memory B cells established in lungs in allergic asthma. *J Immunol.* (2017) 198:71.3

17

Extracellular Vesicle: An Emerging Mediator of Intercellular Crosstalk in Lung Inflammation and Injury

Heedoo Lee[1†], Eric Abston[1†], Duo Zhang[1], Ashish Rai[2] and Yang Jin[1]*

[1] *Division of Pulmonary and Critical Care Medicine, Department of Medicine, Boston University Medical Campus, Boston, MA, United States,* [2] *Department of Internal Medicine, North Shore Medical Center, Boston, MA, United States*

*Correspondence:
Yang Jin
yjin1@bu.edu

[†]*These authors have contributed equally to this work.*

Inflammatory lung responses are one of the characterized features in the pathogenesis of many lung diseases, including acute respiratory distress syndrome (ARDS) and chronic obstructive pulmonary disease (COPD). Alveolar macrophages (AMs) and alveolar epithelial cells are the first line of host defense and innate immunity. Due to their central roles in both the initiation and resolution of inflammatory lung responses, AMs constantly communicate with other lung cells, including the alveolar epithelial cells. In the past, emerging evidence suggests that extracellular vesicles play an essential role in cell–cell crosstalk. In this review, we will discuss the recent findings on the intercellular communications between lung epithelial cells and alveolar macrophages, *via* EV-mediated signal transfer.

Keywords: macrophage-epithelium crosstalk, lung injury and inflammation, extracellular vesicles, exosome, microvesicle, apoptosis, apoptotic bodies, microRNA

INTRODUCTION

Acute respiratory distress syndrome (ARDS) and acute lung injury (ALI) is fundamentally a syndrome characterized with an intense inflammatory response, severe injury to the epithelial/endothelial barrier, and alveolar edema (1–3). Overwhelming inflammatory responses cause collateral damage in lung tissue irrespective of the initial cause, patients with ARDS universally have high levels of inflammation and circulating cytokines. However, clinical trials using anti-inflammatory agents, such as glucocorticoids to treat ARDS have failed to improve outcomes (4). Chronic obstructive pulmonary disease (COPD) is also characterized by a heterogeneous lung inflammation (5) involving epithelial cells, alveolar macrophages (AMs), neutrophils, and T cells (6). To date, the knowledge on how pulmonary cells communicate with each other and subsequently trigger an inflammatory cascade remains incompletely understood.

Alveolar macrophages are a distinct resident population that comprises the majority of inflammatory cells in the healthy lung. They form the first line of host defense against inhaled dust and/or infection, working as antigen-presenting cells and releasing powerful pro-inflammatory cytokines to drive the inflammatory response required to fight infection. Macrophages are capable to directing the type and severity of inflammatory response based on the type of injury to the lung, and also plays an important role in the resolution of inflammation and lung injury. Due to its central roles in both the initiation and resolution of inflammatory lung responses, AMs constantly communicate with other lung cells. The interactions between macrophage–neutrophil, macrophage-recruited macrophages, macrophage-lymphocyte, and macrophage-mesenchymal stem cell have been well described previously (7–10). In this review, we will discuss a novel paradigm on how macrophage–epithelial cell crosstalk occurs *via* extracellular vesicles (EVs) and EV-containing microRNAs (miRNAs).

The alveolar epithelium, with their large surface area acts as the first-line defense against insult, and contribute to the integrity and function of the lungs during the development of ALI (11, 12). Two major cell types populate the alveolar epithelium, alveolar epithelial cell type I (AECI) and type II (AECII) cells. AECII cells cover 2–5% of the surface area and have many known functions, including the secretion of surfactant (13, 14). AECI cells constitute the vast majority of the internal surface area (approximately 95%) of the lung, and interact with noxious stimuli during the development of ALI (13, 14). Recent evidence suggests that ATI cells have important functions in innate immunity and are under-appreciated players in lung cell–cell crosstalk (15).

Alveolar Macrophage Polarization, Activation, and Function in the Pathogenesis of Lung Injury

As a first-line defender, AMs are armed with high levels of pathogen-associated molecular pattern and danger-associated molecular pattern receptors in order to initiate necessary immune response (16). In response to the stimulation of microenvironmental signals, AMs often display the M1 macrophage phenotype (classically activated macrophage) or M2 phenotype (alternatively activated macrophage). M1-activated AMs produce high levels of proinflammatory cytokines, including IL-1β, tumor necrosis factor (TNF)-α, IL-12, and iNOS in the presence of IFN-γ or IFN-β (17). M2 macrophages produce anti-inflammatory cytokines, IL-10 and IL-1ra in response to IL-4 and IL-13. M1-activated macrophages often express MHC II (IA/IE), CD80, CD86, and CCR2, while M2-macrophages express mannose receptor, dectin-1, TfR (transferrin receptor), and CD200R (17).

During the development of ALI in animals, AMs are thought to play essential roles in both the acute inflammatory phase and resolution phase. Macrophage-derived cytokines are viewed as the major mediators. Resident AMs generate IL-8 and TNF-α, and subsequently stimulate neighboring cells to propagate the inflammatory responses (18). Increased BAL IL-8 level and increased IL-8 expression in AMs are associated with increased mortality in ARDS patients (18, 19). Additionally, macrophages secrete epithelial growth factor and GM-CSF to promote epithelial repair (20), an example of macrophage–epithelial communications. In order to achieve classical activation (M1) or alternative activation (M2), macrophages constantly receive signals from surrounding or other distant cells. A crosstalk has been reported between AMs and epithelial cells, in particular AECII cells, primarily *via* an autocrine and/or paracrine manner (21). The paracrine communication network between AMs and epithelial cells has been reported to affect alveolar fluid clearance in influenza virus-induced lung injury (22), *via* epithelial type I IFN and especially the IFN-dependent, macrophage-expressed TNF-related apoptosis-inducing ligand (TRAIL). TRAIL determines Na, K-ATPase plasma membrane protein abundance and, thus, edema clearance during IAV infection (22). Appropriate modulation of the epithelial–macrophage crosstalk might represent a novel strategy to improve the unchecked balance of lung inflammation, epithelial damage, and fluid absorption, thus alter the outcomes in lung injury. However, the trials of cytokine suppression or antibody administration have not resulted in any favorable outcomes (23), suggesting unrecognized mechanisms that remain to be explored. For example, the minimum amount of cytokine required to maintain a concentration in the lung microenvironment, the mechanism by which the released cytokines are guided to their target cells. And how are the signaling molecules, including cytokines, proteins, and DNA/RNAs protected from degradation or inactivation by extracellular enzymes?

Recently, emerging evidence suggest that EVs provide further understandings in addition to what we have known on the macrophage–epithelial crosstalk *via* cytokines and chemokines.

EVs: Newly Recognized "Organelles"

Extracellular vesicle-like molecules were initially described by Chargaff and West in 1946 (24). Currently, EVs have been isolated from almost all cell types and biological fluids, including broncho-alveolar lavage fluid (BALF). The morphology and structure of EVs can be visualized under transmission electron microscopy (Figure 1A) and 2D view (Figure 1B). In the past decade, accumulating evidence suggests that EVs play a crucial role in intercellular communication and inter-organ crosstalk.

CLASSIFICATIONS, NOMENCLATURE, AND BIOGENESIS OF EVs

According to the International Society of EVs, three main subgroups of EVs have been classified based on the size of EVs, the membrane compositions, and the mechanisms of formation (25). As illustrated in Figure 1C, apoptotic bodies (ABs) are the largest EVs and formed in the process of undergoing apoptosis. Microvesicles (MVs) are the second subgroup measuring approximately 200–500 nm in diameter, comprising of different sized vesicles directly protruding from plasma membranes. Exosomes are the smallest subgroup among EVs measuring approximately 30–100 nm, and are released after multiple vesicular bodies (MVBs) fuse with the plasma membrane [Figure 1C; (26)]. The mechanisms of formation of EVs are also heterogeneous. ABs are generated by cell membrane-blebbing resulting from systematic cellular breakdown during the process of apoptosis. The generation of exosomes is tightly associated with the dynamic homeostasis of endosomes/lysosomes, trans-Golgi network, the MVBs, and intra luminal vesicles. ESCRT machinery plays an essential role in the formation of polymeric filaments and subsequently results in ILV formation, once released, called exosomes. ESCRT protein components have been confirmed in exosomes. Furthermore, ESCRT-independent mechanisms involving ceramide and tetraspanin CD63 have been reported in the exosome biogenesis and release (27–29). Fusion machinery, such as the SNARE proteins and GTPases, has been shown to regulate the ILV-plasma membrane fusion. Examples of such machineries are SNARE proteins and Rab GTPases (30, 31). As shown in Figure 1C, MVs are formed *via* the outward budding and expulsion of plasma membrane directly from the cell surface. This process of vesicle formation is often triggered by translocation of phosphatidylserine to the outer-membrane leaflet through aminophospholipid translocase activity (32, 33). MV formation is an energy-consuming process and requires ATP (34, 35).

Extracellular Vesicle: An Emerging Mediator of Intercellular Crosstalk in Lung Inflammation and Injury

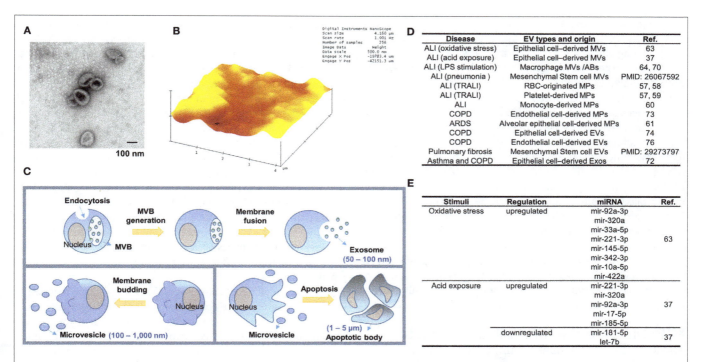

FIGURE 1 | Extracellular vesicle (EV) generation during lung inflammation. (A,B) Transmission electron microscopy (TEM)-based (A) and atomic force microscopy (AFM)-based (B) structure images of EVs derived from bronchoalveolar lavage fluid. EVs were fixed and dried on the formvar coated TEM grids (Ted Pella, Redding, CA, USA) and the cleaved mica sheets (Grade V-1, thickness 0.15 mm, size 15 × 15 mm) for TEM and AFM analysis, respectively. (C) Three main types of EVs. Exosome generation is initiated by membrane-endocytosis and inward-budding of the endosomal membranes to form multiple vesicular bodies (MVBs). Exosomes are then released when the MVBs are fused with the plasma membrane of the cells. Meanwhile, microvesicles (MVs) are formed by outward-budding of the plasma membrane. The size of MVs (100 nm–1 μm) is bigger than exosomes (50–100 nm) and their production is stimulated in various cell-stress conditions. Apoptotic bodies (ABs) are formed by membrane-blebbing of apoptotic cells. ABs are the largest EVs (1–5 μm) and contain nuclear fragments. (D) The type of EVs released during the development of lung inflammation and injury. (E) Epithelial MV-containing miRNAs altered in sterile ALIs.

EV COMPOSITIONS

Microvesicles and exosomes are highly enriched with a variety of components and surface marker. A subset of marker proteins derived from parent cells is often detectable in EVs. Surfactant proteins, marker of alveolar type II cells (AECII), and caveolin-1, marker of alveolar type I cells (AECI) can be detected in the EVs derived from lung epithelial cells (34–37). MVs and exosomes also carry distinct proteins which can be used to differentiate the two types of EVs. Vesicle-associated membrane protein 3 can be found in the MVs while transferrin receptors are highly enriched in exosomes, but not in the MVs (38, 39). The marker proteins of MVs or exosomes are related to the parent cells and mechanism of secretion, thus can be used to distinguish the types of EVs, i.e., MVs vs exosomes vs ABs, as well as their origins. EV-encapsulated cytokines are a group of key proteins which potentially transmit inflammatory signals among cells. Examples of the EV-carrying cytokines include but not limit to interleukin 1β (IL-1β), IL1α, IL-18, macrophage migration inhibitory factor, IL-32, TNF, IL-6, vascular endothelial growth factor, IL-8 (CXCL8), fractalkine (CX3CL1), CCL2, CCL3, CCL4, CCL5, and CCL20 (40). Identifications of these important immune-modulatory cytokines/chemokines in EVs strongly indicate that EVs carry crucial cellular functions and mediate intercellular communication.

RNAs detected in EVs generally are much smaller than cellular RNAs [less than 700 nucleotides (nt)]. Despite the smaller sizes of EV-RNAs, long non-coding RNAs, Ribosomal RNA, and the fragments of these intact RNA molecules have all been found in EVs (26, 41, 42). A large amount of 3′UTR mRNA fragments have been identified in EVs (43). There are multiple microRNA (miRNA) binding sites on the 3′UTR mRNAs (44) and a variety of miRNAs have been identified in EVs, suggesting that EVs serve as a cargo for circulating miRNAs. However, MVs appear to be the main cargo carrying majority of miRNAs, recent studies have highlighted that there are various number of copies of "highly up-regulated" miRNAs found in tumor cells, and very low exosome detected in plasma (45).

EV FUNCTIONS AND THEIR SIGNIFICANCE

Current understanding on EVs facilitates to fill the knowledge gap on cell–cell communications. For example, EVs may partially answer the questions on how cytokines/chemokines achieve the needed concentration in the microenvironment and reach their target cells. It has been reported that cytokines are not transmitted in free forms, but appear to be associated with EVs (46). Cytokines, chemokines, protein, and miRNAs are markedly enriched inside

EVs, suggesting that EV function as a vehicle to concentrate and transport these signaling molecules. Additionally, EV-encapsulating RNAs are protected from RNaseA, and thus EVs provide a consistent source of miRNAs for therapeutic delivery and disease biomarker detection (47). EV-based drug delivery offers several advantages over conventional drug delivery systems: EVs exhibit increased stability in the blood that allows them to travel long distances within the body under both physiological and pathological conditions (48, 49). For example, EVs in plasma are stable up to 90 days under various storage conditions (50). In contrast, peak concentrations of TNF-alpha occur approximately 2 h after administration followed by a rapid decline of free TNF-alpha concentration in plasma (half-life approximately 18.2 min) (5). Moreover, EVs express the same surface markers as their "mother" cells. This feature potentially provides an opportunity to deliver EV-containing molecules in a cell type-specific manner. Furthermore, EVs carrying cell type-specific markers may serve as a diagnostic agent referring as "liquid biopsy" to avoid invasive tissue diagnosis. In fact, many EV-containing molecules have been reported to potentially serve as biomarkers as shown in **Figure 2A** (51–54).

MVs Mediate the Intercellular Crosstalk
The Type of EVs Released During the Development of Lung Inflammation and Injury

Extracellular vesicle-mediated signal transfer among lung cells is increasingly recognized as a novel mechanism by which the innate immune response is initiated (**Figure 1D**). A decade ago, scattered reports have shown the association between ALI and the generation of "microparticles" (MPs) derived from platelets, neutrophils, monocytes, lymphocytes, red blood cells, and endothelial and epithelial cells (55, 56). The MPs are now believed to be replaced with the term of MVs.

Initial observations on the potential roles of MPs were made in the transfusion-associated acute lung injury (TRALI) (57). Stored packed RBCs release MPs and these RBC-originated MPs contribute to neutrophil priming, activation, and transfusion-associated ALI (TRALI) (57, 58). Platelet-derived microparticles (PMPs) which carry the sCD40L increase during the storage period. PMPs may contribute to the occurrence of TRALI (57, 59). Furthermore, the signal transmission from monocyte/macrophage to epithelial cells has also been identified. Monocyte-derived MPs upregulate the synthesis of pro-inflammatory factors in lung epithelial cells *via* NF-κB activation through a PPAR-γ-dependent pathway (60).

Alveolar epithelial cell-derived "MPs" have been reported to be the main source of tissue factor procoagulant activity in ARDS (61). EVs detected in BALF may be derived from multiple different cell types, including but not limited to alveolar and bronchial epithelial cells, endothelial cells, AMs, neutrophils, lymphocytes fibroblasts, and the above-mentioned blood cells. The type of EVs detected in BALF, i.e., MVs, exosomes, or ABs, may be dependent on the type of noxious stimuli

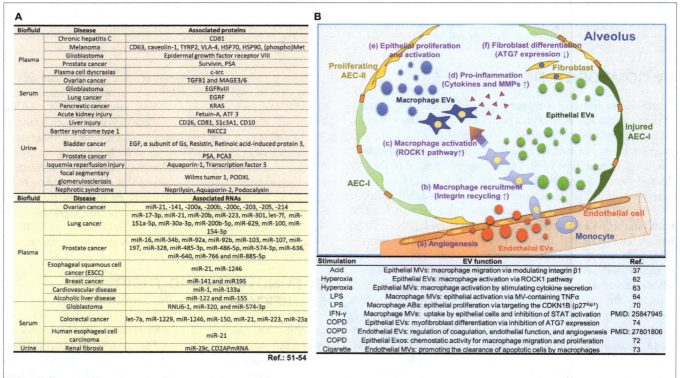

FIGURE 2 | Roles of extracellular vesicles (EVs) in lung injury. **(A)** EV-containing molecules reported to potentially serve as biomarkers. **(B)** The current reports on EVs and their functions involved in lung injury and inflammation. Schematic illustration and the summarized table for the biological pathways by which EVs contribute to the alveolar inflammatory process.

and the severity of diseases in a time/dose-dependent dynamic manner. Moon and Lee et al. recently described that MVs form the dominant type of EVs in BALF after exposure to oxidative stress (62, 63). Lee et al. further reported that MVs are also the main type of EVs detected in BALF after exposure to acid inhalation (37). Approximately, 70% of BALF-EVs are MVs based on the size and marker analysis, using Nano Tracking Analysis (NTA) and Western Blot Analysis, respectively (37, 63). In the setting of hyperoxia or acid exposure, the second largest group of EVs is composed of exosomes, followed by a small amount of ABs. Apparently, Moon and Lee et al. focused on the early stage of exposure to noxious stimuli, whether the MVs remain dominant type of EVs after prolonged exposure to oxidative stress or acid requires further investigation. Interestingly, in LPS-induced lung injury model, a fair amount of large size vesicles are detected in BALF (64). Since the size of EVs in this study is not analyzed using NTA, the current "state of the art" analysis used in EV research, one potentially argues that the EVs studied in this report are composed of AB and MV mixture.

The Source of MVs Detected in BALF During the Development of Lung Inflammation and Injury

Moon et al. also report that at the usual state of mice, i.e., without exposure to noxious stimuli, AMs are the main sources of the MVs detected in BALF (62) (**Figure 1D**). After exposure to hyperoxia-associated oxidative stress, MVs derived from alveolar epithelial cells increase robustly in BALF. On the other hand, AM-derived MVs remain at a steady level (62). MVs derived from other cells failed to increase as robust as the epithelial cell-derived MVs (62). Lee et al. further confirmed this observation in the setting of acid-exposure induced lung injury (37). In both studies, the type of EVs was analyzed using FACS analysis *via* a bead-based antibody conjugation against the surface markers of interested cells, such as AMs, AECI, or AECII cells.

These studies used non-infectious or sterile stimuli (hyperoxia or acid inhalation). Alveolar epithelium has a large surface area which is exposing to the inhaled stimulators. Hyperoxia-induced oxidative stress and acid inhalation are both known to cause diffuse alveolar cell damage (65–69). Therefore, it is expected that majority of MVs in BALF are derived from lung epithelial cells. On the other hand, bacterial infection often triggers extensive pro-inflammatory responses to induce bactericidal effects. Presumably, after inhaled bacteria or LPS, the first responder which is AM may be responsible for the release of EVs into BALF. Furthermore, Moon and Lee et al. focus on the MV release in BALF at the early stage of exposure rather than prolonged treatment. All the above noxious stimuli, including both sterile and the infectious, potentially induce the generation of ABs after prolonged exposure. Zhu et al. reported recently that AM-derived ABs exert a functional role on the epithelial cells and potentially promote epithelium proliferation (70). Their work confirmed that there is a mutual communication between epithelial cells and AMs, rather than a single direction crosstalk.

The Compositions of MVs During the Development of Lung Inflammation and Injury

Microvesicles are highly enriched with proteins, lipids, DNA, and RNA molecules (63, 71). Lee et al. first determine the amount of protein and RNAs in the isolated MVs. Although both components are highly upregulated in the presence of noxious stimuli, only RNA components are robustly increased in each individual MV after normalization with the number of MVs. Furthermore, Lee et al. demonstrated that small RNA molecules are elevated much more significantly than the large RNAs (63). Subsequent miRNA profiles and RT-PCR confirmation suggest that after oxidative stress, epithelial MV-containing miRNAs are dramatically altered (**Figure 1E**).

Functionally, Lee et al. showed that MV-miRNAs promote macrophage migration and infiltration *in vitro* and *in vivo*. After exposure to acid, epithelial MV-containing miR-17 and miR-221 exert the effects on promoting macrophage migration *via* modulating integrin β1 (37). After exposure to hyperoxia, MV-containing miR-221 and miR-320 activate AMs by stimulating pro-inflammatory cytokine secretion (63). It appears that after specific stimuli, different MV-containing miRNAs exert specific functional roles. Collectively, in response to sterile stimuli such as hyperoxia or acid inhalation, AMs receive "pro-inflammatory" signals from the epithelial MV-containing miRNAs and subsequently respond by classical activation (M1) and increased migration.

Macrophage-Derived EV-Containing miRNAs Regulate Lung Epithelial Cell Proliferation and Cell Cycle

The EV research focused on the roles of MVs or Exos, Zhu et al. recently demonstrate that after LPS stimulation, ABs derived from macrophages exert a functional role in maintaining lung epithelial cell growth *via* their regulation of cell cycle (70). Although AB is significantly larger in size and contains more diverse contents than MV and exosome, Zhu et al. demonstrated that AB-containing miR-221/222 confer robust effects on promoting epithelial cell proliferation *via* targeting the CDKN1B (p27Kip1) gene (70). This observation demonstrates that under certain condition, an EV-mediated macrophage-epithelium crosstalk exists in both directions, further confirming a constant and dynamic intercellular communication among different cell types in the microenvironment of lungs.

EVs Play a Role in Other Inflammatory Lung Responses

Apart from ALI and inflammation, the generation and function of EVs in the pathogenesis of other lung disease have gained increasing attention. For example, in the development of COPD, EV-mediated signaling transport has been widely reported (72–74). Epithelial cell-derived exosomes have been detected from BALF of control and asthmatic mice (72), in response to IL-13. These epithelial exosomes induce chemotaxis of undifferentiated macrophages and confer proliferative effects (72). Despite that in this report, due to the lack of NTA analysis of the sizes of EVs, the term "exosome" here may represent the three groups of EVs.

Cigarette smoke has been reported to induce the endothelial cell-derived MVs and MV-containing miRNAs, such as miR-191, miR-126, and miR125a. These miRNAs are transferred to macrophages in an EV-mediated manner, subsequently promoting the clearance of apoptotic cells (73). Interestingly, besides AMs, lung epithelial EVs can also transport EV-containing miRNA, miR-210, into lung fibroblasts, resulting in the inhibition of ATG7 expression and promotion of myofibroblast differentiation (74).

In addition to the EVs derived from lung epithelial cells, endothelial cells also generate a significant amount of EVs. Takahashi et al. have demonstrated that endothelial cell-derived MVs increase robustly in COPD patients compared to those in healthy volunteers (75). Furthermore, the injured endothelial cells release a significant amount of EVs, which regulate the process of coagulation, inflammation, endothelial function, and angiogenesis (76). The current reports on EVs and their functions involved in lung injury and inflammation are summarized in **Figure 2B**.

Pitfalls and Further Directions

Many questions remain to be answered on the role of EVs in the cell–cell crosstalk during the development of lung inflammation and injury. These questions include but are not limited to the concentration and amount of specific miRNAs in each MVs, exosomes or ABs after noxious stimuli; the effective "dose" or "amount" of MV/AB-shuttling miRNAs to trigger cellular effects;

the efficacy and pathway of MV or AB-shuttling miRNAs to enter the recipient cells. There is yet to be a study on the underlying mechanisms by which EV-shuttling miRNAs exert functions in the recipient cells.

In summary, EVs (MVs, exosomes, or ABs) play an essential role in mediating epithelial–macrophage crosstalk in the absence and presence of noxious stimuli. EV-containing miRNAs are the likely emerging targets for the development of novel therapeutic and/or diagnostic agents.

AUTHOR CONTRIBUTIONS

YJ designed, wrote, and supervised this manuscript. HL and EA wrote the manuscript, drew the schema. DZ and AR participated in the writing of the manuscript. HL and EA contributed equally to this work.

REFERENCES

1. Martin TR. Cytokines and the acute respiratory distress syndrome (ARDS): a question of balance. *Nat Med* (1997) 3(3):272–3. doi:10.1038/nm0397-272
2. Matthay MA, Ware LB, Zimmerman GA. The acute respiratory distress syndrome. *J Clin Invest* (2012) 122(8):2731–40. doi:10.1172/JCI60331
3. Ashbaugh DG, Bigelow DB, Petty TL, Levine BE. Acute respiratory distress in adults. *Lancet* (1967) 2(7511):319–23. doi:10.1016/S0140-6736(67)90168-7
4. Steinberg KP, Hudson LD, Goodman RB, Hough CL, Lanken PN, Hyzy R, et al. Efficacy and safety of corticosteroids for persistent acute respiratory distress syndrome. *N Engl J Med* (2006) 354(16):1671–84. doi:10.1056/NEJMoa051693
5. Fabbri LM, Rabe KF. From COPD to chronic systemic inflammatory syndrome? *Lancet* (2007) 370(9589):797–9. doi:10.1016/S0140-6736(07)61383-X
6. Chung KF, Adcock IM. Multifaceted mechanisms in COPD: inflammation, immunity, and tissue repair and destruction. *Eur Respir J* (2008) 31(6):1334–56. doi:10.1183/09031936.00018908
7. Lefkowitz DL, Lefkowitz SS. Macrophage-neutrophil interaction: a paradigm for chronic inflammation revisited. *Immunol Cell Biol* (2001) 79(5):502–6. doi:10.1046/j.1440-1711.2001.01020.x
8. Rosenthal AS, Lipsky PE, Shevach EM. Macrophage-lymphocyte interaction and antigen recognition. *Fed Proc* (1975) 34(8):1743–8.
9. Mao F, Kang JJ, Cai X, Ding NF, Wu YB, Yan YM, et al. Crosstalk between mesenchymal stem cells and macrophages in inflammatory bowel disease and associated colorectal cancer. *Contemp Oncol (Pozn)* (2017) 21(2):91–7. doi:10.5114/wo.2017.68616
10. Mortha A, Chudnovskiy A, Hashimoto D, Bogunovic M, Spencer SP, Belkaid Y, et al. Microbiota-dependent crosstalk between macrophages and ILC3 promotes intestinal homeostasis. *Science* (2014) 343(6178):1249288. doi:10.1126/science.1249288
11. Whitsett JA, Alenghat T. Respiratory epithelial cells orchestrate pulmonary innate immunity. *Nat Immunol* (2015) 16(1):27–35. doi:10.1038/ni.3045
12. Nold MF, Nold-Petry CA, Zepp JA, Palmer BE, Bufler P, Dinarello CA. IL-37 is a fundamental inhibitor of innate immunity. *Nat Immunol* (2010) 11(11):1014–22. doi:10.1038/ni.1944
13. Gonzalez RF, Dobbs LG. Isolation and culture of alveolar epithelial type I and type II cells from rat lungs. *Methods Mol Biol* (2013) 945:145–59. doi:10.1007/978-1-62703-125-7_10
14. Castranova V, Rabovsky J, Tucker JH, Miles PR. The alveolar type II epithelial cell: a multifunctional pneumocyte. *Toxicol Appl Pharmacol* (1988) 93(3): 472–83. doi:10.1016/0041-008X(88)90051-8

15. Yamamoto K, Ferrari JD, Cao Y, Ramirez MI, Jones MR, Quinton LJ, et al. Type I alveolar epithelial cells mount innate immune responses during pneumococcal pneumonia. *J Immunol* (2012) 189(5):2450–9. doi:10.4049/jimmunol.1200634
16. Miyata R, van Eeden SF. The innate and adaptive immune response induced by alveolar macrophages exposed to ambient particulate matter. *Toxicol Appl Pharmacol* (2011) 257(2):209–26. doi:10.1016/j.taap.2011.09.007
17. Arango Duque G, Descoteaux A. Macrophage cytokines: involvement in immunity and infectious diseases. *Front Immunol* (2014) 5:491. doi:10.3389/fimmu.2014.00491
18. Vlahos R, Bozinovski S. Role of alveolar macrophages in chronic obstructive pulmonary disease. *Front Immunol* (2014) 5:435. doi:10.3389/fimmu.2014.00435
19. Bouros D, Alexandrakis MG, Antoniou KM, Agouridakis P, Pneumatikos I, Anevlavis S, et al. The clinical significance of serum and bronchoalveolar lavage inflammatory cytokines in patients at risk for acute respiratory distress syndrome. *BMC Pulm Med* (2004) 4:6. doi:10.1186/1471-2466-4-6
20. D'Angelo F, Bernasconi E, Schafer M, Moyat M, Michetti P, Maillard MH, et al. Macrophages promote epithelial repair through hepatocyte growth factor secretion. *Clin Exp Immunol* (2013) 174(1):60–72. doi:10.1111/cei.12157
21. Tao F, Kobzik L. Lung macrophage-epithelial cell interactions amplify particle-mediated cytokine release. *Am J Respir Cell Mol Biol* (2002) 26(4):499–505. doi:10.1165/ajrcmb.26.4.4749
22. Peteranderl C, Morales-Nebreda L, Selvakumar B, Lecuona E, Vadasz I, Morty RE, et al. Macrophage-epithelial paracrine crosstalk inhibits lung edema clearance during influenza infection. *J Clin Invest* (2016) 126(4):1566–80. doi:10.1172/JCI83931
23. Marshall E. Clinical research. Lessons from a failed drug trial. *Science* (2006) 313(5789):901. doi:10.1126/science.313.5789.901a
24. Chargaff E, West R. The biological significance of the thromboplastic protein of blood. *J Biol Chem* (1946) 166(1):189–97.
25. Yanez-Mo M, Siljander PRM, Andreu Z, Zavec AB, Borras FE, Buzas EI, et al. Biological properties of extracellular vesicles and their physiological functions. *J Extracell Vesicles* (2015) 4:27066. doi:10.3402/jev.v4.27066
26. Crescitelli R, Lasser C, Szabo TG, Kittel A, Eldh M, Dianzani I, et al. Distinct RNA profiles in subpopulations of extracellular vesicles: apoptotic bodies, microvesicles and exosomes. *J Extracell Vesicles* (2013) 2:20677. doi:10.3402/jev.v2i0.20677
27. van Niel G, Charrin S, Simoes S, Romao M, Rochin L, Saftig P, et al. The tetraspanin CD63 regulates ESCRT-independent and -dependent endosomal

sorting during melanogenesis. *Dev Cell* (2011) 21(4):708–21. doi:10.1016/j.devcel.2011.08.019

28. Colombo M, Moita C, van Niel G, Kowal J, Vigneron J, Benaroch P, et al. Analysis of ESCRT functions in exosome biogenesis, composition and secretion highlights the heterogeneity of extracellular vesicles. *J Cell Sci* (2013) 126(Pt 24):5553–65. doi:10.1242/jcs.128868

29. Andreu Z, Yanez-Mo M. Tetraspanins in extracellular vesicle formation and function. *Front Immunol* (2014) 5:442. doi:10.3389/fimmu.2014.00442

30. Duman JG, Forte JG. What is the role of SNARE proteins in membrane fusion? *Am J Physiol Cell Physiol* (2003) 285(2):C237–49. doi:10.1152/ajpcell.00091.2003

31. Piper RC, Katzmann DJ. Biogenesis and function of multivesicular bodies. *Annu Rev Cell Dev Biol* (2007) 23:519–47. doi:10.1146/annurev.cellbio.23.090506.123319

32. Devaux PF, Herrmann A, Ohlwein N, Kozlov MM. How lipid flippases can modulate membrane structure. *Biochim Biophys Acta* (2008) 1778(7–8):1591–600. doi:10.1016/j.bbamem.2008.03.007

33. Tuck S. Extracellular vesicles: budding regulated by a phosphatidylethanolamine translocase. *Curr Biol* (2011) 21(24):R988–90. doi:10.1016/j.cub.2011.11.009

34. Prado N, Marazuela EG, Segura E, Fernandez-Garcia H, Villalba M, Thery C, et al. Exosomes from bronchoalveolar fluid of tolerized mice prevent allergic reaction. *J Immunol* (2008) 181(2):1519–25. doi:10.4049/jimmunol.181.2.1519

35. Carrasco-Ramirez P, Greening DW, Andres G, Gopal SK, Martin-Villar E, Renart J, et al. Podoplanin is a component of extracellular vesicles that reprograms cell-derived exosomal proteins and modulates lymphatic vessel formation. *Oncotarget* (2016) 7(13):16070–89. doi:10.18632/oncotarget.7445

36. Aliotta JM, Pereira M, Sears EH, Dooner MS, Wen S, Goldberg LR, et al. Lung-derived exosome uptake into and epigenetic modulation of marrow progenitor/stem and differentiated cells. *J Extracell Vesicles* (2015) 4:26166. doi:10.3402/jev.v4.26166

37. Lee H, Zhang D, Wu J, Otterbein LE, Jin Y. Lung epithelial cell-derived microvesicles regulate macrophage migration via MicroRNA-17/221-induced integrin beta1 recycling. *J Immunol* (2017) 199(4):1453–64. doi:10.4049/jimmunol.1700165

38. Muralidharan-Chari V, Clancy J, Plou C, Romao M, Chavrier P, Raposo G, et al. ARF6-regulated shedding of tumor cell-derived plasma membrane microvesicles. *Curr Biol* (2009) 19(22):1875–85. doi:10.1016/j.cub.2009.09.059

39. Akers JC, Gonda D, Kim R, Carter BS, Chen CC. Biogenesis of extracellular vesicles (EV): exosomes, microvesicles, retrovirus-like vesicles, and apoptotic bodies. *J Neurooncol* (2013) 113(1):1–11. doi:10.1007/s11060-013-1084-8

40. Keerthikumar S, Chisanga D, Ariyaratne D, Al Saffar H, Anand S, Zhao K, et al. ExoCarta: a web-based compendium of exosomal cargo. *J Mol Biol* (2016) 428(4):688–92. doi:10.1016/j.jmb.2015.09.019

41. Mittelbrunn M, Sanchez-Madrid F. Intercellular communication: diverse structures for exchange of genetic information. *Nat Rev Mol Cell Biol* (2012) 13(5):328–35. doi:10.1038/nrm3335

42. Kogure T, Yan IK, Lin WL, Patel T. Extracellular vesicle-mediated transfer of a novel long noncoding RNA TUC339: a mechanism of intercellular signaling in human hepatocellular cancer. *Genes Cancer* (2013) 4(7–8):261–72. doi:10.1177/1947601913499020

43. Batagov AO, Kurochkin IV. Exosomes secreted by human cells transport largely mRNA fragments that are enriched in the 3'-untranslated regions. *Biol Direct* (2013) 8:12. doi:10.1186/1745-6150-8-12

44. Lee I, Ajay SS, Yook JI, Kim HS, Hong SH, Kim NH, et al. New class of microRNA targets containing simultaneous 5'-UTR and 3'-UTR interaction sites. *Genome Res* (2009) 19(7):1175–83. doi:10.1101/gr.089367.108

45. Chevillet JR, Kang Q, Ruf IK, Briggs HA, Vojtech LN, Hughes SM, et al. Quantitative and stoichiometric analysis of the microRNA content of exosomes. *Proc Natl Acad Sci U S A* (2014) 111(41):14888–93. doi:10.1073/pnas.1408301111

46. Konadu KA, Chu J, Huang MB, Amancha PK, Armstrong W, Powell MD, et al. Association of cytokines with exosomes in the plasma of HIV-1-seropositive individuals. *J Infect Dis* (2015) 211(11):1712–6. doi:10.1093/infdis/jiu676

47. Cheng L, Sharples RA, Scicluna BJ, Hill AF. Exosomes provide a protective and enriched source of miRNA for biomarker profiling compared to intracellular and cell-free blood. *J Extracell Vesicles* (2014) 3:23743. doi:10.3402/jev.v3.23743

48. Jiang XC, Gao JQ. Exosomes as novel bio-carriers for gene and drug delivery. *Int J Pharm* (2017) 521(1–2):167–75. doi:10.1016/j.ijpharm.2017.02.038

49. Yousefpour P, Chilkoti A. Co-opting biology to deliver drugs. *Biotechnol Bioeng* (2014) 111(9):1699–716. doi:10.1002/bit.25307

50. Kalra H, Adda CG, Liem M, Ang CS, Mechler A, Simpson RJ, et al. Comparative proteomics evaluation of plasma exosome isolation techniques and assessment of the stability of exosomes in normal human blood plasma. *Proteomics* (2013) 13(22):3354–64. doi:10.1002/pmic.201300282

51. Lin J, Li J, Huang B, Liu J, Chen X, Chen XM, et al. Exosomes: novel biomarkers for clinical diagnosis. *ScientificWorldJournal* (2015) 2015:657086. doi:10.1155/2015/657086

52. Properzi F, Logozzi M, Fais S. Exosomes: the future of biomarkers in medicine. *Biomark Med* (2013) 7(5):769–78. doi:10.2217/bmm.13.63

53. Gamez-Valero A, Lozano-Ramos SI, Bancu I, Lauzurica-Valdemoros R, Borras FE. Urinary extracellular vesicles as source of biomarkers in kidney diseases. *Front Immunol* (2015) 6:6. doi:10.3389/fimmu.2015.00006

54. Zocco D, Ferruzzi P, Cappello F, Kuo WP, Fais S. Extracellular vesicles as shuttles of tumor biomarkers and anti-tumor drugs. *Front Oncol* (2014) 4:267. doi:10.3389/fonc.2014.00267

55. Barteneva NS, Fasler-Kan E, Bernimoulin M, Stern JN, Ponomarev ED, Duckett L, et al. Circulating microparticles: square the circle. *BMC Cell Biol* (2013) 14:23. doi:10.1186/1471-2121-14-23

56. Lacedonia D, Carpagnano GE, Trotta T, Palladino GP, Panaro MA, Zoppo LD, et al. Microparticles in sputum of COPD patients: a potential biomarker of the disease? *Int J Chron Obstruct Pulmon Dis* (2016) 11:527–33. doi:10.2147/COPD.S99547

57. Xie RF, Hu P, Li W, Ren YN, Yang J, Yang YM, et al. The effect of platelet-derived microparticles in stored apheresis platelet concentrates on polymorphonuclear leucocyte respiratory burst. *Vox Sang* (2014) 106(3):234–41. doi:10.1111/vox.12092

58. Belizaire RM, Prakash PS, Richter JR, Robinson BR, Edwards MJ, Caldwell CC, et al. Microparticles from stored red blood cells activate neutrophils and cause lung injury after hemorrhage and resuscitation. *J Am Coll Surg* (2012) 214(4):648–55; discussion 56–7. doi:10.1016/j.jamcollsurg.2011.12.032

59. Xie RF, Hu P, Wang ZC, Yang J, Yang YM, Gao L, et al. Platelet-derived microparticles induce polymorphonuclear leukocyte-mediated damage of human pulmonary microvascular endothelial cells. *Transfusion* (2015) 55(5):1051–7. doi:10.1111/trf.12952

60. Neri T, Armani C, Pegoli A, Cordazzo C, Carmazzi Y, Brunelleschi S, et al. Role of NF-kappaB and PPAR-gamma in lung inflammation induced by monocyte-derived microparticles. *Eur Respir J* (2011) 37(6):1494–502. doi:10.1183/09031936.00023310

61. Bastarache JA, Fremont RD, Kropski JA, Bossert FR, Ware LB. Procoagulant alveolar microparticles in the lungs of patients with acute respiratory distress syndrome. *Am J Physiol Lung Cell Mol Physiol* (2009) 297(6):L1035–41. doi:10.1152/ajplung.00214.2009

62. Moon HG, Cao Y, Yang J, Lee JH, Choi HS, Jin Y. Lung epithelial cell-derived extracellular vesicles activate macrophage-mediated inflammatory responses via ROCK1 pathway. *Cell Death Dis* (2015) 6:e2016. doi:10.1038/cddis.2015.282

63. Lee H, Zhang D, Zhu Z, Dela Cruz CS, Jin Y. Epithelial cell-derived microvesicles activate macrophages and promote inflammation via microvesicle-containing microRNAs. *Sci Rep* (2016) 6:35250. doi:10.1038/srep35250

64. Soni S, Wilson MR, O'Dea KP, Yoshida M, Katbeh U, Woods SJ, et al. Alveolar macrophage-derived microvesicles mediate acute lung injury. *Thorax* (2016) 71(11):1020–9. doi:10.1136/thoraxjnl-2015-208032

65. Bhandari V, Choo-Wing R, Lee CG, Zhu Z, Nedrelow JH, Chupp GL, et al. Hyperoxia causes angiopoietin 2-mediated acute lung injury and necrotic cell death. *Nat Med* (2006) 12(11):1286–93. doi:10.1038/nm1494

66. Clement A, Edeas M, Chadelat K, Brody JS. Inhibition of lung epithelial cell proliferation by hyperoxia. Posttranscriptional regulation of proliferation-related genes. *J Clin Invest* (1992) 90(5):1812–8. doi:10.1172/JCI116056

67. Ray P, Devaux Y, Stolz DB, Yarlagadda M, Watkins SC, Lu Y, et al. Inducible expression of keratinocyte growth factor (KGF) in mice inhibits lung epithelial cell death induced by hyperoxia. *Proc Natl Acad Sci U S A* (2003) 100(10):6098–103. doi:10.1073/pnas.1031851100

68. Corne J, Chupp G, Lee CG, Homer RJ, Zhu Z, Chen Q, et al. IL-13 stimulates vascular endothelial cell growth factor and protects against hyperoxic acute lung injury. *J Clin Invest* (2000) 106(6):783–91. doi:10.1172/JCI9674

69. Matute-Bello G, Frevert CW, Martin TR. Animal models of acute lung injury. *Am J Physiol Lung Cell Mol Physiol* (2008) 295(3):L379–99. doi:10.1152/ajplung.00010.2008

70. Zhu Z, Zhang D, Lee H, Menon AA, Wu J, Hu K, et al. Macrophage-derived apoptotic bodies promote the proliferation of the recipient cells via shuttling microRNA-221/222. *J Leukoc Biol* (2017) 101(6):1349–59. doi:10.1189/jlb.3A1116-483R

71. Balaj L, Lessard R, Dai L, Cho YJ, Pomeroy SL, Breakefield XO, et al. Tumour microvesicles contain retrotransposon elements and amplified oncogene sequences. *Nat Commun* (2011) 2:180. doi:10.1038/ncomms1180

72. Kulshreshtha A, Ahmad T, Agrawal A, Ghosh B. Proinflammatory role of epithelial cell-derived exosomes in allergic airway inflammation. *J Allergy Clin Immunol* (2013) 131(4):1194–203, 1203.e1–14. doi:10.1016/j.jaci.2012.12.1565

73. Serban KA, Rezania S, Petrusca DN, Poirier C, Cao D, Justice MJ, et al. Structural and functional characterization of endothelial microparticles released by cigarette smoke. *Sci Rep* (2016) 6:31596. doi:10.1038/srep31596

74. Fujita Y, Araya J, Ito S, Kobayashi K, Kosaka N, Yoshioka Y, et al. Suppression of autophagy by extracellular vesicles promotes myofibroblast differentiation in COPD pathogenesis. *J Extracell Vesicles* (2015) 4:28388. doi:10.3402/jev.v4.28388

75. Takahashi T, Kobayashi S, Fujino N, Suzuki T, Ota C, He M, et al. Increased circulating endothelial microparticles in COPD patients: a potential biomarker for COPD exacerbation susceptibility. *Thorax* (2012) 67(12):1067–74. doi:10.1136/thoraxjnl-2011-201395

76. Kadota T, Fujita Y, Yoshioka Y, Araya J, Kuwano K, Ochiya T. Extracellular vesicles in chronic obstructive pulmonary disease. *Int J Mol Sci* (2016) 17(11):1801. doi:10.3390/ijms17111801

18

Mechanisms of Virus-Induced Airway Immunity Dysfunction in the Pathogenesis of COPD Disease, Progression and Exacerbation

Hong Guo-Parke[1], Dermot Linden[1], Sinéad Weldon[1], Joseph C. Kidney[2†] and Clifford C. Taggart[1*†]

[1] Airway Innate Immunity Research Group, Wellcome Wolfson Institute for Experimental Medicine, School of Medicine, Dentistry & Biomedical Sciences, Queens University Belfast, Belfast, United Kingdom, [2] Department of Respiratory Medicine Mater Hospital Belfast, Belfast, United Kingdom

*Correspondence:
Clifford C. Taggart
c.taggart@qub.ac.uk

[†] These authors share
senior authorship

Chronic obstructive pulmonary disease (COPD) is the integrated form of chronic obstructive bronchitis and pulmonary emphysema, characterized by persistent small airway inflammation and progressive irreversible airflow limitation. COPD is characterized by acute pulmonary exacerbations and associated accelerated lung function decline, hospitalization, readmission and an increased risk of mortality, leading to huge social-economic burdens. Recent evidence suggests ~50% of COPD acute exacerbations are connected with a range of respiratory viral infections. Nevertheless, respiratory viral infections have been linked to the severity and frequency of exacerbations and virus-induced secondary bacterial infections often result in a synergistic decline of lung function and longer hospitalization. Here, we review current advances in understanding the cellular and molecular mechanisms underlying the pathogenesis of COPD and the increased susceptibility to virus-induced exacerbations and associated immune dysfunction in patients with COPD. The multiple immune regulators and inflammatory signaling pathways known to be involved in host-virus responses are discussed. As respiratory viruses primarily target airway epithelial cells, virus-induced inflammatory responses in airway epithelium are of particular focus. Targeting virus-induced inflammatory pathways in airway epithelial cells such as Toll like receptors (TLRs), interferons, inflammasomes, or direct blockade of virus entry and replication may represent attractive future therapeutic targets with improved efficacy. Elucidation of the cellular and molecular mechanisms of virus infections in COPD pathogenesis will undoubtedly facilitate the development of these potential novel therapies that may attenuate the relentless progression of this heterogeneous and complex disease and reduce morbidity and mortality.

Keywords: chronic obstructive pulmonary disease, virus, inflammation, infection, lung damage, acute pulmonary exacerbation

INTRODUCTION

Chronic obstructive pulmonary disease (COPD) is the umbrella term for chronic obstructive bronchitis and pulmonary emphysema, and is characterized by persistent small airway inflammation and progressive irreversible airflow limitation (1–5). COPD is associated with acute pulmonary exacerbations, accelerated lung function decline and increased risk of mortality (6, 7). As a common global epidemic, COPD affects 10% of the population and is the third leading cause of death worldwide (3). Viral and bacterial infections are key elements in the pathogenesis of exacerbations (5–9). Recent evidence suggests respiratory viral infections cause ~50% of COPD acute exacerbations (5, 6, 10). Secondary bacterial infections often ensue with pronounced illness (6).

However, the underlying mechanisms of how viruses subvert host immune defense systems in COPD exacerbations are not completely understood. Herein, we review current advances in understanding the cellular and molecular mechanisms associated with the increased susceptibility to virus infections. As respiratory viruses preferentially infect airway epithelial cells, we focus on virus-induced inflammatory responses in airway epithelium. Understanding these pathogenic pathways may facilitate the development of potential novel therapies to attenuate the relentless progression of the disease.

COPD PATHOGENESIS

Cigarette smoking is the predominant etiologic factor in the development of COPD (3–5). Other risk factors include host genetic factors, which is most evident in alpha-1 antitrypsin (AAT) deficiency (11–13). Recently, childhood respiratory viral infections have been postulated as an independent risk factor associated with COPD later in life (14). Other environmental factors such as pollutant and occupational exposure to dusts or fumes, particularly organic dusts are strongly associated with COPD (4, 13, 15, 16). Social deprivation is also a factor in the development of COPD (6, 17, 18).

Cigarette smoke and other inhale noxious gases induce an abnormal inflammatory response, that is further amplified by protease and oxidative stress, which are central to COPD pathogenesis (8, 11). Persistent small airway inflammation and the resulting destruction of the lung architecture leads to emphysema and loss of lung elastic recoil, chronic bronchitis induced mucus hypersecretion and airflow obstruction, as well as peribronchial fibrosis (11, 19, 20). Excessive neutrophilic infiltration and associated proteolytic enzymes including neutrophil elastase are hallmark features of smoke-induced inflammation (19, 21–25). Consequently, the protease/antiprotease imbalance contributes to the pathogenesis of emphysema due to the increased breakdown of elastin and loss of elastic recoil in the lung parenchyma (19, 21–24). Diminished activity of protein phosphatase 2A (PP2A), a regulator of the inflammatory response in the airways, has been demonstrated in COPD and upregulation of PP2A activity can ameliorate inflammation in a cigarette smoke model of COPD by reducing activity of the cysteine protease, cathepsin S (26). Recent

research has proposed a role for formylated peptides and formyl peptide receptor (FPR) receptor signaling in the initiation and progression of lung disease in current and former smokers (27, 28). These peptides are present in tobacco leaves and are actively secreted by bacteria or passively released from dead and dying host cells after tissue injury (29). FPR1 and FPR2 activation may play a role in neutrophil migration, degranulation, reactive oxygen species (ROS) production, and phagocytosis (29, 30). A novel cross-talk mechanism was identified in neutrophils, by which signals generated by the purinergic receptor for ATP (P2Y$_2$) reactivate ligand-bound inactive FPRs, which resume signaling (31). Furthermore, a role for purinergic receptors in the pathophysiology of COPD has been demonstrated in human and experimental models (32–35), however, further work is needed to elucidate its role in the immune dysfunction associated with COPD (36). Excessive production of ROS results in an oxidant-antioxidant imbalance leading to oxidative stress and is a major predisposing feature in the development of the disease (37–41). Therefore, a vicious cycle is created in which inflammation drives a protease-antiprotease and oxidant-antioxidant imbalance, as well as multiple intracellular cell signaling mechanisms, which potentiate inflammation, goblet cell hyperplasia and mucus hypersecretion (8, 40).

Chronic low-grade respiratory syncytial virus (RSV) infection has also been implicated in COPD pathogenesis (42–45). However, the detection of RSV infection in stable COPD remains controversial (46, 47). Hogg and colleagues showed that the E1A region of the adenovirus may contribute to COPD pathogenesis by enhancing soluble ICAM-1 expression and inflammatory cells infiltration (48). In contrast, another study failed to demonstrate the persistent presence of adenovirus V or E1A (49). Polosukhin at al. detected Epstein Barr Virus (EBV) positive cells in COPD lung tissue sections by immunochemistry staining (50). Consistent with this finding, we have demonstrated that EBV DNA is frequently present in COPD sputum compared with unaffected smokers (51). Latent viral infections and cigarette smoke may synergistically contribute to the chronic inflammation in COPD (52). COPD is a heterogeneous disease with a complex etiology, however, acute and chronic lower respiratory tract infections occur with increased frequency in patients with COPD. Whatever the cause, it is clear that a defective host response plays an important role and improving our understanding of the mechanisms involved is essential to improving prevention and treatment strategies.

AIRWAY EPITHELIUM DYSFUNCTION IN COPD

Normal airway epithelial cells play a pivotal role in innate immune defense. They act as a barrier to pathogens and noxious stimuli and produce mediators and enzymes to orchestrate and maintain proper functioning of the innate and adaptive immune responses (24, 53, 54). As illustrated in **Figure 1**, the COPD airway epithelium responds to cigarette smoke by secreting inflammatory mediators and recruiting immune cells to the site of damage to orchestrate the inflammatory response. A robust infiltration of macrophages and CD8[+] T cells, and to a lesser extent CD4[+] T cells, in the airway mucosa as well as elevated neutrophils in the airway lumen are the hallmark features of COPD inflammation, the degree of which correlates to disease severity (46, 55). Increased levels of epithelial-derived CXCL9 (MIG), CXCL10 (IP-10), and CXCL11 (I-TAC) and their receptor CXCR3 has been demonstrated to contribute, in part, to the mechanism of CD8[+] cellular accumulation (40, 53, 54). CD8[+] T cells release IP-10, TNF-α, IFN-γ, perforins, and granzyme, and have been associated with alveolar epithelial cell apoptosis (19, 37, 56, 57). As COPD progresses, elevated numbers of dendritic cells and B lymphocytes also appear in the airways and alveolar walls. CD8[+] T cells and B cells organize into lymphoid follicles and may contribute to increased "immune surveillance" in COPD (19, 37, 39). The airway epithelium also releases a cascade of secondary mediators including cytokines, lipid mediators, growth factors, proteases, antiproteases and ROS to escalate COPD inflammation (53, 54, 58). Cigarette smoke and other irritants also activate epithelial cells and macrophages to release neutrophil and macrophage chemoattractants, such as LTB4, IL-8, and related CXC chemokines (MCP-1, GRO-α and GM-CSF), which contribute to the development of emphysema (39, 46, 59, 60).

The mechanism of neutrophilic inflammation has been linked to CD11b/CD18 on neutrophils binding to ICAM-1 on bronchial epithelium, which is up-regulated in COPD (54, 61–63). Neutrophils migrate to the respiratory tract and release serine proteases, matrix metalloproteinases (MMPs) and oxidants (24, 40, 46). Neutrophil serine proteases are associated with emphysema, mucus hypersecretion, increased risk of exacerbation and accelerated forced expiratory volume in 1 s (FEV$_1$) decline (64–66). Subsequently, these proteases degrade extracellular matrix components leading to the destruction of the alveolar wall, epithelial barrier dysfunction, reduction in mucociliary clearance, mucus hypersecretion and goblet cell metaplasia through activation of the epidermal growth factor receptor (EGFR) (37, 59, 64). Moreover, alveolar epithelial cells also secrete transforming growth factor-β (TGF-β) which may contribute to small airway fibrosis and emphysema (67).

MOLECULAR MECHANISMS ASSOCIATED WITH VIRAL-INDUCED COPD EXACERBATIONS

Viral-Induced COPD Exacerbations

Acute exacerbations of COPD are characterized by a sudden decline in lung function, hospitalization and high mortality (7, 9, 46). The complicated interaction between the host and viral or bacterial infections or co-infection, as well as environmental factors, precipitate the onset of exacerbations. These factors amplify the inflammatory burden in the small airway, overpowering host anti-inflammatory mechanisms leading to profound airway obstruction in COPD (46, 68–70). Severe virus-associated exacerbations also induce elevated levels of CD8[+] T cells, neutrophils, eosinophils, TNF-α and IL-6 in the sputum of COPD patients (68–70).

Exacerbations often occur seasonally accompanied by common cold-like symptoms implicating respiratory viral infections rather than hitherto suspected bacterial infection (43, 44). Respiratory virus infection, including human rhinovirus (HRV), influenza virus (IAV), coronavirus, RSV, human parainfluenza, metapneumovirus (hMPV) and adenovirus initiate nearly 50% of COPD exacerbations often with more severe symptoms (69–73). Viruses have developed a myriad of aversion strategies to subvert and manipulate host immune responses and these have been recently reviewed elsewhere (74, 75). Most respiratory viruses target airway epithelial cells leading to epithelial barrier destruction, microvascular dilatation, oedema and immune cell infiltration (58, 70–72). These viruses are associated with small airway secondary bacterial infection, thus magnifying the inflammatory response in COPD leading to a synergistic deterioration in lung function and prolonged hospitalization (42, 44, 71).

As detailed below, recent research has focused on immune regulators and inflammatory signaling pathways orchestrating the underlying mechanisms of increased susceptibility to virus-associated exacerbation and the exaggerated inflammatory response in COPD airways and potential therapeutic inventions.

T Cell Exhaustion

Although accumulated CD8[+] T cells are present in greater numbers in severe COPD, a diminished CD8[+] T cell antiviral response, worsened airflow limitation and respiratory symptoms have been reported in IAV and HRV-induced COPD exacerbations (68, 71, 76, 77). As a result, CD8[+] cells potentially amplify airway epithelium destruction and promote tissue injury through mechanisms including direct cytotoxic effects, pro-inflammatory signaling and recruitment of other immune cells, leading to increased susceptibility to virus infections of airway epithelium (42–44, 69).

In COPD, prolonged receptor–ligand interaction during T cell activation may be linked to T cell exhaustion. McKendry and colleagues investigated increased CD8[+] activation through the programmed cell death protein (PD)-1 exhaustion pathway as a potential mechanism of viral-induced COPD exacerbations (76). Dysregulation of T-cell cytotoxicity was associated with elevated levels of PD-1, which further increased following influenza infection in COPD patients (76). In contrast, infection-induced expression of the ligand PD-L1 on COPD macrophages was diminished, with a concomitant increase in IFN-γ release. These synergistic effects may cause excessive T-cell inflammation in response to virus infection.

The NF-κB Pathway

The NF-κB pathway is consistently activated in COPD macrophages and airway epithelium, in particular, during bacterial or viral infections (78). Upon pathogen stimulation, the canonical pathway is mainly triggered by Toll like receptors (TLRs) and pro-inflammatory cytokines such as TNFα and IL-1 leading to the activation of the RelA containing NF-κB complexes. This initiates the translocation of RelA (p65)/p50 to the nucleus, where it induces the transcriptional response of pro-inflammatory and cell survival genes (78–80). The alternative

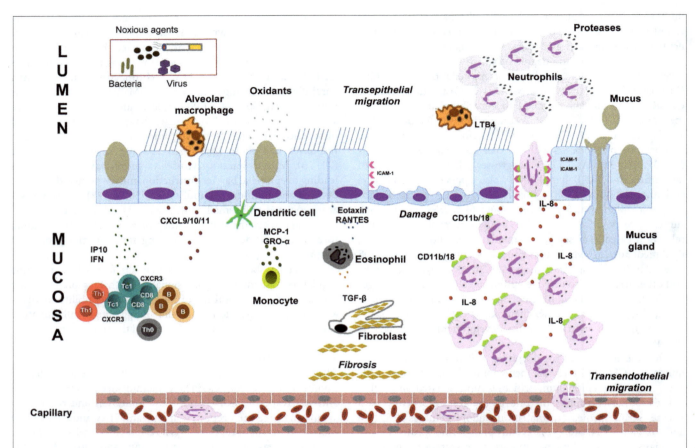

FIGURE 1 | Mechanisms of airway immunity dysfunction in COPD. Cigarette smoke and noxious agents activate epithelial cells and macrophages to release chemotactic factors such as CXCL9 (MIG), CXCL10 (IP10), and CXCL11 (I-TAC), which increase CD8+ T cells, dendritic cells, B lymphocytes and eosinophil infiltration into the airway mucosa. These inflammatory cells together with macrophages and epithelial cells initiate an inflammatory cascade that triggers the release of inflammatory mediators such as TNF-α, IFN-γ, proteases (such as MMPs), inflammatory cytokines and chemokines (IL-1, IL-6, IL-8) and growth factors. These inflammatory mediators sustain the airway mucosal inflammatory process in COPD, which cause elastin degradation and emphysema. Epithelial cells and macrophages also release TGF-β, which stimulates fibroblast proliferation resulting in small airway fibrosis. During exacerbation, the inflammatory burden in the small airways over-powers host anti-inflammatory mechanisms leading to profound alveolar damage and inflammation. Cigarette smoke and other irritants activate epithelial cells and macrophages to release neutrophil chemoattractants, such as LTB4, IL-8, TNFα, CXC chemokines (MCP-1, GRO-α, and GM-CSF). CXC chemokines also act as chemoattractants for monocytes. Cigarette smoke causes increased level of ROS produced in the airways is reflected by increased markers of oxidative stress. Oxidative stress is involved in several events in the pathogenesis of COPD including oxidative inactivation of anti-proteases and surfactants, mucus hypersecretion, alveolar epithelial injury, remodeling of extracellular matrix and apoptosis. Neutrophils bind to ICAM-1, the level of which has been found to upregulated in bronchial epithelial cells in COPD. Neutrophils migrate to the respiratory tract under the control of IL8/LTB4 chemotactic gradient. These cells then release proteases that break down connective tissue in the lung parenchyma, resulting in emphysema. Neutrophil elastase release in airway induces epithelial barrier dysfunction, mucus hypersecretion and reduces mucociliary clearance. GM-CSF, Granulocyte-macrophage colony-stimulating factor: GRO-α, Growth-regulated oncogene-α; ICAM-1, epithelial intercellular adhesion molecule-1; LTB4, leukotriene B4; IL, interleukin; IP10, CXCL10, interferon g-induced protein 10; I-TAC, CXCL11, interferon-inducible T-cell α chemoattractant; MCP-1, monocyte chemoattractant protein-1; MIG, CXCL9, monokine induced by g interferon; MMPs, matrix metalloproteinases; RANTES, regulated on activation, normal T cell expressed and secreted; ROS: reactive oxygen species; TGF, transforming growth factor; TNF-α, Tumor necrosis factor-α; IFN, interferon.

non-canonical NF-κB pathway signals through a subset of receptors to activate the kinase NIK and IKKα complexes and downstream NF-κB2 p100 leading to the p52/RelB nucleus translocation and lymphoid organogenesis and B cell activation (78, 79).

Persistent or prolonged activation of NF-κB may contribute to COPD pathogenesis by switching on the transcriptional response of pro-inflammatory cytokines, chemokines, cell adhesion molecules (CAMs), proteases, and inhibitors of apoptosis to amplify inflammation. Therefore, strategies, which block the activation of NF-κB, offer attractive therapeutic options to regulate COPD inflammation. Several IKK-β inhibitors have been identified to inhibit p65 nuclear translocation and exert anti-inflammatory effects (81, 82). Lung-targeted overexpression of RelB has also been demonstrated to protect against cigarette smoke–induced inflammation by reducing inflammatory mediator production (83). In COPD airway epithelium, influenza virus infection increased microRNA-125a/b, which directly inhibits A20 and mitochondrial antiviral-signaling protein (MAVS) to promote inflammation and impair antiviral responses in COPD (84). Thus, miR-125a/b may provide a potential therapeutic target for both inflammation and antiviral responses in COPD.

TLR Sensing and EGFR Signaling

Figure 2 illustrates key virus innate recognition signaling pathways in COPD airway epithelium. Briefly, ssRNAs of HRV, RSV, and IAV are recognized by TLR3 in the endosomes which consequently activate IRF-3 via the Toll/IL-1 receptor domain-containing adaptor (TRIF), leading to the induction of IFN-β and IFN-λ1. Other endosomal TLRs (TLR7/8 and TLR7/9) recognize the dsRNAs of IAV and adenovirus through MyD88-dependent pathway to activate NF-κB and IRF-7 to secrete pro-inflammatory mediators and IFNs, respectively. TLR4 expressed on the cell surface senses RSV and IAV, signaling through both the MyD88 and TRIF pathways to activate NF-κB and IRF-7. The airway epithelium may recognize EBV by endosomal TLRs and TLR2 at the cell surface to activate downstream pathways (85, 86). As a risk factor for RSV-induced COPD exacerbations, TLR3 activation has been found to correlate with lung function deterioration during exacerbations highlighting TLR3 blockade as a therapeutic target (87). However, Silkoff et al. showed that TLR3 inhibition was inefficient in attenuating HRV-induced experimental asthma exacerbation (88).

Many TLRs recognize pathogen-associated molecular patterns (PAMPs) to activate airway epithelial EGFR signaling cascades. Aberrant EGFR signaling promotes progressive lung fibrosis and mucus hypersecretion; characteristic features of COPD, asthma and cystic fibrosis pathogenesis (24, 89). The EGFR cascade consists of multiple receptors and extracellular ligands that function via receptor auto-phosphorylation and cytoplasmic protein binding of four downstream complexes including the mitogen-activated protein kinases/extracellular signal–regulated kinases (MEK/ERK), phosphatidylinositol 3-kinases/protein kinase B (PKB) (PI3K/AKT), Just Another Kinase/signal transducer and activator of transcription (JAK/STAT) and mammalian target of rapamycin (mTOR) pathways (89). In a murine COPD model, EGFR activation through PI3K inhibited ciliated cell apoptosis and allowed IL-13 to stimulate the trans-differentiation of ciliated to goblet cell metaplasia (90). HRV infection induced the phosphorylation of PKD, a downstream kinase of PI3K. PKD inhibitors have been reported to effectively block HRV, poliovirus (PV) and foot-and-mouth disease virus (FMDV) replication at an early stage of infection, highlighting the potential of PKD inhibition in anti-HRV therapy in COPD (91). Chronic inflammation can also induce ICAM-1 and its ligand fibrinogen has been shown to promote EGFR-dependent mucin production in the airways of subjects with mucus hypersecretion (92).

EGF and the EGFR ligand, TGF-α, have been reported to directly enhance TNF-α-induced IL-8 secretion in airway inflammation (93). Ganesan et al. found that abnormal EGFR activation contributed to enhanced IL-8 expression in COPD airways via the NF-κB regulator, FoxO3A (94). Interestingly, TLR3 also induced EGFR activation and EGFR ligands (TGF-α and amphiregulin), which in turn promote EGFR-ERK signaling and mucin production through an autocrine/paracrine loop (95).

Collectively, TLR antiviral defense mechanisms integrate with the EGFR mediated epithelial proliferation/repair pathways and may play an important role in viral-induced airway remodeling and airway disease exacerbations (93, 95, 96).

Viral infection *per se* also activates EGFR and EGFR signaling to ERK1/2, while STATs control the severity of HRV mediated airway inflammation. *In vitro*, HRV induced goblet cell hyperplasia was demonstrated to function through NF-κB-dependent MMP-mediated TGF-α release, leading to EGFR activation and mucus secretion (97). Interestingly, virus-induced EGFR activation suppressed interferon regulatory factor 1 (IRF1)-dependent IFN-λ airway epithelial antiviral signaling (98, 99). Inhibiting virus-mediated EGFR signaling augmented IRF1, IFN-λ secretion and viral clearance, indicating EGFR pathways as potential therapeutic targets in viral-induced COPD exacerbations (99).

Cytoplasmic-Sensing Pathways

As shown in **Figure 2**, the airway epithelium also detects viral invasion through cytoplasmic pathogen recognition receptors. DNA and RNA viruses release their genomes into cytoplasm, which are detected by the host through cytoplasmic retinoic acid-inducible gene I/melanoma differentiation-associated protein 5-mitochondrial antiviral-signaling protein (RIG-I/MDA5–MAVS) RNA-sensing and the cyclic GMP–AMP synthase- signaling effector stimulator of interferon genes (cGAS–STING) DNA-sensing pathways, respectively (100). Upon ss/dsRNA binding, the RNA helicases, RIG-I and MDA5, interact with the adaptor protein MAVS on the mitochondrial outer membrane to activate the downstream signaling of type I interferon antiviral responses (100, 101). In contrast, the cGAS receptor senses retroviral replication products, dsDNA and RNA/DNA hybrids, to induce the synthesis of cGAMP which binds and activates STING (100). Interferon γ-inducible protein 16 (IFI16), a novel DNA sensor, has been found to recruit STING to activate type I IFN signaling through an unknown molecular mechanism (102). STING and MAVS also stimulate downstream multiple kinase signaling cascades resulting in IRF3 phosphorylation and NF-κB nuclear translocation (101, 102).

The primary consequence of these virus-sensing pathways is the induction of type I/type III IFNs and IFN stimulated genes as well as the production of inflammatory cytokines and chemokines. Attenuation of the IFN response following virus infection could result in uncontrolled viral replication and an escalated inflammatory response, a potential mechanism of virus-induced exacerbations in COPD. IFNα/β deficiency has been demonstrated in bronchial biopsies of asthmatic patients with rhinovirus-induced exacerbations and smoking-induced COPD (103). Farazuddin et al. have demonstrated that quercetin, a potent antioxidant and anti-inflammatory agent with antiviral properties, effectively mitigates rhinovirus-induced COPD exacerbation in a mouse model (104). Elevated ICAM-1 expression on the surface of airway epithelium has been directly linked to the mechanism of increased susceptibility of HRV-induced acute exacerbation. As the receptor of the major group of HRV and a ligand of lymphocyte function-associated antigen 1 (LFA-1) on neutrophils, ICAM-1 over-expression has been

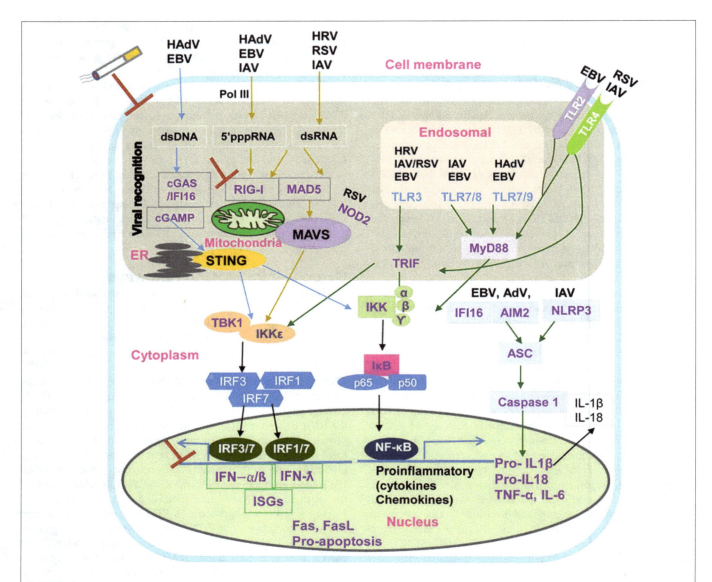

FIGURE 2 | Intracellular Viral Sensing Pathways. DNA and RNA viruses release their genomes in the cytoplasm, where host innate sensors for nucleic acids reside. Upon ss/dsRNA binding, RIG-I engages the adaptor protein MAVS on the mitochondrial outer membrane. The cGAS receptor recognizes dsDNA and the RNA:DNA hybrids generated during retroviral replication and catalyzes the synthesis of cGAMP, which is the primary agonist of the adaptor protein STING. Another sensor, IFI16 can recruit STING in response to cytoplasmic DNA through a molecular mechanism yet to be described. Both STING and MAVS stimulate downstream signaling cascades that involve multiple kinases and finally lead to IRF3 phosphorylation and nuclear translocation. The primary consequence of these virus sensing pathways is the induction of type I IFN and IFN stimulated genes. cGAS, cyclic GMP-AMP synthase; cGAMP, 2'3'guanosine-adenosine monophosphate; IFI16, interferon-g inducible protein 16; IKK, IkB kinase; IRF3, interferon regulatory factor 3; MAVS, mitochondrial antiviral-signaling protein; RIG-I, retinoic acid inducible gene-I; ss/dsRNA, single-stranded/double-stranded RNA; vRNA/DNA, viral RNA/DNA; STING, stimulator of interferon genes; TANK, TRAF-associated NF-kB activator; TBK1, TANK binding kinase 1.

shown on epithelial cells in smokers and patients with COPD (63, 105, 106). Blocking ICAM-1 may also represent as a potential therapeutic option in HRV-induced exacerbations.

Direct Targeting of Viral Binding, Entry, and Replication

Strategies that directly prevent virus binding, entry and replication may provide attractive alternatives in the treatment of COPD exacerbations (107). Capsid binders represent attractive potential inhibitors of HRV entry, however, they are strain-specific and have shown no effect on improving lung function and exacerbation in clinical trials to date (106). Mousnier and colleagues demonstrated that a dual inhibitor of human N-myristoyltransferases NMT1 and NMT2 can inhibit host-cell N-myristoylation and completely prevent rhinoviral replication, highlighting the therapeutic potential of targeting myristoylation in blocking rhinovirus infection in COPD (108). Short palate, lung, nasal epithelium clone 1 (SPLUNC1), a multifunctional host defense protein, was demonstrated to inhibit IAV binding and entry into airway epithelial cells, indicating an antiviral role for this protein in the airways (109). Therefore, in the COPD lung, SPLUNC1 degradation by proteases such as neutrophil elastase and/or inactivation by cigarette smoke may increase susceptibility to viral as well as bacterial infections, in addition to airway dehydration (110, 111). Recent research suggests that, in addition to modulating neutrophil chemotaxis, FPR2 signaling may be an important player in viral replication and IAV pathogenesis (30, 112, 113).

Inflammasome

The inflammasome is a multiprotein pro-inflammatory complex and serves as an important link between the innate and adaptive immune responses. Inflammasomes that are activated by IAV RNA, EBV and adenoviral DNA include the nucleotide binding and oligomerization domain (NOD)-like receptor family pyrin domain-containing 3 (NLRP3) protein, absent in melanoma 2 (AIM2) protein and IFI16 protein (114). The inflammasome complexes assemble after recognition of PAMPs or danger-associated molecular patterns (DAMPs) induced by virus-killed cells or tissue damage and interact with apoptosis-associated speck like protein containing a caspase recruitment domain (ASC) via caspase activation and recruitment domains (CARD)-CARD/caspase-1 pathway (115–117). Activation of the inflammasome complex results in the autocatalytic cleavage of caspase-1 and ultimately leads to the production of pro-inflammatory cytokines including IL-1β, IL-18 and pro-IL-33 (116, 117). Upon maturation, these cytokines

mediate inflammatory responses by activating lymphocytes and facilitating their infiltration to the site of primary infection and by inducing IFNs and other pro-inflammatory cytokines secretions (116).

CONCLUDING REMARKS

COPD is a heterogeneous and complex disease resulting from the deregulation of multiple immune regulators and inflammatory signaling pathways. Significant progress has been made to elucidate the causative mechanism of COPD pathophysiology including viral infection in disease development, severity and exacerbations. Targeting virus-induced inflammatory pathways such as T cell exhaustion, NF-κB, TLRs, EGFR, interferons and the inflammasome provide attractive future therapeutic options. Understanding the cellular and molecular mechanisms of virus-induced COPD pathogenesis could potentially limit pathogen-mediated disease exacerbations and minimize viral-associated inflammation, tissue destruction and pulmonary function deterioration.

AUTHOR CONTRIBUTIONS

All authors listed have made a substantial, direct and intellectual contribution to the work, and approved it for publication.

REFERENCES

1. Buist AS, McBurnie MA, Vollmer WM, Gillespie S, Burney P, Mannino DM, et al. International variation in the prevalence of COPD (the BOLD study): a population-based prevalence study. Lancet. (2007) 370:741–50. doi: 10.1016/S0140-6736(07)61377-4
2. Mirza S, Clay RD, Koslow MA, Scanlon PD. COPD guidelines: a review of the 2018. GOLD Report. Mayo Clin Proc. (2018) 93:1488–502. doi: 10.1016/j.mayocp.2018.05.026
3. Barnes PJ. Chronic obstructive pulmonary disease: a growing but neglected global epidemic. PLoS Med. (2007) 4:e112. doi: 10.1371/journal.pmed.0040112
4. Salvi S. Tobacco smoking and environmental risk factors for chronic obstructive pulmonary disease. Clin Chest Med. (2014) 35:17–27. doi: 10.1016/j.ccm.2013.09.011
5. Bauer CMT, Morissette MC, Stämpfli MR. The influence of cigarette smoking on viral infections. Chest. (2013) 143:196–206. doi: 10.1378/chest.12-0930
6. Mohan A, Chandra S, Agarwal D, Guleria R, Broor S, Gaur B, et al. Prevalence of viral infection detected by PCR and RT-PCR in patients with acute exacerbation of COPD: a systematic review. Respirology. (2010) 15:536–42. doi: 10.1111/j.1440-1843.2010.01722.x
7. Merinopoulou E, Raluy-Callado M, Ramagopalan S, MacLachlan S, Khalid JM. COPD exacerbations by disease severity in England. Int J Chron Obstruct Pulmon Dis. (2016) 11:697–709. doi: 10.2147/COPD.S100250
8. Sethi S, Murphy TF. Infection in the pathogenesis and course of chronic obstructive pulmonary disease. N Engl J Med. (2008) 359:2355–65. doi: 10.1056/NEJMra0800353

9. Ko FW, Chan KP, Hui DS, Goddard JR, Shaw JG, Reid DW, et al. Acute exacerbation of COPD. Respirology. (2016) 21:1152–65. doi: 10.1111/resp.12780
10. Linden D, Guo-Parke H, Coyle P V., Fairley D, McAuley DF, Taggart CC, et al. Respiratory viral infection: a potential "missing link" in the pathogenesis of COPD. Eur Respir Rev. (2019) 28:180063. doi: 10.1183/16000617.0063-2018
11. Calverley PMA, Walker P. Chronic obstructive pulmonary disease. Lancet. (2003) 362:1053–61. doi: 10.1016/S0140-6736(03)14416-9
12. Pauwels RA, Rabe KF. Burden and clinical features of chronic obstructive pulmonary disease (COPD). Lancet. (2004) 364:613–20. doi: 10.1016/S0140-6736(04)16855-4
13. Mannino DM, Buist AS. Global burden of COPD: risk factors, prevalence, and future trends. Lancet. (2007) 370:765–73. doi: 10.1016/S0140-6736(07)61380-4
14. Marsico S, Caccuri F, Mazzuca P, Apostoli P, Roversi S, Lorenzin G, et al. Human lung epithelial cells support human metapneumovirus persistence by overcoming apoptosis. Pathog Dis. (2018) 76:fty013. doi: 10.1093/femspd/fty013
15. Marsh S, Aldington S, Shirtcliffe P, Weatherall M, Beasley R. Smoking and COPD: what really are the risks? Eur Respir J. (2006) 28:883–4. doi: 10.1183/09031936.06.00074806
16. Lundbäck B, Lindberg A, Lindström M, Rönmark E, Jonsson AC, Jönsson E, et al. Obstructive lung disease in northern Sweden studies. Not 15 but 50% of smokers develop COPD?–Report from the obstructive lung disease in northern Sweden studies. Respir Med. (2003) 97:115–22. doi: 10.1053/rmed.2003.1446

17. GBD 2015 Chronic Respiratory Disease Collaborators. Global, regional, and national deaths, prevalence, disability-adjusted life years, and years lived with disability for chronic obstructive pulmonary disease and asthma, 1990-2015: a systematic analysis for the global burden of disease study 2015. *Lancet Respir Med.* (2017) 5:691–706. doi: 10.1016/S2213-2600(17)30293-X

18. Rycroft CE, Heyes A, Lanza L, Becker K. Epidemiology of chronic obstructive pulmonary disease: a literature review. *Int J Chron Obstruct Pulmon Dis.* (2012) 7:457–94. doi: 10.2147/COPD.S32330

19. Hogg JC, Chu F, Utokaparch S, Woods R, Elliott WM, Buzatu L, et al. The nature of small-airway obstruction in chronic obstructive pulmonary disease. *N Engl J Med.* (2004) 350:2645–53. doi: 10.1056/NEJMoa032158

20. Kim V, Criner GJ. Chronic bronchitis and chronic obstructive pulmonary disease. *Am J Respir Crit Care Med.* (2013) 187:228–37. doi: 10.1164/rccm.201210-1843CI

21. Navratilova Z, Kolek V, Petrek M. Matrix metalloproteinases and their inhibitors in chronic obstructive pulmonary disease. *Arch Immunol Ther Exp.* (2016) 64:177–93. doi: 10.1007/s00005-015-0375-5

22. Owen CA. Roles for proteinases in the pathogenesis of chronic obstructive pulmonary disease. *Int J Chron Obstruct Pulmon Dis.* (2008) 3:253–68. doi: 10.2147/COPD.S2089

23. Shapiro SD. Proteolysis in the lung. *Eur Respir J.* (2003) 22:30s–2. doi: 10.1183/09031936.03.00000903a

24. Bagdonas E, Raudoniute J, Bruzauskaite I, Aldonyte R. Novel aspects of pathogenesis and regeneration mechanisms in COPD. *Int J Chron Obstruct Pulmon Dis.* (2015) 10:995–1013. doi: 10.2147/COPD.S82518

25. Hoenderdos K, Condliffe A. The neutrophil in chronic obstructive pulmonary disease. Too Little, Too Late or Too Much, Too Soon? *Am J Respir Cell Mol Biol.* (2013) 48:531–9. doi: 10.1165/rcmb.2012-0492TR

26. Doherty DF, Nath S, Poon J, Foronjy RF, Ohlmeyer M, Dabo AJ, et al. Protein phosphatase 2a reduces cigarette smoke-induced cathepsin s and loss of lung function. *Am J Respir Crit Care Med.* (2019) 200:51–62. doi: 10.1164/rccm.201808-1518OC

27. Cardini S, Dalli J, Fineschi S, Perretti M, Lungarella G, Lucattelli M. Genetic ablation of the fpr1 gene confers protection from smoking-induced lung emphysema in mice. *Am J Respir Cell Mol Biol.* (2012) 47:332–9. doi: 10.1165/rcmb.2012-0036OC

28. De Cunto G, Bartalesi B, Cavarra E, Balzano E, Lungarella G, Lucattelli M. Ongoing lung inflammation and disease progression in mice after smoking cessation: beneficial effects of formyl-peptide receptor blockade. *Am J Pathol.* (2018) 188:2195–206. doi: 10.1016/j.ajpath.2018.06.010

29. Dorward DA, Lucas CD, Chapman GB, Haslett C, Dhaliwal K, Rossi AG. The role of formylated peptides and formyl peptide receptor 1 in governing neutrophil function during acute inflammation. *Am J Pathol.* (2015) 185:1172–84. doi: 10.1016/j.ajpath.2015.01.020

30. Bozinovski S, Anthony D, Anderson GP, Irving LB, Levy BD, Vlahos R. Treating neutrophilic inflammation in COPD by targeting ALX/FPR2 resolution pathways. *Pharmacol Ther.* (2013) 140:280–9. doi: 10.1016/j.pharmthera.2013.07.007

31. Önnheim K, Christenson K, Gabl M, Burbiel JC, Müller CE, Oprea TI, et al. A novel receptor cross-talk between the ATP receptor P2Y2 and formyl peptide receptors reactivates desensitized neutrophils to produce superoxide. *Exp Cell Res.* (2014) 323:209–17. doi: 10.1016/j.yexcr.2014.01.023

32. Lommatzsch M, Cicko S, Müller T, Lucattelli M, Bratke K, Stoll P, et al. Extracellular adenosine triphosphate and chronic obstructive pulmonary disease. *Am J Respir Crit Care Med.* (2010) 181:928–34. doi: 10.1164/rccm.200910-1506OC

33. Lazar Z, Müllner N, Lucattelli M, Ayata CK, Cicko S, Yegutkin GG, et al. NTPDase1/CD39 and aberrant purinergic signalling in the pathogenesis of COPD. *Eur Respir J.* (2016) 47:254–63. doi: 10.1183/13993003.02144-2014

34. Cicko S, Lucattelli M, Müller T, Lommatzsch M, De Cunto G, Cardini S, et al. Purinergic receptor inhibition prevents the development of smoke-induced lung injury and emphysema. *J Immunol.* (2010) 185:688–97. doi: 10.4049/jimmunol.0904042

35. Lucattelli M, Cicko S, Müller T, Lommatzsch M, De Cunto G, Cardini S, et al. P2X7 receptor signaling in the pathogenesis of smoke-induced lung inflammation and emphysema. *Am J Respir Cell Mol Biol.* (2011) 44:423–9. doi: 10.1165/rcmb.2010-0038OC

36. Antonioli L, Blandizzi C, Pacher P, Haskó G. The purinergic system as a pharmacological target for the treatment of immune-mediated inflammatory diseases. *Pharmacol Rev.* (2019) 71:345–82. doi: 10.1124/pr.117.014878

37. Barnes PJ. Cellular and molecular mechanisms of asthma and COPD. *Clin Sci.* (2017) 131:1541–58. doi: 10.1042/CS20160487

38. Eapen MS, Myers S, Walters EH, Sohal SS. Airway inflammation in chronic obstructive pulmonary disease (COPD): a true paradox. *Expert Rev Respir Med.* (2017) 11:827–39. doi: 10.1080/17476348.2017.1360769

39. Barnes PJ, Shapiro SD, Pauwels RA. Chronic obstructive pulmonary disease: molecular and cellular mechanisms. *Eur Respir J.* (2003) 22:672–88. doi: 10.1183/09031936.03.00040703

40. MacNee W. Pathogenesis of chronic obstructive pulmonary disease. *Proc Am Thorac Soc.* (2005) 2:258–66. doi: 10.1513/pats.200504-045SR

41. McGuinness A, Sapey E. Oxidative stress in COPD: sources, markers, and potential mechanisms. *J Clin Med.* (2017) 6:21. doi: 10.3390/jcm6020021

42. Sikkel MB, Quint JK, Mallia P, Wedzicha JA, Johnston SL. Respiratory syncytial virus persistence in chronic obstructive pulmonary disease. *Pediatr Infect Dis J.* (2008) 27:S63–70. doi: 10.1097/INF.0b013e3181684d67

43. Seemungal T, Harper-Owen R, Bhowmik A, Moric I, Sanderson G, Message S, et al. Respiratory viruses, symptoms, and inflammatory markers in acute exacerbations and stable chronic obstructive pulmonary disease. *Am J Respir Crit Care Med.* (2001) 164:1618–23. doi: 10.1164/ajrccm.164.9.2105011

44. Singanayagam A, Joshi P V, Mallia P, Johnston SL. Viruses exacerbating chronic pulmonary disease: the role of immune modulation. *BMC Med.* (2012) 10:27. doi: 10.1186/1741-7015-10-27

45. Wilkinson TMA, Donaldson GC, Johnston SL, Openshaw PJM, Wedzicha JA. Respiratory syncytial virus, airway inflammation, and FEV1 decline in patients with chronic obstructive pulmonary disease. *Am J Respir Crit Care Med.* (2006) 173:871–6. doi: 10.1164/rccm.200509-1489OC

46. Papi A, Bellettato CM, Braccioni F, Romagnoli M, Casolari P, Caramori G, et al. Infections and airway inflammation in chronic obstructive pulmonary disease severe exacerbations. *Am J Respir Crit Care Med.* (2006) 173:1114–21. doi: 10.1164/rccm.200506-859OC

47. Falsey AR, Formica MA, Hennessey PA, Criddle MM, Sullender WM, Walsh EE. Detection of respiratory syncytial virus in adults with chronic obstructive pulmonary disease. *Am J Respir Crit Care Med.* (2006) 173:639–43. doi: 10.1164/rccm.200510-1681OC

48. Matsuse T, Hayashi S, Kuwano K, Keunecke H, Jefferies WA, Hogg JC. Latent adenoviral infection in the pathogenesis of chronic airways obstruction. *Am Rev Respir Dis.* (1992) 146:177–84. doi: 10.1164/ajrccm/146.1.177

49. McManus TE, Marley A-M, Baxter N, Christie SN, Elborn JS, Heaney LG, et al. Acute and latent adenovirus in COPD. *Respir Med.* (2007) 101:2084–90. doi: 10.1016/j.rmed.2007.05.015

50. Polosukhin VV, Cates JM, Lawson WE, Zaynagetdinov R, Milstone AP, Massion PP, et al. Bronchial secretory immunoglobulin a deficiency correlates with airway inflammation and progression of chronic obstructive pulmonary disease. *Am J Respir Crit Care Med.* (2011) 184:317–27. doi: 10.1164/rccm.201010-1629OC

51. McManus TE, Marley A-M, Baxter N, Christie SN, Elborn JS, O'Neill HJ, et al. High levels of epstein-barr virus in COPD. *Eur Respir J.* (2008) 31:1221–6. doi: 10.1183/09031936.00107507

52. Foronjy RF, Dabo AJ, Taggart CC, Weldon S, Geraghty P. Respiratory syncytial virus infections enhance cigarette smoke induced COPD in Mice. *PLoS ONE.* (2014) 9:e90567. doi: 10.1371/journal.pone.0090567

53. Gao W, Li L, Wang Y, Zhang S, Adcock IM, Barnes PJ, et al. Bronchial epithelial cells: the key effector cells in the pathogenesis of chronic obstructive pulmonary disease? *Respirology.* (2015) 20:722–9. doi: 10.1111/resp.12542

54. Vareille M, Kieninger E, Edwards MR, Regamey N. The airway epithelium: soldier in the fight against respiratory viruses. *Clin Microbiol Rev.* (2011) 24:210–29. doi: 10.1128/CMR.00014-10

55. O'Shaughnessy TC, Ansari TW, Barnes NC, Jeffery PK. Inflammation in bronchial biopsies of subjects with chronic bronchitis: inverse relationship of CD8+ T lymphocytes with FEV1. *Am J Respir Crit Care Med.* (1997) 155:852–7. doi: 10.1164/ajrccm.155.3.9117016

56. Kim W-D, Chi H-S, Choe K-H, Oh Y-M, Lee S-D, Kim K-R, et al. A possible role for CD8 + and non-CD8 + cell granzyme B in early small

airway wall remodelling in centrilobular emphysema. *Respirology*. (2013) 18:688–96. doi: 10.1111/resp.12069

57. Majo J, Ghezzo H, Cosio MG. Lymphocyte population and apoptosis in the lungs of smokers and their relation to emphysema. *Eur Respir J*. (2001) 17:946–53. doi: 10.1183/09031936.01.17509460

58. Aghapour M, Raee P, Moghaddam SJ, Hiemstra PS, Heijink IH. Airway epithelial barrier dysfunction in chronic obstructive pulmonary disease: role of cigarette smoke exposure. *Am J Respir Cell Mol Biol*. (2018) 58:157–69. doi: 10.1165/rcmb.2017-0200TR

59. Barnes PJ. Inflammatory mechanisms in patients with chronic obstructive pulmonary disease. *J Allergy Clin Immunol*. (2016) 138:16–27. doi: 10.1016/j.jaci.2016.05.011

60. Wang Y, Xu J, Meng Y, Adcock IM, Yao X. Role of inflammatory cells in airway remodeling in COPD. *Int J Chron Obstruct Pulmon Dis*. (2018) 13:3341–8. doi: 10.2147/COPD.S176122

61. Lopez-Campos JL, Calero C, Arellano-Orden E, Marquez-Martín E, Cejudo-Ramos P, Ortega Ruiz F, et al. Increased levels of soluble ICAM-1 in chronic obstructive pulmonary disease and resistant smokers are related to active smoking. *Biomark Med*. (2012) 6:805–11. doi: 10.2217/bmm.12.64

62. Kidney JC, Proud D. Neutrophil transmigration across human airway epithelial monolayers: mechanisms and dependence on electrical resistance. *Am J Respir Cell Mol Biol*. (2000) 23:389–95. doi: 10.1165/ajrcmb.23.3.4068

63. Shukla SD, Mahmood MQ, Weston S, Latham R, Muller HK, Sohal SS, et al. The main rhinovirus respiratory tract adhesion site (ICAM-1) is upregulated in smokers and patients with chronic airflow limitation (CAL). *Respir Res*. (2017) 18:6. doi: 10.1186/s12931-016-0483-3

64. Dey T, Kalita J, Weldon S, Taggart CC. Proteases and their inhibitors in chronic obstructive pulmonary disease. *J Clin Med*. (2018) 7:244. doi: 10.3390/jcm7090244

65. Sommerhoff CP, Nadel JA, Basbaum CB, Caughey GH. Neutrophil elastase and cathepsin G stimulate secretion from cultured bovine airway gland serous cells. *J Clin Invest*. (1990) 85:682–9. doi: 10.1172/JCI114492

66. Weiss SJ. Tissue destruction by neutrophils. *N Engl J Med*. (1989) 320:365–76. doi: 10.1056/NEJM198902093200606

67. Aschner Y, Downey GP. Transforming growth factor-β: master regulator of the respiratory system in health and disease. *Am J Respir Cell Mol Biol*. (2016) 54:647–55. doi: 10.1165/rcmb.2015-0391TR

68. Kurai D, Saraya T, Ishii H, Takizawa H. Virus-induced exacerbations in asthma and COPD. *Front Microbiol*. (2013) 4:293. doi: 10.3389/fmicb.2013.00293

69. Frickmann H, Jungblut S, Hirche TO, Groß U, Kuhns M, Zautner AE. The influence of virus infections on the course of COPD. *Eur J Microbiol Immunol*. (2012) 2:176–85. doi: 10.1556/EuJMI.2.2012.3.2

70. Allie SR, Randall TD. Pulmonary immunity to viruses. *Clin Sci*. (2017) 131:1737–62. doi: 10.1042/CS20160259

71. Schneider D, Ganesan S, Comstock AT, Meldrum CA, Mahidhara R, Goldsmith AM, et al. Increased cytokine response of rhinovirus-infected airway epithelial cells in chronic obstructive pulmonary disease. *Am J Respir Crit Care Med*. (2010) 182:332–40. doi: 10.1164/rccm.200911-1673OC

72. Potena A, Caramori G, Casolari P, Contoli M, Johnston SL, Papi A. Pathophysiology of viral-induced exacerbations of COPD. *Int J Chron Obstruct Pulmon Dis*. (2007) 2:477–83.

73. Jafarinejad H, Moghoofei M, Mostafaei S, Salimian J, Azimzadeh Jamalkandi S, Ahmadi A. Worldwide prevalence of viral infection in AECOPD patients: a meta-analysis. *Microb Pathog*. (2017) 113:190–6. doi: 10.1016/j.micpath.2017.10.021

74. Christiaansen A, Varga SM, Spencer J V. Viral manipulation of the host immune response. *Curr Opin Immunol*. (2015) 36:54–60. doi: 10.1016/j.coi.2015.06.012

75. Moreno-Altamirano MMB, Kolstoe SE, Sánchez-García FJ. Virus control of cell metabolism for replication and evasion of host immune responses. *Front Cell Infect Microbiol*. (2019) 9:95. doi: 10.3389/fcimb.2019.00095

76. McKendry RT, Spalluto CM, Burke H, Nicholas B, Cellura D, Al-Shamkhani A, et al. Dysregulation of antiviral function of cd8(+) t cells in the chronic obstructive pulmonary disease lung. Role of the PD-1-PD-L1 Axis. *Am J Respir Crit Care Med*. (2016) 193:642–51. doi: 10.1164/rccm.201504-0782OC

77. Singanayagam A, Loo S-L, Calderazzo MA, Finney LJ, Trujillo Torralbo M-B, Bakhsoliani E, et al. Anti-viral immunity is impaired in COPD patients with frequent exacerbations. *Am J Physiol Lung Cell Mol Physiol*. (2019) 317:L893–903. doi: 10.1101/632372

78. Schuliga M. NF-kappaB signaling in chronic inflammatory airway disease. *Biomolecules*. (2015) 5:1266–83. doi: 10.3390/biom5031266

79. Lawrence T. The nuclear factor NF-B pathway in inflammation. *Cold Spring Harb Perspect Biol*. (2009) 1:a001651. doi: 10.1101/cshperspect.a001651

80. Zhou L, Liu Y, Chen X, Wang S, Liu H, Zhang T, et al. Over-expression of nuclear factor-κB family genes and inflammatory molecules is related to chronic obstructive pulmonary disease. *Int J Chron Obstruct Pulmon Dis*. (2018) 13:2131–8. doi: 10.2147/COPD.S164151

81. Gagliardo R, Chanez P, Profita M, Bonanno A, Albano GD, Montalbano AM, et al. IκB kinase-driven nuclear factor-κB activation in patients with asthma and chronic obstructive pulmonary disease. *J Allergy Clin Immunol*. (2011) 128:635–45.e1-2. doi: 10.1016/j.jaci.2011.03.045

82. Banerjee A, Koziol-White C, Panettieri R. p38 MAPK inhibitors, IKK2 inhibitors, and TNFα inhibitors in COPD. *Curr Opin Pharmacol*. (2012) 12:287–92. doi: 10.1016/j.coph.2012.01.016

83. McMillan DH, Baglole CJ, Thatcher TH, Maggirwar S, Sime PJ, Phipps RP. Lung-targeted overexpression of the NF-κB member RelB inhibits cigarette smoke-induced inflammation. *Am J Pathol*. (2011) 179:125–33. doi: 10.1016/j.ajpath.2011.03.030

84. Hsu AC-Y, Dua K, Starkey MR, Haw T-J, Nair PM, Nichol K, et al. MicroRNA-125a and -b inhibit A20 and MAVS to promote inflammation and impair antiviral response in COPD. *JCI Insight*. (2017) 2:e90443. doi: 10.1172/jci.insight.90443

85. Shehab M, Sherri N, Hussein H, Salloum N, Rahal EA. Endosomal toll-like receptors mediate enhancement of interleukin-17a production triggered by Epstein-Barr virus DNA in mice. *J Virol*. (2019) 93:e00987–19. doi: 10.1128/JVI.00987-19

86. West JA, Gregory SM, Damania B. Toll-like receptor sensing of human herpesvirus infection. *Front Cell Infect Microbiol*. (2012) 2:122. doi: 10.3389/fcimb.2012.00122

87. Liu D, Chen Q, Zhu H, Gong L, Huang Y, Li S, et al. Association of respiratory syncytial virus toll-like receptor 3-mediated immune response with COPD exacerbation frequency. *Inflammation*. (2018) 41:654–66. doi: 10.1007/s10753-017-0720-4

88. Silkoff PE, Flavin S, Gordon R, Loza MJ, Sterk PJ, Lutter R, et al. Toll-like receptor 3 blockade in rhinovirus-induced experimental asthma exacerbations: a randomized controlled study. *J Allergy Clin Immunol*. (2018) 141:1220–30. doi: 10.1016/j.jaci.2017.06.027

89. Vallath S, Hynds RE, Succony L, Janes SM, Giangreco A. Targeting EGFR signalling in chronic lung disease: therapeutic challenges and opportunities. *Eur Respir J*. (2014) 44:513–22. doi: 10.1183/09031936.00146413

90. Tyner JW, Kim EY, Ide K, Pelletier MR, Roswit WT, Morton JD, et al. Blocking airway mucous cell metaplasia by inhibiting EGFR antiapoptosis and IL-13 transdifferentiation signals. *J Clin Invest*. (2006) 116:309–21. doi: 10.1172/JCI25167

91. Guedán A, Swieboda D, Charles M, Toussaint M, Johnston SL, Asfor A, et al. Investigation of the role of protein kinase D in human rhinovirus replication. *J Virol*. (2017) 91:e00217–17. doi: 10.1128/JVI.00217-17

92. Kim S, Nadel JA. Fibrinogen binding to ICAM-1 promotes EGFR-dependent mucin production in human airway epithelial cells. *Am J Physiol Lung Cell Mol Physiol*. (2009) 297:L174–83. doi: 10.1152/ajplung.00032.2009

93. Subauste MC, Proud D. Effects of tumor necrosis factor-α, epidermal growth factor and transforming growth factor-α on interleukin-8 production by, and human rhinovirus replication in, bronchial epithelial cells. *Int Immunopharmacol*. (2001) 1:1229–34. doi: 10.1016/S1567-5769(01)00063-7

94. Ganesan S, Unger BL, Comstock AT, Angel KA, Mancuso P, Martinez FJ, et al. Aberrantly activated EGFR contributes to enhanced IL-8 expression in COPD airways epithelial cells via regulation of nuclear FoxO3A. *Thorax*. (2013) 68:131–41. doi: 10.1136/thoraxjnl-2012-201719

95. Zhu L, Lee P-K, Lee W-M, Zhao Y, Yu D, Chen Y. Rhinovirus-induced major airway mucin production involves a novel TLR3-EGFR-dependent pathway. *Am J Respir Cell Mol Biol*. (2009) 40:610–9. doi: 10.1165/rcmb.2008-0223OC

96. Hewson CA, Haas JJ, Bartlett NW, Message SD, Laza-Stanca V, Kebadze T, et al. Rhinovirus induces MUC5AC in a human infection model and

in vitro via NF-κB and EGFR pathways. *Eur Respir J.* (2010) 36:1425–35. doi: 10.1183/09031936.00026910

97. Stolarczyk M, Scholte BJ. The EGFR-ADAM17 axis in chronic obstructive pulmonary disease and cystic fibrosis lung pathology. *Mediators Inflamm.* (2018) 2018:1067134. doi: 10.1155/2018/1067134

98. Ueki IF, Min-Oo G, Kalinowski A, Ballon-Landa E, Lanier LL, Nadel JA, et al. Respiratory virus-induced EGFR activation suppresses IRF1-dependent interferon λ and antiviral defense in airway epithelium. *J Exp Med.* (2013) 210:1929–36. doi: 10.1084/jem.20121401

99. Kalinowski A, Galen BT, Ueki IF, Sun Y, Mulenos A, Osafo-Addo A, et al. Respiratory syncytial virus activates epidermal growth factor receptor to suppress interferon regulatory factor 1-dependent interferon-lambda and antiviral defense in airway epithelium. *Mucosal Immunol.* (2018) 11:958–67. doi: 10.1038/mi.2017.120

100. Abe T, Marutani Y, Shoji I. Cytosolic DNA-sensing immune response and viral infection. *Microbiol Immunol.* (2019) 63:51–64. doi: 10.1111/1348-0421.12669

101. Chan YK, Gack MU. Viral evasion of intracellular DNA and RNA sensing. *Nat Rev Microbiol.* (2016) 14:360–73. doi: 10.1038/nrmicro.2016.45

102. Orzalli MH, Broekema NM, Diner BA, Hancks DC, Elde NC, Cristea IM, et al. cGAS-mediated stabilization of IFI16 promotes innate signaling during herpes simplex virus infection. *Proc Natl Acad Sci USA.* (2015) 112:E1773–81. doi: 10.1073/pnas.1424637112

103. Zhu J, Message SD, Mallia P, Kebadze T, Contoli M, Ward CK, et al. Bronchial mucosal IFN-α/β and pattern recognition receptor expression in patients with experimental rhinovirus-induced asthma exacerbations. *J Allergy Clin Immunol.* (2019) 143:114–25.e4. doi: 10.1016/j.jaci.2018.04.003

104. Farazuddin M, Mishra R, Jing Y, Srivastava V, Comstock AT, Sajjan US. Quercetin prevents rhinovirus-induced progression of lung disease in mice with COPD phenotype. *PLoS ONE.* (2018) 13:e0199612. doi: 10.1371/journal.pone.0199612

105. Traub S, Nikonova A, Carruthers A, Dunmore R, Vousden KA, Gogsadze L, et al. An anti-human ICAM-1 antibody inhibits rhinovirus-induced exacerbations of lung inflammation. *PLoS Pathog.* (2013) 9:e1003520. doi: 10.1371/journal.ppat.1003520

106. Mirabelli C, Scheers E, Neyts J. Novel therapeutic approaches to simultaneously target rhinovirus infection and asthma/COPD pathogenesis. *F1000Res.* (2017) 6:1860. doi: 10.12688/f1000research.11978.1

107. Beigel JH, Nam HH, Adams PL, Krafft A, Ince WL, El-Kamary SS, et al. Advances in respiratory virus therapeutics - a meeting report from the 6th isirv antiviral group conference. *Antiviral Res.* (2019) 167:45–67. doi: 10.1016/j.antiviral.2019.04.006

108. Mousnier A, Bell AS, Swieboda DP, Morales-Sanfrutos J, Pérez-Dorado I, Brannigan JA, et al. Fragment-derived inhibitors of human N-myristoyltransferase block capsid assembly and replication of the common cold virus. *Nat Chem.* (2018) 10:599–606. doi: 10.1038/s41557-018-0039-2

109. Schaefer N, Li X, Seibold MA, Jarjour NN, Denlinger LC, Castro M, et al. The effect of BPIFA1/SPLUNC1 genetic variation on its expression and function in asthmatic airway epithelium. *JCI Insight.* (2019) 4:e127237. doi: 10.1172/jci.insight.127237

110. Jiang D, Wenzel SE, Wu Q, Bowler RP, Schnell C, Chu HW. Human neutrophil elastase degrades SPLUNC1 and impairs airway epithelial defense against bacteria. *PLoS ONE.* (2013) 8:e64689. doi: 10.1371/journal.pone.0064689

111. Seys LJM, Verhamme FM, Dupont LL, Desauter E, Duerr J, Seyhan Agircan A, et al. Airway surface dehydration aggravates cigarette smoke-induced hallmarks of COPD in mice. *PLoS ONE.* (2015) 10:e0129897. doi: 10.1371/journal.pone.0129897

112. Tcherniuk S, Cenac N, Comte M, Frouard J, Errazuriz-Cerda E, Galabov A, et al. Formyl peptide receptor 2 plays a deleterious role during influenza a virus infections. *J Infect Dis.* (2016) 214:237–47. doi: 10.1093/infdis/jiw127

113. Ampomah PB, Moraes LA, Lukman HM, Lim LHK. Formyl peptide receptor 2 is regulated by RNA mimics and viruses through an IFN-b-STAT3-dependent pathway. *FASEB J.* (2018) 32:1468–78. doi: 10.1096/fj.201700584RR

114. Lupfer C, Malik A, Kanneganti T-D. Inflammasome control of viral infection. *Curr Opin Virol.* (2015) 12:38–46. doi: 10.1016/j.coviro.2015.02.007

115. Chen I-Y, Ichinohe T. Response of host inflammasomes to viral infection. *Trends Microbiol.* (2015) 23:55–63. doi: 10.1016/j.tim.2014.09.007

116. Colarusso C, Terlizzi M, Molino A, Pinto A, Sorrentino R. Role of the inflammasome in chronic obstructive pulmonary disease (COPD). *Oncotarget.* (2017) 8:81813–24. doi: 10.18632/oncotarget.17850

117. Hikichi M, Mizumura K, Maruoka S, Gon Y. Pathogenesis of chronic obstructive pulmonary disease (COPD) induced by cigarette smoke. *J Thorac Dis.* (2019) 11:S2129–40. doi: 10.21037/jtd.2019.10.43

19

Epigenetic Regulation of Airway Epithelium Immune Functions in Asthma

Bilal Alashkar Alhamwe [1,2,3], Sarah Miethe [1,4], Elke Pogge von Strandmann [3], Daniel P. Potaczek [1,5†] and Holger Garn [1,4*†]

[1] Institute of Laboratory Medicine, Philipps-University Marburg, Member of the German Center for Lung Research (DZL), Universities of Giessen and Marburg Lung Center, Marburg, Germany, [2] College of Pharmacy, International University for Science and Technology (IUST), Daraa, Syria, [3] Center for Tumor Biology and Immunology, Institute of Tumor Immunology, Philipps University Marburg, Marburg, Germany, [4] Translational Inflammation Research Division & Core Facility for Single Cell Multiomics, Philipps University Marburg, Marburg, Germany, [5] John Paul II Hospital, Kraków, Poland

*Correspondence:
Holger Garn
garn@staff.uni-marburg.de

[†] These authors have contributed equally to this work

Asthma is a chronic inflammatory disease of the respiratory tract characterized by recurrent breathing problems resulting from airway obstruction and hyperresponsiveness. Human airway epithelium plays an important role in the initiation and control of the immune responses to different types of environmental factors contributing to asthma pathogenesis. Using pattern recognition receptors airway epithelium senses external stimuli, such as allergens, microbes, or pollutants, and subsequently secretes endogenous danger signaling molecules alarming and activating dendritic cells. Hence, airway epithelial cells not only mediate innate immune responses but also bridge them with adaptive immune responses involving T and B cells that play a crucial role in the pathogenesis of asthma. The effects of environmental factors on the development of asthma are mediated, at least in part, by epigenetic mechanisms. Those comprise classical epigenetics including DNA methylation and histone modifications affecting transcription, as well as microRNAs influencing translation. The common feature of such mechanisms is that they regulate gene expression without affecting the nucleotide sequence of the genomic DNA. Epigenetic mechanisms play a pivotal role in the regulation of different cell populations involved in asthma pathogenesis, with the remarkable example of T cells. Recently, however, there is increasing evidence that epigenetic mechanisms are also crucial for the regulation of airway epithelial cells, especially in the context of epigenetic transfer of environmental effects contributing to asthma pathogenesis. In this review, we summarize the accumulating evidence for this very important aspect of airway epithelial cell pathobiology.

Keywords: airway, allergy, asthma, epigenetic, epithelium, histone, methylation, microRNA (miRNA)

INTRODUCTION

Asthma is a chronic inflammatory disease of the airways, in which airway obstruction and hyperresponsiveness underlie recurrent breathing problems, with symptoms being especially pronounced during disease exacerbations (1, 2). Respiratory tract epithelium plays an important role in asthma by initiating and controlling immune responses to different types of pathogenic environmental factors, including allergens, viruses, pollutants, and others. The biology of the airway epithelium in health and its pathobiology in asthma are regulated by epigenetic mechanisms forming the intercellular homeostatic system responding to internal as well as external changing conditions on the level of transcriptional and posttranscriptional regulation of gene expression (3, 4).

AIRWAY EPITHELIUM AND ASTHMA

The airway epithelium is the first structure of the body getting into contact with inhaled air with all its containing environmental components. Initially, it was thought to just constitute a mechanical barrier to enable the bidirectional transfer of air to and from the gas-exchanging alveolar structures. Over the last years, it turned out, however, that the airway epithelium in general and the bronchial epithelium as a major part of it in particular represent a much more complex tissue fulfilling a variety of additional functions such as retrograde transport of inhaled particles, establishment of a biochemical barrier system, and initiation and regulation of innate and adaptive immune mechanisms by release of various cytokines and chemokines. By this, it represents an integrative part of the innate immune system, the coordinated activity of which is essential for maintaining the local tissue and even systemic body integrity (5). To exert these diverse functions, the bronchial epithelium is composed of multiple structurally and/or functionally differing cell types, such as ciliated cells (mucociliary transport), goblet cells (mucus secretion), tuft and M cells (luminal signal sampling and antigen presentation), ionocytes (water regulation), and club cells (mucus and surfactant protein production) (6). All these cell types develop from local stem cell precursors, called basal cells (7). It is quite obvious that the continuous development of the different cell types from such precursors, as well as their concerted action under healthy conditions, requires a high level of control and regulation (8). In asthma, the underlying control mechanisms are disturbed by both external (environmental factors such as allergens, pollen, bacteria, viruses) and internal (i.e., cytokines, chemokines, low-molecular-weight mediators produced by innate and adaptive immune cells) influences, resulting in dysregulated activities of the bronchial epithelium (9). This includes hypersecretion of mucus, release of epithelial-derived cytokines called alarmins [e.g., interleukin 25 (IL-25), IL-33, thymic stromal lymphopoietin], chemokines, and antimicrobial peptides, as well as uncontrolled proliferation and differentiation processes, altogether leading to functional [e.g., airway hyperresponsiveness(AHR)] and structural (e.g., airway remodeling) changes that represent characteristic features of asthma pathology (10). Not unexpectedly, because of the close relation to environmental influences and their changes, epigenetic regulation processes are crucially involved in the appropriate development, maintenance, and functionality of the different components of the airway epithelium (11). Chronic inflammatory processes such as in asthma are expected to interfere with these well-balanced epigenetic mechanisms in

the epithelium of the airways. This may happen at the level of the aforementioned finally differentiated cell types and by changing related gene expression patterns that influence their functional behavior. It is also conceivable that epigenetic changes occur already at the level of the basal cells, which would then be inherited to all kinds of cells developing from the affected precursors with multiple functional consequences (12). It needs to be considered that these mechanisms may either lead to further perpetuation of the disease process or, alternatively, represent repair activities initiated to get the complex system back to steady state, that is, healthy conditions.

EPIGENETIC MECHANISMS

Epigenetics comprises molecular mechanisms of inheritable but reversible phenotypic changes that lead to modified gene expression without alterations at the level of the DNA sequence (13). In the human genome, 80% of the DNA is packed into nucleosomes, and the rest forms linkers between nucleosomes. The nucleosomes are further packed into dense three-dimensional structures called chromosomes (14). The core components of the nucleosome are histone proteins, which are accessible to different types of posttranslational modifications (PTMs), including acetylation, methylation, phosphorylation, sumoylation, and ubiquitination. Posttranslational modifications, especially if occurring at important regulatory genomic regions such as enhancers or promoters, are able to change the accessibility of the DNA to the transcriptional machinery, which is associated with active, poised, or silenced status of transcriptional activity. For example, histone acetylations, the changes introduced by histone acetyltransferases (HATs) and removed by histone deacetylases (HDACs), are usually associated with transcriptional activation of the gene (15, 16). DNA methylation, in which a methyl group is enzymatically added to the cytosine ring of DNA, is another type of the epigenetic modification. While the methylation reaction is catalyzed by DNA methyltransferases, ten-eleven translocation (TET) methylcytosine dioxygenase family proteins mediate DNA demethylation. DNA methylation is typically associated with gene repression (3, 17). In addition to the classical epigenetic modifications mentioned above, different types of the non-coding RNAs such as microRNAs (miRNAs) and others, for instance, piwi-interacting RNAs or small nucleolar RNAs, are involved in the epigenetic regulation of gene expression. Briefly, miRNAs exert their silencing effects through the binding to the mature mRNA molecules in the cytosol that leads to mRNA degradation or reduction in the translational efficiency of the ribosomes (18, 19) (**Figure 1**).

DNA METHYLATION

DNA methylation is probably the best studied epigenetic modification in general but also in relation to asthma. Although studies conducted so far on the involvement of DNA methylation in asthma have mostly used already available DNA samples and/or DNA extracted from easily available tissues, also

Epigenetic Regulation of Airway Epithelium Immune Functions in Asthma

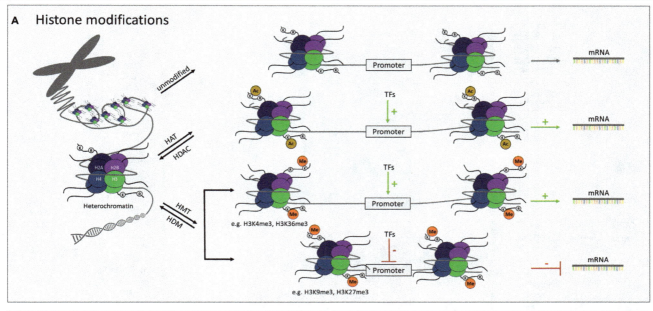
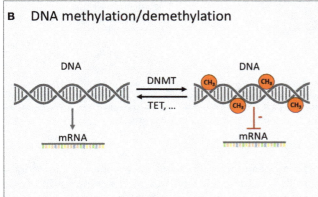
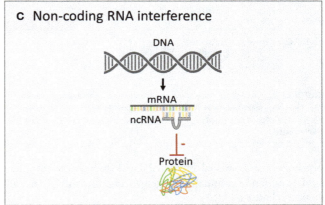

FIGURE 1 | Schematic illustration of major epigenetic modifications. **(A)** Modification of histones such as histone acetylation/deacetylation via histone acetyltransferases (HATs)/histone deacetylases (HDAC) and methylation/demethylation via histone methyltransferases (HMT)/histone demethylases (HDM) can either activate or repress the target gene transcription. Histone acetylation is typically associated with higher expression of the gene. Histone methylation can be related to either higher or lower transcriptional activity, depending on the amino acid residue modified and the number of methyl groups added. **(B)** DNA methylation or demethylation of genomic DNA through DNA methyltransferases (DNMT) or ten-eleven translocation (TET) enzymes and others, respectively. Higher level of DNA methylation is typically associated with lower transcriptional activity of the respective gene. **(C)** MicroRNAs (miRNAs) and further small non-coding RNAs can interfere with gene expression through base pairing with messenger RNAs and thus inhibiting their translation into the encoded protein.

lower airway epithelial cells (AECs) have been investigated (**Figure 2**). Stefanowicz et al. (20) performed a comparative DNA methylation analysis of 807 genes in bronchial AECs and peripheral blood mononuclear cells (PBMCs) obtained from atopics, atopic asthmatics, non-atopic asthmatics, or healthy controls. They identified signature sets of CpG sites differentially methylated between AECs and PBMCs, which were either independent of the disease phenotype or specific to healthy controls, atopics, or asthmatics. Although no differences in the DNA methylation status were found between disease phenotypes in PBMCs, they were observed between asthmatics and atopics in AECs (20). Kim et al. (21) comparatively analyzed genome-wide DNA methylation levels in bronchial mucosa tissues obtained from atopic and non-atopic asthmatics and healthy controls. Although the methylation levels were similar between asthmatics and controls, a set of loci has been identified with significant differences in DNA methylation between atopic and non-atopic asthmatics (21). Clifford et al. (22) investigated in turn the effects of experimental respiratory tract exposure to allergen, diesel exhaust, or both as a coexposure, always observing only minimal resulting changes in the bronchial epithelial DNA methylome of the participating individuals. They found, however, that if any of the two insults occurs in advance of the other (crossover exposure with a 4-week interval), the initial

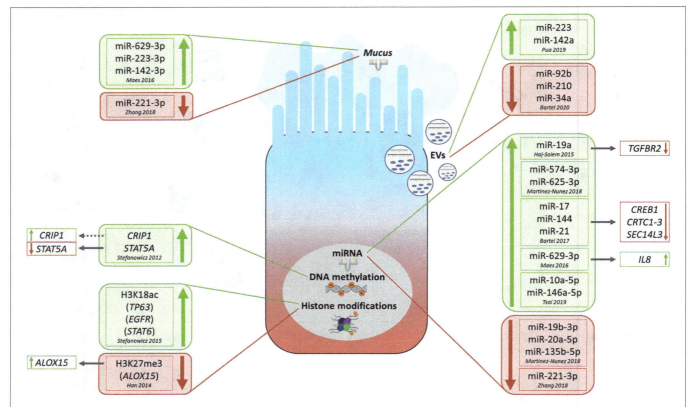

FIGURE 2 | Overview of currently known key epigenetic modifications observed in lower airway epithelial cells from asthma/allergic airway inflammation conditions and—if known—associated functional consequences. The green color always indicates upregulation of the respective modification in asthmatics vs. healthy while red color identifies opposite regulation. EVs, extracellular vesicles; miRNA, microRNA; H3K18ac, histone H3K18 acetylation; H3K27me3, histone H3K27me3 trimethylation.

one primes the bronchial epithelial DNA methylome for the second, resulting in cumulative epigenetic changes with potential biological relevance (22).

In most cases, however, DNA methylation studies conducted in airway tissue in the context of asthma have not been performed in bronchial or lung ACEs but rather in nasal epithelial cells (NECs) due to easier accessibility (23–28). Cardenas et al. (23) conducted an epigenome-wide study on DNA methylation using nasal swabs collected in a large group of early teenagers deriving from a birth cohort. They identified multiple DNA methylation loci associated with asthma, allergies, and related clinical or laboratory parameters (23). In another cohort of adolescents, Forno et al. (24) performed in turn an epigenome-wide analysis of DNA methylation in nasal epithelium. The major findings of this study, replicated in two independent cohorts, comprised the identification of specific DNA methylation profiles associated with atopy and atopic asthma and a nasal methylation panel that could classify children by atopy or atopic asthma (24). Reese et al. (25) sought to identify differential DNA methylation related to pediatric asthma in blood from newborns and school-aged children. Interestingly, they were able to replicate in eosinophils or nasal respiratory epithelium most of the asthma-related differential methylation signatures initially detected in blood (25). Brugha et al. (29) comparatively analyzed DNA methylation in airway and surrogate tissues. They found that the methylation profile in nasal epithelium was most representative of that in the airway epithelium, whereas the profile in buccal cells was moderately and that in blood was least similar (29). In our view, these results clearly suggest that DNA methylation studies performed in the context of asthma as an airway disease should preferentially be conducted using AECs or NECs. Although beyond the scope of this review, we would like to mention that, in our view, sorted specific white blood cell populations would be highly valuable to study systemic adaptive immunity DNA methylation patterns underlying asthma. However, how well those signatures correspond to local lung DNA methylation patterns would need to be assessed in separate studies. Back to NECs, Xiao et al. (27) showed that nasal DNA methylation at the promoter of the vanin 1 gene (*VNN1*) might be a clinically useful biomarker of corticosteroid treatment response in asthmatic children. Another study from the same group demonstrated in turn that DNA methylation at the TET methylcytosine dioxygenase 1 gene (*TET1*) contributes to traffic-related air pollution and asthma (26).

Finally, allelic differences in DNA methylation and thus gene expression in AECs can mediate the effects of certain genetic variants known to be associated with susceptibility to childhood asthma, such as those in chromosome 17q21 (30, 31).

HISTONE MODIFICATIONS

In addition to DNA methylation, also histone modifications participate in epithelial (patho-) mechanisms related to asthma (**Figure 2**). Stefanowicz et al. (32) compared global and gene-specific alveolar epithelial cells histone acetylation and methylation status between asthmatics and healthy subjects. Generally, they observed higher global H3K18ac and H3K9me3 levels in asthmatic subjects. In more detail, they found in asthmatics a higher association of H3K18ac (but not H3K9me3) around the transcription start sites of *TP63* (tumor protein p63, ΔNp63 isoform), *EGFR* (epidermal growth factor receptor), and *STAT6* (signal transducer and activator of transcription 6) genes. Finally, they detected a non-significant increase in protein expression of those three genes in AECs treated with trichostatin A, an HDAC inhibitor (HDACi) (32). In another work, the same group comparatively analyzed the expression of 82 epigenetic modifying enzymes in AECs and bronchial fibroblasts obtained from asthmatics and healthy controls (33). Thirty-nine enzymes were differentially expressed between AECs and bronchial fibroblasts, 24 of which passed the correction for multiple testing. Six histone modifiers turned out to be differentially expressed in AECs between asthmatics and non-asthmatics, however, mostly not significantly when corrected for multiple testing (33).

Beneficial effects of HDACi have been observed in murine models of allergic airway inflammation (AAI) mimicking features of human allergic asthma (34, 35). Application of HDACi in an ovalbumin (OVA)–based model reduced airway inflammation, remodeling, and AHR. In addition, HDACi treatment was associated with lower expression of transforming growth factor β1 (TGF-β1) in AECs and diminished synthesis of contractile proteins by airway smooth muscle cells (34). HDACi treatment in mice subjected to a house dust mite (HDM)–based model was in turn able to prevent them from developing AHR and AAI. Moreover, HDACi restored the integrity of the *ex vivo*–cultured NECs isolated from AR patients (35). Significantly lower H3K27me3 levels at the promoter of the arachidonate 15-lipoxygenase (ALOX15) gene (*ALOX15*) were observed in human lung epithelial A549 cells after the treatment with IL-4, which coincided with higher *ALOX15* mRNA levels (36).

Targeting histone modification—related mechanisms turned out to be effective also in a cockroach allergen extract–induced mouse model of mixed granulocytic (eosinophilic and neutrophilic), T_H2/T_H17-driven asthma (37). Specifically, whereas a bromo- and extraterminal (BET) inhibitor was already alone able to abolish T_H17-driven neutrophilic inflammation, in combination with dexamethasone it completely blocked both T_H2- and T_H17-driven immune responses in the lung, which was associated with reductions in lung eosinophilia and neutrophilia, and mucin secretion. Furthermore, BET inhibition improved cockroach allergen extract– or IL-17A–induced increase in markers of glucocorticoid insensitivity [i.e., decrease in HDAC2 expression (38)] in murine or human AECs, respectively (37). In another study, $Hdac2^{+/-}$ mice subjected to an HDM-induced AAI model demonstrated stronger inflammatory infiltration as well as higher expression of type 2 cytokines and IL-17A in the lung tissue compared to wild-type animals. Additional IL-17A depletion was able to reverse these HDAC2 impairment-induced effects (39). In turn, HDM and IL-17A synergistically reduced HDAC2 expression in human bronchial epithelial cells (BECs) *in vitro*. Besides, silencing the HDAC2-encoding gene further enhanced HDM- and/or IL-17A–induced inflammatory cytokines in human BECs, whereas HDAC2 overexpression or knockdown of the gene encoding IL-17A was able to reduce the release of such inflammatory cytokines (39). Taken together, original findings by Zijlstra et al. (38), who first discovered IL-17A–induced steroid resistance mediated by a reduction of HDAC2 activity, have thus been corroborated and expanded.

MICRORNA

Several recent studies have highlighted the importance of miRNAs in the regulation of epithelial pathobiology in asthma (**Figure 2**). Bartel et al. (40) combined different approaches such as *in vivo* studies in mice with OVA- or HDM-induced AAI, *ex vivo/in vitro* experiments including luciferase reporter assay and stimulation–expression analyses, miRNA/mRNA microarrays, and *in silico* approaches. This composed strategy enabled the authors to identify the transcription factor cAMP-responsive element binding protein (*Creb1*) and its transcriptional coactivators (*Crtc1-3*) as targets for miR-17, miR-144, and miR-21, all three deregulated in lungs of mice with AAI. Moreover, they observed downregulation of Sec14-like 3 (*Sec14l3*), a putative target of Creb1, in both AAI models and in primary normal human BECs upon IL-13 treatment suggesting that miRNA-regulated Crtc1-3 and Sec14l3 play a role in early epithelial responses to type 2 stimuli (40). Microarray analysis of miRNA expression in bronchoscopy-isolated human BECs showed in turn an upregulation of miR-19a in samples obtained from severe asthmatic subjects compared to those from mild asthmatics and healthy controls (41). Furthermore, luciferase reporter assay- and Western blot–based functional studies demonstrated miR-19a to enhance proliferation of BECs in severe asthma through targeting TGF-β receptor 2 gene (*TGFBR2*) mRNA (41). Using subcellular fractionation and RNA sequencing (Frac-seq) in human primary BECs from healthy controls and severe asthmatics, Martinez-Nunez et al. (42) assessed paired genome-wide expression of miRNAs along with cytoplasmic (total) and polyribosome-bound (translational) mRNA levels. They identified a hub of six dysregulated miRNAs, displaying preference for polyribosome-bound mRNAs, which accounted for ~90% of whole miRNA targeting. Interestingly, transfection of such miRNAs into BECs obtained from healthy subjects turned them into cells mimicking features of those obtained from severe asthmatics (42).

Recently, extracellular vesicles (EVs) transferring miRNAs between cells have been identified as a novel mechanism of intercellular communication (3, 43, 44). Of note, the composition of the extracellular miRNA pool in the lung of mice was very similar to that of the airway epithelium, and ~80% of the detected EVs were of epithelial origin (45). However, following the induction of AAI, the presence of miRNAs preferentially expressed by immune cells, such as miR-223 and miR-142a, and hematopoietic cell–derived EVs increased also substantially, indicating an importance of the extracellular miRNA pool for the development of local allergic inflammatory processes (45). Gupta et al. (46) focused on EVs secreted by two kinds of human airway cell cultures, that is, primary tracheobronchial cells and a cultured AEC line (Calu-3). Their data suggest that cellular information can be transferred between AECs via miRNA-containing EVs, which may thereby contribute to epithelial biology and remodeling (46). Another study profiled the expression of miRNAs in EVs secreted from the apical and basal sides by normal human BECs treated with IL-13 in order to induce an asthma-like response (47). Significant candidates were then confirmed in EVs isolated from nasal lavages obtained from children with mild to moderate or severe asthma and healthy control subjects. Interestingly, levels of miR-92b, miR-210, and miR-34a turned out to correlate with lung function measures (47).

Two studies investigated miRNAs in asthmatic sputum (48, 49). In two independent cohorts, Maes et al. (48) found a significant upregulation of miR-629-3p, miR-223-3p, and miR-142-3p in sputum of severe asthmatics compared to healthy controls, with the highest levels in patients with neutrophilic asthma. Of those three miRNAs associated with sputum neutrophilia and airway obstruction, miR-629-3p was expressed in BECs. Interestingly, transfection of human BECs with a miR-629-3p mimic induced expression of IL-8, the sputum levels of which were significantly increased and positively correlated with sputum neutrophilia in severe asthmatics (48). Zhang et al. (49) found in turn that epithelial, sputum, and plasma miR-221-3p levels were significantly lower in asthmatics compared to healthy controls. In addition, levels of epithelial and sputum miR-221-3p inversely correlated with airway eosinophilia (49).

Finally, Tsai et al. (50) sought to find the common miRNA-related effects in BECs obtained from subjects with asthma and chronic obstructive pulmonary disease (COPD). First detected with next-generation sequencing, the upregulation of miR-10a-5p and miR-146a-5p in BECs obtained from both asthma and COPD patients was subsequently confirmed by quantitative polymerase chain reaction. Moreover, compared to healthy controls, also serum miR-146a-5p levels were higher in asthma and COPD subjects (50). Further research will establish whether miRNAs mediating intercellular communication can be used for clinical applications as biomarkers or therapeutic targets.

SPECIAL ASPECTS

Airborne viruses, for instance, human rhinoviruses (HRVs), stimulate asthma exacerbations. In addition, repeated early life infections with such viruses can lead to the development of a persistent asthma phenotype, especially in children with atopic susceptibility (3, 51). Interestingly, some studies suggest that the effects of respiratory viral infections are at least partly mediated by epigenetic changes in airway epithelial cells. It has been demonstrated that *ex vivo* experimental HRV infection of NECs obtained from asthmatic children significantly changes patterns of DNA methylation and mRNA expression (52). Moreover, HRV infection in young children has been associated with changes in the airway secretory miRNome, characterized by a highly specific additional appearance of miR-155 in nasal secretion EVs (53). In turn, BECs obtained from asthmatics have been shown to be characterized by dysregulated miR-22 expression after experimental *ex vivo* infection with influenza A virus (IAV) (54). Other epigenetic modifications, specifically histone methylations, also seem to be involved in the regulation of epithelial antiviral responses (55).

Dysregulated epithelial–mesenchymal transition (EMT) is the process driven mostly by TGF-β1, which strongly contributes to the establishment of the persistent asthma phenotype, that is, to disease chronification (56). Epigenetic mechanisms seem to play an important role in EMT. It has been demonstrated in mouse models mimicking allergic asthma that miR-448-5p can inhibit TGF-β1–induced EMT and pulmonary fibrosis (57). Applying an epigenome-wide approach in a human study, McErlean et al. (58) identified in turn multiple loci showing differential H3K27ac enrichment in asthma, which clustered at genes associated with type 2–driven asthma and EMT.

CONCLUSIONS AND PERSPECTIVES

Epigenetic mechanisms play a very important role in the epithelial pathobiology of asthma. While histone modifications seem to be especially interesting as possible therapeutic targets, DNA methylation and miRNAs, also from the easily accessible nasal epithelium, show a substantial diagnostic potential. Although the data gathered by now (for overview, see also **Supplementary Table 1**) already strongly suggest a usefulness of epigenetics in the asthma management, further studies, especially those considering the complex interplay of different epigenetic mechanisms and those focusing on a single-cell type or investigations on the single cell level, are needed.

AUTHOR CONTRIBUTIONS

BA: draft writing and figure drafts. SM: draft writing and final figures. ES: editing and reviewing. DP: conceptualization, draft writing, and reviewing. HG: conceptualization, coordination, draft writing, and reviewing. All authors contributed to the article and approved the submitted version.

REFERENCES

1. Miethe S, Guarino M, Alhamdan F, Simon H-U, Renz H, Dufour J-F, et al. Effects of obesity on asthma: immunometabolic links. *Polish Arch Internal Med.* (2018) 128:469–77. doi: 10.20452/pamw.4304
2. Koczulla AR, Vogelmeier CF, Garn H, Renz H. New concepts in asthma: clinical phenotypes and pathophysiological mechanisms. *Drug Discov Today.* (2017) 22:388–96. doi: 10.1016/j.drudis.2016.11.008
3. Potaczek DP, Harb H, Michel S, Alhamwe BA, Renz H, Tost J. Epigenetics and allergy: from basic mechanisms to clinical applications. *Epigenomics.* (2017) 9:539–71. doi: 10.2217/epi-2016-0162
4. Pepper AN, Renz H, Casale TB, Garn H. Biologic therapy and novel molecular targets of severe asthma. *J Allergy Clin Immunol Pract.* (2017) 5:909–16. doi: 10.1016/j.jaip.2017.04.038
5. Potaczek DP, Miethe S, Schindler V, Alhamdan F, Garn H. Role of airway epithelial cells in the development of different asthma phenotypes. *Cell Signal.* (2020) 69:109523. doi: 10.1016/j.cellsig.2019.109523
6. Plasschaert LW, Žilionis R, Choo-Wing R, Savova V, Knehr J, Roma G, et al. A single-cell atlas of the airway epithelium reveals the CFTR-rich pulmonary ionocyte. *Nature.* (2018) 560:377–81. doi: 10.1038/s41586-018-0394-6
7. Watson JK, Rulands S, Wilkinson AC, Wuidart A, Ousset M, van Keymeulen A, et al. Clonal dynamics reveal two distinct populations of basal cells in slow-turnover airway epithelium. *Cell Rep.* (2015) 12:90–101. doi: 10.1016/j.celrep.2015.06.011
8. Loxham M, Davies DE. Phenotypic and genetic aspects of epithelial barrier function in asthmatic patients. *J Allergy Clin Immunol.* (2017) 139:1736–51. doi: 10.1016/j.jaci.2017.04.005
9. Holgate ST. The sentinel role of the airway epithelium in asthma pathogenesis. *Immunol Rev.* (2011) 242:205–19. doi: 10.1111/j.1600-065X.2011.01030.x
10. Lloyd CM, Saglani S. Epithelial cytokines and pulmonary allergic inflammation. *Curr Opin Immunol.* (2015) 34:52–8. doi: 10.1016/j.coi.2015.02.001
11. Wawrzyniak P, Wawrzyniak M, Wanke K, Sokolowska M, Bendelja K, Rückert B, et al. Regulation of bronchial epithelial barrier integrity by type 2 cytokines and histone deacetylases in asthmatic patients. *J Allergy Clin Immunol.* (2017) 139:93–103. doi: 10.1016/j.jaci.2016.03.050
12. Ordovas-Montanes J, Dwyer DF, Nyquist SK, Buchheit KM, Vukovic M, Deb C, et al. Allergic inflammatory memory in human respiratory epithelial progenitor cells. *Nature.* (2018) 560:649–54. doi: 10.1038/s41586-018-0449-8
13. Lacal I, Ventura R. Epigenetic inheritance: concepts, mechanisms and perspectives. *Front Mol Neurosci.* (2018) 11:292. doi: 10.3389/fnmol.2018.00292
14. Alberts B, Johnson A, Lewis J, Raff M, Roberts K, Walter P. *Molecular Biology of the Cell: Chromosomal DNA and Its Packaging in the Chromatin Fiber.* 4th ed. New York, NY: Garland Science (2002).
15. Harb H, Alashkar Alhamwe B, Garn H, Renz H, Potaczek DP. Recent developments in epigenetics of pediatric asthma. *Curr Opin Pediatr.* (2016) 28:754–63. doi: 10.1097/MOP.0000000000000424
16. Alaskhar Alhamwe B, Khalaila R, Wolf J, Bülow V, von Harb H, Alhamdan F, et al. Histone modifications and their role in epigenetics of atopy and allergic diseases. *Allergy Asthma Clin Immunol.* (2018) 14:39. doi: 10.1186/s13223-018-0259-4
17. Alashkar Alhamwe B, Alhamdan F, Ruhl A, Potaczek DP, Renz H. The role of epigenetics in allergy and asthma development. *Curr Opin Allergy Clin Immunol.* (2020) 20:48–55. doi: 10.1097/ACI.0000000000000598
18. Hu G, Niu F, Humburg BA, Liao K, Bendi S, Callen S, et al. Molecular mechanisms of long noncoding RNAs and their role in disease pathogenesis. *Oncotarget.* (2018) 9:18648–63. doi: 10.18632/oncotarget.24307
19. Karlsson O, Baccarelli AA. Environmental health and long non-coding RNAs. *Curr Environ Health Rep.* (2016) 3:178–87. doi: 10.1007/s40572-016-0092-1
20. Stefanowicz D, Hackett T-L, Garmaroudi FS, Günther OP, Neumann S, Sutanto EN, et al. DNA methylation profiles of airway epithelial cells and PBMCs from healthy, atopic and asthmatic children. *PLoS ONE.* (2012) 7:e44213. doi: 10.1371/journal.pone.0044213
21. Kim Y-J, Park S-W, Kim T-H, Park J-S, Cheong HS, Shin HD, et al. Genome-wide methylation profiling of the bronchial mucosa of asthmatics: relationship to atopy. *BMC Med Genet.* (2013) 14:39. doi: 10.1186/1471-2350-14-39
22. Clifford RL, Jones MJ, MacIsaac JL, McEwen LM, Goodman SJ, Mostafavi S, et al. Inhalation of diesel exhaust and allergen alters human bronchial epithelium DNA methylation. *J Allergy Clin Immunol.* (2017) 139:112–21. doi: 10.1016/j.jaci.2016.03.046
23. Cardenas A, Sordillo JE, Rifas-Shiman SL, Chung W, Liang L, Coull BA, et al. The nasal methylome as a biomarker of asthma and airway inflammation in children. *Nat Commun.* (2019) 10:3095. doi: 10.1038/s41467-019-11058-3
24. Forno E, Wang T, Qi C, Yan Q, Xu C-J, Boutaoui N, et al. DNA methylation in nasal epithelium, atopy, and atopic asthma in children: a genome-wide study. *Lancet Respir Med.* (2019) 7:336–46. doi: 10.1016/S2213-2600(18)30466-1
25. Reese SE, Xu C-J, den Dekker HT, Lee MK, Sikdar S, Ruiz-Arenas C, et al. Epigenome-wide meta-analysis of DNA methylation and childhood asthma. *J Allergy Clin Immunol.* (2019) 143:2062–74. doi: 10.1016/j.jaci.2018.11.043
26. Somineni HK, Zhang X, Biagini Myers JM, Kovacic MB, Ulm A, Jurcak N, et al. Ten-eleven translocation 1 (TET1) methylation is associated with childhood asthma and traffic-related air pollution. *J Allergy Clin Immunol.* (2016) 137:797–805.e5. doi: 10.1016/j.jaci.2015.10.021
27. Xiao C, Biagini Myers JM, Ji H, Metz K, Martin LJ, Lindsey M, et al. Vanin-1 expression and methylation discriminate pediatric asthma corticosteroid treatment response. *J Allergy Clin Immunol.* (2015) 136:923–31.e3. doi: 10.1016/j.jaci.2015.01.045
28. Zhang X, Biagini Myers JM, Burleson JD, Ulm A, Bryan KS, Chen X, et al. Nasal DNA methylation is associated with childhood asthma. *Epigenomics.* (2018) 10:629–41. doi: 10.2217/epi-2017-0127
29. Brugha R, Lowe R, Henderson AJ, Holloway JW, Rakyan V, Wozniak E, et al. DNA methylation profiles between airway epithelium and proxy tissues in children. *Acta Paediatr.* (2017) 106:2011–6. doi: 10.1111/apa.14027
30. Moussette S, Al Tuwaijri A, Kohan-Ghadr H-R, Elzein S, Farias R, Bérubé J, et al. Role of DNA methylation in expression control of the IKZF3-GSDMA region in human epithelial cells. *PLoS ONE.* (2017) 12:e0172707. doi: 10.1371/journal.pone.0172707
31. Toncheva AA, Potaczek DP, Schedel M, Gersting SW, Michel S, Krajnov N, et al. Childhood asthma is associated with mutations and gene expression differences of ORMDL genes that can interact. *Allergy.* (2015) 70:1288–99. doi: 10.1111/all.12652
32. Stefanowicz D, Lee JY, Lee K, Shaheen F, Koo H-K, Booth S, et al. Elevated H3K18 acetylation in airway epithelial cells of asthmatic subjects. *Respir Res.* (2015) 16:95. doi: 10.1186/s12931-015-0254-y
33. Stefanowicz D, Ullah J, Lee K, Shaheen F, Olumese E, Fishbane N, et al. Epigenetic modifying enzyme expression in asthmatic airway epithelial cells and fibroblasts. *BMC Pulm Med.* (2017) 17:24. doi: 10.1186/s12890-017-0371-0
34. Ren Y, Su X, Kong L, Li M, Zhao X, Yu N, et al. Therapeutic effects of histone deacetylase inhibitors in a murine asthma model. *Inflamm Res.* (2016) 65:995–1008. doi: 10.1007/s00011-016-0984-4
35. Steelant B, Wawrzyniak P, Martens K, Jonckheere A-C, Pugin B, Schrijvers R, et al. Blocking histone deacetylase activity as a novel target for epithelial barrier defects in patients with allergic rhinitis. *J Allergy Clin Immunol.* (2019) 144:1242–53.e7. doi: 10.1016/j.jaci.2019.04.027
36. Han H, Xu D, Liu C, Claesson H-E, Björkholm M, Sjöberg J. Interleukin-4-mediated 15-lipoxygenase-1 trans-activation requires UTX recruitment and H3K27me3 demethylation at the promoter in A549 cells. *PLoS ONE.* (2014) 9:e85085. doi: 10.1371/journal.pone.0085085
37. Nadeem A, Ahmad SF, Al-Harbi NO, Siddiqui N, Ibrahim KE, Attia SM. Inhibition of BET bromodomains restores corticosteroid responsiveness in a mixed granulocytic mouse model of asthma. *Biochem Pharmacol.* (2018) 154:222–33. doi: 10.1016/j.bcp.2018.05.011
38. Zijlstra GJ, Hacken NHT, ten Hoffmann RF, van Oosterhout AJM, Heijink IH. Interleukin-17A induces glucocorticoid insensitivity in human bronchial epithelial cells. *Eur Respir J.* (2012) 39:439–45. doi: 10.1183/09031936.00017911
39. Lai T, Wu M, Zhang C, Che L, Xu F, Wang Y, et al. HDAC2 attenuates airway inflammation by suppressing IL-17A production in HDM-challenged mice. *Am J Physiol Lung Cell Mol Physiol.* (2019) 316:L269–79. doi: 10.1152/ajplung.00143.2018
40. Bartel S, Schulz N, Alessandrini F, Schamberger AC, Pagel P, Theis FJ, et al. Pulmonary microRNA profiles identify involvement of Creb1 and Sec14l3

in bronchial epithelial changes in allergic asthma. *Sci Rep.* (2017) 7:46026. doi: 10.1038/srep46026

41. Haj-Salem I, Fakhfakh R, Bérubé J-C, Jacques E, Plante S, Simard MJ, et al. MicroRNA-19a enhances proliferation of bronchial epithelial cells by targeting TGFβR2 gene in severe asthma. *Allergy.* (2015) 70:212–9. doi: 10.1111/all.12551

42. Martinez-Nunez RT, Rupani H, Platé M, Niranjan M, Chambers RC, Howarth PH, et al. Genome-wide posttranscriptional dysregulation by MicroRNAs in human asthma as revealed by Frac-seq. *J Immunol.* (2018) 201:251–63. doi: 10.4049/jimmunol.1701798

43. Tost J. A translational perspective on epigenetics in allergic diseases. *J Allergy Clin Immunol.* (2018) 142:715–26. doi: 10.1016/j.jaci.2018.07.009

44. Guiot J, Struman I, Louis E, Louis R, Malaise M, Njock M-S. Exosomal miRNAs in lung diseases: from biologic function to therapeutic targets. *J Clin Med.* (2019) 8:1345. doi: 10.3390/jcm8091345

45. Pua HH, Happ HC, Gray CJ, Mar DJ, Chiou N-T, Hesse LE, et al. Increased hematopoietic extracellular RNAs and vesicles in the lung during allergic airway responses. *Cell Rep.* (2019) 26:933–44.e4. doi: 10.1016/j.celrep.2019.01.002

46. Gupta R, Radicioni G, Abdelwahab S, Dang H, Carpenter J, Chua M, et al. Intercellular communication between airway epithelial cells is mediated by exosome-like vesicles. *Am J Respir Cell Mol Biol.* (2019) 60:209–20. doi: 10.1165/rcmb.2018-0156OC

47. Bartel S, La Grutta S, Cilluffo G, Perconti G, Bongiovanni A, Giallongo A, et al. Human airway epithelial extracellular vesicle miRNA signature is altered upon asthma development. *Allergy.* (2020) 75:346–56. doi: 10.1111/all.14008

48. Maes T, Cobos FA, Schleich F, Sorbello V, Henket M, Preter K, et al. Asthma inflammatory phenotypes show differential microRNA expression in sputum. *J Allergy Clin Immunol.* (2016) 137:1433–46. doi: 10.1016/j.jaci.2016.02.018

49. Zhang K, Liang Y, Feng Y, Wu W, Zhang H, He J, et al. Decreased epithelial and sputum miR-221-3p associates with airway eosinophilic inflammation and CXCL17 expression in asthma. *Am J Physiol Lung Cell Mol Physiol.* (2018) 315:L253–L264. doi: 10.1152/ajplung.00567.2017

50. Tsai M-J, Tsai Y-C, Chang W-A, Lin Y-S, Tsai P-H, Sheu C-C, et al. Deducting microRNA-mediated changes common in bronchial epithelial cells of asthma and chronic obstructive pulmonary disease-a next-generation sequencing-guided bioinformatic approach. *Int J Mol Sci.* (2019) 20:553. doi: 10.3390/ijms20030553

51. Potaczek DP, Unger SD, Zhang N, Taka S, Michel S, Akdag N, et al. Development and characterization of DNAzyme candidates demonstrating significant efficiency against human rhinoviruses. *J Allergy Clin Immunol.* (2019) 143:1403–15. doi: 10.1016/j.jaci.2018.07.026

52. Pech M, Weckmann M, König IR, Franke A, Heinsen F-A, Oliver B, et al. Rhinovirus infections change DNA methylation and mRNA expression in children with asthma. *PLoS ONE.* (2018) 13:e0205275. doi: 10.1371/journal.pone.0205275

53. Gutierrez MJ, Gomez JL, Perez GF, Pancham K, Val S, Pillai DK, et al. Airway secretory microRNAome changes during rhinovirus infection in early childhood. *PLoS ONE.* (2016) 11:e0162244. doi: 10.1371/journal.pone.0162244

54. Moheimani F, Koops J, Williams T, Reid AT, Hansbro PM, Wark PA, et al. Influenza A virus infection dysregulates the expression of microRNA-22 and its targets; CD147 and HDAC4, in epithelium of asthmatics. *Respir Res.* (2018) 19:145. doi: 10.1186/s12931-018-0851-7

55. Spalluto CM, Singhania A, Cellura D, Woelk CH, Sanchez-Elsner T, Staples KJ, et al. IFN-γ influences epithelial antiviral responses via histone methylation of the RIG-I promoter. *Am J Respir Cell Mol Biol.* (2017) 57:428–38. doi: 10.1165/rcmb.2016-0392OC

56. Rout-Pitt N, Farrow N, Parsons D, Donnelley M. Epithelial mesenchymal transition (EMT): a universal process in lung diseases with implications for cystic fibrosis pathophysiology. *Respir Res.* (2018) 19:136. doi: 10.1186/s12931-018-0834-8

57. Yang Z-C, Qu Z-H, Yi M-J, Shan Y-C, Ran N, Xu L, et al. MiR-448-5p inhibits TGF-β1-induced epithelial-mesenchymal transition and pulmonary fibrosis by targeting Six1 in asthma. *J Cell Physiol.* (2019) 234:8804–14. doi: 10.1002/jcp.27540

58. McErlean P, Kelly A, Dhariwal J, Kirtland M, Watson J, Ranz I, et al. Genome-wide profiling of an enhancer-associated histone modification reveals the influence of asthma on the epigenome of the airway epithelium. *bioRxiv.* (2018) 6. doi: 10.1101/282889

20

Genetic Ablation of CXCR2 Protects against Cigarette Smoke-Induced Lung Inflammation and Injury

Chad A. Lerner, Wei Lei [†], Isaac K. Sundar and Irfan Rahman *

Department of Environmental Medicine, University of Rochester Medical Center, Rochester, NY, USA

*Correspondence:
Irfan Rahman
irfan_rahman@urmc.rochester.edu

[†] Present Address:
Wei Lei,
Department of Respiratory Medicine,
The First Affiliated Hospital of
Soochow University, Suzhou, China

Antagonism of CXCR2 receptors, predominately located on neutrophils and critical for their immunomodulatory activity, is an attractive pharmacological therapeutic approach aimed at reducing the potentially damaging effects of heightened neutrophil influx into the lung. The role CXCR2 in lung inflammation in response to cigarette smoke (CS) inhalation using the mutant mouse approach is not known. We hypothesized that genetic ablation of CXCR2 would protect mice against CS-induced inflammation and DNA damage response. We used CXCR2$^{-/-}$ deficient/mutant (knock-out, KO) mice, and assessed the changes in critical lung inflammatory NF-κB-driven chemokines released from the parenchyma of CS-exposed mice. The extent of tissue damage was assessed by the number of DNA damaging γH2AX positive cells. CXCR2 KO mice exhibited protection from heightened levels of neutrophils measured in BALF taken from mice exposed to CS. IL-8 (KC mouse) levels in the BALF from CS-exposed CXCR2 KO were elevated compared to WT. IL-6 levels in BALF were refractory to increase by CS in CXCR2 KO mice. There were no significant changes to MIP-2, MCP-1, or IL-1β. Total levels of NF-κB were maintained at lower levels in CS-exposed CXCR2 KO mice compared to WT mice exposed to CS. Finally, CXCR2 KO mice were protected from lung cells positive for DNA damage response and senescence marker γH2AX. CXCR2 KO mice are protected from heightened inflammatory response mediated by increased neutrophil response as a result of acute 3 day CS exposure. This is also associated with changes in pro-inflammatory chemokines and reduced incursion of γH2AX indicating CXCR2 deficient mice are protected from lung injury. Thus, CXCR2 may be a pharmacological target in setting of inflammation and DNA damage in the pathogenesis of COPD.

Keywords: cigarette smoke, inflammation, DNA damage, NF-κB, emphysema

INTRODUCTION

Cigarette smoke (CS) is predominately the driving factor in the etiology of chronic obstructive pulmonary disease (COPD). COPD is characterized by destruction of alveolar wall, inflammatory response, and premature lung aging or cellular senescence (Nyunoya et al., 2006; Moriyama et al., 2010; Yao et al., 2012; Ahmad et al., 2015). Pro-inflammatory mediators such as IL-8 (mouse KC) and MIP-2, act as CXCR2 ligands, which are critical for recruitment of peripheral neutrophils. Elevated neutrophil exudate found in bronchoalveolar lavage fluid (BALF) or neutrophils observed amongst the parenchyma in histological sections are a feature of COPD and may contribute to tissue destruction due to lack of inflammatory resolution. The CXCR2 chemokine receptor is differentially expressed on the surface of certain myeloid and lymphoid cell types and plays a major role in peripheral neutrophil mediated inflammation. Chemotactic cytokines that bind to CXC family receptors mediate recruitment of the immune cells expressing them toward the injured or infected tissue (Belperio et al., 2002; Wareing et al., 2007; Nagarkar et al., 2009). The CXCR2$^{-/-}$ deficient/mutant (knock-out, KO) mouse is defective in neutrophil function and exhibits reduced neutrophil lung infiltration following infection, injury, and exposure to ozone (Johnston et al., 2005; Reutershan et al., 2006). Thus, targeting of CXCR2 has been sought after as a potential therapy to quell inflammation in response to lung injury and infection in order to reduce the potential for excessive tissue damage mediated by neutrophil inflammation (Lomas-Neira et al., 2004; Nomellini et al., 2008; Zarbock et al., 2008; Russo et al., 2009; Leaker et al., 2013). However, the role of CXCR2 in mediating neutrophil inflammatory response to CS is not well understood. We hypothesize exposure of lungs to CS lays the ground work for progression toward COPD through activation of CXCR2 and excessive recruitment of neutrophils. To elucidate the role of CXCR2 in neutrophil recruitment and lung damage in response to CS, we utilized CXCR2$^{-/-}$ mice in our experiments. This model allowed us to further assess the CS mediated response of critical lung inflammatory cytokines, the γH2AX DNA damage signal in the CXCR2$^{-/-}$ background, and examine how NF-κB as a master regulator of lung inflammatory cytokines, is affected by CS in the absence of CXCR2 expression *in vivo*.

MATERIALS AND METHODS

Ethics Statement and Scientific Rigor/Reproducibility

All experiments for animal studies were performed in accordance with the standards established by the United States Animal Welfare Act, as set forth by the National Institutes of Health guidelines. The research protocol for mouse studies was approved by the University Committee on Animal Research Committee of the University of Rochester.

We used a rigorous/robust and unbiased approach throughout the experimental plans (e.g., *in vivo* mouse model) and during data analysis so as to ensure that our data are reproducible along with full and detailed reporting of both methods and raw/analyzed data. All the key biological and/or chemical resources that are used in this study were validated and authenticated (methods and resources) and are of scientific standard from commercial sources. Our results adhere to NIH standards of reproducibility and scientific rigor.

Animals

Male C57BL/6J (C57) and CXCR2 knockout/deficient (referred to as CXCR2$^{-/-}$ or KO) mice were purchased from the Jackson Laboratory (Bar Harbor, ME). These mice were housed under a 12:12 light-dark (LD) cycle with lights on at 6 a.m. and fed with a regular diet and water *ad libitum* unless otherwise indicated. For CS exposure, mice were kept in a standard 12:12 (LD) cycle with lights on from 6 a.m. to 6 p.m. throughout the experiment. All of the procedures described in this study were approved by the University Committee on Animal Research at the University of Rochester, Rochester, NY.

CS exposure

Eight to ten weeks old mice were exposed to acute (3 days) CS using Baumgartner-Jaeger CSM2082i cigarette smoking machine (CH Technologies, Westwood, NJ) in the Inhalation Core Facility at the University of Rochester. For acute CS exposure, mice were placed in individual compartments of a wire cage, which was placed inside a closed plastic box connected to the smoke source. The smoke was generated from 3R4F research cigarettes containing 10.9 mg of total particulate matter (TPM), 9.4 mg of tar, and 0.726 mg of nicotine, and carbon monoxide 11.9 mg per cigarette (University of Kentucky, Lexington, KY). Mice received two 1-h exposures per day, 1 h apart, according to the Federal Trade Commission protocol (1 puff/min of 2-s duration and 35 mL volume) for 3 days (acute exposure). Mainstream CS was diluted along with filtered air and directed into the exposure chamber. Monitoring of CS exposure (TPM per cubic meter of air) was done in real time using a MicroDust Pro-aerosol monitor (Casella CEL, Bedford, UK) and verified daily by gravimetric sampling immediately after the exposure was completed. By adjusting the number of cigarettes used to produce smoke and the flow rate of the dilution air, the concentration of smoke was set at a nominal value ($\sim$300 mg/m^3 TPM).

Tissue Harvest and Differential Cell Count in Bronchoalveolar Lavage (BAL) Fluid

Mice were injected intraperitoneally with 100 mg/kg body weight of pentobarbiturate (Abbott laboratories, Abbott Park, IL) and then sacrificed by exsanguination. The lungs were lavaged 3 times with 0.6 ml of saline via a cannula inserted into the trachea. The aliquots were combined, centrifuged, and the BAL inflammatory cell pellet was resuspended in saline. The total cell number was determined with a hemocytometer, and cytospin slides (Thermo Shandon, Pittsburgh, PA) were prepared using 50,000 cells per slide. Differential cell counts ($\sim$500 cells/slide) were performed on cytospin-prepared slides stained with Diff-Quik (Dade Behring, Newark, DE).

Cytokine Analysis in Bronchoalveolar Lavage

The level of proinflammatory mediators, such as the chemokine keratinocyte chemoattractant (KC), macrophage inflammatory protein 2 (MIP-2), interleukin 6 (IL-6), monocyte chemotatic protein (MCP)-1 and, interleukin 1 beta (IL-1β) in BAL fluid were measured by enzyme-linked immunosorbent assay (ELISA) using respective dual-antibody kits (R&D Systems, Minneapolis, MN) according to the manufacturer's instructions. The results were expressed as pg/ml.

Protein Extraction from Lung Tissues and Quantification

One lobe of the lung tissue (~50 mg) was homogenized (Pro 200 homogenizer, at maximum speed, 5th gear for 40 s) in 0.5 mL of ice-cold RIPA buffer containing complete protease inhibitor cocktail (Sigma). The tissue homogenate was then incubated on ice for 45 min to allow total cell lysis. The homogenate was then centrifuged at 13,000 × g for 5 min at 4°C to separate the protein fraction from the cell/tissue debris. The supernatant containing protein was aliquoted and stored at −80°C for Western blotting. This fraction was taken for protein analysis by bicinchoninic acid (BCA) colorimetric assay (Thermo Scientific, Rockford, IL) using BSA as a standard.

Western Blot Analysis for NF-κB Levels in the Lungs

Proteins (25 μg) from lung tissue homogenates, were separated on a 7.5% sodium dodecyl sulfate (SDS)-polyacrylamide gel, transferred onto nitrocellulose membranes (Amersham, Arlington Heights, IL), and blocked using 5% bovine serum albumin (BSA) for 1 h at room temperature. The membranes were then probed with NF-κB (sc-109, Santa Cruz, CA), NF-κB-Phospho-serine536 (sc-101752, Santa Cruz, CA), and GAPDH (sc-365062, Santa Cruz, CA) primary antibody (1:1000 dilution in 5% BSA in phosphate-buffered saline [PBS] containing 0.1% Tween 20) at 4°C for overnight. After three 10-min washing steps, the membrane was probed with suitable secondary anti-rabbit, or anti-mouse, or anti-goat antibody (1:10,000 dilution in 5% BSA) linked to horseradish peroxidase for 1 h, and detected using the enhanced chemiluminescence method (Perkin Elmer, Waltham, MA) and images were taken with Bio-Rad ChemiDoc MP, Imaging system. Equal loading of the gel was determined by quantitation of protein as well as by reprobing the same membranes for GAPDH.

Immunohistochemistry for γH2AX Levels in the Lungs

Immunostaining was performed on formalin-fixed, paraffin-embedded lung tissue. Paraffin sections (4 μm thick) were deparaffinized and then rehydrated through series of xylene and graded ethanol. Antigen retrieval was performed by heating in citrate buffer (10 mM Citric acid, 0.05% Tween 20, pH 6.0). Primary antibody was incubated overnight at 4°C with rabbit anti-γH2AX antibody (05-636, EMD Millipore, Darmstadt, Germany) Appropriate fluorescently labeled secondary antibodies (FITC-conjugated anti-mouse 2° antibodies) were used to detect the immune complexes before tissues sections were counterstained with 4′,d-diamidino-2-phenylindole (dapi).

Statistical Analysis

Statistical analysis of significance was calculated using one-way analysis of variance (ANOVA) followed by Tukey's *post-hoc* test for multigroup comparisons using the StatView software or GraphPad Prism. Image J software (Version 1.47, National Institutes of Health, Bethesda, MD) was used for quantification of the number of fluorescent punctate nuclei present in γH2AX immunohistochemistry, and densitometry of Western blot analysis. These results are shown as the mean ± SEM. $^{*}P < 0.05$, $^{**}P < 0.01$, $^{***}P < 0.001$ which were considered as statistically significant.

RESULTS

Neutrophil Influx in CXCR2$^{-/-}$ Mouse Exposed to Acute Cigarette Smoke

CXCR2$^{-/-}$ mice exposed with CS for 3 days are refractory to neutrophil influx into the BALF. In contrast, wild type (WT) mice exposed to acute CS exhibit robust neutrophil transmigration into BAL fluid in the lungs compared to WT air group. These results show that CS is a potent activator of neutrophil recruitment to the lung and the process is highly dependent on the expression of CXCR2 (**Figure 1**).

Level of Pro-Inflammatory Cytokines in CXCR2$^{-/-}$ Mice Exposed to Acute Cigarette Smoke

To assess if the absence of CXCR2 influences levels of pro-inflammatory cytokines that may play a role in neutrophil recruitment in response to acute CS exposure, the Cxcr2 ligands KC and MIP2 were measured in BALF. CXCR2$^{-/-}$ mice exposed to CS exhibit increased levels of KC compared to CXCR2$^{-/-}$ air group and WT air group. Levels of MIP2 are not significantly affected by CS in the WT and CXCR2$^{-/-}$ mice. IL-6 was significantly increased in WT mice exposed to CS. However, in CXCR2$^{-/-}$ mice, IL-6 is resistant to increase by

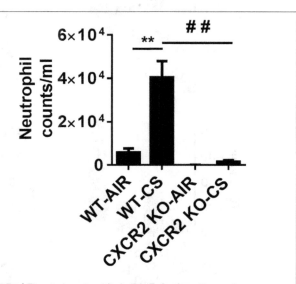

FIGURE 1 | Elevated neutrophils in BALF via cigarette smoke are blocked in CXCR2$^{-/-}$ mice. Mice were exposed to acute CS [300 mg/m^3; total particulate matter (TPM)] for 2 h per day for 3 days. Mice were sacrificed 24 h following last day of CS exposure. Data are shown as the mean ± SEM (WT-Air; n = 4, WT-CS; n = 5, CXCR2; KO-Air n = 3, CXCR2 KO-CS; n = 3). $^{**}P < 0.01$ significant for WT-CS compared to WT-Air; $^{\#\#}P < 0.01$ significant for CXCR2 KO-CS compared to WT-CS.

CS. Levels of MCP-1 and IL-1β in CS-exposed CXCR2$^{-/-}$ was not significantly different compared to CS or air exposed WT mice and this was confirmed for IL-1β in plasma (**Figure 2**). We conclude key cytokines IL-6 and KC both involved in mediating inflammation and neutrophil activity in response to acute CS exposure are altered due to the absence of CXCR2. Lack of neutrophil influx in response to CS results in enhanced KC and blunted IL-6.

NF-κB Expression in CXCR2$^{-/-}$ Mouse Lung Homogenates Exposed to Acute Cigarette Smoke

To determine if NF-κB is affected in CXCR2$^{-/-}$ mouse lung as it is a master regulator of IL-6, we prepared whole lung homogenates after acute air and CS exposure and measured both the relative levels of total NF-κB and phospho-Ser536 on NF-κB to assess its activation. Following CS exposure in WT mice, total NF-κB levels are increased compared to air group. Conversely, CS is not able to induce lung NF-κB expression to similar levels in CXCR2$^{-/-}$ mice compared to WT CS-exposed mice (**Figures 3A,B**). Levels of Ser536 phospho-NF-κB relative to total NF-κB remained unchanged between air and CS-exposed WT or CXCR2$^{-/-}$ mice (data not shown). These results suggest that by ablating CXCR2, NF-κB expression in response to CS exposure is attenuated.

DNA Damage Signaling in CXCR2$^{-/-}$ Mouse Lung

Lung tissue is prone to DNA damage by exposure to CS. In addition, since neutrophil influx is suggested to contribute lung DNA damage through inducing genotoxic stress (van Berlo et al., 2010), we sought to determine if CXCR2 status, in its ability to influence CS mediated neutrophil influx into BALF (**Figure 1**) might affect DNA damage response, which also intersects inflammatory signaling pathways (McCool and Miyamoto, 2012). In lung tissue sections from mice exposed to acute CS, WT mice exhibit an increased number of γH2AX positive cells by immunofluorescence compared to air group. The CXCR2$^{-/-}$ mouse lung was highly devoid of γH2AX positive cells following CS exposure and exhibited only a marginal increase in γH2AX compared to CXCR2$^{-/-}$ air group (**Figures 4A,B**). These data indicate the γH2AX DNA damage signal is associated with increased BALF neutrophils in response to CS exposure, which are both dependent on expression of CXCR2.

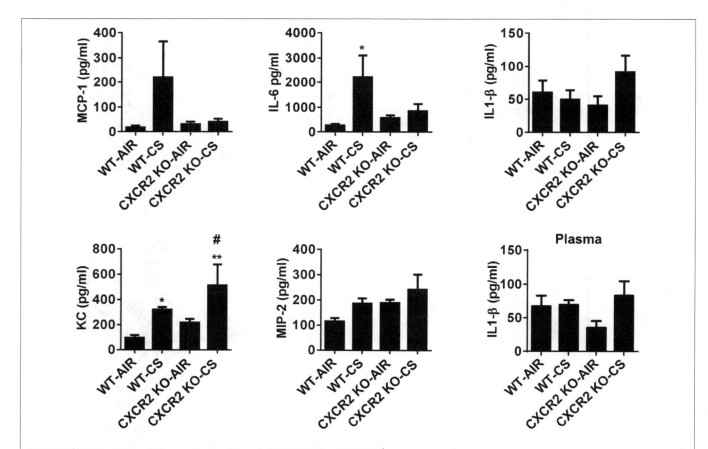

FIGURE 2 | The levels of proinflammatory mediators in BALF of WT and CXCR2$^{-/-}$ after acute CS exposure. Mice were exposed to acute CS [300 mg/m^3; total particulate matter (TPM)] for 2 h per day for 3 days. The levels of proinflammatory mediators in BALF; MCP-1, IL-6, IL-1β, KC, and MIP-2 after 3 days CS exposure and IL-1β in plasma were measured by ELISA. Data are shown as the mean ± SEM (WT-Air; $n = 3$–4, WT-CS; $n = 5$, CXCR2 KO-Air; $n = 3$, CXCR2 KO-CS; $n = 3$). *$P < 0.05$, **$P < 0.01$ significant for WT-CS compared to WT-Air; #$P < 0.05$ significant for CXCR2 KO-CS compared to WT-CS.

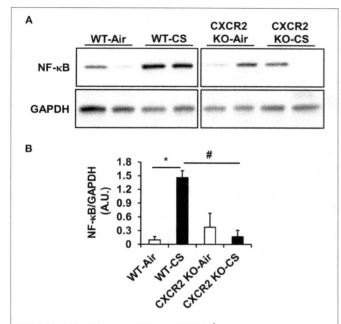

FIGURE 3 | NF-κB levels in WT and CXCR2$^{-/-}$ mice after acute CS exposure. Mice were exposed to acute CS [300 mg/m^3; total particulate matter (TPM)] for 2 h per day for 3 days. Total proteins isolated from lung homogenates were resolved on SDS-PAGE gel for immunoblotting. **(A)** Immunoblot of total NF-κB. GAPDH was used as a housekeeping control. Immunoblots are representative of 2 independent experiments. **(B)** Densitometry for quantitation of relative differences in band intensity for total NF-κB normalized to GAPDH in **(A)**. Measurements are shown as arbitrary units (A.U.). Data are shown as the mean ± SEM. *$P < 0.05$ significant for WT-CS compared to WT-Air; #$P < 0.05$ significant for CXCR2 KO-CS compared to WT-CS.

DISCUSSION

The increased neutrophilic environment induced by CS may contribute to COPD etiology which is typically associated with COPD. COPD is frequently accompanied by bacterial and viral infections that further exacerbate symptoms and accelerate pathogenesis. We utilized CXCR2$^{-/-}$ mice to assess neutrophil recruitment, pro-inflammatory cytokines, NF-κB activity, and the DNA damage signal γH2AX in mouse lungs exposed to acute CS. MIP-2 and KC are primarily CXCR2 ligands. In our CXCR2$^{-/-}$ mice exposed to acute CS, KC levels were significantly altered. The up-regulation of KC in CXCR2$^{-/-}$ mice exposed to CS is consistent with a previous report which showed inhibition of CS-induced lung inflammation by a CXCR2 antagonist (Thatcher et al., 2005), though no gene deletion approach was used without implicating DNA damaging response. CXCR2 is desensitized by very high levels of KC, which may allude to its regulation under inflammatory states where KC is potentially internalized (Wiekowski et al., 2001; Rose et al., 2004). We indeed observed KC increase in CS-exposed WT mice. However, in the CXCR2$^{-/-}$ background, we find KC expression increases further in response to CS which may allude to the possibility that KC levels are regulated by receptor-ligand complex dynamics during heightened tissue inflammation. CXCR2 internalization in addition to canonical G-protein coupled receptor desensitization mechanisms and autocrine feedback responses may further limit excessive immunological activity on cells expressing CXC family receptors, a dynamic that requires further investigation.

Although IL-6 is not a CXCR2 ligand, the CXCR2$^{-/-}$ mice when exposed to either air or CS exhibited reduced IL-6 in the BALF which may extend anti-inflammatory effects beyond limited neutrophil recruitment. An interesting dynamic between IL-6 expression and CXCR2 activity is beginning to emerge in studies involving modulating CXC type receptor activity. The CXCR2 antagonist SCH-N is predominantly a CXCR2 antagonist with partial CXCR1 antagonism in primates and almost exclusively a CXCR2 antagonist in rodent (Chapman et al., 2007). Though SCH-N CXCR2 antagonism did not appreciably affect CS-exposed mouse BALF IL-6 levels (Thatcher et al., 2005), mice treated with a nasal instillation of barn dust in conjunction with the dual CXCR1/CXCR2 antagonist CXCL8 (3-74) K11R/G31P exhibited similar results to CXCR2$^{-/-}$ mice BALF IL-6 levels (Schneberger et al., 2015). Thus, it is possible dual CXCR1/2 antagonism is affecting IL-6 regulation and requires more extensive characterization of how other CXC receptors are affected in the CXCR2$^{-/-}$ mice models. The interesting effect of CXCR2 antagonism by antileukinate on PMN extravasation to the lung under septic challenge leads to reduced IL-6 plasma levels (Lomas-Neira et al., 2004). Thus, further assessment will require optimizing therapeutic approaches for CXC receptor family targeting different inflammatory insults in context with cytokine tissue locale.

IL-β is a potent inflammatory mediator. Stevenson et al. observed a time-dependent increase in IL-1β in BALF in rat model at 24 h post-CS exposure (Stevenson et al., 2005). In our mice, 3 days acute CS exposure did not elicit an appreciable increase in IL-1β in the lavage fluid in WT mice and there were no remarkable changes in the CXCR2$^{-/-}$ mice exposed to air or CS. We cannot conclude for certain IL-β response is unaffected by CS or deficiency in CXCR2, rather the acute exposure we employed in this study, may lead to acclimation or impairment for certain inflammatory targets.

The major role NF-κB plays in modulating inflammation in response to injury and infection in multiple tissues was of interest to us in the CXCR2$^{-/-}$ mice exposed to CS, particularly since we observed differential regulation in KC and IL-6. In NF-κB deficient mice, CXCR2 mediated neutrophil influx into the lung, is reported to be enhanced indicating a regulatory interaction (though potentially indirect) may exist between CXCR2 and NF-κB (von Vietinghoff et al., 2010). Prostate cancer cells cultured under hypoxia, also appear to require NF-κB to upregulate CXCR2 RNA (Maxwell et al., 2007). The CXCR2$^{-/-}$ in our study appears to have a reduced capacity to express total levels of NF-κB, however, the activity of NF-κB indicated by phosphorylation of Serine 536 shows it retains competency in its ability to modulate signaling effects despite reduced total expression levels.

The γH2AX DNA damage signal is frequently associated with senescent positive cell. CXCR2 signaling essentially promotes senescence which is hypothesized to be a factor in the

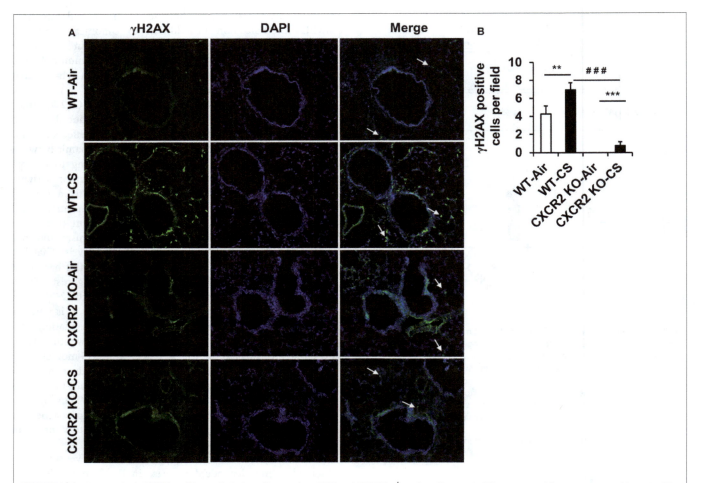

FIGURE 4 | Assessment of γH2AX positive cells in lung tissues from WT and CXCR2$^{-/-}$ mice after acute CS exposure. Mice were exposed to acute CS [300 mg/m^3; total particulate matter (TPM)] for 2 h per day for 3 days. Paraffin embedded lung tissue sections from 24 h following last day of CS exposure were used for immunohistochemistry. (A) Representative immunofluorescent images at 20x showing γH2AX positive nuclei (green) overlaid with DAPI stained nuclei (Blue). White arrows point to γH2AX positive regions. (B) Quantitation of the number of γH2AX positive nuclei per image for each condition. Data are shown as the mean ± SEM (WT-Air; n = 14, WT-CS; n = 15, CXCR2 KO-Air; n = 10, CXCR2 KO-CS; n = 5). **$P < 0.01$ significant for WT-CS compared to WT-Air; ***$P < 0.001$ significant for CXCR2 KO-CS compared to CXCR2 KO-Air; ###$P < 0.001$ significant for CXCR2 KO-CS compared to WT-CS.

pathogenesis of COPD and lung cancer (Acosta et al., 2008). The γH2AX signal is one facet of DNA damage response (DDR), and is frequently used as a corollary to other senescence assays. The hypothesis that COPD etiology integrates accumulation of senescent cells through aging, smoking, or a combination of both explains that the senescent associated secretory phenotype (SASP) contributes to onset or progression of COPD. CXCR2 has been shown to be critical for senescence as many of the SASP factors are CXCR2 ligands (Acosta et al., 2008). More recently CXCR2 is shown to be involved in DDR mediated senescence (Guo et al., 2013). Our results along with others indicate DDR is engaged within the WT lung parenchyma by CS exposure as indicated by increased γH2AX, increased p53 activity, and changes to CXCR2 dynamics and their ligands (Tiwari et al., 2016). The CXCR2-DDR-senescence connection is intriguing and our results show CXCR2 deficiency may protect from DDR in response to acute CS exposure. However, it is not clear how

targeting this axis influences the pathogenesis of COPD (along with overcoming steroid resistance) as it is difficult to target CXCR2 while retaining critical host defense and tissue repair capacity.

Other CXC family members such as CXCR3 have also been shown to attenuate CS mediated lung inflammation in a CXCR3$^{-/-}$ mouse model by reducing CD8$^+$ T cell toxicity which further suggests targeting of multiple CXC family members may be an approach to optimize in treatment of inflammatory lung diseases (Nie et al., 2008a,b). In the CXCR2$^{-/-}$ background, neutrophils are further impaired from extravasation from bone marrow into circulation which underscores the severity of the genetic deficit (Eash et al., 2010). In contrast, the pharmacological targeting and new precise genetic methods such as CRISPR/Cas9 models of CXCR2 allows direct oversight into dose, location of administration, protein activity, and timing which will also help to determine how chemokine profiles are affected by CXCR2 antagonism and which are most therapeutic while retaining host immune defenses. Nevertheless, our data show that CXCR2 may be a pharmacological target in setting of inflammation and DNA damage in the pathogenesis of COPD.

AUTHOR CONTRIBUTIONS

CL, WL, IS, and IR conceived and designed the experiments; WL, IS, and CL performed the experiments; IS and WL analyzed the data; CL, WL, IS, and IR wrote and revised/edited the manuscript.

ACKNOWLEDGMENTS

We thank Ms. Janice Gerloff for her technical assistance. This study was supported by the NIH 1R01HL085613 (to IR), American Lung Association RG-305393 (to IS), pulmonary training grant T32 HL066988, and NIEHS Environmental Health Science Center grant P30-ES01247.

REFERENCES

1. Acosta, J. C., O'Loghlen, A., Banito, A., Guijarro, M. V., Augert, A., Raguz, S., et al. (2008). Chemokine signaling via the CXCR2 receptor reinforces senescence. *Cell* 133, 1006–1018. doi: 10.1016/j.cell.2008.03.038
2. Ahmad, T., Sundar, I. K., Lerner, C. A., Gerloff, J., Tormos, A. M., Yao, H., et al. (2015). Impaired mitophagy leads to cigarette smoke stress-induced cellular senescence: implications for chronic obstructive pulmonary disease. *FASEB J.* 29, 2912–2929. doi: 10.1096/fj.14-268276
3. Belperio, J. A., Keane, M. P., Burdick, M. D., Londhe, V., Xue, Y. Y., Li, K., et al. (2002). Critical role for CXCR2 and CXCR2 ligands during the pathogenesis of ventilator-induced lung injury. *J. Clin. Invest.* 110, 1703–1716. doi: 10.1172/JCI0215849
4. Chapman, R. W., Minnicozzi, M., Celly, C. S., Phillips, J. E., Kung, T. T., Hipkin, R. W., et al. (2007). A novel, orally active CXCR1/2 receptor antagonist, Sch527123, inhibits neutrophil recruitment, mucus production, and goblet cell hyperplasia in animal models of pulmonary inflammation. *J. Pharmacol. Exp. Ther.* 322, 486–493. doi: 10.1124/jpet.106.119040
5. Eash, K. J., Greenbaum, A. M., Gopalan, P. K., and Link, D. C. (2010). CXCR2 and CXCR4 antagonistically regulate neutrophil trafficking from murine bone marrow. *J. Clin. Invest.* 120, 2423–2431. doi: 10.1172/JCI41649
6. Guo, H., Liu, Z., Xu, B., Hu, H., Wei, Z., Liu, Q., et al. (2013). Chemokine receptor CXCR2 is transactivated by p53 and induces p38-mediated cellular senescence in response to DNA damage. *Aging Cell.* 12, 1110–1121. doi: 10.1111/acel.12138
7. Johnston, R. A., Mizgerd, J. P., and Shore, S. A. (2005). CXCR2 is essential for maximal neutrophil recruitment and methacholine responsiveness after ozone exposure. *Am. J. Physiol. Lung Cell. Mol. Physiol.* 288, L61–L67. doi: 10.1152/ajplung.00101.2004
8. Leaker, B. R., Barnes, P. J., and O'Connor, B. (2013). Inhibition of LPS-induced airway neutrophilic inflammation in healthy volunteers with an oral CXCR2 antagonist. *Respir. Res.* 14:137. doi: 10.1186/1465-9921-14-137
9. Lomas-Neira, J. L., Chung, C. S., Grutkoski, P. S., Miller, E. J., and Ayala, A. (2004). CXCR2 inhibition suppresses hemorrhage-induced priming for acute lung injury in mice. *J. Leukoc. Biol.* 76, 58–64. doi: 10.1189/jlb. 1103541
10. Maxwell, P. J., Gallagher, R., Seaton, A., Wilson, C., Scullin, P., Pettigrew, J., et al. (2007). HIF-1 and NF-κB-mediated upregulation of CXCR1 and CXCR2 expression promotes cell survival in hypoxic prostate cancer cells. *Oncogene* 26, 7333–7345. doi: 10.1038/sj.onc.1210536
11. McCool, K. W., and Miyamoto, S. (2012). DNA damage-dependent NF-κB activation: NEMO turns nuclear signaling inside out. *Immunol. Rev.* 246, 311–326. doi: 10.1111/j.1600-065X.2012.01101.x
12. Moriyama, C., Betsuyaku, T., Ito, Y., Hamamura, I., Hata, J., Takahashi, H., et al. (2010). Aging enhances susceptibility to cigarette smoke-induced inflammation through bronchiolar chemokines. *Am. J. Respir. Cell Mol. Biol.* 42, 304–311. doi: 10.1165/rcmb.2009-0025OC
13. Nagarkar, D. R., Wang, Q., Shim, J., Zhao, Y., Tsai, W. C., Lukacs, N. W., et al. (2009). CXCR2 is required for neutrophilic airway inflammation and hyperresponsiveness in a mouse model of human rhinovirus infection. *J. Immunol.* 183, 6698–6707. doi: 10.4049/jimmunol.0900298
14. Nie, L., Xiang, R. L., Liu, Y., Zhou, W. X., Jiang, L., Lu, B., et al. (2008a). Acute pulmonary inflammation is inhibited in CXCR3 knockout mice after short-term cigarette smoke exposure. *Acta Pharmacol. Sin.* 29, 1432–1439. doi: 10.1111/j.1745-7254.2008.00899.x

15. Nie, L., Xiang, R., Zhou, W., Lu, B., Cheng, D., and Gao, J. (2008b). Attenuation of acute lung inflammation induced by cigarette smoke in CXCR3 knockout mice. *Respir. Res.* 9:82. doi: 10.1186/1465-9921-9-82
16. Nomellini, V., Faunce, D. E., Gomez, C. R., and Kovacs, E. J. (2008). An age-associated increase in pulmonary inflammation after burn injury is abrogated by CXCR2 inhibition. *J. Leukoc. Biol.* 83, 1493–1501. doi: 10.1189/jlb.1007672
17. Nyunoya, T., Monick, M. M., Klingelhutz, A., Yarovinsky, T. O., Cagley, J. R., and Hunninghake, G. W. (2006). Cigarette smoke induces cellular senescence. *Am. J. Respir. Cell Mol. Biol.* 35, 681–688. doi: 10.1165/rcmb.2006-0169OC
18. Reutershan, J., Morris, M. A., Burcin, T. L., Smith, D. F., Chang, D., Saprito, M. S., et al. (2006). Critical role of endothelial CXCR2 in LPS-induced neutrophil migration into the lung. *J. Clin. Invest.* 116, 695–702. doi: 10.1172/JCI27009
19. Rose, J. J., Foley, J. F., Murphy, P. M., and Venkatesan, S. (2004). On the mechanism and significance of ligand-induced internalization of human neutrophil chemokine receptors CXCR1 and CXCR2. *J. Biol. Chem.* 279, 24372–24386. doi: 10.1074/jbc.M401364200
20. Russo, R. C., Guabiraba, R., Garcia, C. C., Barcelos, L. S., Roffê, E., Souza, A. L., et al. (2009). Role of the chemokine receptor CXCR2 in bleomycin-induced pulmonary inflammation and fibrosis. *Am. J. Respir. Cell Mol. Biol.* 40, 410–421. doi: 10.1165/rcmb.2007-0364OC
21. Schneberger, D., Gordon, J. R., DeVasure, J. M., Boten, J. A., Heires, A. J., Romberger, D. J., et al. (2015). CXCR1/CXCR2 antagonist CXCL8(3- 74) K11R/G31P blocks lung inflammation in swine barn dust-instilled mice. *Pulm. Pharmacol. Ther.* 31, 55–62. doi: 10.1016/j.pupt.2015.02.002
22. Stevenson, C. S., Coote, K., Webster, R., Johnston, H., Atherton, H. C., Nicholls, A., et al. (2005). Characterization of cigarette smoke-induced inflammatory and mucus hypersecretory changes in rat lung and the role of CXCR2 ligands in mediating this effect. *Am. J. Physiol. Lung Cell. Mol. Physiol.* 288, L514–L522. doi: 10.1152/ajplung.00317.2004
23. Thatcher, T. H., McHugh, N. A., Egan, R. W., Chapman, R. W., Hey, J. A., Turner, C. K., et al. (2005). Role of CXCR2 in cigarette smoke-induced lung inflammation. *Am. J. Physiol. Lung Cell. Mol. Physiol.* 289, L322–L328. doi: 10.1152/ajplung.00039.2005
24. Tiwari, N., Marudamuthu, A. S., Tsukasaki, Y., Ikebe, M., Fu, J., and Shetty, S. (2016). p53- and PAI-1-mediated induction of C-X-C chemokines and CXCR2: importance in pulmonary inflammation due to cigarette smoke exposure. *Am. J. Physiol. Lung Cell. Mol. Physiol.* 310, L496–L506. doi: 10.1152/ajplung.00290.2015
25. van Berlo, D., Wessels, A., Boots, A. W., Wilhelmi, V., Scherbart, A. M., Gerloff, K., et al. (2010). Neutrophil-derived ROS contribute to oxidative DNA damage induction by quartz particles. *Free Radic. Biol. Med.* 49, 1685–1693. doi: 10.1016/j.freeradbiomed.2010.08.031
26. von Vietinghoff, S., Asagiri, M., Azar, D., Hoffmann, A., and Ley, K. (2010). Defective regulation of CXCR2 facilitates neutrophil release from bone marrow causing spontaneous inflammation in severely NF-κB-deficient mice. *J. Immunol.* 185, 670–678. doi: 10.4049/jimmunol.1000339
27. Wareing, M. D., Shea, A. L., Inglis, C. A., Dias, P. B., and Sarawar, S. R. (2007). CXCR2 is required for neutrophil recruitment to the lung during influenza virus infection, but is not essential for viral clearance. *Viral Immunol.* 20, 369–378. doi: 10.1089/vim.2006.0101
28. Wiekowski, M. T., Chen, S. C., Zalamea, P., Wilburn, B. P., Kinsley, D. J., Sharif, W. W., et al. (2001). Disruption of neutrophil migration in a conditional transgenic model: evidence for CXCR2 desensitization *in vivo*. *J. Immunol.* 167, 7102–7110. doi: 10.4049/jimmunol.167.12.7102

29. Yao, H., Chung, S., Hwang, J. W., Rajendrasozhan, S., Sundar, I. K., Dean, D. A., et al. (2012). SIRT1 protects against emphysema via FOXO3-mediated reduction of premature senescence in mice. *J. Clin. Invest.* 122, 2032–2045. doi: 10.1172/JCI60132

30. Zarbock, A., Allegretti, M., and Ley, K. (2008). Therapeutic inhibition of CXCR2 by Reparixin attenuates acute lung injury in mice. *Br. J. Pharmacol.* 155, 357–364. doi: 10.1038/bjp.2008.270

Permissions

All chapters in this book were first published by Frontiers; hereby published with permission under the Creative Commons Attribution License or equivalent. Every chapter published in this book has been scrutinized by our experts. Their significance has been extensively debated. The topics covered herein carry significant findings which will fuel the growth of the discipline. They may even be implemented as practical applications or may be referred to as a beginning point for another development.

The contributors of this book come from diverse backgrounds, making this book a truly international effort. This book will bring forth new frontiers with its revolutionizing research information and detailed analysis of the nascent developments around the world.

We would like to thank all the contributing authors for lending their expertise to make the book truly unique. They have played a crucial role in the development of this book. Without their invaluable contributions this book wouldn't have been possible. They have made vital efforts to compile up to date information on the varied aspects of this subject to make this book a valuable addition to the collection of many professionals and students.

This book was conceptualized with the vision of imparting up-to-date information and advanced data in this field. To ensure the same, a matchless editorial board was set up. Every individual on the board went through rigorous rounds of assessment to prove their worth. After which they invested a large part of their time researching and compiling the most relevant data for our readers.

The editorial board has been involved in producing this book since its inception. They have spent rigorous hours researching and exploring the diverse topics which have resulted in the successful publishing of this book. They have passed on their knowledge of decades through this book. To expedite this challenging task, the publisher supported the team at every step. A small team of assistant editors was also appointed to further simplify the editing procedure and attain best results for the readers.

Apart from the editorial board, the designing team has also invested a significant amount of their time in understanding the subject and creating the most relevant covers. They scrutinized every image to scout for the most suitable representation of the subject and create an appropriate cover for the book.

The publishing team has been an ardent support to the editorial, designing and production team. Their endless efforts to recruit the best for this project, has resulted in the accomplishment of this book. They are a veteran in the field of academics and their pool of knowledge is as vast as their experience in printing. Their expertise and guidance has proved useful at every step. Their uncompromising quality standards have made this book an exceptional effort. Their encouragement from time to time has been an inspiration for everyone.

The publisher and the editorial board hope that this book will prove to be a valuable piece of knowledge for researchers, students, practitioners and scholars across the globe.

List of Contributors

Monika Malczyk, Alexandra Erb, Christine Veith, Hossein Ardeschir Ghofrani, Ralph T. Schermuly, Norbert Weissmann and Akylbek Sydykov
Excellence Cluster Cardio-Pulmonary System, Universities of Giessen and Marburg Lung Center (UGMLC), German Center for Lung Research (DZL), Justus Liebig University of Giessen, Giessen, Germany

Thomas Gudermann and Alexander Dietrich
Walther Straub Institute for Pharmacology and Toxicology, Ludwig Maximilian University of Munich, German Center for Lung Research (DZL), Munich, Germany

Jürg Hamacher
Internal Medicine and Pneumology, Lindenhofspital, Bern, Switzerland
Internal Medicine V – Pneumology, Allergology, Respiratory and Environmental Medicine, Faculty of Medicine, Saarland University, Saarbrücken, Germany
Lungen- und Atmungsstiftung Bern, Bern, Switzerland

Yalda Hadizamani and Michèle Borgmann
Internal Medicine and Pneumology, Lindenhofspital, Bern, Switzerland
Lungen- und Atmungsstiftung Bern, Bern, Switzerland

Markus Mohaupt
Internal Medicine, Sonnenhofspital Bern, Bern, Switzerland

Daniela Narcissa Männel
Faculty of Medicine, Institute of Immunology, University of Regensburg, Regensburg, Germany

Ueli Moehrlen
Paediatric Visceral Surgery, Universitäts-Kinderspital Zürich, Zürich, Switzerland

Uz Stammberger
Lungen- und Atmungsstiftung Bern, Bern, Switzerland
Novartis Institutes for Biomedical Research, Translational Clinical Oncology, Novartis Pharma AG, Basel, Switzerland

Christin Peteranderl and Susanne Herold
Department of Internal Medicine II, University of Giessen and Marburg Lung Center (UGMLC), Member of the German Center for Lung Research (DZL), Giessen, Germany

Jacob I. Sznajder and Emilia Lecuona
Division of Pulmonary and Critical Care Medicine, Feinberg School of Medicine, Northwestern University, Chicago, IL, USA

Anita Willam and Waheed Shabbir
Department of Pharmacology and Toxicology, University of Vienna, Vienna, Austria
APEPTICO GmbH, Vienna, Austria

Mohammed Aufy, Dina El-Malazi, Franziska Poser, Alina Wagner, Birgit Unterköfler, Didja Gurmani, David Martan, Shahid Muhammad Iqbal and Rosa Lemmens-Gruber
Department of Pharmacology and Toxicology, University of Vienna, Vienna, Austria

Susan Tzotzos, Bernhard Fischer, Hendrik Fischer and Helmut Pietschmann
APEPTICO GmbH, Vienna, Austria

Sarah Weidenfeld
Keenan Research Centre for Biomedical Science, St. Michael's Hospital, Toronto, ON, Canada
Institute of Physiology, Charité-Universitätsmedizin Berlin, Berlin, Germany

Wolfgang M. Kuebler
Keenan Research Centre for Biomedical Science, St. Michael's Hospital, Toronto, ON, Canada
Institute of Physiology, Charité-Universitätsmedizin Berlin, Berlin, Germany
Department of Surgery and Physiology, University of Toronto, Toronto, ON, Canada

Laura A. Huppert
Department of Medicine, University of California, San Francisco, CA, USA

Michael A. Matthay
Departments of Medicine and Anesthesia, UCSF School of Medicine, Cardiovascular Research Institute, San Francisco, CA, USA

Bria M. Coates
Department of Pediatrics, Feinberg School of Medicine, Northwestern University, Chicago, IL, United States
Ann & Robert H. Lurie Children's Hospital of Chicago, Chicago, IL, United States

List of Contributors

Kelly L. Staricha and Nandini Ravindran
Department of Pediatrics, Feinberg School of Medicine, Northwestern University, Chicago, IL, United States

Clarissa M. Koch, Yuan Cheng, Jennifer M. Davis and Dale K. Shumaker
Department of Medicine, Feinberg School of Medicine, Northwestern University, Chicago, IL, United States

Karen M. Ridge
Department of Medicine, Feinberg School of Medicine, Northwestern University, Chicago, IL, United States
Department of Cell and Molecular Biology, Feinberg School of Medicine, Northwestern University, Chicago, IL, United States

Istvan Czikora, Supriya Sridhar and Boris Gorshkov
Vascular Biology Center, Medical College of Georgia, Augusta University, Augusta, GA, United States

Abdel A. Alli
Department of Physiology and Functional Genomics, University of Florida College of Medicine, Gainesville, FL, United States
Division of Nephrology, Hypertension, and Renal Transplantation, Department of Medicine, University of Florida College of Medicine, Gainesville, FL, United States

Helena Pillich, Martina Hudel, Besim Berisha and Trinad Chakraborty
Institute for Medical Microbiology, Justus-Liebig University, Giessen, Germany

Maritza J. Romero and David Fulton
Vascular Biology Center, Medical College of Georgia, Augusta University, Augusta, GA, United States
Department of Pharmacology and Toxicology, Medical College of Georgia, Augusta University, Augusta, GA, United States

Joyce Gonzales
Department of Medicine, Medical College of Georgia, Augusta University, Augusta, GA, United States

Guangyu Wua and Yunchao Su
Department of Pharmacology and Toxicology, Medical College of Georgia, Augusta University, Augusta, GA, United States

Yuqing Huo and Alexander D. Verin
Vascular Biology Center, Medical College of Georgia, Augusta University, Augusta, GA, United States
Department of Medicine, Medical College of Georgia, Augusta University, Augusta, GA, United States

Douglas C. Eaton
Department of Physiology, Emory University School of Medicine, Atlanta, GA, United States

Rudolf Lucas
Vascular Biology Center, Medical College of Georgia, Augusta University, Augusta, GA, United States
Department of Pharmacology and Toxicology, Medical College of Georgia, Augusta University, Augusta, GA, United States
Department of Medicine, Medical College of Georgia, Augusta University, Augusta, GA, United States

Patricia L. Brazee, Pritin N. Soni, Natalia Magnani, Alex Yemelyanov, Karen M. Ridge and Laura A. Dada
Pulmonary and Critical Care Division, Feinberg School of Medicine, Northwestern University, Chicago, IL, United States

Elmira Tokhtaeva and Olga Vagin
Department of Physiology, David Geffen School of Medicine, UCLA, Los Angeles, CA, United States
Veterans Administration Greater Los Angeles Healthcare System, Los Angeles, CA, United States

Harris R. Perlman
Division of Rheumatology, Feinberg School of Medicine, Northwestern University, Chicago, IL, United States

Paulina Gwoździńska, Benno A. Buchbinder, Konstantin Mayer and István Vadász
Department of Internal Medicine, Justus Liebig University, Universities of Giessen and Marburg Lung Center, German Center for Lung Research, Giessen, Germany

Rory E. Morty and Werner Seeger
Department of Internal Medicine, Justus Liebig University, Universities of Giessen and Marburg Lung Center, German Center for Lung Research, Giessen, Germany
Max Planck Institute for Heart and Lung Research, Bad Nauheim, Germany

István Vadász
Department of Internal Medicine, Justus Liebig University, Universities of Giessen and Marburg Lung Center, Giessen, Germany

Zaher S. Azzam
Department of Physiology and Biophysics, Technion, Israel Institute of Technology, Haifa, Israel
Internal Medicine "B", Rambam Health Care Campus, Haifa, Israel

Safa Kinaneh, Fadel Bahouth, Reem Ismael-Badarneh, Emad Khoury and Zaid Abassi
Department of Physiology and Biophysics, Technion, Israel Institute of Technology, Haifa, Israel

Michael R. Wilson, Szabolcs Bertok, Charlotte M. Oakley, Brijesh V. Patel, Kieran P. O'Dea and Masao Takata
Section of Anaesthetics, Pain Medicine and Intensive Care, Faculty of Medicine, Imperial College London, Chelsea and Westminster Hospital, London, UK

Kenji Wakabayashi
Section of Anaesthetics, Pain Medicine and Intensive Care, Faculty of Medicine, Imperial College London, Chelsea and Westminster Hospital, London, UK
Department of Intensive Care Medicine, Tokyo Medical and Dental University, Tokyo, Japan

Joanna C. Cordy, Peter J. Morley and Andrew I. Bayliffe
Biopharm Molecular Discovery, GlaxoSmithKline R&D, Stevenage, UK

Brandi M. Wynne
Department of Medicine, Nephrology, Emory University, Atlanta, GA, United States
Department of Physiology, Emory University, Atlanta, GA, United States
The Center for Cell and Molecular Signaling, Emory University, Atlanta, GA, United States

Li Zou and Valerie Linck
Department of Physiology, Emory University, Atlanta, GA, United States

Robert S. Hoover
Department of Medicine, Nephrology, Emory University, Atlanta, GA, United States
Department of Physiology, Emory University, Atlanta, GA, United States
Research Service, Atlanta Veteran's Administration Medical Center, Decatur, GA, United States

He-Ping Ma and Douglas C. Eaton
Department of Physiology, Emory University, Atlanta, GA, United States
The Center for Cell and Molecular Signaling, Emory University, Atlanta, GA, United States

Rachel G. Scheraga, Brian D. Southern, Lisa M. Grove and Mitchell A. Olman
Cleveland Clinic, Department of Pathobiology, Lerner Research Institute, Cleveland, OH, USA

Jacob D. Painter, Lauriane Galle-Treger and Omid Akbari
Department of Molecular Microbiology and Immunology, Keck School of Medicine, University of Southern California, Los Angeles, CA, United States

Heedoo Lee, Eric Abston, Duo Zhang and Yang Jin
Division of Pulmonary and Critical Care Medicine, Department of Medicine, Boston University Medical Campus, Boston, MA, United States

Ashish Rai
Department of Internal Medicine, North Shore Medical Center, Boston, MA, United States

Hong Guo-Parke, Dermot Linden, Sinéad Weldon and Clifford C. Taggart
Airway Innate Immunity Research Group, Wellcome Wolfson Institute for Experimental Medicine, School of Medicine, Dentistry & Biomedical Sciences, Queens University Belfast, Belfast, United Kingdom

Joseph C. Kidney
Department of Respiratory Medicine Mater Hospital Belfast, Belfast, United Kingdom

Bilal Alashkar Alhamwe
Institute of Laboratory Medicine, Philipps-University Marburg, Member of the German Center for Lung Research (DZL), Universities of Giessen and Marburg Lung Center, Marburg, Germany
College of Pharmacy, International University for Science and Technology (IUST), Daraa, Syria
Center for Tumor Biology and Immunology, Institute of Tumor Immunology, Philipps University Marburg, Marburg, Germany

Sarah Miethe
Institute of Laboratory Medicine, Philipps-University Marburg, Member of the German Center for Lung Research (DZL), Universities of Giessen and Marburg Lung Center, Marburg, Germany
Translational Inflammation Research Division & Core Facility for Single Cell Multiomics, Philipps University Marburg, Marburg, Germany

Elke Pogge von Strandmann
Center for Tumor Biology and Immunology, Institute of Tumor Immunology, Philipps University Marburg, Marburg, Germany

List of Contributors

Daniel P. Potaczek
Institute of Laboratory Medicine, Philipps-University Marburg, Member of the German Center for Lung Research (DZL), Universities of Giessen and Marburg Lung Center, Marburg, Germany
John Paul II Hospital, Kraków, Poland

Holger Garn
Institute of Laboratory Medicine, Philipps-University Marburg, Member of the German Center for Lung Research (DZL), Universities of Giessen and Marburg Lung Center, Marburg, Germany

Translational Inflammation Research Division & Core Facility for Single Cell Multiomics, Philipps University Marburg, Marburg, Germany

Chad A. Lerner, Wei Lei, Isaac K. Sundar and Irfan Rahman
Department of Environmental Medicine, University of Rochester Medical Center, Rochester, NY, USA

Index

A

Acid Aspiration, 83, 161-163, 166, 168, 170

Acidification, 26, 50, 112, 114, 201

Acute Lung Injury, 1, 6, 11-12, 19, 44-45, 47-50, 52, 54, 56-58, 61-64, 66, 85-86, 90-94, 106-107, 112-116, 118, 122, 125-126, 128, 138-141, 146-147, 151, 157-158, 171, 173-174, 176, 178, 180-184, 186-188, 207, 210, 213-214, 240

Adenosine, 15, 19, 34, 36, 60, 142, 220, 222

Adhesion, 18, 28-30, 33, 57, 59, 62, 125-127, 149, 154-155, 157-158, 176, 180, 184, 186, 203, 218, 223

Adhesion Molecules, 29-30, 59, 62, 125, 149, 154-155, 158, 176

Albumin, 37, 50, 90, 97, 235

Alveolar Epithelium, 12-13, 17, 21-22, 25, 27, 30, 33-34, 37, 43-45, 54, 58-59, 62, 78, 81, 83-84, 86, 88-91, 112-113, 115-116, 124-125, 128-129, 135, 141-142, 144, 146, 148, 157-158, 173, 179-180, 208, 211

Alveolar Fluid Clearance, 13, 24, 29, 44, 46, 48-50, 55, 57-58, 61-63, 82, 85, 88-91, 128-129, 139, 141-143, 146-148, 150, 157, 170-171, 176, 178, 180, 208

Alveolar Liquid Clearance, 12, 46, 53, 55, 66, 86, 106, 151, 158, 176, 180

Alveolar Space, 7, 13, 16, 21-22, 24, 36-37, 81-82, 86, 92, 94, 102-103, 119, 122, 129, 141, 150, 164-165, 167, 169-170, 173, 175, 180, 183

B

Barrier Dysfunction, 12, 18, 23, 32, 34, 41, 43, 45-46, 48-50, 53, 62, 106, 109-110, 125, 138, 147, 184, 217-218, 223

Barrier Function, 6, 10, 14-18, 21, 23, 27, 30, 32, 36, 41, 43, 45, 48-51, 84, 86, 91, 106-114, 125, 129, 141, 157, 170, 173, 175, 186

C

Cardiac Function, 104, 149, 156, 171

Cardiogenic Edema, 19, 43, 80

Cell Death, 22, 32-33, 39, 59-60, 89, 101, 107, 127, 171, 192-193, 197, 202-204, 206, 213, 217

Cell Growth, 3, 5, 33, 55, 205, 211, 213

Cell Surface, 7, 14, 24, 33, 35, 45, 47, 54, 60, 67, 71, 77, 79, 119, 128-132, 135-136, 138-140, 142-147, 162, 208, 219

Chemokine, 7, 19, 22, 26-27, 29-31, 34-35, 52, 115-116, 125-127, 151, 153, 167, 173, 176, 234, 238-239

Cystic Fibrosis, 3, 15, 25, 27, 34, 36, 38-39, 43, 46, 51, 55, 57-59, 61-63, 80-81, 83, 87, 89, 104, 126, 138-140, 173, 175, 178, 182-183, 186-187, 219, 224, 232

Cytokine Secretion, 27, 115, 124-125, 182, 186, 190, 194, 196-197, 200, 211

Cytokines, 9, 12-13, 19, 23, 27-28, 31-32, 35, 39, 41-44, 49, 52-55, 57, 59-63, 73, 78, 80-87, 89-90, 94-95, 97, 101, 103, 115-118, 120-122, 124-125, 144, 148-151, 153-156, 158, 162, 164, 169, 173-179, 182-187, 191, 193-194, 197-198, 204, 207-209, 226, 229, 231, 234-237

D

Deglycosylation, 66, 71-72

E

Edema, 1, 6-7, 12-13, 16-17, 19, 21-22, 24-25, 27-34, 36-38, 41-64, 66, 73, 78-92, 106-107, 111-113, 116, 122, 126-128, 138-139, 141-142, 144-146, 148-154, 157-159, 161-162, 164-165, 167-168, 170-180, 183-184, 186-187, 207-208, 212

Endocytosis, 24, 37, 45, 50, 59, 62, 77, 89, 109, 126, 128-129, 131-134, 136-139, 142-147, 178, 209

Endothelial Dysfunction, 7, 19, 41, 112, 152-153

Epithelial Permeability, 17-18, 21, 49, 54, 88, 115, 118, 177

Epithelial Sodium Channel, 12, 25, 29, 45-47, 51, 53, 55, 57-59, 62-63, 65-66, 68, 70, 72-74, 78-79, 86, 89, 106-107, 109, 111, 113-114, 128-129, 131, 133-134, 136-137, 139-140, 171, 173-174, 178-181

F

Fistula, 151, 159

Fluid Balance, 22, 32, 35, 43-44, 48, 61-62, 66, 78, 80-81, 113, 128-129, 138, 141-142, 144, 148, 155, 158, 170, 173, 175, 180

Furosemide, 16, 31, 42-44, 81, 83, 86

G

Gestation, 38, 41

Glycerol, 3, 130

H

Heart Disease, 3, 16, 149, 199, 206

Heart Failure, 13, 16, 18-19, 42, 44, 50, 80, 88, 148-149, 151-160, 186

Hydrostatic Edema, 13, 16, 80, 152

Hypercapnia, 24-25, 45, 57, 89, 128-129, 131-139, 141-142, 144-147, 150

Hypertonicity, 38, 55, 84

Hypoxia, 3-10, 14, 18-19, 24-25, 31, 35, 38, 43, 45, 47, 51, 55, 66, 78, 89, 91, 114, 126, 136, 140-147, 149, 178, 187, 237

I

Immune Cell, 19, 62, 103, 127, 151, 182, 190, 199-201, 217

Inflammasome, 18, 50, 61, 94-97, 99-104, 189, 194, 198-199, 203-204, 221, 224

Influenza, 16-17, 33, 48-50, 53, 57-64, 90-96, 99-105, 125, 127, 151, 158, 176, 179, 198, 204, 206, 208, 212, 217-218, 224, 230, 232, 239

Injured Lungs, 52, 62, 91, 140, 152, 158, 180

Interleukin, 14-15, 17-18, 34-35, 38, 46-50, 52-54, 57, 59, 62-63, 78, 81, 86-87, 90, 92, 94-96, 99-100, 102, 104, 127, 136, 140, 147-149, 157-160, 163, 166, 171, 179-181, 188, 201-205, 209, 218, 223, 226, 231, 234

Interstitium, 7, 13, 16, 19, 23-25, 33, 58, 88, 129, 141, 150, 173-174

Index

Intratracheal Instillation, 115-116, 118

Ion Channel, 11-13, 25-26, 28, 33, 38, 40-43, 45-46, 51, 57, 63, 68-69, 73, 75, 78-79, 83, 94, 104, 106, 111-114, 126, 147-148, 173, 175, 179, 184, 186

Ion Translocation, 23, 83

Ischemia-reperfusion Injury, 12, 23, 30-31, 39, 83, 159

L

Lectin-like Domain, 13-15, 17-18, 28-32, 43, 46, 48-49, 59, 62, 64-66, 68-69, 72-75, 77-79, 107, 113, 152, 158, 176

Lung Inflammation, 7, 30, 49, 59-60, 63, 66, 75, 80, 84, 87, 115-116, 121-122, 126, 180, 183, 189-194, 197-201, 204, 207-213, 222, 224, 233, 237-239

Lung Injury, 1, 6-7, 11-12, 19, 21-22, 24, 26, 28, 30-37, 39-40, 44-64, 66, 78-86, 90-95, 97, 101-103, 106-107, 112-116, 118, 120, 122-123, 125-126, 128-129, 138-141, 144, 146-147, 151, 157-159, 161-164, 166-167, 170-171, 173-174, 176-178, 210-214, 222, 233, 239-240

Lung Transplantation, 8, 12, 19, 21, 30-31, 39-40, 43-45, 49, 52, 56, 66, 86

M

Monocyte, 53, 62-63, 97, 99-100, 116, 124-125, 127, 149, 153, 156, 164, 169-171, 192, 194, 204, 206, 210, 213, 218, 234

Myocardial Infarction, 16, 35, 86, 90, 104, 149, 156-160, 171

Myocarditis, 149, 156, 160

O

Osmotic Gradient, 58, 88-91, 141, 150, 173

P

Pathophysiology, 30, 40, 52, 82, 85, 87, 90-91, 104, 149, 154-155, 159, 165, 171, 175, 177, 187, 202, 204, 216, 221, 223, 232

Peptide, 12-13, 19, 26-27, 29, 31-32, 37, 40-43, 46-47, 52, 59, 61, 64, 66, 68-69, 71-72, 74-75, 78-79, 104, 106-113, 152-155, 159-160, 176-178, 206, 216, 222, 224

Phagocytes, 30, 59-60

Phagocytic Process, 184

Phosphatidylinositol, 2, 4, 7, 33, 113, 219

Phosphorylation, 18, 24-25, 27, 34, 36, 50, 83-84, 86, 106-107, 109-113, 118, 121, 125, 127-130, 132, 134, 136-140, 142-143, 145, 147-148, 183, 195, 205, 219-220, 226, 237

Plasma Levels, 22, 35, 37, 158, 237

Pneumolysin, 14, 17, 32, 43, 46-47, 66, 106-108, 110-113

Pneumonia, 12, 19, 21-23, 29, 32, 39, 48, 52-53, 59-60, 62-63, 82, 86-87, 89-90, 92, 106-107, 111-112, 139, 158, 171, 174, 180, 183, 188, 206, 212

Pulmonary Circulation, 8-9, 13, 24, 141, 174, 178

Pulmonary Edema, 13, 16, 19, 21-22, 24-25, 27-34, 37, 41-45, 47, 51-55, 59-62, 64, 66, 78-82, 84-86, 88-92, 113, 122, 126, 128, 139, 141, 144, 146, 151, 157-158, 161-162, 164-165, 170-171, 173-180, 184, 186

Pulmonary Hypertension, 1-2, 8-10, 28, 51, 114, 175, 187

R

Renal Tissue, 153, 155

Respiratory Mechanics, 161-163, 166, 170

S

Sodium Transport, 30-31, 42, 47, 54, 58, 60-61, 66, 78, 80, 86, 91-92, 128-129, 141-142, 146, 153, 158, 173, 179-180

Solnatide, 13, 29, 31-32, 43, 46, 65-78, 107, 113

T

Tumor Necrosis Factor, 6, 12-14, 17, 21, 28-30, 43-46, 48-49, 52-53, 57, 59, 61-62, 64-66, 68-70, 72, 75, 77-79, 81, 85-87, 92, 113, 127, 147-149, 153, 156-158, 160-162, 170-172, 176, 179-180, 218, 223

U

Ubiquitination, 24, 47, 77, 107, 128-132, 134-136, 138-140, 143-144, 147, 198, 206, 226

V

Vascular Cell, 3, 5, 176

Vascular Leak, 17, 38, 184

Vascular Permeability, 1, 6-7, 11, 16, 18, 27-28, 30-32, 49-50, 60, 80-81, 184

Vasoconstriction, 1, 3-4, 8-10, 19, 28, 31, 37, 42, 55, 149, 153, 155, 159

Vectorial Ion Transport, 88-89

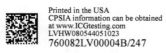